J. W. Rohen
C. Yokochi
E. Lütjen-Drecoll

# Color Atlas
# of Anatomy

A Photographic Study
of the Human Body

Sixth Edition

Coeditions
in 17 Languages

Johannes W. Rohen
Chihiro Yokochi
Elke Lütjen-Drecoll

# Color Atlas of Anatomy

## A Photographic Study of the Human Body

## Sixth Edition

with 1258 Figures,
1147 in Color,
and 111 Radiographs,
CT and MRI Scans

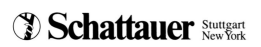
**Schattauer** Stuttgart New York

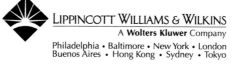
LIPPINCOTT WILLIAMS & WILKINS
**A Wolters Kluwer** Company
Philadelphia • Baltimore • New York • London
Buenos Aires • Hong Kong • Sydney • Tokyo

**Prof. em. Dr. med. Dr. med. h. c. Johannes W. Rohen**
Anatomisches Institut II der Universität Erlangen-Nürnberg
Universitätsstr. 19, D-91054 Erlangen, Germany

**Chihiro Yokochi, M.D.**
Professor Emeritus, Department of Anatomy
Kanagawa Dental College, Yokosuka, Kanagawa, Japan
Correspondence to:
Prof. Chihiro Yokochi, c/o Igaku-Shoin Ltd., 5-24-3 Hongo,
Bunkyo-ku, Tokyo 113-8719, Japan

**Prof. Dr. med. Elke Lütjen-Drecoll**
Head of the Department of Anatomy
Anatomisches Institut II der Universität Erlangen-Nürnberg
Universitätsstr. 19, D-91054 Erlangen, Germany

**Acknowledgements**

We would like to express our great gratitude to all coworkers
who helped to make the *Atlas* a success. We are particularly indebted to those who dissected new specimens with great skill and
knowledge, particularly to Jeff Bryant (member of our staff) and
Dr. Martin Rexer (now Klinikum Fürth), who prepared most of
the new specimens of the fifth and sixth edition. We would also
like to thank Dr. K. Okamoto (now Nagasaki, Japan), who dissected many excellent specimens of the fourth edition, also included in the fifth edition. Furthermore, we are greatly indebted
to Prof. Winfried Neuhuber and his coworkers for their great
efforts in supporting our work.

The specimens of the previous editions also depicted in this volume were dissected with great skill and enthusiasm by Prof. Dr. S.
Nagashima (now Nagasaki, Japan), Dr. Mutsuko Takahashi (now
Tokyo), Dr. Gabriele Lindner-Funk (Erlangen), Dr. P. Landgraf (Erlangen), and Miss Rachel M. McDonnell (now Dallas, Texas, USA).

We would also like to express our many thanks to Prof. W.
Bautz (Radiologisches Institut, Universität Erlangen-Nürnberg)
and Prof. A. Heuck (Radiologisches Zentrum, München-Pasing),
who provided the newly included excellent CT and MRI scans.

We are also greatly indebted to Mr. Hans Sommer (SOMSO
Co., Coburg), who kindly provided a number of excellent bone specimens.

Finally, we would like to express our great gratitude to our
photographer, Mr. Marco Gößwein, who contributed the very excellent macrophotos. Excellent and untiring work was done by
our secretaries, Mrs. Lis Köhler and Elisabeth Glas, as well by
our artists, Mr. Jörg Pekarsky and Mrs. Annette Gack, who not
only performed excellent new drawings but revised effectively
the layout of the new edition.

Last but not least, we would like to express our sincere thanks
to all scientists, students, and other coworkers, particularly to the
ones at the publishing companies themselves.

J. W. Rohen
C. Yokochi
E. Lütjen-Drecoll

***Visit Lippincott Williams & Wilkins on the Internet:***
*http://www.LWW.com.* Lippincott Williams & Wilkins customer ser-
vice representatives are available from 8:30 am to 6:00 pm, EST.

**Library of Congress Cataloging-in-Publication Data has been ap-
plied for.**

Composing, printing, and binding:
Mayr Miesbach, Druckerei und Verlag GmbH,
Am Windfeld 15, D-83714 Miesbach, Germany
Printed in Germany

1 2 3 4 5 6 7 8 9 10

ISBN 0-7817-9013-1

# Preface to the Sixth Edition

Twenty-three years after its first edition the *Atlas* was again thoroughly revised and modernized. Numerous new figures were incorporated. Nearly 30 new photographs taken from newly dissected specimens, many new drawings, and, for the first time, photographs of the surface anatomy of the human body were added. To avoid an undesirable increase in volume size we omitted all figures of minor quality from the previous editions and revised thoroughly the layout of the book. To provide a more detailed outline on cross sectional and regional anatomy which becomes increasingly important to clinical work, we added a great number of CT and MRI scans taken with latest modern techniques.

Each chapter of this edition consists of two parts. The first part describes the anatomical structure of the organs in a systemic manner, e.g., in the case of an extremity: bones, joints, ligaments, muscles, blood vessels, and nerves. In the second part, the regional anatomy is depicted, so that the description of the superficial layers is followed by the deeper and deepest layers; thus the student in the lab can find the orientation needed for the dissection of the cadaver. When viewing the photographs, the use of a magnifier is strongly recommended in order to identify more precisely the three-dimensional structure of the tissues and organs depicted.

While preparing this new edition, the authors were reminded of how precisely, beautifully, and admirably the human body is constructed. If this book helps the student or medical doctor to appreciate the overwhelming beauty of the anatomical architecture of tissues and organs in the human, then it greatly fulfills its task. Deep interest and admiration of the anatomical structures may create the "love for man", which alone can be considered of primary importance for daily medical work.

We would like to express our great gratitude to all coworkers for their skilled work. Without their help the improvement of the *Atlas* would not have been possible. We would also like to express our sincere thanks to those at Schattauer GmbH, Stuttgart, Germany, Lippincott, Williams & Wilkins, Baltimore, Maryland, USA, and Igaku-Shoin, Tokyo, Japan, who always listened to our suggestions and invested again a great deal of their effort into improving this book.

March 2006

J. W. Rohen
C. Yokochi
E. Lütjen-Drecoll

# Preface to the First Edition

Today there exist any number of good anatomic atlases. Consequently, the advent of a new work requires justification. We found three main reasons to undertake the publication of such a book. First of all, most of the previous atlases contain mainly schematic or semischematic drawings which often reflect reality only in a limited way; the third dimension, i.e., the spatial effect, is lacking. In contrast, the photo of the actual anatomic specimen has the advantage of conveying the reality of the object with its proportions and spatial dimensions in a more exact and realistic manner than the "idealized", colored "nice" drawings of most previous atlases. Furthermore, the photo of the human specimen corresponds to the student's observations and needs in the dissection courses. Thus he has the advantage of immediate orientation by photographic specimens while working with the cadaver. Secondly, some of the existing atlases are classified by systemic rather than regional aspects. As a result, the student needs several books each supplying the necessary facts for a certain region of the body. The present atlas, however, tries to portray macroscopic anatomy with regard to the regional and stratigraphic aspects of the object itself as realistically as possible. Hence it is an immediate help during the dissection courses in the study of medical and dental anatomy.

Another intention of the authors was to limit the subject to the essential and to offer it didactically in a way that is self-explanatory. To all regions of the body we added schematic drawings of the main tributaries of nerves and vessels, of the course and mechanism of the muscles, of the nomenclature of the various regions, etc. This will enhance the understanding of the details seen in the photographs. The complicated architecture of the skull bones, for example, was not presented in a descriptive way, but rather through a series of figures revealing the mosaic of bones by adding one bone to another, so that ultimately the composition of skull bones can be more easily understood.

Finally, the authors also considered the present situation in medical education. On one hand there is a universal lack of cadavers in many departments of anatomy, while on the other hand there has been a considerable increase in the number of students almost everywhere. As a consequence, students do not have access to sufficient illustrative material for their anatomic studies. Of course, photos can never replace the immediate observation, but we think the use of a macroscopic photo instead of a painted, mostly idealized picture is more appropriate and is an improvement in anatomic study over drawings alone.

The majority of the specimes depicted in the atlas were prepared by the authors either in the Dept. of Anatomy in Erlangen, Germany, or in the Dept. of Anatomy, Kanagawa Dental College, Yokosuka, Japan. The specimens of the chapter on the neck and those of the spinal cord demonstrating the dorsal branches of the spinal nerves were prepared by Dr. K. Schmidt with great skill and enthusiasm. The specimens of the ligaments of the vertebral column were prepared by Dr. Th. Mokrusch, and a great number of specimens in the chapter of the upper and lower limb was very carefully prepared by Dr. S. Nagashima, Kurume, Japan.

Once again, our warmest thanks go out to all of our co-workers for their unselfish, devoted and highly qualified work.

Erlangen, Spring 1983

J.W. Rohen
C. Yokochi

# Contents

# 3 Trunk

# 4 Thoracic Organs 243

# 5 Abdominal Organs 291

# 8 Lower Limb    431

## List of Figures

# 1 General Anatomy

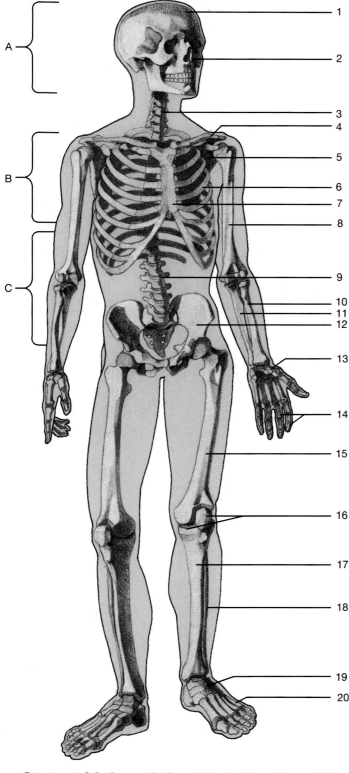

In contrast to most other mammals the human body is adapted for bipedal locomotion. Three general principles in the architecture of the human organism are recognizable:

1. The principle of **segmentation,** which dominates in the trunk. The vertebral column and the thorax consist of relatively equal, segmentally arranged elements.
2. The principle of **bilateral symmetry.** Both sides of the body are separated by a midsagittal plane and resemble each other like image and mirror-image.
3. The principle of **polarity** between the head at one end of the body and the lower extremities at the other. As the center of the information system the head contains the main sensory organs and the brain. The head has a predominantly spherical form, while the extremities consist of radially formed skeletal elements, the number of which increases distally.

A. The **skull** consists of two parts:
   1. a **cranial part** containing mainly the brain and the sensory organs and
   2. a **facial part** containing the nasal and oral cavities and the chewing apparatus. The cranial cavity is continuous with the vertebral canal, which contains the spinal cord.

B. The **thorax** contains the respiratory and circulatory organs (lung, heart, etc.) but also some of the abdominal organs, which are located underneath the diaphragm.

C. The **abdominal cavity** contains the organs of metabolism such as the liver, the stomach, and the intestinal tract as well as the excretory and genital organs (kidney, uterus, urinary bladder, etc.). The latter are located primarily in the **pelvic cavity** with the exception of the testes.

**Structure of the human body and the skeleton.** Blue = joints.

A: Head (caput)
B: Thorax (thoracic cavity)
C: Abdominal and pelvic cavities

1 Cranial part } of the skull
2 Facial part }
3 Vertebral column (cervical part)
4 Clavicle
5 Scapula
6 Ribs
7 Sternum
8 Arm (humerus)
9 Vertebral column (lumbar part)

10 Radius } forearm
11 Ulna }
12 Pelvis
13 Wrist (carpals) } hand
14 Fingers (phalanges) }
15 Thigh (femur)
16 Patella and knee joint
17 Tibia } leg
18 Fibula }
19 Tarsals } foot
20 Metatarsals }

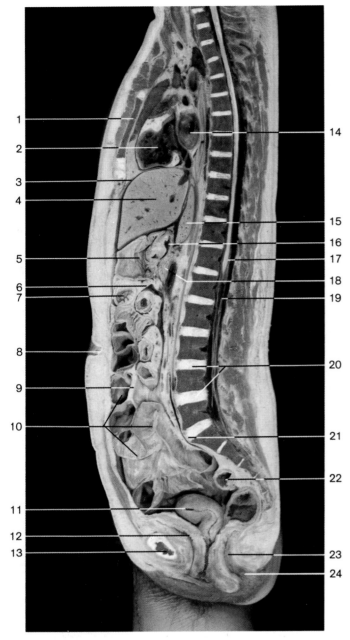

**Median section through the trunk** (female).

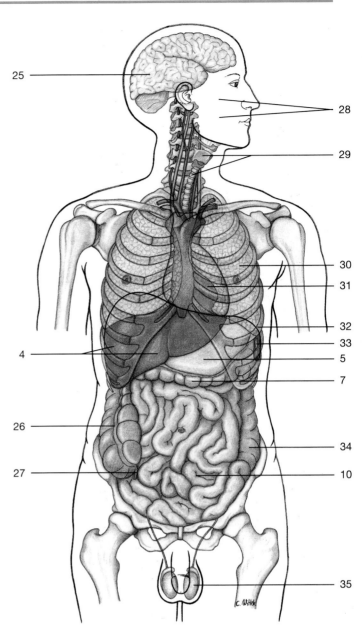

**Position of the inner organs of the human body** (anterior aspect).
The main cavities of the body and their contents.

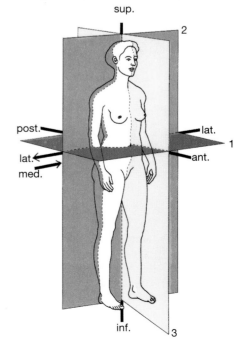

| | | | |
|---|---|---|---|
| 1 | Sternum | 21 | Sacral promontory |
| 2 | Right ventricle of heart | 22 | Sigmoid colon |
| 3 | Diaphragm | 23 | Anal canal |
| 4 | Liver | 24 | Anus |
| 5 | Stomach | 25 | Head (neurocranium) with brain |
| 6 | Transverse mesocolon | 26 | Ascending colon |
| 7 | Transverse colon | 27 | Appendix |
| 8 | Umbilicus | 28 | Facial region (viscerocranium) |
| 9 | Mesentery | | with oral and nasal cavities |
| 10 | Small intestine | 29 | Trachea and larynx |
| 11 | Uterus | 30 | Thorax with the lungs |
| 12 | Urinary bladder | 31 | Heart |
| 13 | Pubic symphysis | 32 | Surface projection of the diaphragm |
| 14 | Left atrium of heart | 33 | Spleen |
| 15 | Caudate lobe of liver | 34 | Descending colon |
| 16 | Omental bursa or lesser sac | 35 | Testis |
| 17 | Conus medullaris | | |
| 18 | Pancreas | | |
| 19 | Cauda equina | | |
| 20 | Intervertebral discs | | |
| | (lumbar vertebral column) | | |

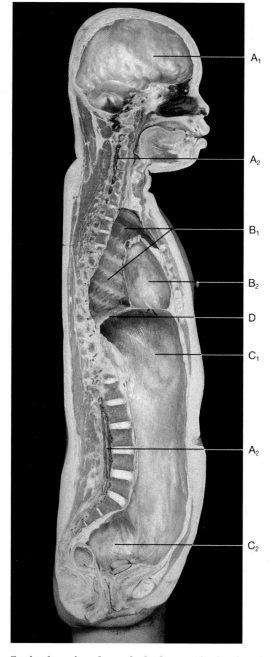

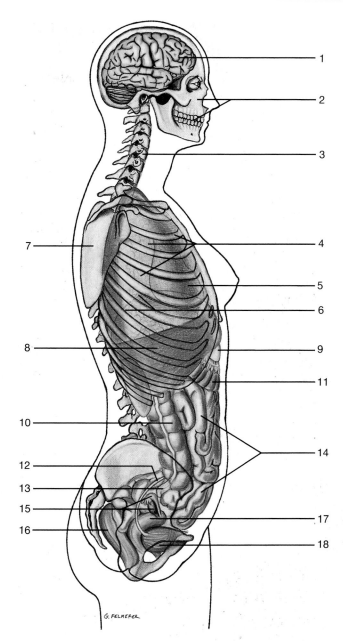

**Sagittal section through the human body** (female).
Demonstration of the main cavities of the body.
Internal organs are removed.

A₁  Cranial cavity
A₂  Vertebral canal
B₁  Thoracic cavity
B₂  Pericardial cavity
C₁  Abdominal cavity
C₂  Pelvic cavity
D   Diaphragm

◁

**Planes of the body**
1  Transverse plane
2  Frontal plane
3  Sagittal plane (midsagittal)

**Lines of direction**
ant.  =  anterior
inf.  =  inferior
lat.  =  lateral
med. =  medial
post. =  posterior
sup.  =  superior

**Position of the inner organs of the human body**
(lateral aspect).
The three main cavities of the body and their contents.

1   Head (neurocranium) with the brain
2   Facial bones with oral and nasal cavities
3   Vertebral column (cervical part)
4   Thorax with the lungs
5   Heart
6   Surface projection of the diaphragm
7   Scapula
8   Liver
9   Stomach
10  Ascending colon
11  Transverse colon
12  Ureter
13  Appendix
14  Small intestine
15  Ovary, uterine tube
16  Rectum
17  Uterus
18  Urinary bladder

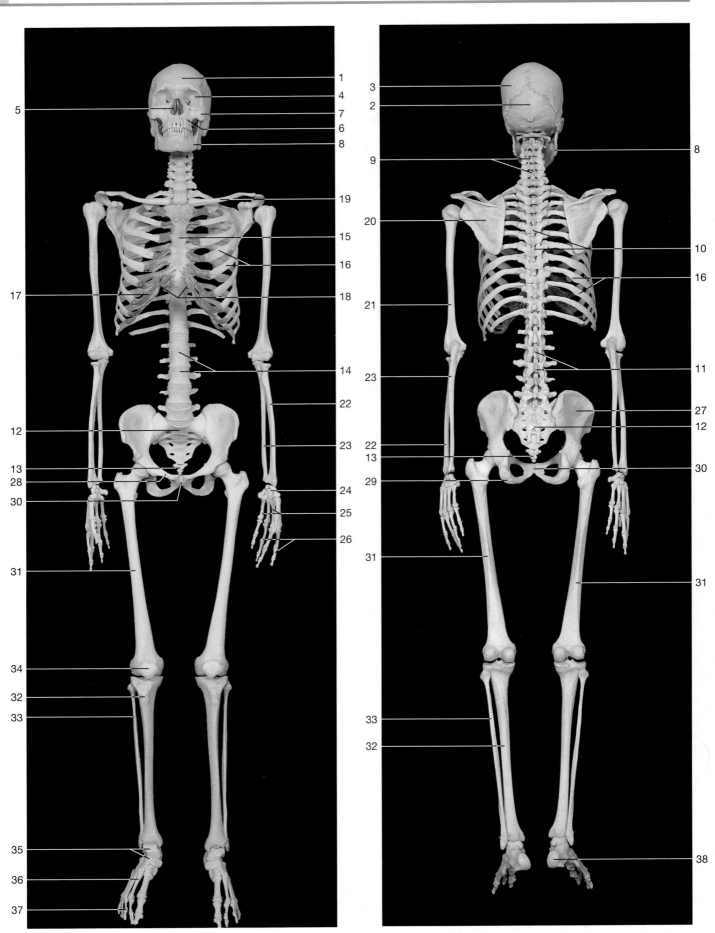

**Skeleton of a female adult** (anterior aspect).

**Skeleton of a female adult** (posterior aspect).

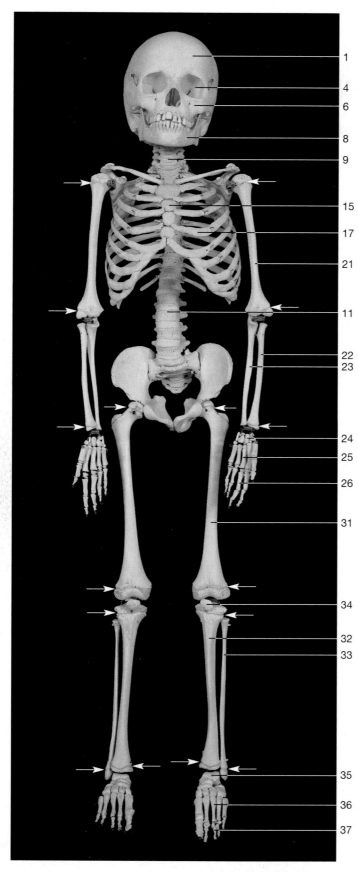

**Skeleton of a 5-year-old child** (anterior aspect).
The zones of the cartilaginous growth plates are seen (arrows).
In contrast to the adult, the ribs show a predominantly
horizontal position.

**Axial skeleton**
**Head**
1 Frontal bone
2 Occipital bone
3 Parietal bone
4 Orbit
5 Nasal cavity
6 Maxilla
7 Zygomatic bone
8 Mandible

**Trunk and thorax**
**Vertebral column**
9 Cervical vertebrae
10 Thoracic vertebrae
11 Lumbar vertebrae
12 Sacrum
13 Coccyx
14 Intervertebral discs

**Thorax**
15 Sternum
16 Ribs
17 Costal cartilage
18 Infrasternal angle

**Appendicular skeleton**
**Upper limb and shoulder girdle**
19 Clavicle
20 Scapula
21 Humerus
22 Radius
23 Ulna
24 Carpal bones
25 Metacarpal bones
26 Phalanges of the hand

**Lower limb and pelvis**
27 Ilium
28 Pubis
29 Ischium
30 Symphysis pubis
31 Femur
32 Tibia
33 Fibula
34 Patella
35 Tarsal bones
36 Metatarsal bones
37 Phalanges of the foot
38 Calcaneus

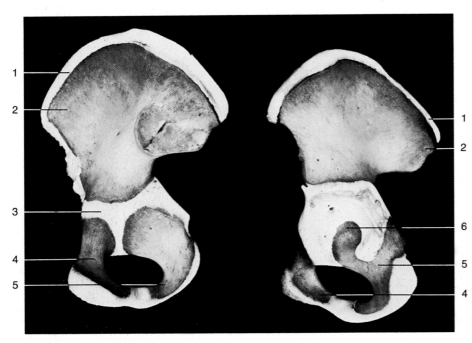

1 Subscapular fossa
2 Coracoid process
3 Glenoid fossa
4 Acromion
5 Spine of scapula
6 Infraspinous fossa

**Ossification of the scapula**
(left: anterior aspect, right: posterior aspect).

1 Cartilage of the iliac crest
2 Ilium
3 Cartilage
4 Pubis
5 Ischium
6 Acetabulum

**Ossification of the hip bone**
(left: medial aspect, right: lateral aspect).

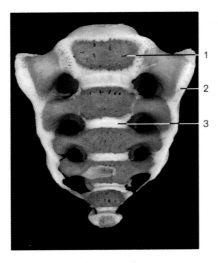

1 Bone tissue
  (vertebral body)
2 Cartilaginous tissue
  (lateral epiphysis)
3 Intervertebral discs

**Ossification of the sacrum** (anterior aspect).
Note the five vertebral bones, which are still separated
from each other.

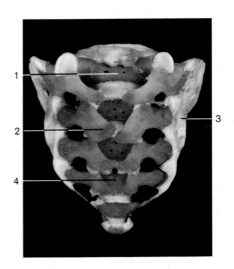

1 Bony tissue
  (center of
  ossification)
2 Vertebral arch
  (not completely
  united)
3 Cartilaginous
  tissue
  (lateral epiphysis)
4 Sacral canal

**Ossification of the sacrum**
(posterior aspect).

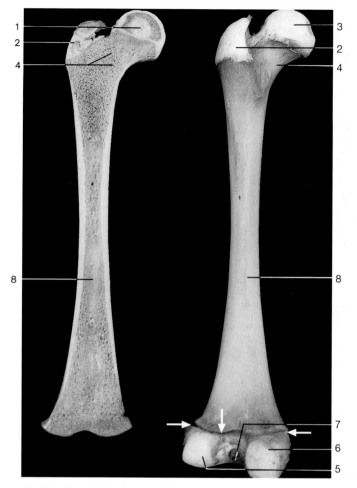

◁ 1  Ossification center in the head of the femur
  2  Greater trochanter
  3  Head of the femur
  4  Neck of the femur
  5  Lateral condyle
  6  Medial condyle
  7  Intercondylar notch
  8  Diaphysis

**Ossification of the femur** (left: coronal section,
right: posterior view of the femur). Arrows: distal epiphysis.

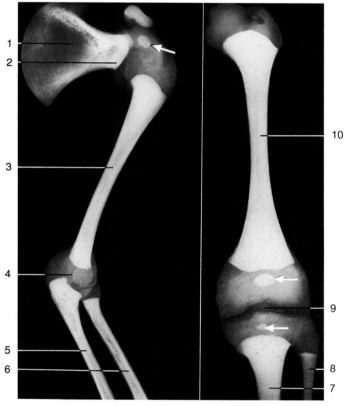

**X-ray of the upper and lower limb of a newborn child**
(left: upper limb, right: lower limb).
Arrows: ossification centers.

| | | | | | |
|---|---|---|---|---|---|
| 1 | Scapula | 4 | Elbow joint | 7 | Tibia |
| 2 | Shoulder joint | 5 | Ulna | 8 | Fibula |
| 3 | Humerus | 6 | Radius | 9 | Knee joint |
| | | | | 10 | Femur |

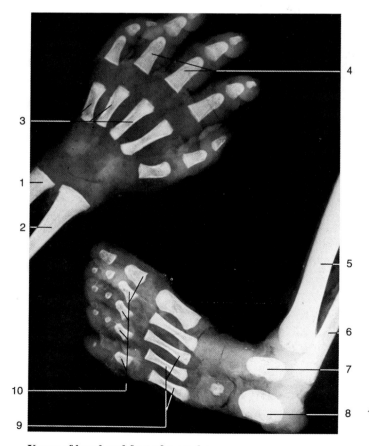

**X-ray of hand and foot of a newborn.**

| | | | | | |
|---|---|---|---|---|---|
| ◁ 1 | Ulna | 4 | Phalanges | 7 | Talus |
| 2 | Radius | 5 | Tibia | 8 | Calcaneus |
| 3 | Metacarpals | 6 | Fibula | 9 | Metatarsals |
| | | | | 10 | Phalanges |

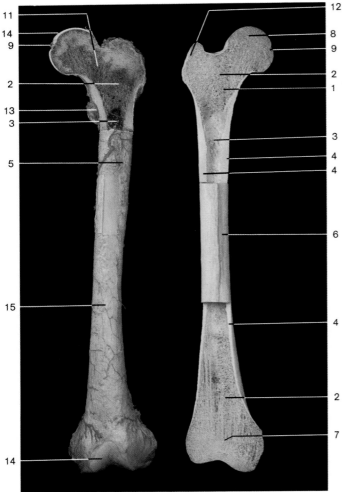

1   Metaphysis
2   Spongy bone
3   Medullary cavity in the diaphysis
4   Compact bone
5   Nutrient canal
6   Diaphysis
7   Epiphyseal line (remnants of the epiphyseal plate)
8   Epiphysis (head of the femur)
9   Fovea of head
10  Trabeculae of spongy bone
11  Neck of the femur
12  Greater trochanter
13  Lesser trochanter
14  Articular surface
15  Periosteum
16  Skin
17  Vastus medialis muscle
18  Sartorius muscle
19  Femoral artery and vein
20  Great saphenous vein
21  Gracilis muscle
22  Adductor longus muscle
23  Adductor magnus muscle
24  Semimembranosus muscle
25  Semitendinosus muscle
26  Rectus femoris muscle
27  Vastus lateralis muscle
28  Femur and medullary cavity
29  Vastus intermedius muscle
30  Sciatic nerve
31  Biceps femoris muscle
32  Spongy bone trabeculae containing bone marrow
33  Compact bone
34  Osteon with Haversian lamellae
35  Periosteum
36  Blood vessels and nerves for periosteum and bone

**Femur of the adult.** Left: the periosteum and the nutrient vessels are preserved. Right: coronal section of the proximal and distal epiphyses to display the spongy bone and the medullary cavity.

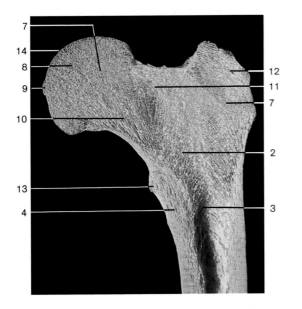

**Coronal section through the proximal end of the adult femur,** revealing the characteristic trajectorial structure of the spongy bone.

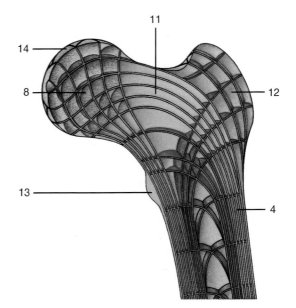

**Threedimensional representation on the trajectorial lines of the femoral head** (according to B. Kummer).

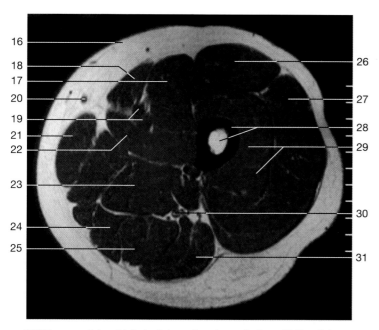

**MRI scan** of the thigh (axial section through the middle of the left thigh, the same level as the CT scan).

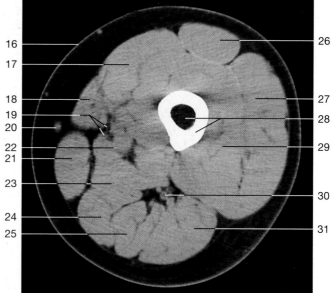

**CT scan** of the section through the middle of the left thigh (axial section). Note the differences between the CT and MRI scan (see text below).

The **bones** of the skeletal system consist of two different parts, the spongy and the compact bone. The spongy bone trabeculae are highly adapted to mechanical forces revealing a trajectorial structure. The intertrabecular spaces are filled with bone marrow, the site of blood formation. The appearance of bones, muscles, and soft tissues is quite different in **CT** and **MRI scans.** The CT scans relate well to radiographs in that areas of great absorption such as bones are white, and those with little absorption such as fat appear black. In contrast, the intensity of signals in MRI scans, obtained without X-rays but by magnetic forces, is different so that dense areas of bones appear black and soft tissues such as bone marrow and fat appear white (for comparison see above figures).

A highly innervated **periosteum** is an essential structure for bone nutrition, blood supply, growth, and bone repair.

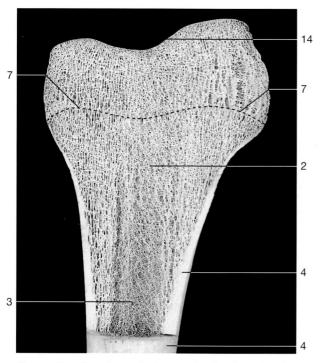

**Coronal section through the proximal epiphysis of the adult tibia.** Note the zone of dense bone at the site of the former epiphyseal plate (dotted line).

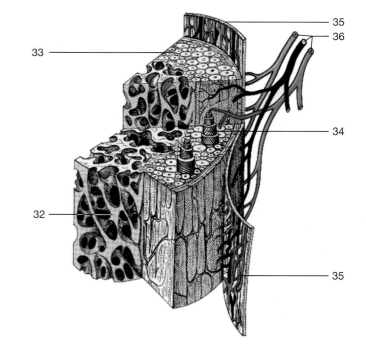

**Structure of bones of the skeletal system** (after Benninghoff). Note that the compact bone reveals a lamellar structure with Haversian lamellae and canals.

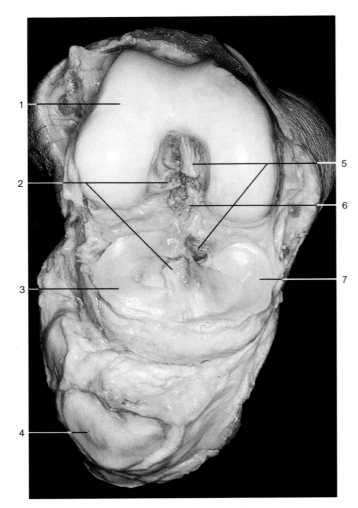

1
2
5
6
3
7
4

**Knee joint.** Anterior aspect, showing menisci and cruciate ligaments (cut). Quadriceps tendon cut and patella reflected distally.

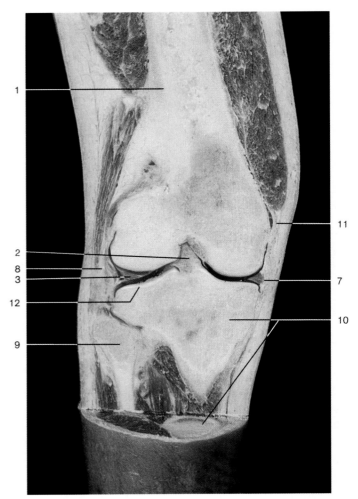

1
11
2
8
3
7
12
10
9

**Coronal section through the knee joint.**
Anterior aspect of the right joint in extension.

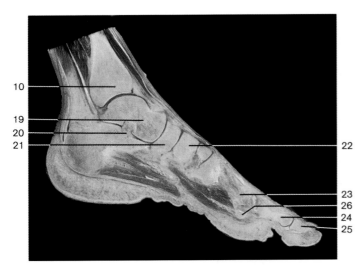

10
19
20
21
22
23
26
24
25

**Sagittal section through the lower limb and the foot.**

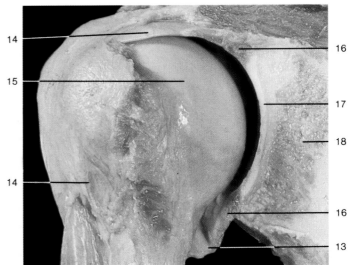

14
16
15
17
14
18
16
13

**Shoulder joint** (anterior view). The anterior part of the articular capsule has been removed.

| | | | |
|---|---|---|---|
| 1 | Femur | 10 | Tibia |
| 2 | Anterior cruciate ligament | 11 | Tibial collateral ligament |
| 3 | Lateral meniscus | 12 | Articular cartilage |
| 4 | Patella | 13 | Articular capsule |
| 5 | Posterior cruciate ligament | 14 | Tendon of long head |
| 6 | Posterior meniscofemoral | | of biceps brachii muscle |
| | ligament | 15 | Head of humerus |
| 7 | Medial meniscus | 16 | Glenoid labrum |
| 8 | Fibular collateral ligament | 17 | Articular cartilage of |
| 9 | Fibula | | glenoid fossa |

| | |
|---|---|
| 18 | Scapula |
| 19 | Talus |
| 20 | Interosseous talocalcaneal ligament |
| 21 | Navicular bone |
| 22 | Medial cuneiform bone |
| 23 | First metatarsal bone |
| 24 | Proximal phalanx of the hallux (great toe) |
| 25 | Distal phalanx of the hallux |
| 26 | Sesamoid bone |

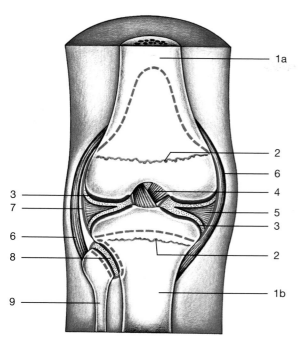

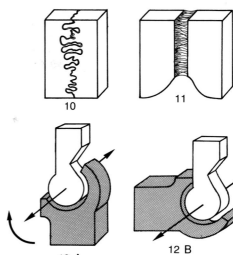

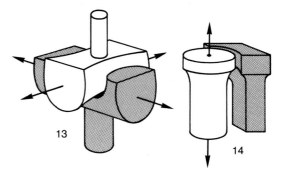

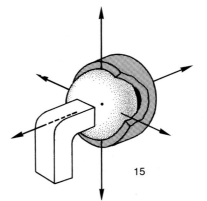

**General architecture of a synovial joint** with two articulating bones and a synovial cavity (right side, anterior view).
**Coronal section through the knee joint.**
Red line = Articular capsule with synovial membrane.
Dotted red line = extension of articular capsule (suprapatellar bursa).

1　Articulating bones: a) Femur, b) Tibia
2　Epiphysial line
3　Articular cartilage
4　Intra-articular ligaments (e. g., cruciate ligaments)
5　Fibrocartilaginous disc (e. g., meniscus)
6　Collateral ligaments
7　Articular capsule with synovial membrane
8　Tibiofibular articulation (example of gliding synovial joint)
9　Fibula

**Main types of joints.** Arrows: axes of movement.

**Fibrous joints (synarthroses)**
10　Serrate suture
11　Syndesmosis

**Synovial joints (diarthroses)**
12　Hinge joints (monaxial) ginglymus
　　A　Extension
　　B　Flexion
13　Saddle joint (biaxial)
14　Pivot joint (monaxial, rotation)
15　Ball-and-socket joint (multiaxial)

|   |   | Movement | Examples |
|---|---|---|---|
| **A** | **Fibrous joints** | | |
| | 1　Sutures | No movements | Sutures of the skull |
| | 2　Syndesmoses | No movements | Distal tibiofibular joint |
| | 3　Gomphosis | No movements | Roots of teeth in alveolar process |
| **B** | **Cartilaginous joints** | | |
| | 1　Synchondroses | No movements | Epiphysial plates |
| | 2　Symphyses | Slight movement | Pubic symphysis Intervertebral discs |
| **C** | **Synovial joints** | | |
| | 1　Gliding | Monaxial | Intercarpal joint Intertarsal joint Sacro-iliac joint |
| | 2　Hinge | Monaxial | Interphalangeal joint Humero-ulnar joint Talocrural joint |
| | 3　Pivot | Monaxial | Atlanto-axial joint Radio-ulnar joint |
| | 4　Ellipsoidal | Biaxial | Radiocarpal joint |
| | 5　Saddle | Biaxial | Carpometacarpal joint of the thumb |
| | 6　Ball-and-socket | Multiaxial | Shoulder and hip joint |

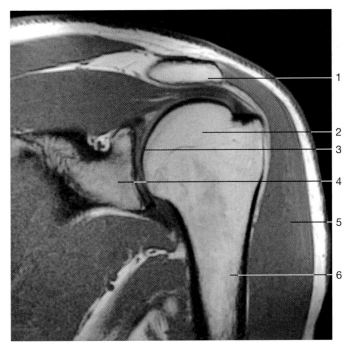

**Shoulder joint** (MRI scan, coronal section, courtesy of Prof. Dr. A. Heuck, Munich).

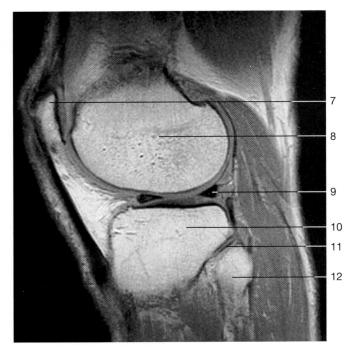

**Knee joint** (MRI scan, sagittal section, courtesy of Prof. Dr. W. Bautz, Erlangen).

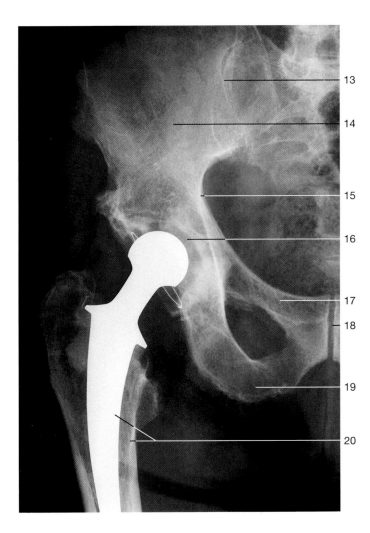

1  Acromion
2  Head of humerus
3  Shoulder joint
4  Scapula
5  Deltoid muscle
6  Humerus
7  Patella
8  Femur
9  Knee joint with menisci
10  Tibia
11  Tibiofibular joint
12  Head of fibula
13  Sacro-iliac joint
14  Iliac fossa
15  Linea terminalis
16  Cavity of hip joint
17  Pectineal line
18  Pubic symphysis
19  Ischial tuberosity
20  Femur with the prosthetic device

**Artificial hip joint.** The prosthesis has been introduced into the cavity of the femur (X-ray, a.-p. direction).

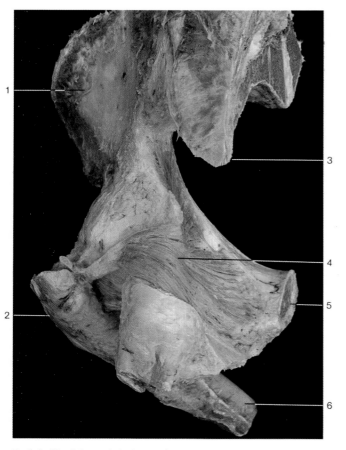

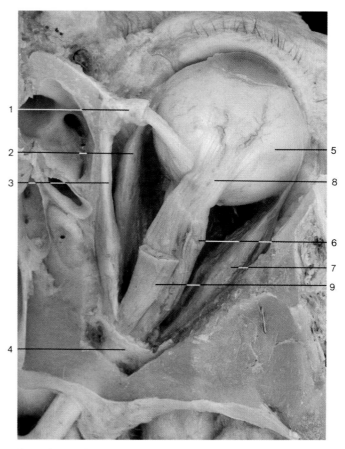

**Left half of the pelvis** (posterior aspect).
**Obturator internus muscle** as an example of a muscle, the tendon of which does not act in the direction of the main muscle fibers. Its fibers originate at the internal aspect of the obturator foramen, turn around the posterior rim of the ischium, and insert at the greater trochanter of the femur. The ischium thereby serves as a pulley.

| | | | | | |
|---|---|---|---|---|---|
| 1 | Ilium | 3 | Coccyx | 5 | Pubis |
| 2 | Greater trochanter | 4 | Obturator internus muscle | 6 | Femur |

**Superior oblique muscle of the eyeball,** right eye (superior aspect). The tendon of this muscle bends over the trochlea, changing its direction so that it becomes attached to the posterior lateral quadrant of the eyeball.

| | | | |
|---|---|---|---|
| 1 | Trochlea | 6 | Superior rectus muscle |
| 2 | Medial rectus muscle | 7 | Lateral rectus muscle |
| 3 | Superior oblique muscle | 8 | Superior rectus muscle (tendon) |
| 4 | Common annular tendon | 9 | Levator palpebrae superioris |
| 5 | Eyeball | | muscle (divided) |

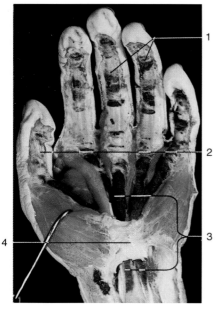

1  Digital synovial sheaths of the tendons of flexor digitorum superficialis and profundus muscles
2  Digital synovial sheaths of the tendon of long flexor pollicis longus muscle
3  Common flexor synovial sheaths of flexor digitorum superficialis and profundus muscles
4  Flexor retinaculum

**The synovial sheaths of the tendons on the palmar aspect of the left wrist** (colored fluid has been injected).

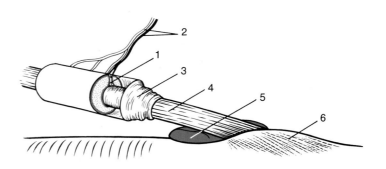

1  Mesotendon
2  Blood vessels
3  Synovial sheath
4  Tendon
5  Synovial bursa
6  Bone (tuberosity)

**Structure of a tendon sheath.** The synovial membrane, which also forms the mesotendon, is indicated in red. (Schematic drawing.)

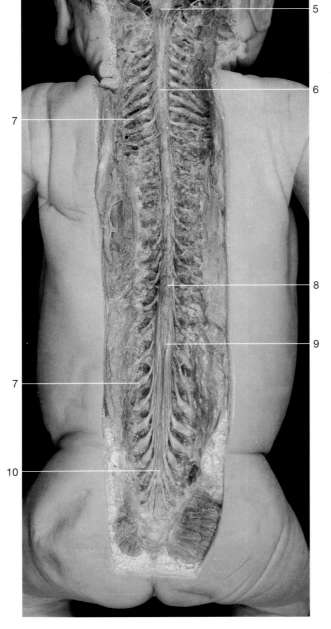

1   Falx cerebri
2   Cerebral hemispheres
3   Tentorium cerebelli
4   Cerebellum
5   Medulla oblongata
6   Spinal cord, cervical enlargement
7   Spinal ganglia
8   Spinal cord, lumbar enlargement
9   Conus medullaris
10  Cauda equina
11  Cervical plexus (formed from ventral rami of $C_1$–$C_4$)
12  Brachial plexus (formed from ventral rami of $C_5$–$T_1$)
13  Lumbosacral plexus (formed from ventral rami of $L_1$–$S_4$)
14  Sympathetic trunk

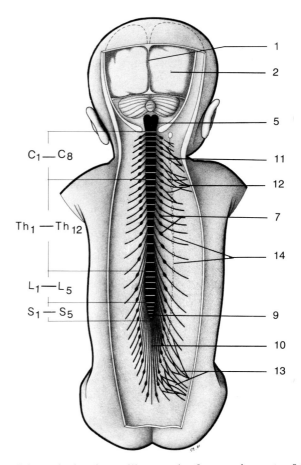

**Brain,** the **spinal cord** and the **spinal nerves** in the fetus (posterior aspect).

Schematic drawing to illustrate the **three main parts of the nervous system** in general.

The **nervous system** can be divided into three, functionally distinct parts:
1.  The cranial part, which comprises the great sensory organs and the brain,
2.  the spinal cord, which shows a segmental structure and serves predominantly as a reflex-organ, and
3.  the autonomic nervous system, which controls the involuntary functions (subconscious control) of organs and tissues. The autonomic part of the nervous system forms many delicate plexus within the organs. At certain places these plexus contain aggregations of nerve cells (prevertebral and intramural ganglia).

The spinal nerves leave the spinal cord at regular intervals, forming the 8 cervical, 12 thoracic, 5 lumbar, 5 sacral, and a varying number of coccygeal segments. The ventral rami of the first four cervical spinal nerves ($C_1$–$C_4$) form the cervical plexus (for innervation of the anterior neck); the ventral rami of the lower cervical spinal nerves ($C_5$–$T_1$) form the brachial plexus, which innervates the upper extremity; and the ventral rami of the lumbar and sacral spinal nerves form the lumbosacral plexus ($L_1$–$S_4$), which innervates the pelvic and genital organs and the lower extremity.

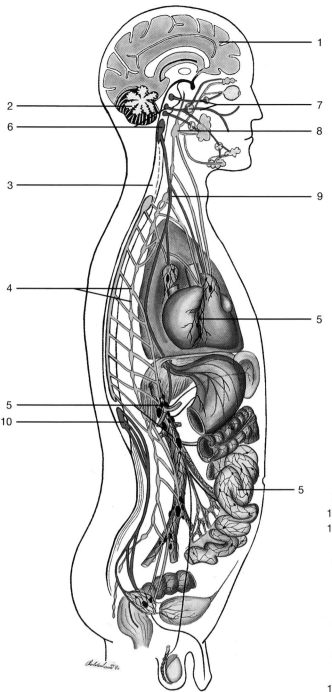

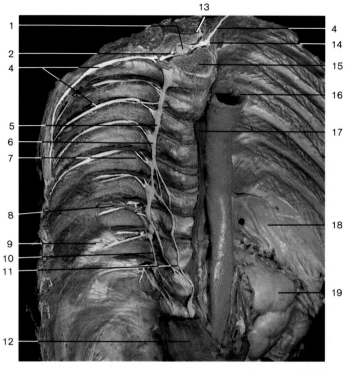

**Posterior part of the thorax.** Cross section at the level of the 5th thoracic segment. Spinal nerves and their connections to the sympathetic trunk.

Diagram illustrating the localization of the
**three functional portions of the nervous system**
(brain, spinal cord and autonomic nervous system).
Yellow = sympathetic system;
red = parasympathetic system.

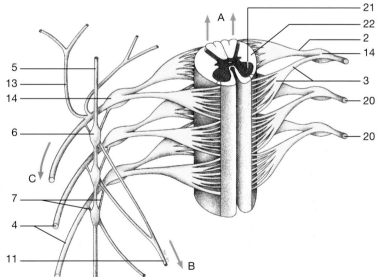

**Organization of the spinal cord** in structurally equal segments that form the paired spinal nerves. A = connections to the brain; B = connections to the autonomic nervous system; C = connections to the trunk and extremities (intercostal nerves and plexus). (Schematic drawing.)

| | | | |
|---|---|---|---|
| 1 | Cerebrum | | |
| 2 | Cerebellum | | |
| 3 | Spinal cord | | |
| 4 | Sympathetic trunk and ganglion | | |
| 5 | Plexus and ganglia of the autonomic nervous system | | |
| 6 | Cranial autonomic system | | |
| 7 | Cranial nerves (n. III and n. VII) | | |
| 8 | Superior cervical ganglion | | |
| 9 | Vagus nerve (n. X) | | |
| 10 | Sacral autonomic system | | |

| | | | |
|---|---|---|---|
| 1 | Spinal cord | 12 | Inferior vena cava |
| 2 | Dorsal root | 13 | Dorsal ramus of spinal nerve |
| 3 | Ventral root | 14 | Spinal (dorsal root) ganglion |
| 4 | Intercostal nerves | 15 | Body of the vertebra |
| 5 | Sympathetic trunk | 16 | Aorta |
| 6 | Ganglia of the sympathetic trunk | 17 | Azygos vein |
| 7 | Rami communicantes | 18 | Diaphragm |
| 8 | Intercostal artery and vein | 19 | Left kidney |
| 9 | Subcostalis muscle | 20 | Spinal nerve |
| 10 | Lesser splanchnic nerve | 21 | Gray matter of the spinal cord |
| 11 | Greater splanchnic nerve | 22 | White matter of the spinal cord |

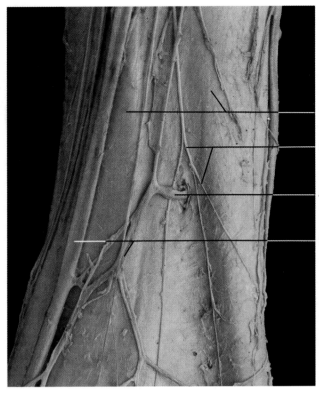

**Superficial nerves and vessels of the lower leg,** illustrating the structural differences between veins and nerves.

| | | | |
|---|---|---|---|
| 1 | Crural fascia (fascia cruris) | 3 | Superficial cutaneous veins |
| 2 | Cutaneous nerves | 4 | Perforating vein |

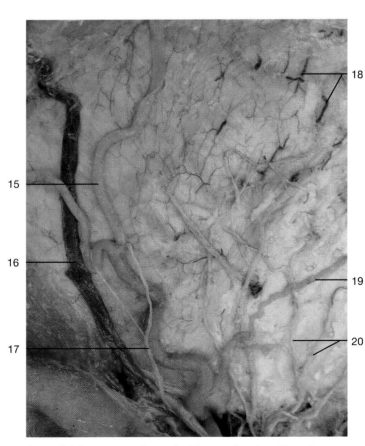

**Superficial nerves and vessels.** Temporal region. Note the differences between arteries, veins, and nerves.

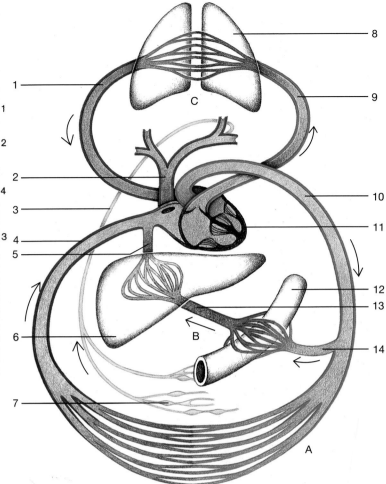

**Organization of the circulatory system.** Arrows: direction of the blood flow.

Vessel wall in red   = Arteries
Vessel wall in blue  = Veins
Yellow               = Lymphatic vessels

A   Systemic circulation
B   Hepatic portal circulation
C   Pulmonary circulation

| | | | |
|---|---|---|---|
| 1 | Pulmonary vein | 12 | Small intestine with capillary network |
| 2 | Superior vena cava | 13 | Portal vein |
| 3 | Thoracic duct | 14 | Mesenteric artery |
| 4 | Inferior vena cava | 15 | Superficial temporal artery |
| 5 | Hepatic vein | 16 | Superficial temporal vein |
| 6 | Liver | 17 | Auriculotemporal nerve |
| 7 | Lymph nodes and lymphatic vessels | 18 | Perforating veins for subcutaneous fatty tissue |
| 8 | Lung | 19 | Small artery |
| 9 | Pulmonary artery | 20 | Small nerves (branches of facial nerve) |
| 10 | Aorta | | |
| 11 | Heart | | |

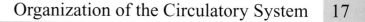

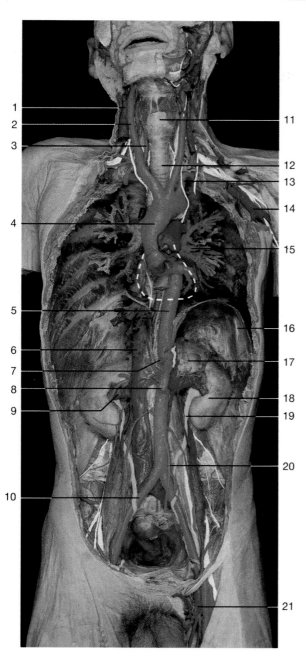

**Major vessels of the trunk.** The position of the heart is indicated by the dotted line.

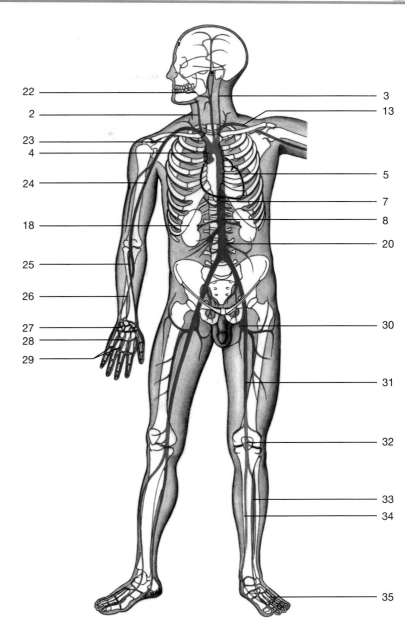

**Major arteries of the human body** (schematic drawing).

| | |
|---|---|
| 1 Internal jugular vein | 19 Ureter |
| 2 Common carotid artery | 20 Inferior mesenteric artery |
| 3 Vertebral artery | 21 Femoral vein |
| 4 Ascending aorta | 22 Facial artery |
| 5 Descending aorta | 23 Axillary artery |
| 6 Inferior vena cava | 24 Brachial artery |
| 7 Celiac trunk | 25 Radial artery |
| 8 Superior mesenteric artery | 26 Ulnar artery |
| 9 Renal vein | 27 Deep palmar arch |
| 10 Common iliac artery | 28 Superficial palmar arch |
| 11 Larynx | 29 Common palmar digital arteries |
| 12 Trachea | 30 Profunda femoris artery |
| 13 Left subclavian artery | 31 Femoral artery |
| 14 Left axillary vein | 32 Popliteal artery |
| 15 Pulmonary veins | 33 Anterior tibial artery |
| 16 Diaphragm | 34 Posterior tibial artery |
| 17 Suprarenal gland | 35 Plantar arch |
| 18 Kidney | |

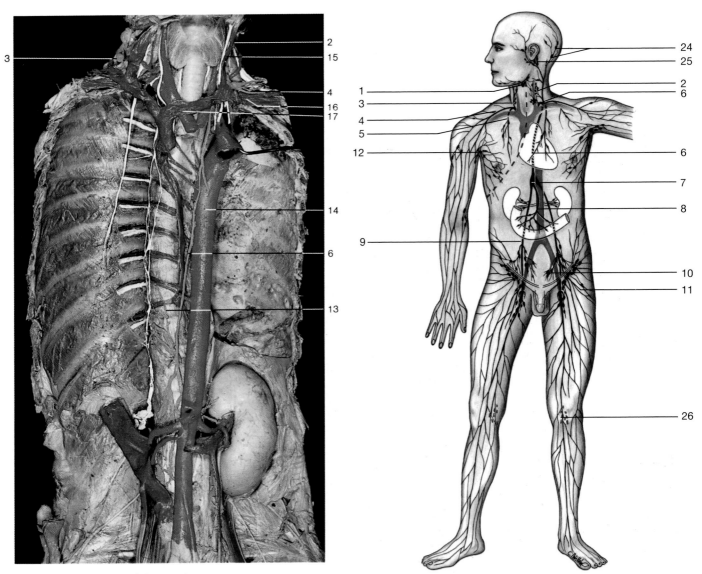

**Major lymph vessels of the trunk.**

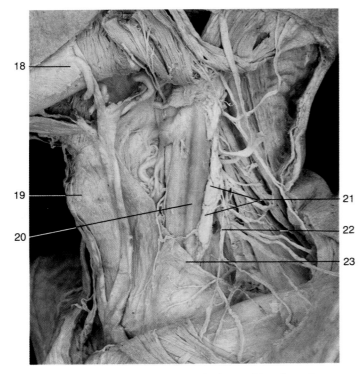

**Deep cervical nodes,** adjacent to the internal jugular vein.

**Lymphatic system.** Course of the main lymphatic vessels and lymph nodes in the body. Dotted line = border between lymphatic vessels draining toward the right venous angle and toward the left.

| | | | |
|---|---|---|---|
| 1 | Submandibular nodes | 14 | Descending aorta |
| 2 | Deep cervical nodes | 15 | Internal jugular vein |
| 3 | Right jugular trunk | 16 | Subclavian vein |
| 4 | Subclavian trunk | 17 | Left brachiocephalic vein |
| 5 | Right bronchomediastinal trunk | 18 | Mandible |
| 6 | Thoracic duct | 19 | Larynx |
| 7 | Cisterna chyli | 20 | Internal jugular vein |
| 8 | Intestinal trunk | 21 | Deep cervical nodes |
| 9 | Right lumbar trunk | 22 | Cervical nerve plexus |
| 10 | Internal iliac nodes | 23 | Superficial layer of deep fascia |
| 11 | Inguinal nodes | 24 | Occipital nodes |
| 12 | Axillary nodes | 25 | Parotid nodes |
| 13 | Descending trunk | 26 | Popliteal nodes |

Lymphatic vessels originate in the tissue spaces (lymph capillaries) and unite to form larger vessels (lymphatics). These resemble veins but have a much thinner wall, more valves, and are interrupted by lymph nodes at various intervals. Large groups of lymph nodes are located in the inguinal and axillary regions, deep to the mandible and sternocleidomastoid muscle, and within the root of the mesentery of the intestine.

# 2 Head and Neck

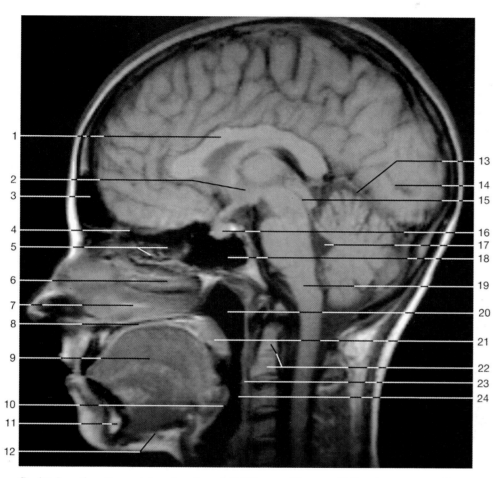

1 Corpus callosum
2 Hypothalamus
3 Frontal sinus
4 Cribriform plate
5 Ethmoidal air cells
6 Middle nasal concha
7 Inferior nasal concha
8 Hard palate
9 Tongue
10 Epiglottis
11 Mandible
12 Mylohyoid muscle
13 Tentorium of cerebellum
14 Calcarine fissure
15 Cerebral aqueduct
16 Pituitary gland
17 Fourth ventricle
18 Sphenoidal sinus
19 Medulla oblongata
20 Nasopharynx
21 Uvula
22 Dens of axis
23 Constrictor muscle of pharynx
24 Oral part of pharynx
25 Cerebrum (right hemisphere)
26 Calvaria
27 Cerebellum

**Sagittal section through head and neck** (MRI scan. 23-year-old female, courtesy of Prof. Dr. A. Heuck, Munich).

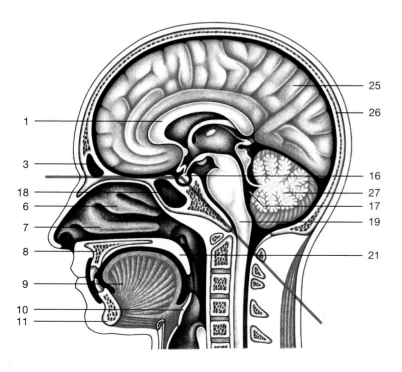

**Sagittal section through the head** (schematic drawing). The red line represents the border between the neurocranium and viscerocranium forming the clivus angle. The neural cavity, contains the brain; the viscerocranium comprises the orbit, the nasal cavity, and the oral cavity arranged one beneath the other.

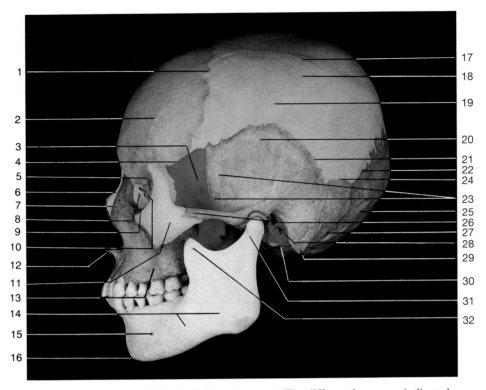

| | |
|---|---|
| 1 | Coronal suture |
| 2 | Frontal bone |
| 3 | Sphenoidal bone |
| 4 | Sphenofrontal suture |
| 5 | Ethmoidal bone |
| 6 | Nasal bone |
| 7 | Nasomaxillary suture |
| 8 | Lacrimal bone |
| 9 | Lacrimomaxillary suture |
| 10 | Ethmoidolacrimal suture |
| 11 | Zygomatic bone |
| 12 | Anterior nasal spine |
| 13 | Maxilla |
| 14 | Mandible |
| 15 | Mental foramen |
| 16 | Mental protuberance |
| 17 | Superior temporal line |
| 18 | Inferior temporal line |
| 19 | Parietal bone |
| 20 | Temporal bone |
| 21 | Squamous suture |
| 22 | Lambdoid suture |
| 23 | Temporal fossa |
| 24 | Parietomastoid suture |
| 25 | Occipital bone |
| 26 | Zygomatic arch |
| 27 | Occipitomastoid suture |
| 28 | External acoustic meatus |
| 29 | Mastoid process |
| 30 | Tympanic portion of temporal bone |
| 31 | Condylar process of mandible |
| 32 | Coronoid process of mandible |

**General architecture of the skull** (lateral aspect). The different bones are indicated in color (numbers cf. table).

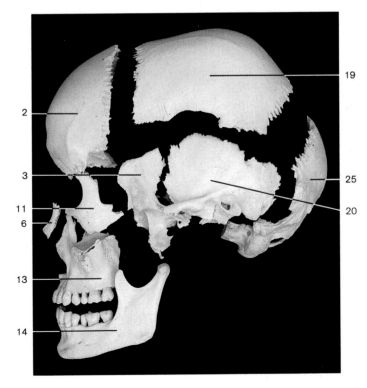

| |  | |
|---|---|---|
| 2 | Frontal bone (orange) | **Cranial bones** |
| 19 | Parietal bone (light yellow) | |
| 3 | Greater wing of sphenoidal bone (red) | |
| 25 | Squama of occipital bone (blue) | |
| 20 | Squama of temporal bone (brown) | |
| 5 | Ethmoidal bone (dark green) | **Base of skull** |
| 3 | Sphenoidal bone (red) | |
| | Temporal bone excluding squama (brown) | |
| 30 | Tympanic portion of temporal bone (dark brown) | |
| | Occipital bone excluding squama (blue) | |
| 6 | Nasal bone (white) | **Facial bones** |
| 8 | Lacrimal bone (light yellow) | |
| | Inferior nasal concha | |
| | Vomer | |
| 11 | Zygomatic bone (dark yellow) | |
| | Palatine bone | |
| 13 | Maxilla (violet) | |
| 14 | Mandible (white) | |
| | Malleus ⎫ within petrous portion of | **Auditory ossicles** |
| | Incus ⎬ temporal bone | |
| | Stapes ⎭ | |
| | Hyoid | |

**Lateral aspect of the disarticulated skull** (palatine bone, lacrimal bone, ethmoidal bone, and vomer are not depicted).

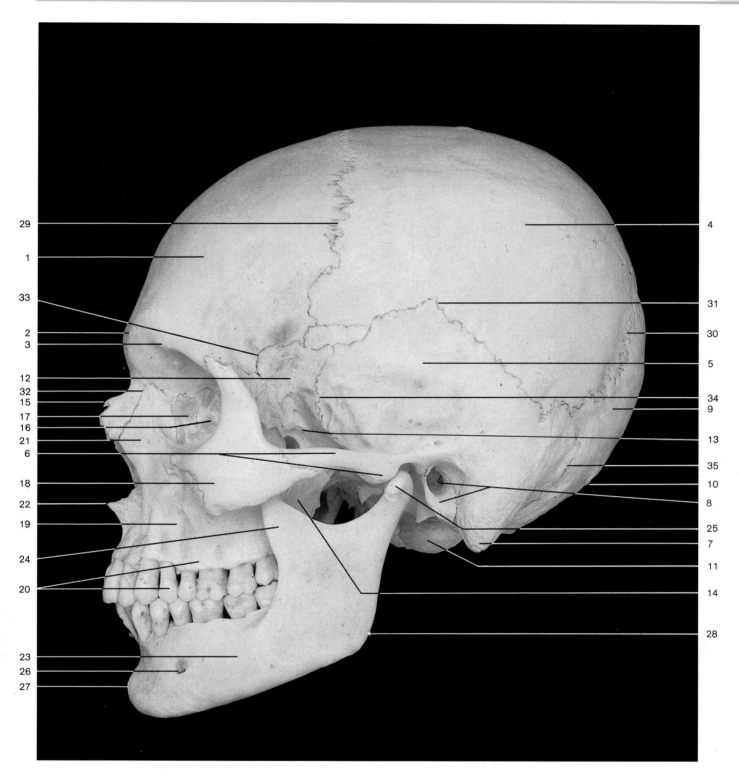

**Lateral aspect of the skull.**

| | | | | | |
|---|---|---|---|---|---|
| 1 | Frontal bone | 12 | Sphenoidal bone (greater wing) | 25 | Condylar process |
| 2 | Glabella | 13 | Infratemporal crest of sphenoid | 26 | Mental foramen |
| 3 | Supraorbital margin | 14 | Pterygoid process (lateral pterygoid plate) | 27 | Mental protuberance |
| 4 | Parietal bone | 15 | Nasal bone | 28 | Angle of the mandible |
| 5 | Temporal bone (squamous part) | 16 | Ethmoidal bone (orbital part) | | |
| 6 | Zygomatic process (articular tubercle) | 17 | Lacrimal bone | **Sutures** | |
| 7 | Mastoid process | 18 | Zygomatic bone | 29 | Coronal suture |
| 8 | Tympanic part (tympanic plate) and external acoustic meatus | 19 | Maxilla (body) | 30 | Lambdoid suture |
| | | 20 | Alveolar process and teeth | 31 | Squamous suture |
| 9 | Occipital bone (squamous part) | 21 | Frontal process | 32 | Nasomaxillary suture |
| 10 | External occipital protuberance | 22 | Anterior nasal spine | 33 | Frontosphenoid suture |
| 11 | Occipital condyle | 23 | Mandible (body) | 34 | Sphenosquamosal suture |
| | | 24 | Coronoid process | 35 | Occipitomastoid suture |

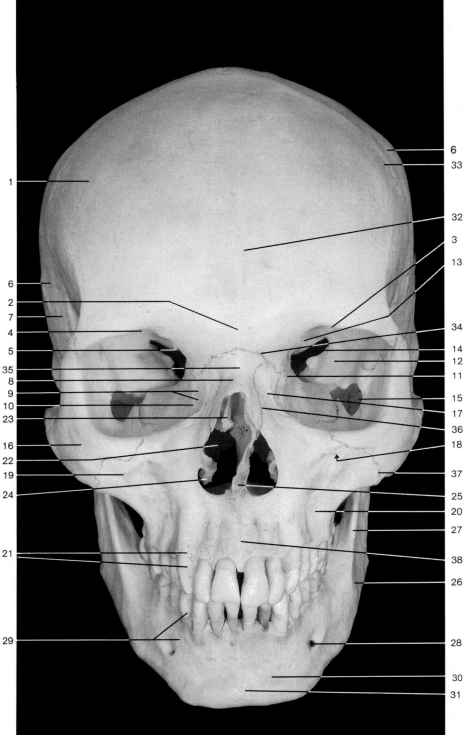

Anterior aspect of the skull.

1   Frontal bone
2   Glabella
3   Supra-orbital margin
4   Supra-orbital notch
5   Trochlear spine
6   Parietal bone
7   Temporal bone
8   Nasal bone

**Orbit**
9   Lacrimal bone
10  Posterior lacrimal crest
11  Ethmoidal bone

**Sphenoidal bone**
12  Greater wing of sphenoidal bone
13  Lesser wing of sphenoidal bone
14  Superior orbital fissure
15  Inferior orbital fissure
16  Zygomatic bone

**Maxilla**
17  Frontal process
18  Infra-orbital foramen
19  Zygomatic process
20  Body of maxilla
21  Alveolar process with teeth

**Nasal cavity**
22  Anterior nasal aperture
23  Middle nasal concha
24  Inferior nasal concha
25  Nasal septum, vomer

**Mandible**
26  Body of mandible
27  Ramus of mandible
28  Mental foramen
29  Alveolar part with teeth
30  Base of mandible
31  Mental protuberance

**Sutures**
32  Frontal suture
33  Coronal suture
34  Frontonasal suture
35  Internasal suture
36  Nasomaxillary suture
37  Zygomaticomaxillary suture
38  Intermaxillary suture

The skull comprises a mosaic of numerous complicated bones that form the cranial cavity protecting the brain (**neurocranium**) and several cavities such as the nasal and oral cavities in the facial region. The neurocranium consists of large bony plates that develop directly from the surrounding sheets of connective tissue (**desmocranium**). The bones of the skull base are formed out of cartilaginous tissue (**chondrocranium**), which ossifies secondarily. The **visceral skeleton,** which in fish gives rise to the gills, has in higher vertebrates been transformed into the bones of the masticatory and auditory apparatus (maxilla, mandible, auditory ossicles, and hyoid bone).

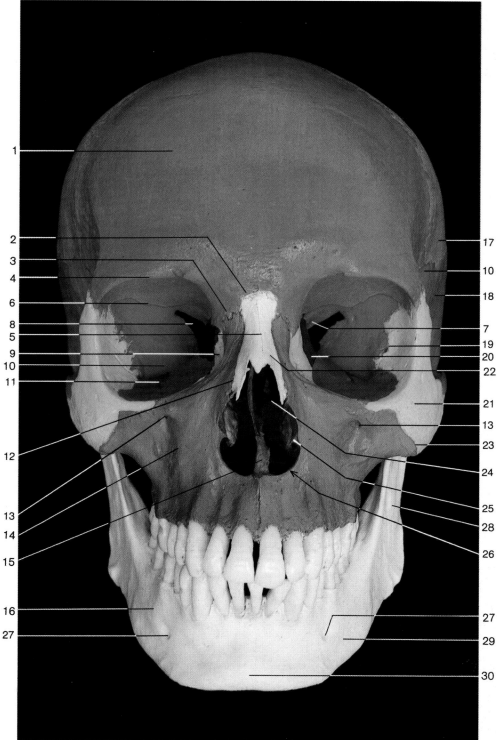

1   Frontal bone
2   Frontonasal suture
3   Frontomaxillary suture
4   Supra-orbital margin
5   Internasal suture
6   Sphenofrontal suture
7   Optic canal in lesser wing
    of sphenoidal bone
8   Superior orbital fissure
9   Lacrimal bone
10  Sphenoidal bone (greater wing)
11  Inferior orbital fissure
12  Nasomaxillary suture
13  Infra-orbital foramen
14  Maxilla
15  Vomer
16  Body of mandible
17  Parietal bone
18  Temporal bone
19  Sphenozygomatic suture
20  Ethmoidal bone
21  Zygomatic bone
22  Nasal bone
23  Zygomaticomaxillary suture
24  Middle nasal concha
25  Inferior nasal concha
26  Anterior nasal aperture
27  Mental foramen
28  Ramus of mandible
29  Base of mandible
30  Mental protuberance

**Bones**
Frontal bone (brown)
Parietal bone (light green)
Temporal bone (dark brown)
Sphenoidal bone (red)
Zygomatic bone (yellow)
Ethmoidal bone (dark green)
Lacrimal bone (yellow)
Vomer (orange)
Maxilla (violet)
Nasal bone (white)
Mandible (white)

**Anterior aspect of the skull** (individual bones indicated by color).

The following series of figures are arranged so that the mosaic-like pattern of the skull becomes understandable. It starts with the bones of the **skull base** (sphenoidal and occipital bones) to which the other bones are added step by step. The facial skeleton is built up by the ethmoidal bone to which the palatine bone and maxilla are attached laterally; the small nasal and lacrimal bones fill the remaining spaces. Cartilages remain only in the external part of the nose.

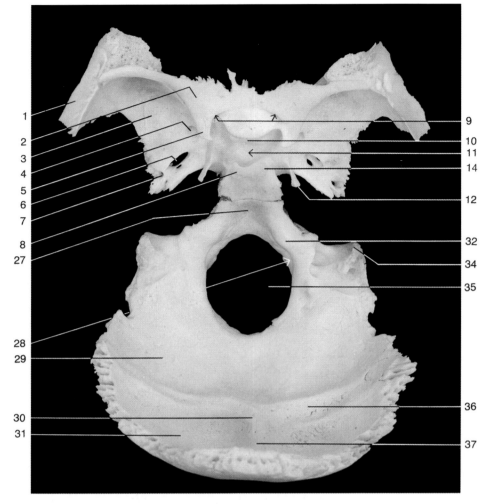

**Sphenoidal and occipital bone** (from above).

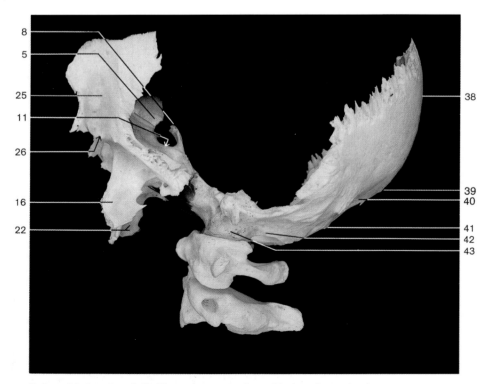

**Sphenoidal and occipital bone** in connection with the atlas and axis
(1st and 2nd cervical vertebrae) (left lateral view).

**Sphenoidal bone**
1 Greater wing
2 Lesser wing
3 Cerebral or superior surface of greater wing
4 Foramen rotundum
5 Anterior clinoid process
6 Foramen ovale
7 Foramen spinosum
8 Dorsum sellae
9 Optic canal
10 Chiasmatic groove (sulcus chiasmatis)
11 Hypophysial fossa (sella turcica)
12 Lingula
13 Opening of sphenoidal sinus
14 Posterior clinoid process
15 Pterygoid canal
16 Lateral pterygoid plate of pterygoid process
17 Pterygoid notch
18 Pterygoid hamulus
19 Orbital surface of greater wing
20 Sphenoidal crest
21 Sphenoidal rostrum
22 Medial pterygoid plate
23 Superior orbital fissure
24 Spine of sphenoid
25 Temporal surface of greater wing
26 Infratemporal crest

**Occipital bone**
27 Clivus with basilar part of occipital bone
28 Hypoglossal canal
29 Fossa for cerebellar hemisphere
30 Internal occipital protuberance
31 Fossa for cerebral hemisphere
32 Jugular tubercle
33 Condylar canal
34 Jugular process
35 Foramen magnum
36 Groove for transverse sinus
37 Groove for superior sagittal sinus
38 Squamous part of the occipital bone
39 External occipital protuberance
40 Superior nuchal line
41 Inferior nuchal line
42 Condylar fossa
43 Condyle
44 Pharyngeal tubercle
45 External occipital crest

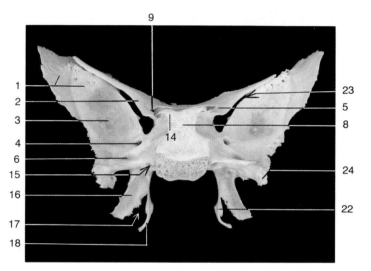

**Sphenoidal bone** (anterior aspect).

**Sphenoidal bone** (posterior aspect).

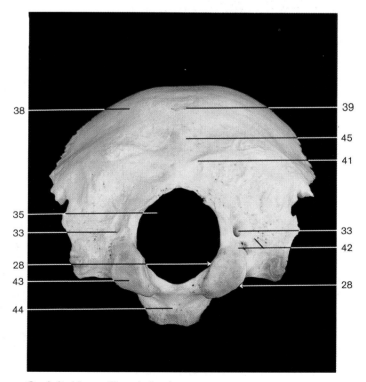

**Occipital bone** (from below).

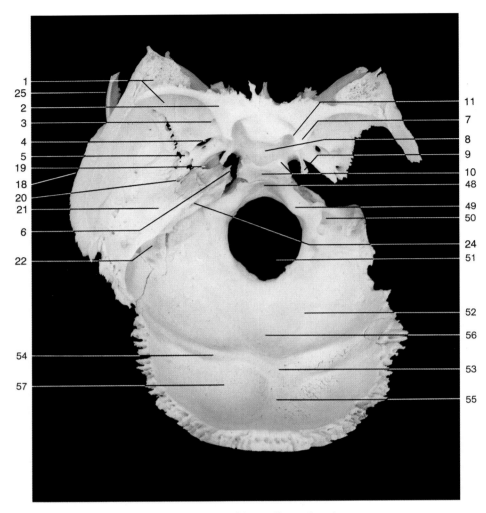

**Sphenoidal, occipital and left temporal bone** (from above).
Internal aspect of the base of the skull. The left temporal
bone has been added to the preceding figure.

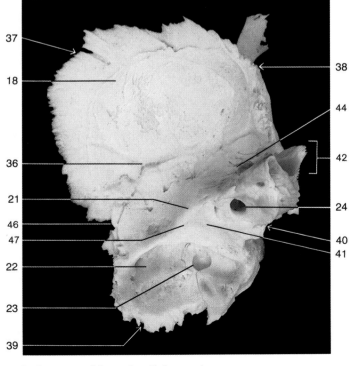

**Left temporal bone** (medial aspect).

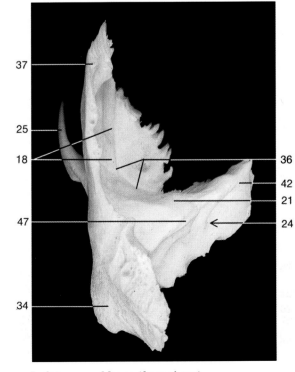

**Left temporal bone** (from above).

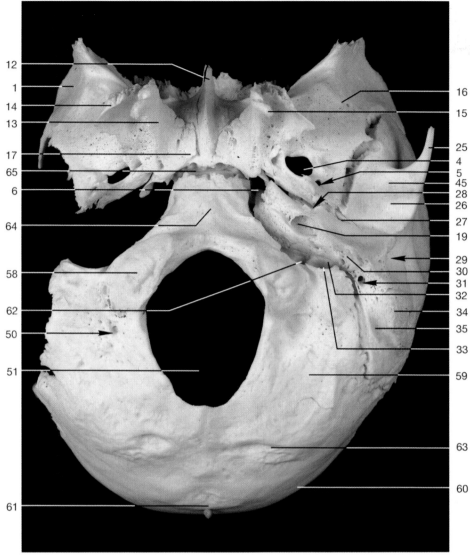

**Sphenoidal, occipital, and left temporal bone.** Base of the skull (external aspect).

**Temporal bone**
18  Squamous part
19  Carotid canal
20  Hiatus of facial canal
    (for the greater petrosal nerve)
21  Arcuate eminence
22  Groove for the sigmoid sinus
23  Mastoid foramen
24  Internal acoustic meatus
25  Zygomatic process
26  Mandibular fossa
27  Petrotympanic fissure
28  Canalis musculotubarius
    (bony part of auditory tube)
29  External acoustic meatus
30  Styloid process (remnant only)
31  Stylomastoid foramen
32  Mastoid canaliculus
33  Jugular fossa
34  Mastoid process
35  Mastoid notch
36  Groove for middle
    meningeal vessels
37  Parietal margin
38  Sphenoidal margin
39  Occipital margin
40  Cochlear canaliculus
41  Aqueduct of the vestibule
42  Apex of the petrous part
43  Tympanic part
44  Trigeminal impression
45  Articular tubercle
46  Parietal notch
47  Groove for the superior
    petrosal sinus

**Occipital bone**
48  Clivus
49  Jugular tubercle
50  Condylar canal
51  Foramen magnum
52  Lower part of squamous
    occipital bone
    (cerebellar fossa)
53  Internal occipital protuberance
54  Groove for the transverse sinus
55  Groove for the superior sagittal sinus
56  Internal occipital crest
57  Upper part of squamous occipital
    bone (cerebral fossa)
58  Condyle
59  Nuchal plane
60  Superior nuchal line
61  External occipital protuberance
62  Jugular foramen
63  Inferior nuchal line
64  Pharyngeal tubercle
65  Spheno-occipital synchondrosis

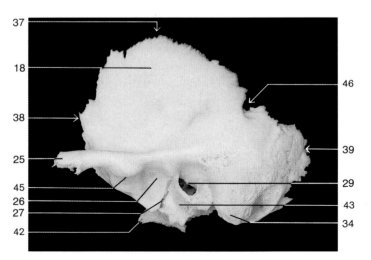

**Left temporal bone** (lateral aspect).

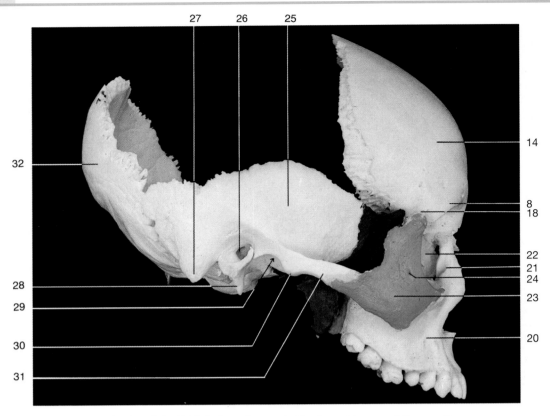

**Part of a disarticulated skull** (right lateral aspect). The frontal bone and the maxilla are connected with the temporal bone by the zygomatic bone (orange). Sphenoidal bone (black), palatine bone (red), lacrimal bone (yellow).

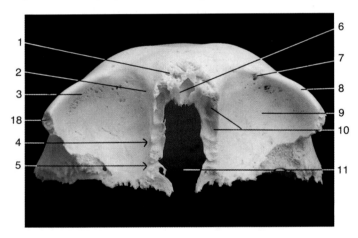

**Frontal bone** (inferior aspect). The ethmoidal foveolae cover the ethmoidal cavities of the ethmoidal bone.

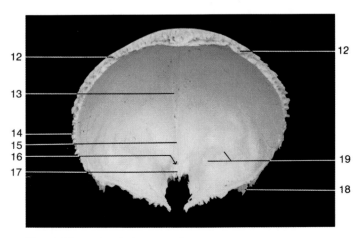

**Frontal bone** (posterior aspect).

**Frontal bone**
1  Nasal margin
2  Trochlear fossa
3  Fossa for lacrimal gland
4  Anterior ethmoidal foramen
5  Posterior ethmoidal foramen
6  Nasal spine
7  Supra-orbital notch
8  Supra-orbital margin
9  Orbital plate
10  Roofs of the ethmoidal air cells
11  Ethmoidal notch
12  Parietal margin
13  Groove for superior sagittal sinus
14  Squamous part of frontal bone
15  Frontal crest
16  Foramen cecum
17  Nasal spine
18  Zygomatic process of frontal bone
19  Juga cerebralia

**Facial bones**
20  Maxilla
21  Frontal process of maxilla
22  Lacrimal bone (yellow)
23  Zygomatic bone (orange)
24  Zygomaticofacial foramen

**Temporal bone**
25  Squamous part of temporal bone
26  External acoustic meatus
27  Mastoid process
28  Styloid process
29  Mandibular fossa
30  Articular tubercle
31  Zygomatic process

**Occipital bone**
32  Squamous part of occipital bone

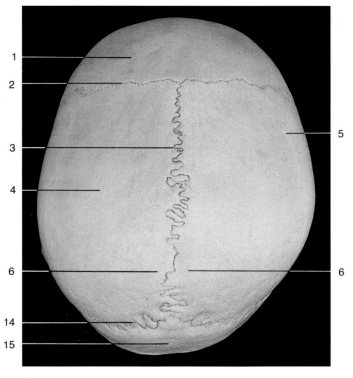

**Calvaria** (superior aspect).

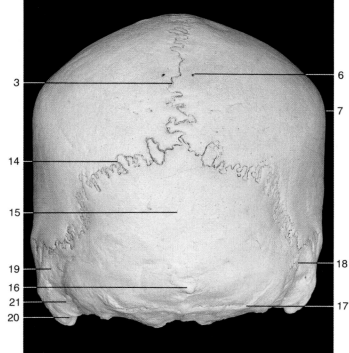

**Calvaria** (posterior aspect).

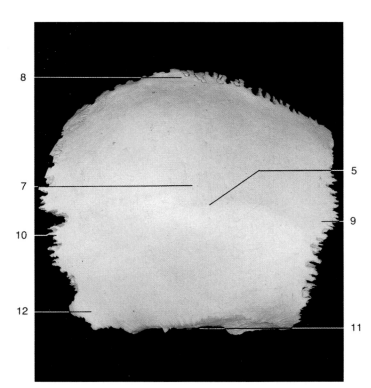

**Left parietal bone** (external aspect).

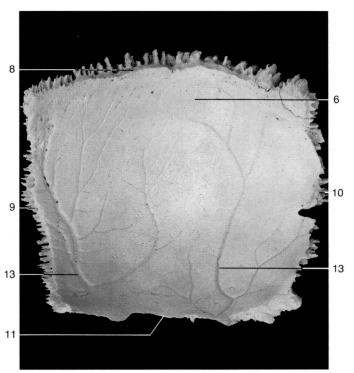

**Left parietal bone** (internal aspect).

| | | |
|---|---|---|
| 1 Frontal bone | 8 Sagittal margin | 15 Occipital bone |
| 2 Coronal suture | 9 Occipital margin | 16 External occipital protuberance |
| 3 Sagittal suture | 10 Frontal margin | 17 Inferior nuchal line |
| 4 Parietal bone | 11 Squamous margin | 18 Occipitomastoid suture |
| 5 Superior temporal line | 12 Sphenoidal angle | 19 Temporal bone |
| 6 Parietal foramen | 13 Groove for middle meningeal artery | 20 Mastoid process |
| 7 Parietal tuber or eminence | 14 Lambdoid suture | 21 Mastoid notch |

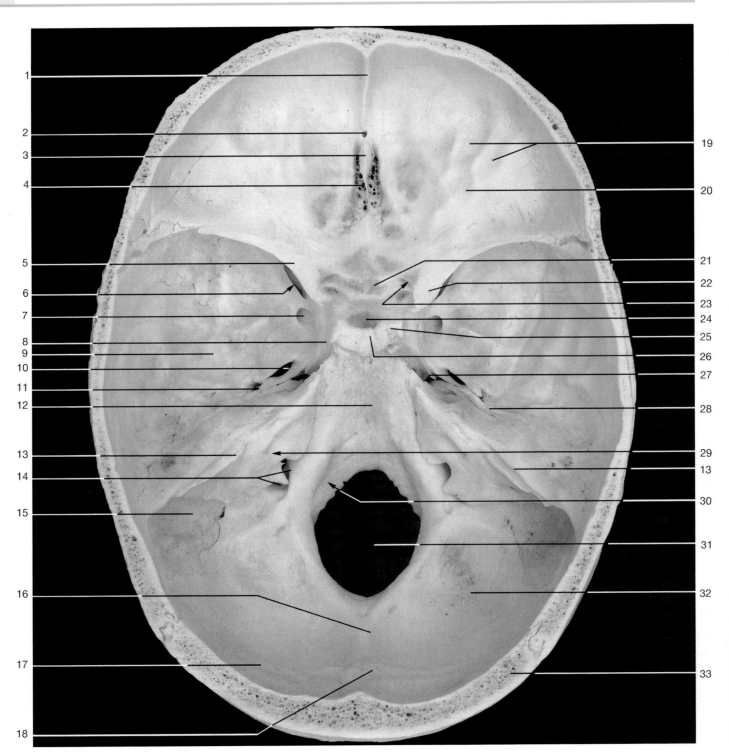

**Base of the skull,** calvaria removed (internal aspect).

| | | |
|---|---|---|
| 1 | Frontal crest | 12 Clivus |
| 2 | Foramen cecum | 13 Groove for superior petrosal sinus |
| 3 | Crista galli | 14 Jugular foramen |
| 4 | Cribriform plate of ethmoidal bone | 15 Groove for sigmoid sinus |
| 5 | Lesser wing of sphenoidal bone | 16 Internal occipital crest |
| 6 | Superior orbital fissure | 17 Groove for transverse sinus |
| 7 | Foramen rotundum | 18 Internal occipital protuberance |
| 8 | Carotid sulcus | 19 Digitate impressions |
| 9 | Middle cranial fossa | 20 Anterior cranial fossa |
| 10 | Foramen ovale | 21 Chiasmatic sulcus |
| 11 | Foramen spinosum | 22 Anterior clinoid process |

23 Optic canal
24 Sella turcica (hypophysial fossa)
25 Posterior clinoid process
26 Dorsum sellae
27 Foramen lacerum
28 Groove for greater petrosal nerve
29 Internal acoustic meatus
30 Hypoglossal canal
31 Foramen magnum
32 Posterior cranial fossa
33 Diploe

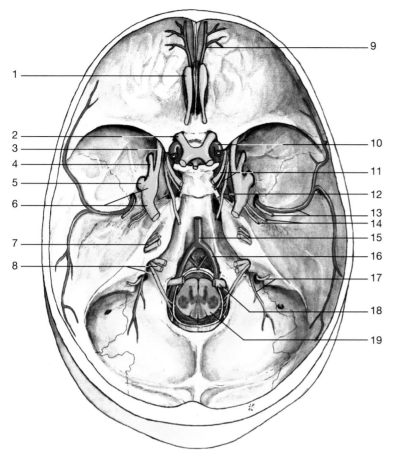

1 Olfactory bulb
2 Optic nerve (n. II)
3 Ophthalmic nerve (n. V$_1$)
4 Maxillary nerve (n. V$_2$)
5 Mandibular nerve (n. V$_3$)
6 Trigeminal nerve (n. V) with trigeminal ganglion
7 Facial nerve (n. VII) and vestibulocochlear nerve (n. VIII)
8 Glossopharyngeal nerve (n. IX), vagus nerve (n. X) and accessory nerve (n. XI)
9 Anterior meningeal artery
10 Internal carotid artery
11 Oculomotor nerve (n. III) and trochlear nerve (n. IV)
12 Abducent nerve (n. VI)
13 Middle meningeal artery and meningeal branch of mandibular nerve
14 Greater and lesser petrosal nerves
15 Basilar artery
16 Vertebral artery
17 Posterior meningeal artery and recurrent meningeal nerve
18 Hypoglossal nerve (n. XII)
19 Medulla oblongata

**Base of the skull** with cranial nerves and meningeal arteries (internal aspect, schematic drawing).

| | Cranial nerves and vessels | Related foramina | Related regions |
|---|---|---|---|
| **Anterior cranial fossa** | Olfactory nerves (n. I), Anterior ethmoidal artery, vein, and nerve, Anterior meningeal artery | Lamina cribrosa | Nasal cavity |
| **Middle cranial fossa** | Optic nerve (n. II), Ophthalmic artery | Optic canal | Orbit |
| | Occulomotor nerve (n. III), Trochlear nerve (n. IV), Abducent nerve (n. VI), Ophthalmic nerve (n. V$_1$), Superior ophthalmic vein | Superior orbital fissure | Orbit |
| | Maxillary nerve (n. V$_2$) | Foramen rotundum | Pterygopalatine fossa |
| | Mandibular nerve (n. V$_3$) | Foramen ovale | Infratemporal fossa |
| | Middle meningeal artery, Meningeal branch of mandibular nerve (n. V$_3$) | Foramen spinosum | Infratemporal fossa |
| | Internal carotid artery | Carotid canal | Cavernous sinus, Base of skull |
| **Posterior cranial fossa** | Facial nerve (n. VII), Vestibulocochlear nerve (n. VIII), Artery and vein of the labyrinth | Internal acoustic meatus, Stylomastoid foramen, Facial canal | Inner ear, Face |
| | Glossopharyngeal nerve (n. IX), Vagus nerve (n. X), Accessory nerve (n. XI), Internal jugular vein, Posterior meningeal artery | Jugular foramen | Parapharyngeal region |
| | Hypoglossal nerve (n. XII) | Hypoglossal canal | Tongue |
| | Accessory nerve (n. XI, spinal root), Vertebral arteries, Anterior and posterior spinal arteries, Medulla oblongata | Foramen magnum | Base of skull |

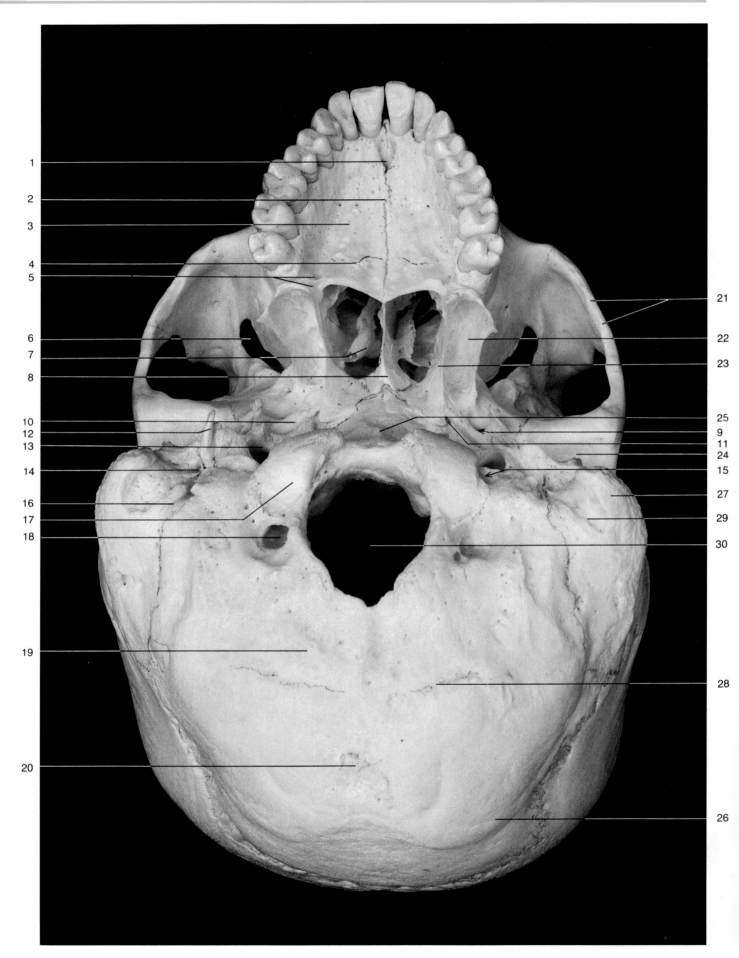

**Base of the skull** (inferior aspect).

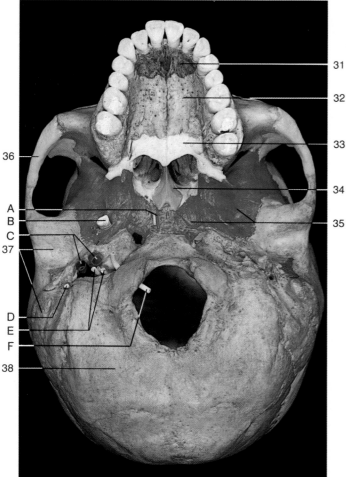

**Base of the skull** (from below). The individual bones are indicated by different colors.

A    **Pterygoid canal**
B    **Foramen ovale**
C    Internal carotid artery within **carotid canal** and internal jugular vein within the venous part of jugular foramen
D    **Stylomastoid foramen** (facial nerve)
E    **Jugular foramen** (glossopharyngeal, vagus and accessory nerves)
F    **Hypoglossal canal** (hypoglossal nerve)

1    Incisive canal
2    Median palatine suture
3    Palatine process of maxilla
4    Palatomaxillary suture
5    Greater and lesser palatine foramina
6    Inferior orbital fissure
7    Middle concha (process of ethmoidal bone)
8    Vomer
9    Foramen ovale
10   Groove for auditory tube
11   Pterygoid canal
12   Styloid process
13   Carotid canal
14   Stylomastoid foramen
15   Jugular foramen
16   Groove for occipital artery
17   Occipital condyle
18   Condylar canal
19   Nuchal plane
20   External occipital protuberance
21   Zygomatic arch
22   Lateral pterygoid plate
23   Medial pterygoid plate
24   Mandibular fossa
25   Pharyngeal tubercle
26   Superior nuchal line
27   Mastoid process
28   Inferior nuchal line
29   Mastoid notch
30   Foramen magnum
31   Incisive bone or premaxilla (dark violet)
32   Maxilla (violet)
33   Palatine bone (white)
34   Vomer (orange)
35   Sphenoidal bone (red)
36   Zygomatic bone (yellow)
37   Temporal bone (brown)
38   Occipital bone (blue)
39   Palatine process of maxilla
40   Vomer
41   Sphenoidal bone
42   Petrous part of temporal bone
43   Basilar part ⎫
44   Lateral part  ⎬ of occipital bone
45   Squamous part ⎭
46   Mandible
47   Zygomatic arch
48   Choana
49   Pterygoid process of sphenoidal bone
50   Carotid canal
51   External acoustic meatus (tympanic anulus)
52   Sphenoidal fontanelle
53   Parietal bone
54   Mastoid fontanelle

**Skull of the newborn** (inferior aspect).

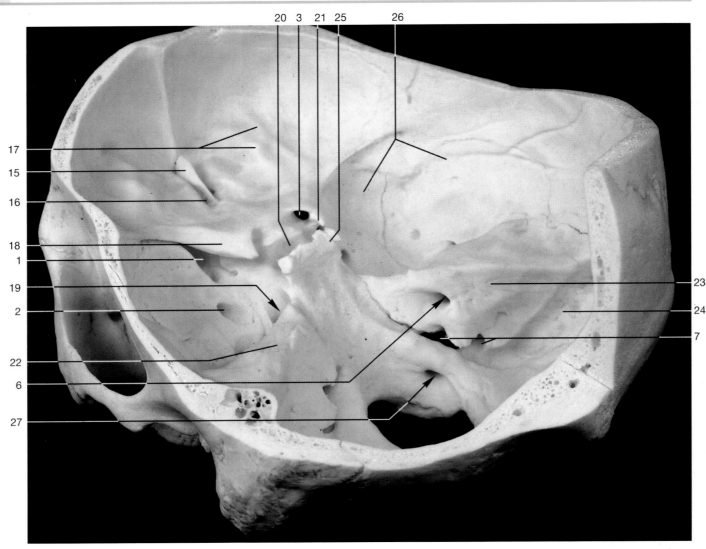

**Base of the skull** (internal aspect, oblique lateral view from left side).

**Canals, fissures and foramina of the base of the skull**

1   Superior orbital fissure
2   Foramen rotundum
3   Optic canal
4   Foramen ovale
5   Foramen spinosum
6   Internal acoustic meatus
7   Jugular foramen
8   Foramen magnum

**Bones**

9   Frontal bone (orange)
10  Ethmoidal bone (dark green)
11  Sphenoidal bone (red)
12  Temporal bone (brown)
13  Parietal bone (yellow)
14  Occipital bone (blue)

**Details of bones**

15  Crista galli
16  Cribriform plate

17  Digitate impressions (frontal bone)
18  Lesser wing of sphenoidal bone
19  Foramen lacerum
20  Hypophysial fossa (sella turcica)
21  Anterior clinoid process
22  Trigeminal impression
23  Petrous part of temporal bone
24  Groove for sigmoid sinus
25  Dorsum sellae (posterior clinoid process)
26  Greater wing of sphenoidal bone, groove for middle meningeal artery
27  Hypoglossal canal

**Base of the skull** (internal aspect, superior view).
Individual bones indicated by color.

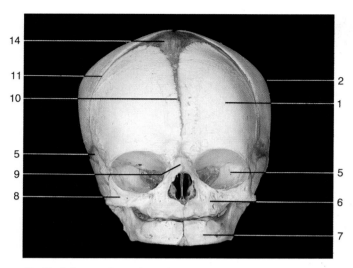

**Skull of the newborn** (anterior aspect).

**Cranial skeleton**
1  Frontal tuber or eminence
2  Parietal tuber or eminence
3  Occipital tuber or eminence
4  Squamous part of temporal bone
5  Greater wing of sphenoidal bone

**Facial skeleton**
6  Maxilla
7  Mandible
8  Zygomatic bone
9  Nasal bone

**Sutures and fontanelles**
10  Frontal suture
11  Coronal suture
12  Sagittal suture
13  Lambdoid suture
14  Anterior fontanelle
15  Posterior fontanelle
16  Sphenoidal (anterolateral) fontanelle
17  Mastoid (posterolateral) fontanelle

**Base of the skull**
18  Frontal bone
19  Ethmoidal bone
20  Sphenoidal bone
21  Hypophysial fossa (sella turcica)
22  Dorsum sellae
23  Temporal bone
24  Mastoid (posterolateral) fontanelle
25  Occipital bone

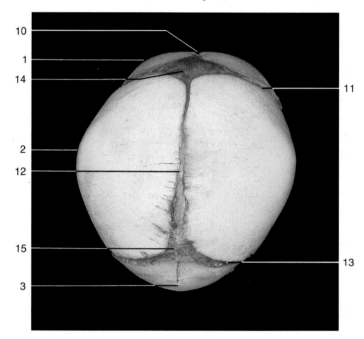

**Skull of the newborn** (superior aspect). Calvaria.

In the newborn the facial skeleton, in contrast to the cranial skeleton, appears relatively small. There are no teeth presenting. The bones of the cranium are separated by wide fontanelles.

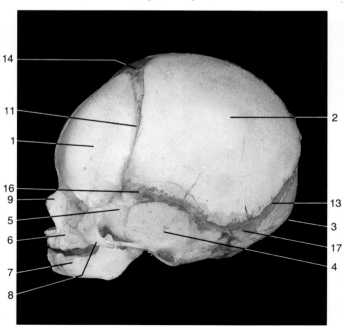

**Skull of the newborn** (lateral aspect).

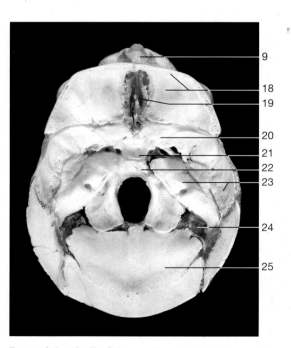

**Base of the skull of the newborn** (internal aspect).

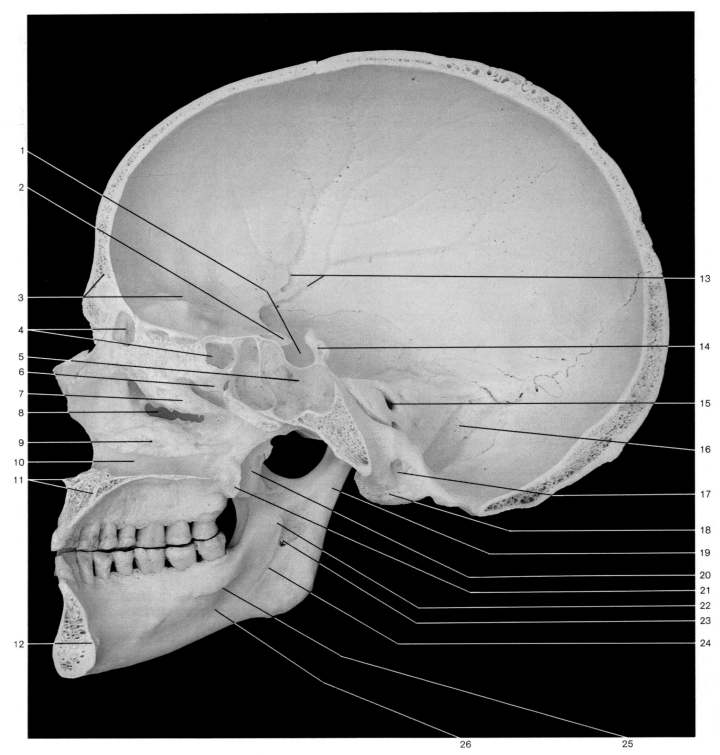

**Median section through the skull,** right half (internal aspect).

| | | | |
|---|---|---|---|
| 1 | Hypophysial fossa (sella turcica) | 14 | Dorsum sellae |
| 2 | Anterior clinoid process | 15 | Internal acoustic meatus |
| 3 | Frontal bone | 16 | Groove for sigmoid sinus |
| 4 | Ethmoidal air cells | 17 | Hypoglossal canal |
| 5 | Sphenoidal sinus | 18 | Occipital condyle |
| 6 | Superior concha | 19 | Condylar process |
| 7 | Middle concha | 20 | Lateral pterygoid plate ⎫ of pterygoid process |
| 8 | Maxillary hiatus | 21 | Medial pterygoid plate ⎬ |
| 9 | Inferior concha | 22 | Lingula of mandible |
| 10 | Inferior meatus | 23 | Mandibular foramen |
| 11 | Anterior nasal spine and maxilla | 24 | Mylohyoid groove |
| 12 | Mental spine or genial tubercle | 25 | Mylohyoid line |
| 13 | Groove for middle meningeal artery | 26 | Submandibular fovea |

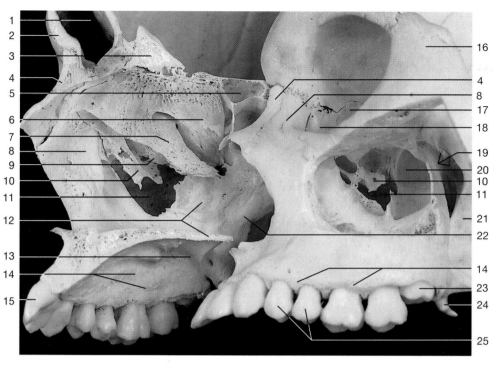

1 Frontal sinus
2 Frontal bone
3 Crista galli
4 Nasal bone
5 Sphenoidal sinus
6 Superior concha } of ethmoidal
7 Middle concha } bone
8 Frontal process
   of maxilla
9 Ethmoidal bulla
10 Uncinate process
11 Maxillary hiatus
12 Palatine bone
13 Greater palatine foramen
14 Alveolar process of maxilla
15 Central incisor
16 Zygomatic bone
17 Ethmoidal bone
18 Lacrimal bone
19 Pterygopalatine fossa
20 Maxillary sinus
21 Lateral pterygoid plate
22 Medial pterygoid plate
23 Third molar tooth
24 Pterygoid hamulus
25 Two premolar teeth

**Facial part of the skull (viscerocranium),** divided in two halves (lateral and medial aspect). Right inferior concha has been removed to show the maxillary hiatus. Left maxillary sinus opened.

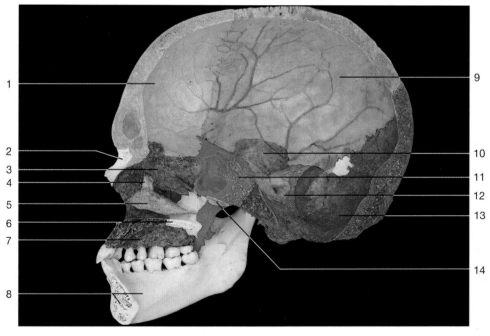

**Bones** (indicated by colors)
1 Frontal bone (yellow)
2 Nasal bone (white)
3 Ethmoidal bone (dark green)
4 Lacrimal bone (yellow)
5 Inferior nasal concha (pink)
6 Palatine bone (white)
7 Maxilla (violet)
8 Mandible (white)
9 Parietal bone (light green)
10 Temporal bone (brown)
11 Sphenoidal bone (red)
12 Petrous part of temporal
   bone (brown)
13 Occipital bone (blue)
14 Ala of vomer (light brown)

**Median section through the skull.** The nasal septum has been removed. Bones indicated by colors.

Because of the upright posture that the human developed in the course of evolution, the cranial cavity greatly increased in size, whereas the facial skeleton decreased. As a result, the base of the skull developed an angulation of about 120° between the clivus and the cribriform plate (see drawing on page 19). The hypophysial fossa containing the pituitary gland lies at the angle formed between these two planes.

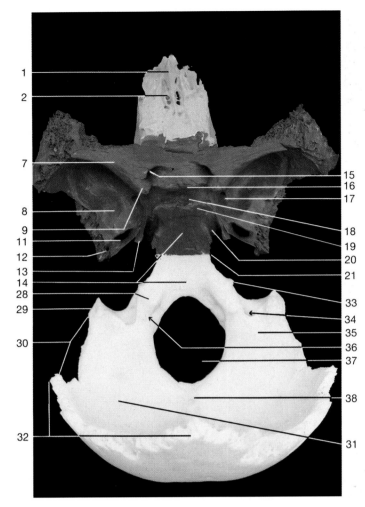

**Ethmoidal bone**
1  Crista galli
2  Cribriform plate
3  Ethmoidal air cells
4  Middle concha
5  Perpendicular plate (part of nasal septum)
6  Orbital plate

**Sphenoidal bone**
7  Lesser wing
8  Greater wing
9  Anterior clinoid process
10  Posterior clinoid process
11  Foramen ovale
12  Foramen spinosum
13  Lingula of the sphenoidal bone
14  Clivus
15  Optic canal
16  Tuberculum sellae
17  Foramen rotundum (right side)
18  Hypophysial fossa (sella turcica)
19  Dorsum sellae
20  Carotid sulcus
21  Spheno-occipital synchondrosis
22  Lateral pterygoid plate
23  Greater wing of sphenoidal bone (orbital surface)
24  Greater wing of sphenoidal bone (maxillary surface)
25  Foramen rotundum (left side)
26  Superior orbital fissure
27  Infratemporal crest of the greater wing

**Part of the disarticulated base of the skull.**
Ethmoidal, sphenoidal and occipital bones (from above).
Green = sphenoidal bone; yellow = ethmoidal bone.

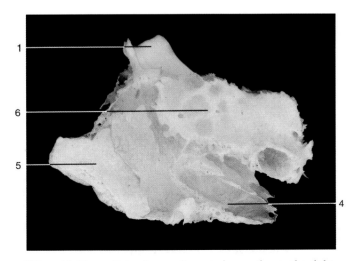

**Ethmoidal bone** (lateral aspect), posterior portion to the right.

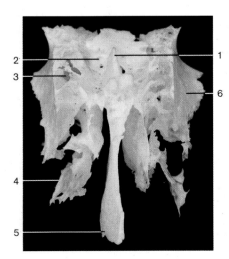

**Ethmoidal bone** (anterior aspect).

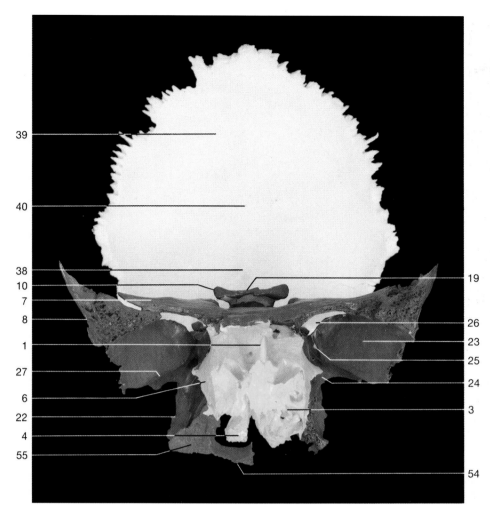

**Occipital bone**
28  Jugular tubercle
29  Jugular process
30  Mastoid margin
31  Posterior cranial fossa
32  Lambdoid margin
33  Intrajugular process
34  Condylar canal
35  Lateral part of occipital bone
36  Hypoglossal canal
37  Foramen magnum
38  Internal occipital crest
39  Squamous part of occipital bone
40  Internal occipital protuberance

**Maxilla**
41  Orbital surface
42  Infra-orbital groove
43  Maxillary tuberosity with foramina
44  Frontal process
45  Nasolacrimal groove
46  Infra-orbital margin
47  Anterior nasal spine
48  Zygomatic process
49  Alveolar process

**Palatine bone**
50  Orbital process
51  Sphenopalatine notch
52  Sphenoidal process
53  Perpendicular plate
54  Horizontal plate
55  Pyramidal process

**Disarticulated base of the skull** (anterior aspect).
Green = sphenoidal bone; yellow = ethmoidal bone; red = palatine bone.

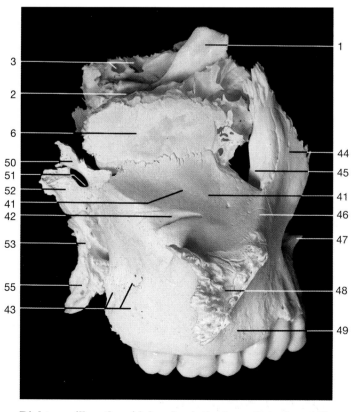

**Right maxilla, ethmoidal and palatine bone** (lateral aspect).

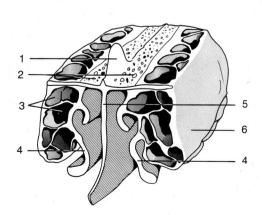

**Ethmoidal bone** (oblique anterior aspect).
(Schematic drawing.)

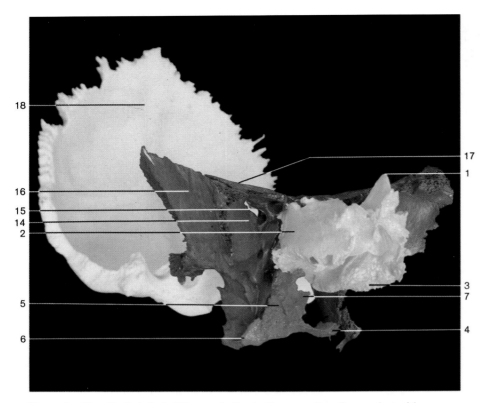

**Ethmoidal bone**
1  Crista galli
2  Orbital plate
3  Middle concha

**Palatine bone**
4  Horizontal plate of palatine bone
5  Greater palatine canal
6  Pyramidal process
7  Maxillary process
8  Orbital process
9  Sphenopalatine notch
10  Perpendicular plate of palatine bone
11  Conchal crest
12  Nasal crest
13  Sphenoidal process

**Sphenoidal bone**
14  Greater wing
15  Superior orbital fissure
16  Greater wing (orbital surface)
17  Lesser wing

**Occipital bone**
18  Squamous part of occipital bone

**Maxilla**
19  Maxillary tuberosity
20  Frontal process
21  Orbital surface
22  Infra-orbital margin
23  Infra-orbital groove
24  Zygomatic process
25  Alveolar process

**Part of a disarticulated skull base,** similar to the preceding figures, but with palatine bone. Green = sphenoidal bone; yellow = ethmoidal bone; red = palatine bone.

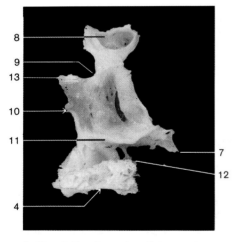

**Left palatine bone** (medial aspect, posterior aspect to the left).

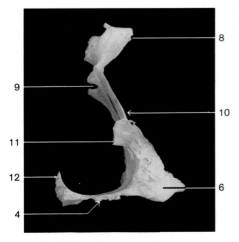

**Left palatine bone** (anterior aspect).

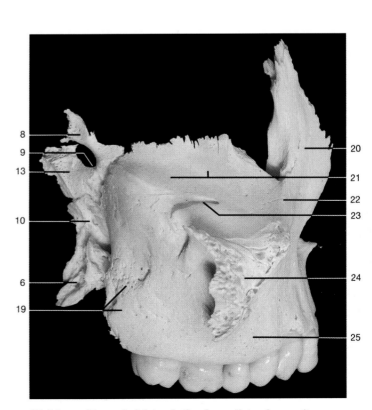

**Right maxilla and right palatine bone** (lateral aspect).

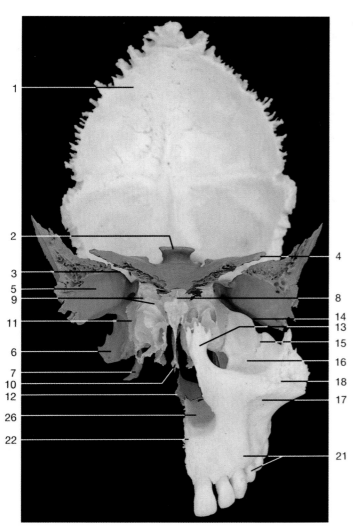

**Occipital bone**
1   Squamous part

**Sphenoidal bone**
2   Dorsum sellae
3   Superior orbital fissure
4   Lesser wing
5   Greater wing (orbital surface)
6   Lateral pterygoid plate
7   Medial pterygoid plate

**Ethmoidal bone**
8   Crista galli
9   Ethmoidal air cells
10   Perpendicular plate
11   Orbital plate

**Palatine bone**
12   Horizontal plate (nasal crest)

**Maxilla**
13   Frontal process
14   Inferior orbital fissure
15   Infra-orbital groove
16   Orbital surface
17   Infra-orbital foramen
18   Zygomatic process
19   Anterior lacrimal crest
20   Canine fossa
21   Alveolar process with teeth
22   Anterior nasal spine
23   Juga alveolaria (elevations formed by roots of teeth)
24   Lacrimal groove
25   Maxillary tuberosity with alveolar foramina
26   Palatine process of maxilla

**Part of a disarticulated skull.**
The left **maxilla** is added to the preceding specimen.

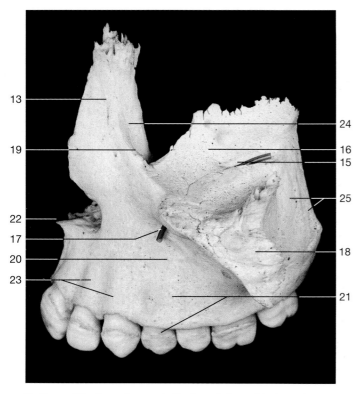

**Left maxilla** (lateral aspect). Probe = infra-orbital canal.

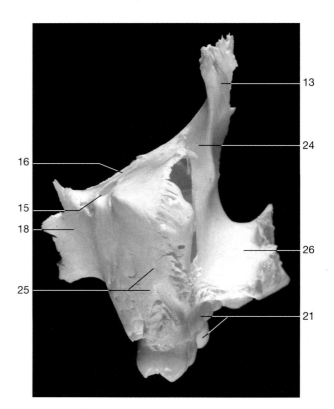

**Left maxilla** (posterior aspect).

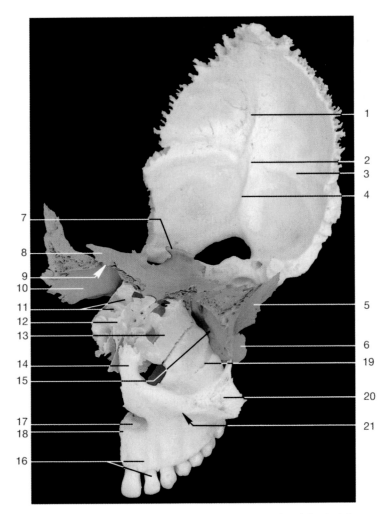

**Part of a disarticulated base of skull.** The mosaic of the facial bones [sphenoidal bone (green), ethmoidal bone (yellow), and palatine bone (red)] is seen from the anterior-lateral aspect.

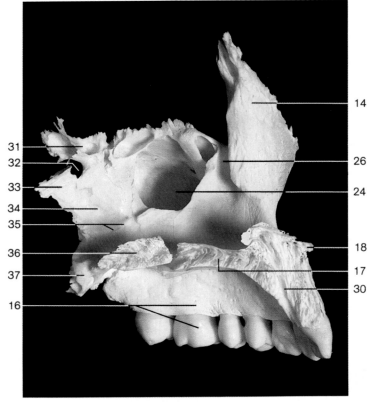

**Left maxilla and palatine bone** (medial aspect).

**Occipital bone**
1  Groove for superior sagittal sinus
2  Internal occipital protuberance
3  Groove for transverse sinus
4  Internal occipital crest

**Sphenoidal bone**
5  Greater wing (temporal surface)
6  Lateral pterygoid plate
7  Dorsum sellae
8  Lesser wing
9  Superior orbital fissure
10  Greater wing (orbital surface)

**Ethmoidal bone**
11  Ethmoidal air cells
12  Crista galli
13  Orbital plate

**Maxilla**
14  Frontal process
15  Inferior orbital fissure
16  Alveolar process with teeth
17  Palatine process
18  Anterior nasal spine
19  Infra-orbital groove
20  Zygomatic process
21  Location of infra-orbital foramen
22  Middle nasal meatus
23  Inferior nasal meatus
24  Maxillary hiatus
    (leading to maxillary sinus)
25  Third molar
26  Lacrimal groove
27  Conchal crest
28  Body of maxilla (nasal surface)
29  Nasal crest
30  Incisive canal

**Palatine bone**
31  Orbital process
32  Sphenopalatine notch
33  Sphenoidal process
34  Perpendicular plate
35  Conchal crest
36  Horizontal plate
37  Pyramidal process

**Frontal bone**
38  Squamous part
39  Supra-orbital foramen
40  Frontal notch
41  Frontal spine

**Inferior nasal concha**
42  Inferior nasal concha
    with maxillary process

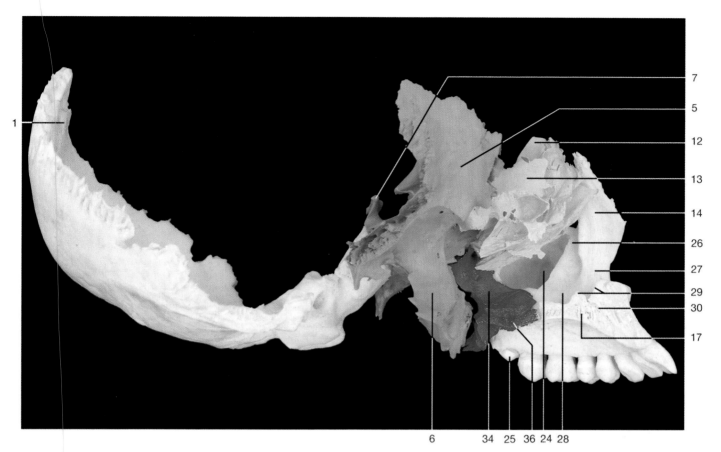

**Part of a disarticulated base of skull** (medial aspect). Green = sphenoidal bone; yellow = ethmoidal bone; red = palatine bone; natural colored = left maxilla.

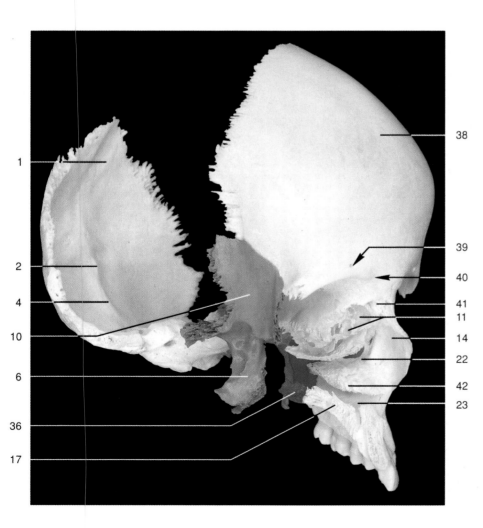

**Part of a disarticulated base of skull.** The same specimen as shown above but with frontal bone (oblique-lateral aspect).

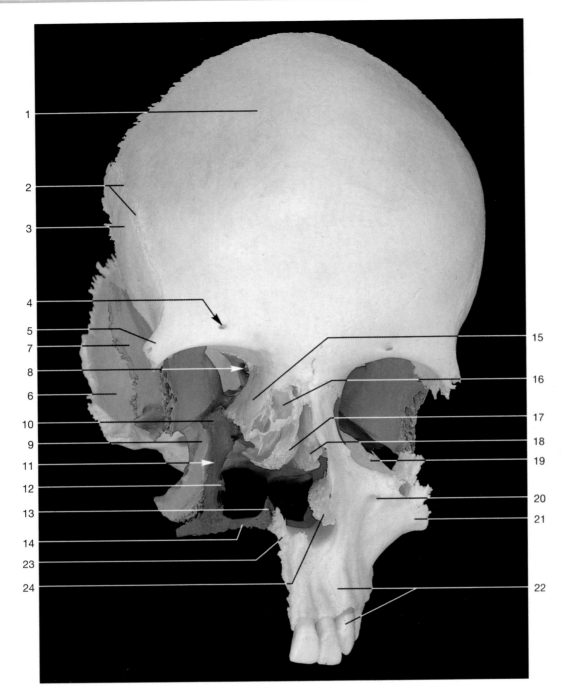

**Part of a disarticulated skull,** showing the connection of the palatine bone (red) and the maxilla with ethmoidal bone (yellow) and sphenoidal bone (light green) (anterior aspect).

**Frontal bone**
1  Squamous part
2  Inferior temporal line
3  Temporal surface
4  Supra-orbital foramen
5  Zygomatic process

**Occipital bone**
6  Squamous part

**Sphenoidal bone**
7  Greater wing (temporal surface)
8  Optic canal within the lesser wing
9  Lateral pterygoid plate

**Palatine bone**
10  Orbital process
11  Perpendicular plate
12  Conchal crest
13  Nasal crest
14  Horizontal plate

**Ethmoidal bone**
15  Orbital plate
16  Ethmoidal air cell
17  Middle concha
18  Perpendicular plate
    (part of bony nasal septum)

**Maxilla**
19  Infra-orbital groove
20  Infra-orbital foramen
21  Zygomatic process
22  Alveolar process with teeth
23  Palatine process

**Left inferior nasal concha**
24  Anterior part of
    inferior concha

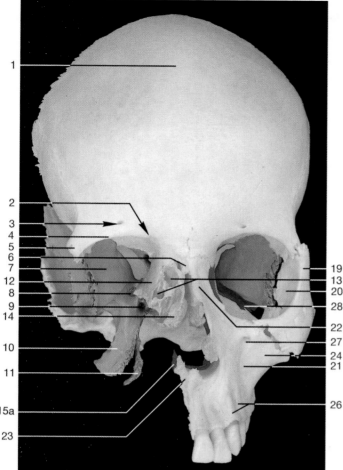

**Frontal bone**
1  Squamous part
2  Frontal notch
3  Supra-orbital foramen
4  Supra-orbital margin
5  Zygomatic process
6  Frontal spine

**Sphenoidal bone**
7  Greater wing (orbital surface)
8  Foramen rotundum
9  Pterygoid or Vidian canal
10  Lateral pterygoid plate
11  Medial pterygoid plate

**Ethmoidal bone**
12  Orbital plate
13  Ethmoidal air cells
14  Middle concha

**Palatine bone**
15  Horizontal plate
15a  Nasal crest
16  Pyramidal process
17  Lesser palatine foramen
18  Greater palatine foramen

**Zygomatic bone**
19  Frontal process
20  Orbital surface

**Maxilla**
21  Canine fossa
22  Frontal process
23  Palatine process
24  Zygomatic process
25  Alveolar process and teeth
26  Juga alveolaria
27  Infra-orbital foramen
28  Infra-orbital groove
29  Anterior nasal aperture
30  Anterior nasal spine

**Incisive bone**
31  Central incisor and incisive bone or premaxilla
32  Incisive fossa

**Vomer**
33  Ala of the vomer

**Sutures and choanae**
34  Median palatine suture
35  Transverse palatine suture
36  Choanae

**Anterior view of a disarticulated skull,** showing the connection of the maxilla with the frontal and zygomatic bones. Yellow = ethmoidal bone; red = palatine bone; green = sphenoidal bone.

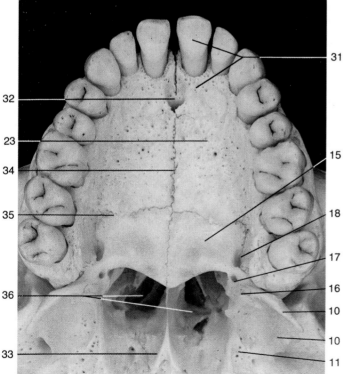

**Bony palate and teeth of the maxillae** (from below).

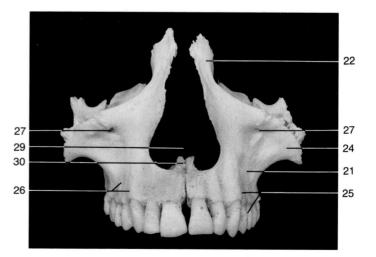

**Anterior view of both maxillae,** forming the anterior bony aperture of the nose.

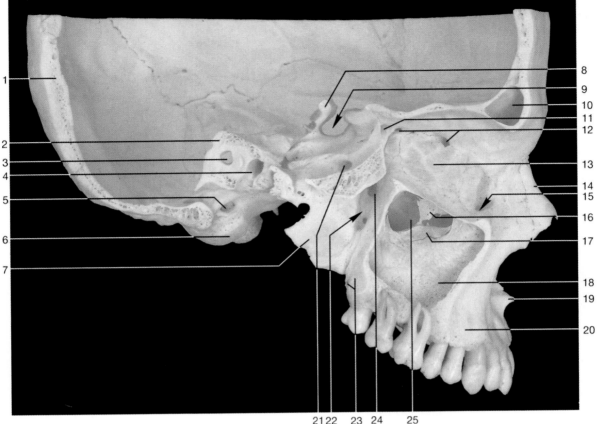

**Paramedian section through the skull,** right side (lateral aspect). Frontal and maxillary sinuses are opened.

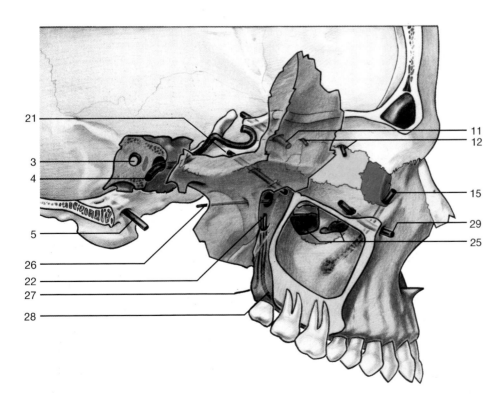

**Illustration of canals and foramina** connected with the right orbit and pterygopalatine fossa (compare the above figure). The greater wing of sphenoidal bone (green) is shown as being transparent. Brown = temporal bone; yellow = ethmoidal bone; red = lacrimal bone; light red = inferior nasal concha; violet = maxilla; red = palatine bone.

1  Occipital bone
2  Temporal bone (petrous part)
3  Internal acoustic meatus
4  Carotid canal
5  Hypoglossal canal
6  Occipital condyle
7  Lateral plate of pterygoid process
8  Dorsum of sella turcica
9  Sella turcica
10  Frontal sinus
11  Optic canal
12  Posterior and anterior
    ethmoidal foramina
13  Orbital plate of ethmoidal bone
14  Nasal bone
15  Nasolacrimal canal
16  Uncinate process
17  Inferior nasal concha
    (maxillary process)
18  Maxillary sinus
19  Anterior nasal spine
20  Alveolar process of maxilla
21  Foramen rotundum
22  Pterygopalatine fossa
23  Tuberosity of maxilla
    with alveolar foramina
24  Sphenopalatine foramen
25  Maxillary hiatus
26  Pterygoid or Vidian canal
27  Lesser palatine canal
28  Greater palatine canal
29  Infra-orbital canal

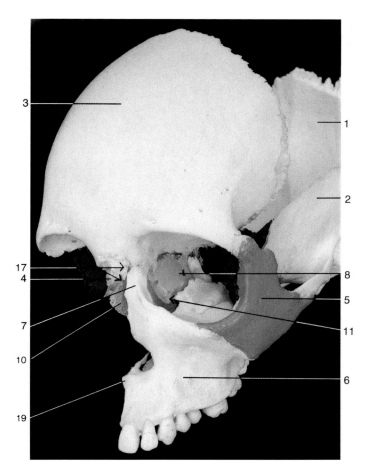

**Anterior part of a disarticulated skull.**
Orange = zygomatic bone; yellow = ethmoidal bone;
brown = sphenoidal bone. The arrows indicate the locations
of the lacrimal bone (11) and the nasal bone (17).

1  Occipital bone
2  Temporal bone
3  Frontal bone
4  Nasal spine of frontal bone
5  Zygomatic bone
6  Maxilla
7  Frontal process of maxilla
8  Ethmoidal bone
9  Orbital plate of ethmoidal bone
10  Perpendicular plate of ethmoidal bone
11  Site of lacrimal bone
12  Lacrimal groove of lacrimal bone
13  Posterior lacrimal crest
14  Fossa for lacrimal sac
15  Lacrimal hamulus
16  Nasolacrimal canal
17  Site of nasal bone
18  Nasal foramina of nasal bone
19  Anterior nasal spine of maxilla
20  Vomer
21  Greater wing of sphenoidal bone
22  Anterior and posterior ethmoidal foramina
23  Optic canal
24  Superior orbital fissure
25  Inferior orbital fissure
26  Infra-orbital groove
27  Infra-orbital foramen

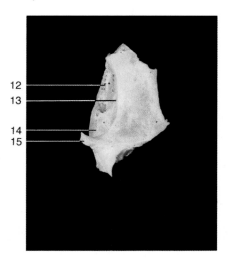

**Left lacrimal bone** (anterior aspect).

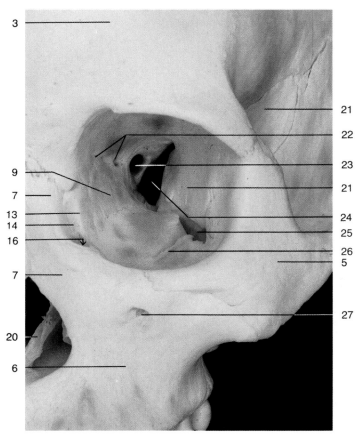

**Left orbit** (anterior aspect).

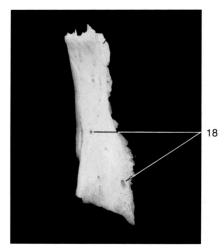

**Left nasal bone** (anterior aspect).

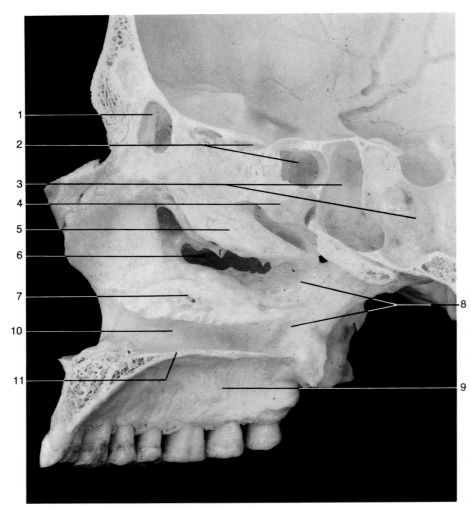

1   Frontal sinus
2   Ethmoidal air cells
3   Sphenoidal sinus
4   Superior nasal concha
5   Middle nasal concha
6   Maxillary hiatus
7   Inferior nasal concha
8   Palatine bone
9   Maxilla
10   Inferior meatus
11   Palatine process of the maxilla

▷

**To page 49:**
| | | |
|---|---|---|
| Blue | = | Occipital bone |
| Light green | = | Parietal bone |
| Yellow | = | Frontal bone |
| Dark brown | = | Temporal bone |
| Red | = | Sphenoidal bone |
| Dark green | = | Ethmoidal bone |
| Light blue | = | Nasal bone |
| Pink | = | Inferior concha |
| Orange | = | Vomer |
| Violet | = | Maxilla |
| White | = | Palatine bone |
| White | = | Mandible |

**Lateral wall of the nasal cavity.** Median section through the skull.

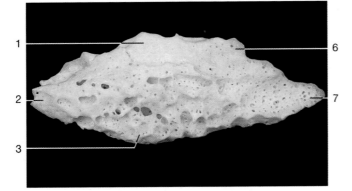

**Inferior concha and vomer**
1   Ethmoidal process
2   Anterior part of concha
3   Inferior border
4   Ala of vomer
5   Posterior border of nasal septum
6   Lacrimal process
7   Posterior part of concha
8   Maxillary process

**Right inferior nasal concha** (medial aspect). Anterior part
to the left.

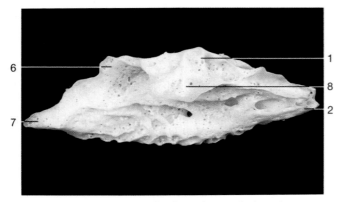

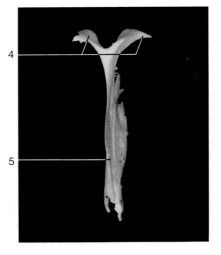

**Right inferior nasal concha** (lateral aspect). Anterior part
to the right.

**Vomer** (posterior aspect).

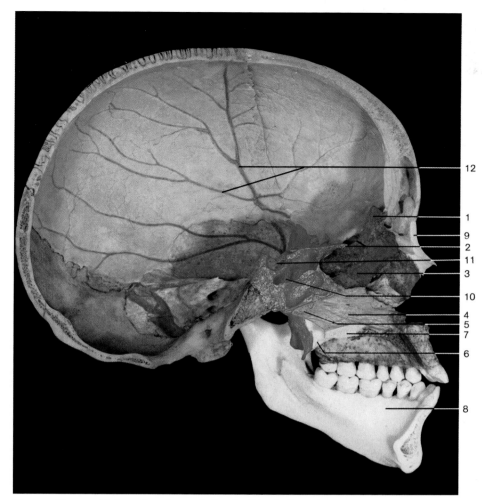

1 Crista galli
2 Cribriform plate
   of ethmoidal bone
3 Perpendicular plate
   of ethmoidal bone
4 Vomer
5 Ala of the vomer
6 Palatine bone
   (perpendicular process)
7 Palatine bone (horizontal plate)
8 Mandible
9 Nasal bone
10 Sphenoidal sinus
11 Hypophysial fossa (sella turcica)
12 Grooves for the middle
    meningeal artery

**Cartilages of the nose**
13 Lateral nasal cartilage
14 Greater alar cartilage
15 Lesser alar cartilages
16 Septal cartilage

17 Location of nasal bone

**Paramedian sagittal section through the skull including the nasal septum.**

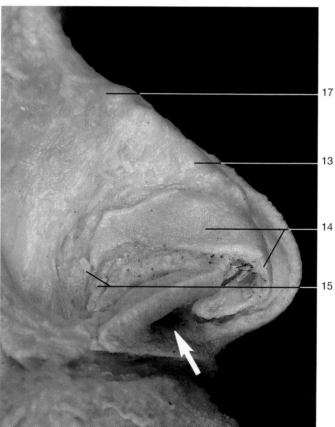

**Cartilages of the nose** (right anterior aspect). Arrow = nostril, framed by nasal wing.

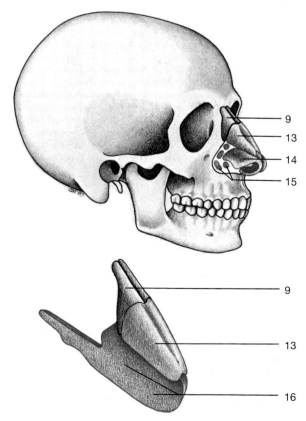

**Cartilages of the nose.**
Schematic diagram of the external nose.

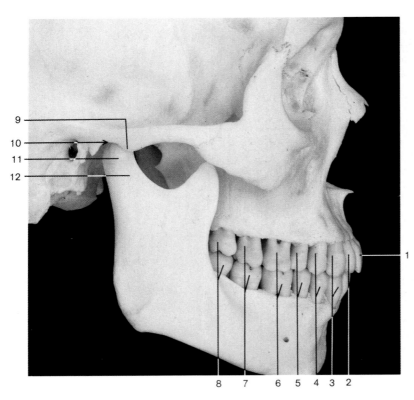

1   Central incisor
2   Lateral incisor
3   Canines
4   First premolars or bicuspids
5   Second premolars or bicuspids
6   First molars
7   Second molars
8   Third molars
9   Articular tubercle
10  Mandibular fossa
11  Head of mandible
12  Condylar process

**Normal position of teeth.** Dentition in centric occlusion (lateral view).

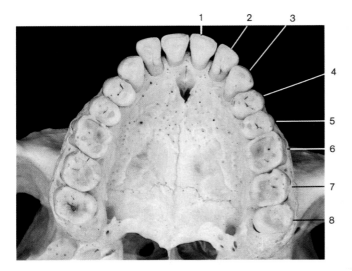

**Upper teeth of the adult** (inferior aspect).

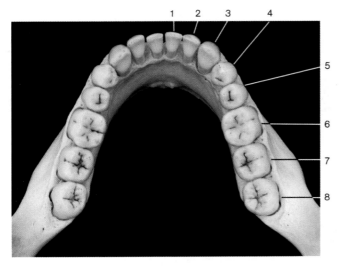

**Lower teeth of the adult** (superior aspect).

**Table of dentition. Eruption of deciduous and permanent teeth** (after C. Röse according to A. Kröncke).

| Primary dentition (Deciduous teeth) | Maxilla months postpartum | Mandible months |
|---|---|---|
| 1. Central incisor | 10.3 | 8.6 |
| 2. Lateral incisor | 12.2 | 14.4 |
| 3. Canine | 19.5 | 20.1 |
| 4. First molar | 15.5 | 16.5 |
| 5. Second molar | 24.8 | 24.5 |

| Secondary dentition (Permanent teeth) | years and months ♂ | ♀ | years and months ♂ | ♀ |
|---|---|---|---|---|
| 1. Central incisor | 7/8 | 7/5 | 6/10 | 6/7 |
| 2. Lateral incisor | 8/11 | 8/6 | 7/11 | 7/7 |
| 3. Canine | 12/2 | 11/7 | 11/12 | 10/3 |
| 4. First premolar | 10/5 | 10/1 | 11/3 | 10/8 |
| 5. Second premolar | 11/4 | 11/1 | 12/0 | 11/7 |
| 6. First molar | 6/7 | 6/6 | 6/5 | 6/3 |
| 7. Second molar | 12/9 | 12/5 | 12/3 | 11/9 |
| 8. Third molar | ~20 (18–30) | | | |

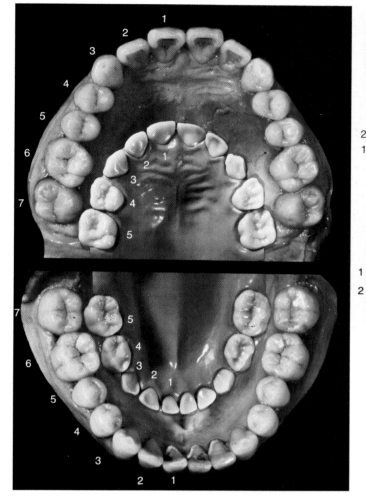

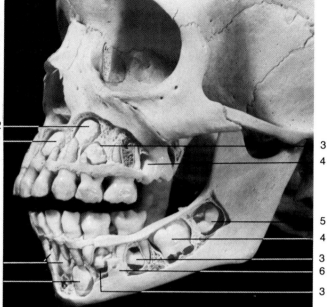

**Deciduous teeth in child's skull.** The developing crowns of the permanent teeth are displayed in their crypts in the maxilla and mandible.

1  Permanent incisors
2  Permanent cuspid (canine)
3  Premolars
4  First permanent molar
5  Second permanent molar
6  Mental foramen

**Comparison of the deciduous and permanent teeth.**
Notice that the breadth of the alveolar arch of the child's mandible and maxilla holding the deciduous teeth is nearly the same as the comparable portion in the jaws of the adult. Note the emergence of the third molars.

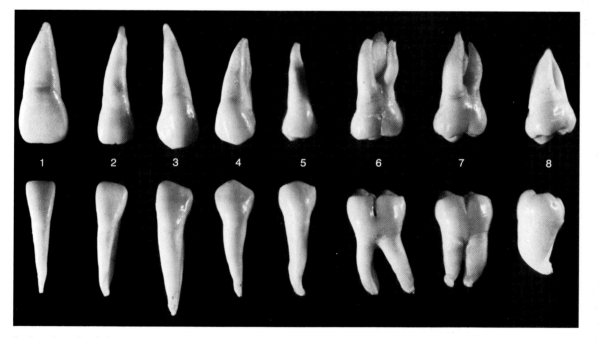

**Isolated teeth of the alveolar part of the maxilla** (top row) and the mandible (lower row), labial surface of the teeth.

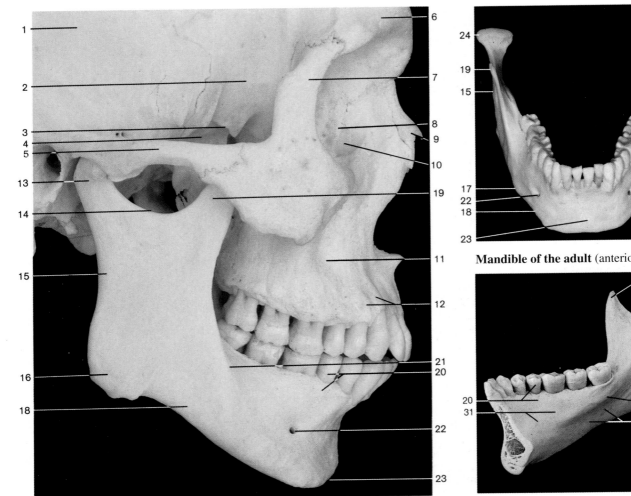

**Lateral aspect of the facial bones.** Mandible and teeth in the position of occlusion. Upper and lower jaw occluded.

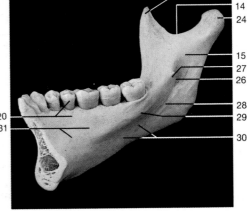

**Mandible of the adult** (anterior aspect).

**Right half of mandible** (medial aspect).

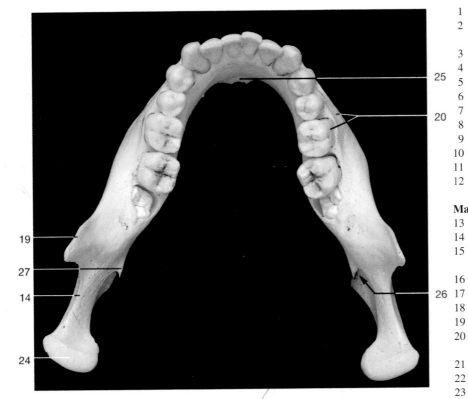

**Mandible of the adult** (superior aspect).

1  Temporal bone
2  Temporal fossa (greater wing of sphenoidal bone)
3  Infratemporal crest
4  Infratemporal fossa
5  Zygomatic arch
6  Frontal bone
7  Zygomatic bone (frontal process)
8  Lacrimal bone
9  Nasal bone
10  Lacrimal groove
11  Maxilla (canine fossa)
12  Alveolar process of maxilla

**Mandible**

| | |
|---|---|
| 13  Condylar process | 25  Genial tubercle or mental spine |
| 14  Mandibular notch | |
| 15  Ramus of the mandible | 26  Mandibular foramen (entrance to mandibular canal) |
| 16  Masseteric tuberosity | |
| 17  Angle of the mandible | 27  Lingula |
| 18  Body of the mandible | 28  Mylohyoid sulcus |
| 19  Coronoid process | 29  Mylohyoid line |
| 20  Alveolar process including teeth | 30  Submandibular fossa |
| 21  Oblique line | 31  Sublingual fossa |
| 22  Mental foramen | |
| 23  Mental protuberance | |
| 24  Head of the mandible | |

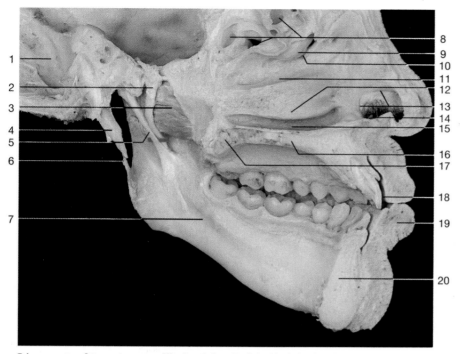

**Ligaments of temporomandibular joint.** Left half of the head (medial aspect).

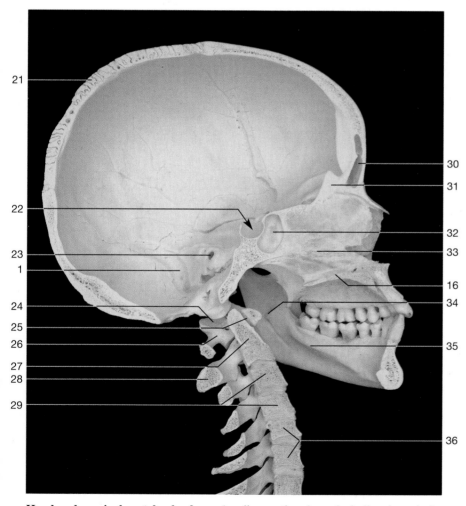

**Head and cervical vertebral column** (median section through skull and cervical vertebrae, medial aspect).

1   Groove for sigmoid sinus
2   Mandibular nerve
3   Lateral pterygoid muscle
4   Styloid process
5   Sphenomandibular ligament
6   Stylomandibular ligament
7   Mylohyoid groove
8   Ethmoidal air cells
9   Ethmoidal bulla
10  Hiatus semilunaris
11  Middle meatus
12  Inferior nasal concha
13  Limen nasi
14  Vestibule with hairs
15  Inferior meatus
16  Hard palate
17  Soft palate
18  Vestibule of oral cavity
19  Lower lip
20  Mandible
21  Calvaria with diploe
22  Sella turcica
23  Internal acoustic meatus
24  Atlanto-occipital articulation
25  Median atlanto-axial articulation
26  Atlas ($C_1$)
27  Dens of axis ($C_2$)
28  Spinous process of axis ($C_2$)
29  Cervical vertebrae ($C_3$, $C_4$)
30  Frontal sinus
31  Crista galli
32  Sphenoidal sinus
33  Nasal septum
34  Mandibular foramen
35  Mylohyoid line
36  Bodies of cervical
    vertebrae ($C_5$, $C_6$)

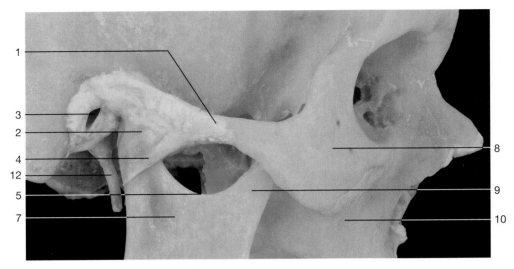

**Temporomandibular joint with ligaments.**

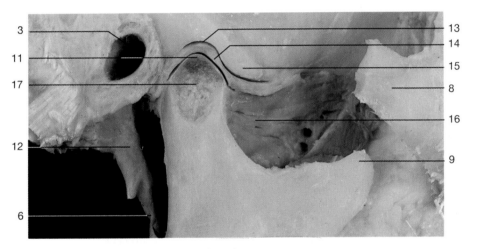

**Temporomandibular joint,** sagittal section.

1  Zygomatic arch
2  Articular capsule
3  External acoustic meatus
4  Lateral ligament
5  Mandibular notch
6  Stylomandibular ligament
7  Ramus of the mandible
8  Zygomatic bone
9  Coronoid process
10  Maxilla
11  Articular cartilage of
    condylar process
12  Styloid process
13  Mandibular fossa
14  Articular disc
15  Articular tubercle
16  Lateral pterygoid muscle
17  Condylar process of mandible
18  Temporalis muscle
19  Digastric muscle, posterior belly
20  Masseter muscle
21  Medial pterygoid muscle
22  Parotid duct
23  Buccinator muscle
24  Mandible

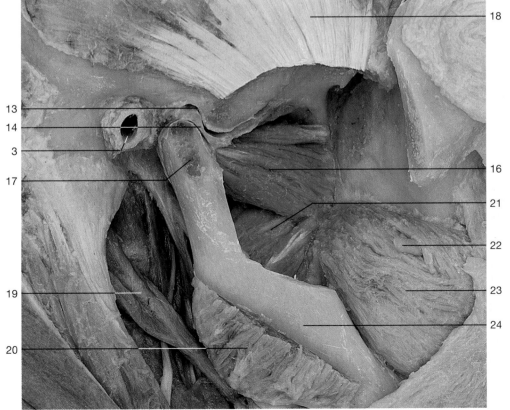

**Temporomandibular joint.**
Dissection of the articular disc
and the related muscles (lateral
aspect).

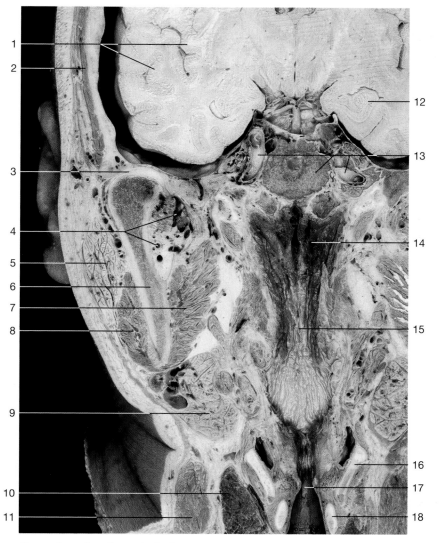

1   Insular lobe and temporal lobe
2   Temporalis muscle
3   Articular disc of
    temporomandibular joint
4   Maxillary artery and pterygoid
    venous plexus
5   Parotid gland
6   Mandible
7   Medial pterygoid muscle
8   Masseter muscle
9   Submandibular gland
10  Thyroid gland
11  Sternocleidomastoid muscle
12  Hippocampus
13  Internal carotid artery and
    sphenoid bone
14  Pharyngeal tonsil
15  Pharynx
16  Thyroid cartilage
17  Rima glottidis
18  Cricoid cartilage
19  Hard palate and palatine glands
20  Oral cavity
21  Upper molar
22  Oral vestibule
23  Lower molar
24  Platysma muscle
25  Maxillary sinus
26  Superior longitudinal muscle of tongue
27  Transverse muscle of tongue
28  Buccinator muscle
29  Inferior longitudinal muscle of tongue
30  Sublingual gland
31  Genioglossus muscle
32  Mastoid process
33  Styloid process
34  Stylomandibular ligament
35  Articular capsule
36  Lateral ligament
37  Zygomatic arch
38  Sphenomandibular ligament
39  Mandibular foramen

**Coronal section through the head at the level of the temporomandibular joint** (right side, anterior aspect).

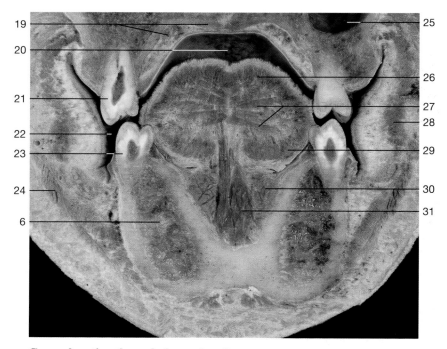

**Coronal section through the oral cavity.**

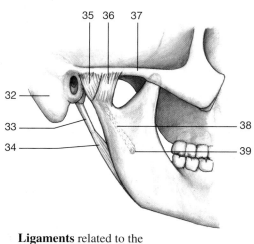

**Ligaments** related to the
**temporomandibular joint.**

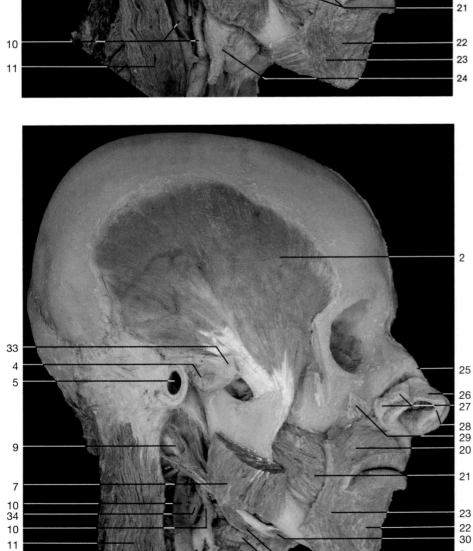

**Temporalis and masseter muscles.**
The temporal fascia has been removed, the temporomandibular joint severed and the zygomatic arch displayed.

1   Galea aponeurotica
2   Temporalis muscle
3   Occipital belly of occipitofrontalis muscle
4   Temporomandibular joint
5   External acoustic meatus
6   Deep layer of masseter muscle
7   Superficial layer of masseter muscle
8   Stylohyoid muscle
9   Posterior belly of digastric muscle
10  Internal jugular vein and external carotid artery
11  Sternocleidomastoid muscle
12  Frontal belly of occipitofrontalis muscle
13  Depressor supercilii muscle
14  Orbicularis oculi muscle
15  Transverse part of nasalis muscle
16  Levator labii superioris alaeque nasi muscle
17  Levator labii superioris muscle
18  Levator anguli oris muscle
19  Zygomaticus major muscle
20  Orbicularis oris muscle
21  Buccinator muscle
22  Depressor labii inferioris muscle
23  Depressor anguli oris muscle
24  Submandibular gland
25  Lateral nasal cartilage
26  Greater alar cartilage (lateral part)
27  Lesser alar cartilages
28  Greater alar cartilage (medial part)
29  Infra-orbital nerve
30  Anterior belly of digastric muscle
31  Hypoglossal nerve and hyoglossus muscle
32  Superior thyroid artery
33  Zygomatic arch
34  Internal carotid artery
35  Common carotid artery

**Temporalis muscle and temporomandibular joint.** The zygomatic arch and the masseter muscle have been partially severed to display the insertion of the temporalis muscle.

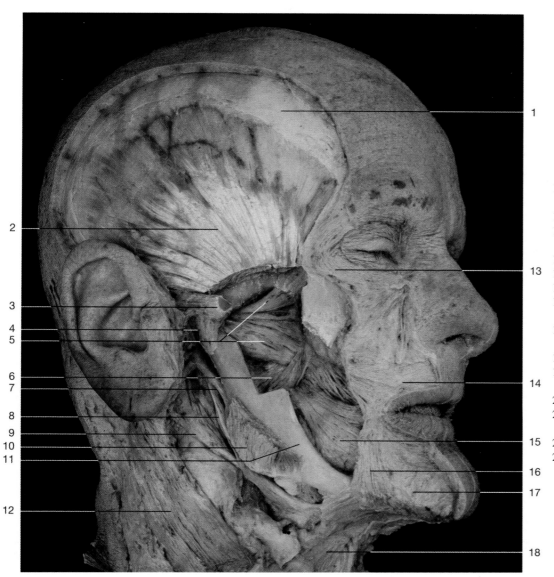

1 Periosteum
2 Temporalis muscle
3 Zygomatic arch
4 Articular capsule of
   temporomandibular joint
5 Lateral pterygoid muscle
   (upper and lower head)
6 Medial pterygoid muscle
7 Styloglossus muscle
8 Stylohyoid muscle
9 Posterior belly of
   digastric muscle
10 Masseter muscle
   (severed)
11 Mandible
12 Sternocleidomastoid
   muscle
13 Orbicularis oculi muscle
14 Orbicularis oris muscle
15 Buccinator muscle
16 Depressor anguli oris
   muscle
17 Depressor labii
   inferioris muscle
18 Platysma muscle
19 Articular disc of
   temporomandibular joint
20 Head of mandible
21 Anterior belly of
   digastric muscle
22 Mylohyoid muscle
23 Hyoid bone

**Medial and lateral pterygoid muscles.** A portion of the mandible and the zygomatic arch has been removed, revealing the pterygoid region or infratemporal fossa.

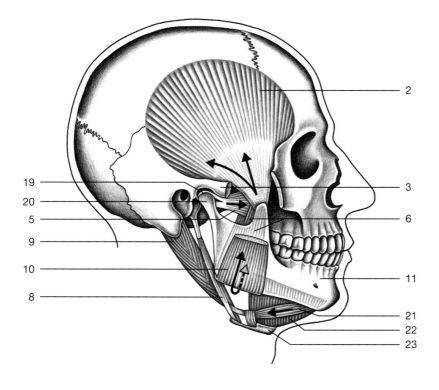

**Effect of the masticatory muscles on the temporomandibular joint** (arrows).

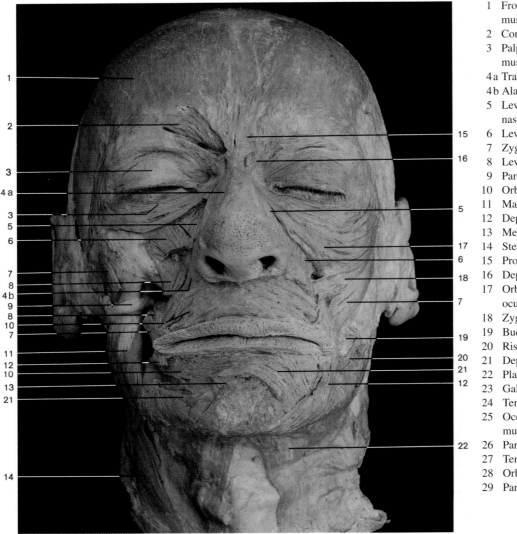

1  Frontal belly of occipitofrontalis
   muscle
2  Corrugator supercilii muscle
3  Palpebral part of orbicularis oculi
   muscle
4a Transverse part of nasalis muscle
4b Alar part of nasalis muscle
5  Levator labii superioris alaeque
   nasi muscle
6  Levator labii superioris muscle
7  Zygomaticus major muscle
8  Levator anguli oris muscle
9  Parotid duct
10 Orbicularis oris muscle
11 Masseter muscle
12 Depressor anguli oris muscle
13 Mentalis muscle
14 Sternocleidomastoid muscle
15 Procerus muscle
16 Depressor supercilii muscle
17 Orbital part of orbicularis
   oculi muscle
18 Zygomaticus minor muscle
19 Buccinator muscle
20 Risorius muscle
21 Depressor labii inferioris muscle
22 Platysma muscle
23 Galea aponeurotica
24 Temporoparietalis muscle
25 Occipital belly of occipitofrontalis
   muscle
26 Parotid gland with fascia
27 Temporal fascia
28 Orbicularis oculi muscle
29 Parotid duct, masseter muscle

**Facial muscles** (anterior aspect). Left side: superficial layer, right side: deeper layer.

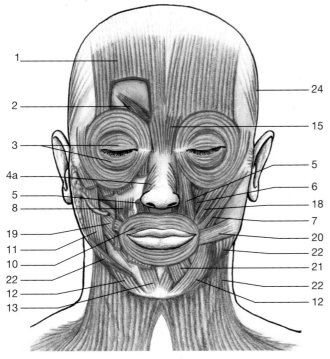

**Facial muscles** (schematic drawing).
Left side: superficial layer, right side: deeper layer.

**Facial muscles.** Sphincter-like muscles surround the orifices of
the head. Radially arranged muscles work as their antagonists.

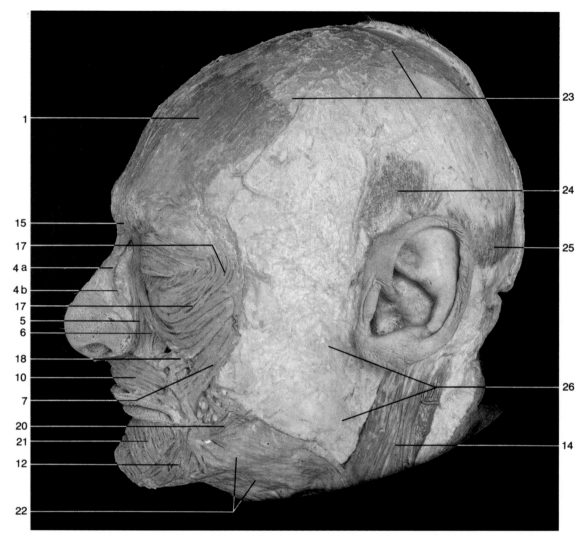

**Facial muscles** (lateral aspect).

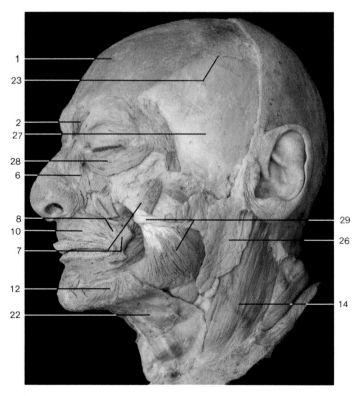

**Facial muscles and parotid gland** (lateral aspect).

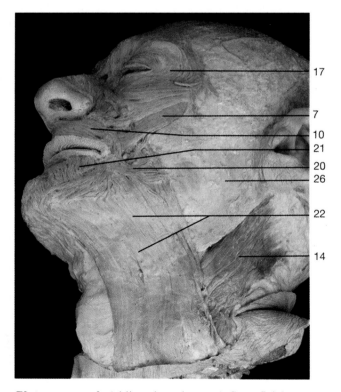

**Platysma muscle** (oblique lateral aspect). Superficial lamina of cervical fascia partly removed.

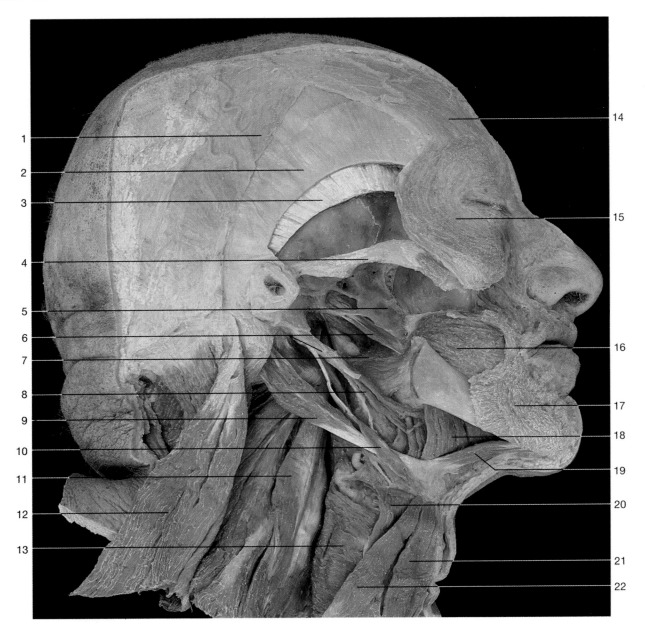

**Supra- and infrahyoid muscles, pharynx I** (lateral aspect). Ramus of mandible, pterygoid muscles, and insertion of temporalis muscle removed.

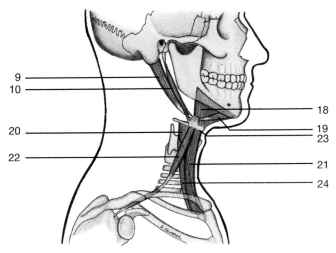

**Supra- and infrahyoid muscles** (schematic drawing).

1   Galea aponeurotica
2   Temporal fascia
3   Tendon of temporalis muscle
4   Zygomatic arch
5   Lateral pterygoid plate
6   Tensor veli palatini muscle (styloid process)
7   Superior constrictor muscle of pharynx
8   Styloglossus muscle
9   Posterior belly of digastric muscle
10  Stylohyoid muscle
11  Longus capitis muscle
12  Sternocleidomastoid muscle (reflected)
13  Inferior constrictor of pharynx
14  Frontal belly of occipitofrontalis muscle
15  Orbital part of orbicularis oculi muscle
16  Buccinator muscle
17  Depressor anguli oris muscle
18  Mylohyoid muscle
19  Anterior belly of digastric muscle
20  Thyrohyoid muscle
21  Sternohyoid muscle
22  Omohyoid muscle
23  Hyoid bone
24  Sternothyroid muscle

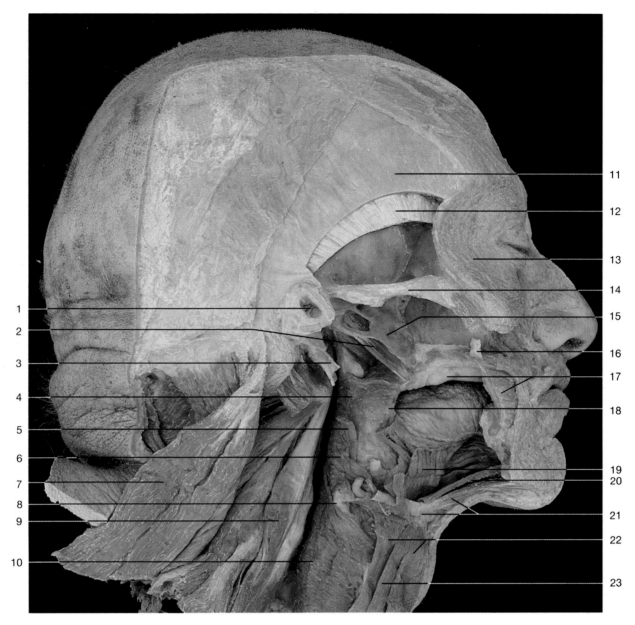

**Supra- and infrahyoid muscles, pharynx II.** Buccinator muscle removed; oral cavity opened.

1   External acoustic meatus
2   Tensor veli palatini muscle
3   Styloid process
4   Superior constrictor muscle of pharynx
5   Stylopharyngeus muscle (divided)
6   Middle constrictor muscle of pharynx
7   Sternocleidomastoid muscle
8   Greater horn of hyoid bone
9   Longus capitis
10  Inferior constrictor muscle of pharynx
11  Temporal fascia
12  Tendon of temporalis muscle
13  Orbicularis oculi muscle
14  Zygomatic arch
15  Lateral pterygoid plate
16  Parotid duct
17  Gingiva of upper jaw (without teeth),
     buccinator muscle (divided)
18  Pterygomandibular raphe
19  Hyoglossus muscle
20  Mylohyoid muscle
21  Anterior belly of digastric muscle (hyoid bone)
22  Sternohyoid and thyrohyoid muscles
23  Omohyoid muscle

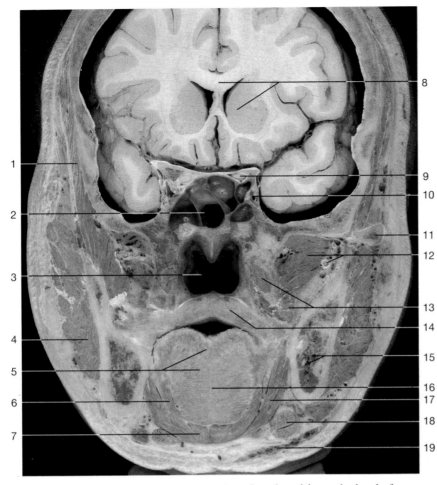

**Coronal section through cranial, nasal, and oral cavities** at the level of sphenoidal sinus.

1 Temporalis muscle
2 Sphenoidal sinus
3 Nasopharynx
4 Masseter muscle
5 Superior longitudinal, transverse and vertical muscles of tongue
6 Hyoglossus muscle
7 Geniohyoid muscle
8 Corpus callosum (caudate nucleus)
9 Optic nerve
10 Cavernous sinus
11 Zygomatic arch
12 Cross section of lateral pterygoid muscle and maxillary artery
13 Section of medial pterygoid muscle
14 Soft palate
15 Mandible and inferior alveolar nerve
16 Septum of the tongue
17 Mylohyoid muscle
18 Submandibular gland
19 Platysma muscle
20 Foramen magnum, vertebral artery and spinal cord
21 Internal carotid artery
22 Head of mandible
23 Styloid process
24 Inferior alveolar nerve
25 Lingual nerve and chorda tympani nerve
26 Medial pterygoid muscle
27 Uvula
28 Anterior belly of digastric muscle (cut)
29 Condyle of occipital bone
30 Mastoid process
31 Lateral pterygoid muscle
32 Auditory tube and levator veli palatini muscle
33 Tensor veli palatini muscle

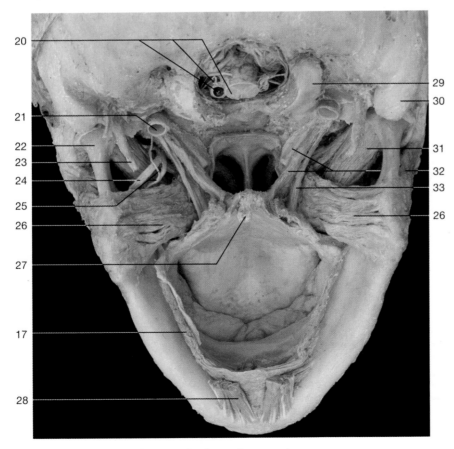

**Pterygoid and palatine muscles** (posterior aspect).

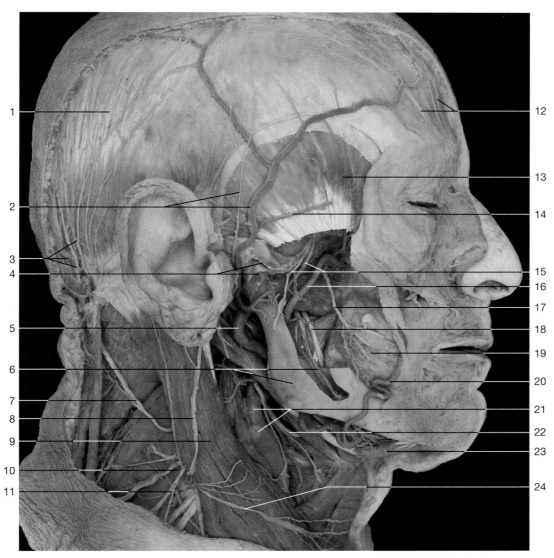

1 Galea aponeurotica
2 Superficial temporal artery and auriculo-temporal nerve
3 Occipital artery and greater occipital nerve (C₂)
4 Temporomandibular joint (opened)
5 External carotid artery
6 Mandible and inferior mandibular artery and nerve
7 Accessory nerve (Var.)
8 Great auricular nerve
9 Sternocleidomastoideus muscle
10 Punctum nervosum
11 Supraclavicular nerves
12 Supra-orbital nerves
13 Temporalis muscle
14 Transverse facial artery
15 Masseteric nerve and deep temporal branch of maxillary artery
16 Maxillary artery
17 Buccal nerve
18 Lingual nerve
19 Buccinator muscle
20 Facial artery
21 External carotid artery and sinus caroticus
22 Hypoglossal nerve
23 Digastric muscle
24 Transverse cervical nerves

**Dissection of maxillary artery** (lateral aspect). Ramus mandibulae partly removed and canalis mandibulae opened.

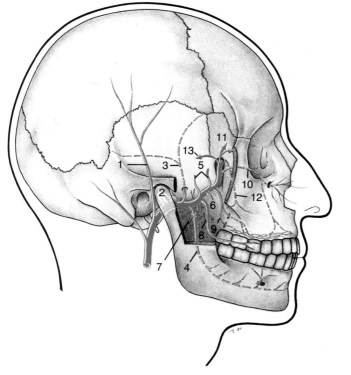

1 Superficial temporal artery

**Branches of the first part**
2 Deep auricular artery and anterior tympanic artery
3 Middle meningeal artery
4 Inferior alveolar artery

**Branches of the second part**
5 Deep temporal branches
6 Pterygoid branches
7 Masseteric artery
8 Buccal artery

**Branches of the third part**
9 Posterior superior alveolar artery
10 Infra-orbital artery
11 Sphenopalatine artery and branches to the nasal cavity
12 Descending palatine artery
13 Artery of the pterygoid canal

**Main branches of maxillary artery** (schematic drawing).

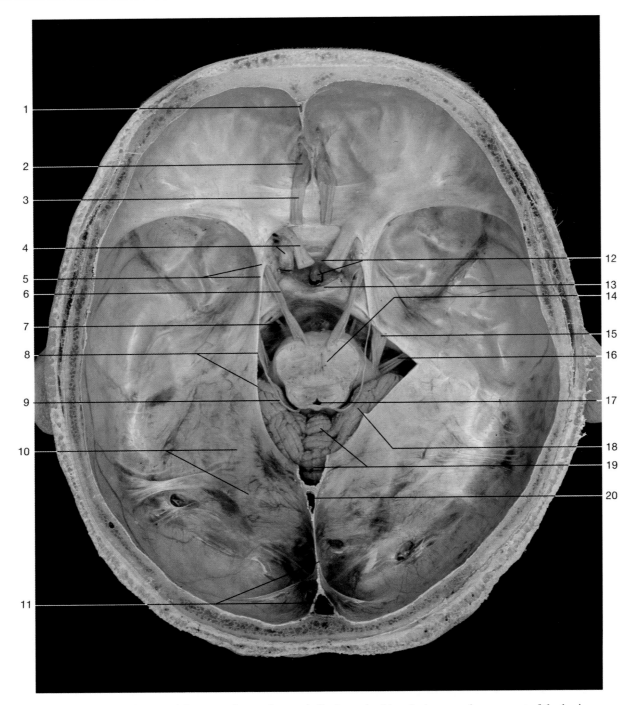

**Base of the skull with cranial nerves** (internal aspect). Both cerebral hemispheres and upper part of the brain stem removed. Incision on the right tentorium cerebelli to display the cranial nerves of the infratentorial space.

1   Superior sagittal sinus with falx cerebri
2   Olfactory bulb
3   Olfactory tract
4   Optic nerve and internal carotid artery
5   Anterior clinoid process and anterior attachment of tentorium cerebelli
6   Oculomotor nerve (n. III)
7   Abducent nerve (n. VI)
8   Tentorial notch (incisura tentorii)
9   Trochlear nerve (n. IV)
10  Tentorium cerebelli
11  Falx cerebri and confluence of sinuses

12  Hypophysial fossa, infundibulum, and diaphragma sellae
13  Dorsum sellae
14  Midbrain (divided)
15  Trigeminal nerve (n. V)
16  Facial nerve (n. VII), nervus intermedius, and vestibulocochlear nerve (n. VIII)
17  Cerebral aqueduct
18  Right hemisphere of cerebellum
19  Vermis of cerebellum
20  Straight sinus

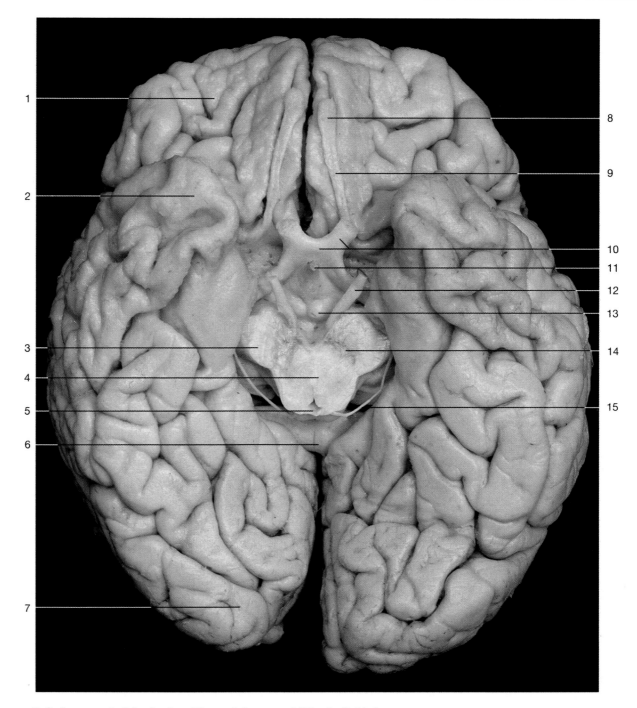

**Inferior aspect of the brain with cranial nerves.** Midbrain divided.

| | | | |
|---|---|---|---|
| 1 | Frontal lobe | 9 | Olfactory tract |
| 2 | Temporal lobe | 10 | Optic nerve and optic chiasma |
| 3 | Pedunculus cerebri | 11 | Infundibulum |
| 4 | Midbrain (divided) | 12 | Oculomotor nerve (n. III) |
| 5 | Cerebral aqueduct | 13 | Mamillary body |
| 6 | Splenium of corpus callosum | 14 | Substantia nigra |
| 7 | Occipital lobe | 15 | Trochlear nerve (n. IV) |
| 8 | Olfactory bulb | | |

| Cranial nerves | | |
|---|---|---|
| I = Olfactory nerves | VII = Facial nerve | |
| II = Optic nerve | VIII = Vestibulocochlear nerve | |
| III = Oculomotor nerve | IX = Glossopharyngeal nerve | |
| IV = Trochlear nerve | X = Vagus nerve | |
| V = Trigeminal nerve | XI = Accessory nerve | |
| VI = Abducent nerve | XII = Hypoglossal nerve | |

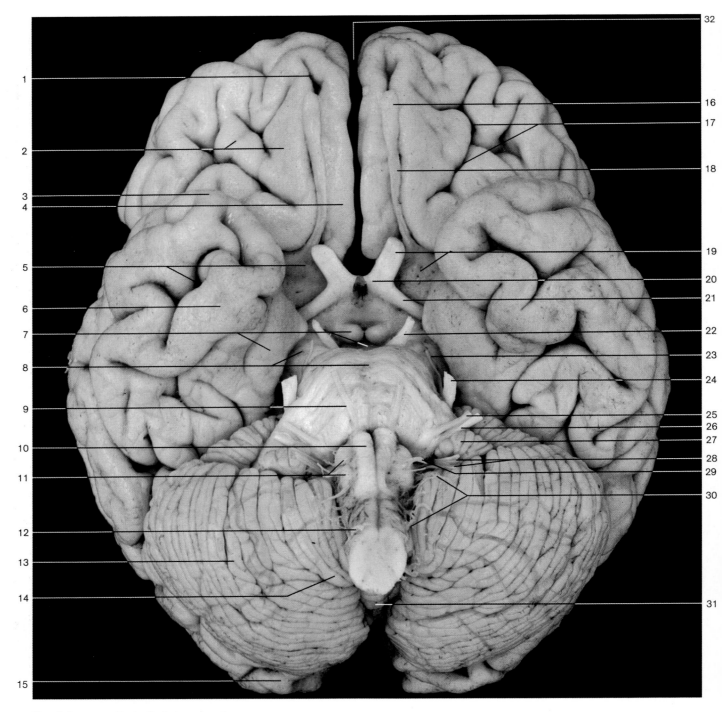

**Cranial nerves.** Brain (inferior aspect).

| | | |
|---|---|---|
| 1 Olfactory sulcus (termination) | 13 Cerebellum | 25 Facial nerve (n. VII) |
| 2 Orbital gyri | 14 Tonsil of cerebellum | 26 Vestibulocochlear nerve (n. VIII) |
| 3 Temporal lobe | 15 Occipital lobe (posterior pole) | 27 Flocculus of cerebellum |
| 4 Straight gyrus | 16 Olfactory bulb | 28 Glossopharyngeal nerve (n. IX) |
| 5 Olfactory trigone and inferior temporal sulcus | 17 Orbital sulci of frontal lobe | and vagus nerve (n. X) |
| 6 Medial occipitotemporal gyrus | 18 Olfactory tract | 29 Hypoglossal nerve (n. XII) |
| 7 Parahippocampal gyrus, mamillary body, and | 19 Optic nerve (n. II) and anterior | 30 Accessory nerve (n. XI) |
| interpeduncular fossa | perforated substance | 31 Vermis of cerebellum |
| 8 Pons and cerebral peduncle | 20 Optic chiasma | 32 Longitudinal fissure |
| 9 Abducent nerve (n. VI) | 21 Optic tract | |
| 10 Pyramid | 22 Oculomotor nerve (n. III) | |
| 11 Inferior olive | 23 Trochlear nerve (n. IV) | |
| 12 Cervical spinal nerves | 24 Trigeminal nerve (n. V) | |

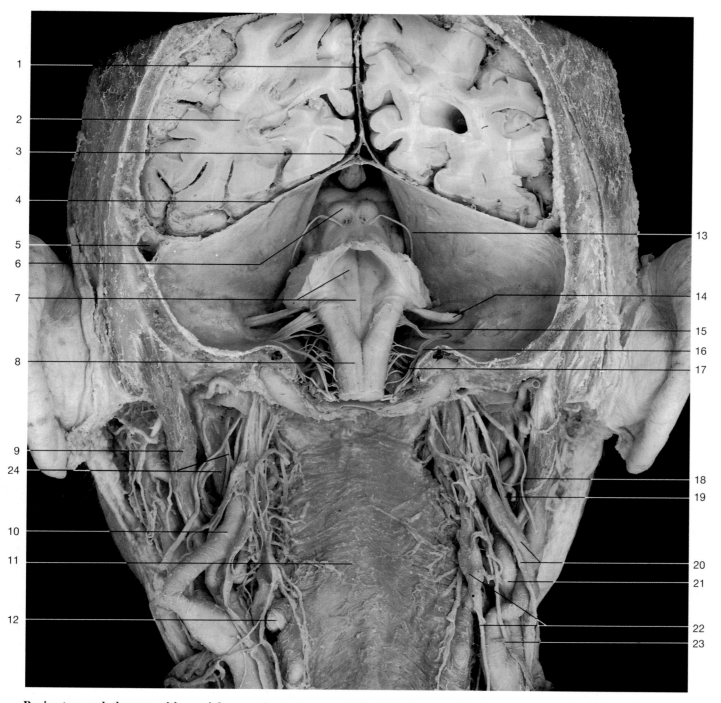

**Brain stem and pharynx with cranial nerves** (posterior aspect). Cranial cavity opened and cerebellum removed.

| | |
|---|---|
| 1 | Falx cerebri |
| 2 | Occipital lobe |
| 3 | Straight sinus |
| 4 | Tentorium cerebelli |
| 5 | Transverse sinus |
| 6 | Inferior colliculus of midbrain |
| 7 | Rhomboid fossa |
| 8 | Medulla oblongata |
| 9 | Posterior belly of digastric muscle |
| 10 | Internal carotid artery |
| 11 | Pharynx (middle constrictor muscle) |
| 12 | Hyoid bone (greater horn) |
| 13 | Trochlear nerve (n. IV) |
| 14 | Facial nerve (n. VII) and vestibulocochlear nerve (n. VIII) |

| | |
|---|---|
| 15 | Glossopharyngeal nerve (n. IX) and vagus nerve (n. X) |
| 16 | Accessory nerve (intracranial portion) (n. XI) |
| 17 | Hypoglossal nerve (intracranial portion) (n. XII) |
| 18 | Accessory nerve (n. XI) |
| 19 | Hypoglossal nerve (n. XII) |
| 20 | Vagus nerve (n. X) and internal carotid artery |
| 21 | External carotid artery |
| 22 | Sympathetic trunk and superior cervical ganglion |
| 23 | Ansa cervicalis (superior root of hypoglossal nerve) |
| 24 | Glossopharyngeal nerve (n. IX) and stylopharyngeus muscle |

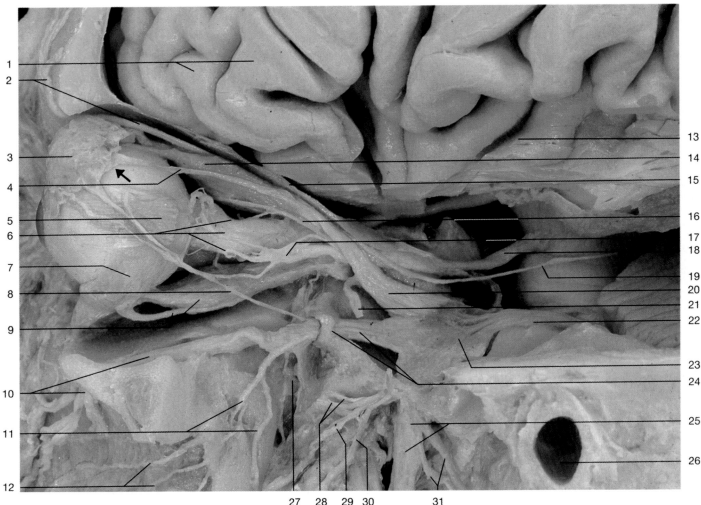

**Cranial nerves of the orbit and pterygopalatine fossa.** Left orbit (lateral aspect). Note the zygomaticolacrimal anastomosis (arrow).

| | | |
|---|---|---|
| 1 Frontal lobe | 6 Optic nerve and short ciliary nerves | 10 Infra-orbital nerve |
| 2 Supra-orbital nerve | 7 Inferior oblique muscle | 11 Posterior superior alveolar nerves |
| 3 Lacrimal gland | 8 Zygomatic nerve | 12 Branches of superior alveolar plexus adjacent to |
| 4 Lacrimal nerve | 9 Inferior branch of oculomotor nerve and | mucous membrane of maxillary sinus |
| 5 Lateral rectus muscle (divided) | inferior rectus muscle | 13 Central sulcus of insula |

14 Superior rectus muscle
15 Periorbita (roof of orbit)
16 Nasociliary nerve
17 Ciliary ganglion
18 Oculomotor nerve (n. III)
19 Trochlear nerve (n. IV)
20 Ophthalmic nerve (n. $V_1$)
21 Abducent nerve (n. VI) (divided)
22 Trigeminal nerve (n. V)
23 Trigeminal ganglion
24 Maxillary nerve (n. $V_2$) and foramen rotundum
25 Mandibular nerve (n. $V_3$)
26 External acoustic meatus
27 Pterygopalatine nerves
28 Deep temporal nerves
29 Buccal nerve
30 Masseteric nerve
31 Auriculotemporal nerve
32 Trochlea and superior oblique muscle

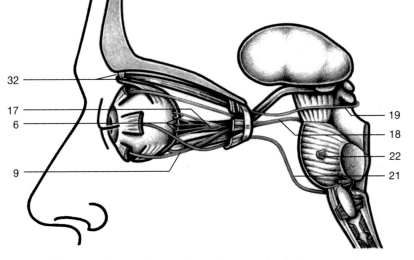

**Cranial nerves innervating extra-ocular muscles** (lateral aspect).
(Schematic drawing.)

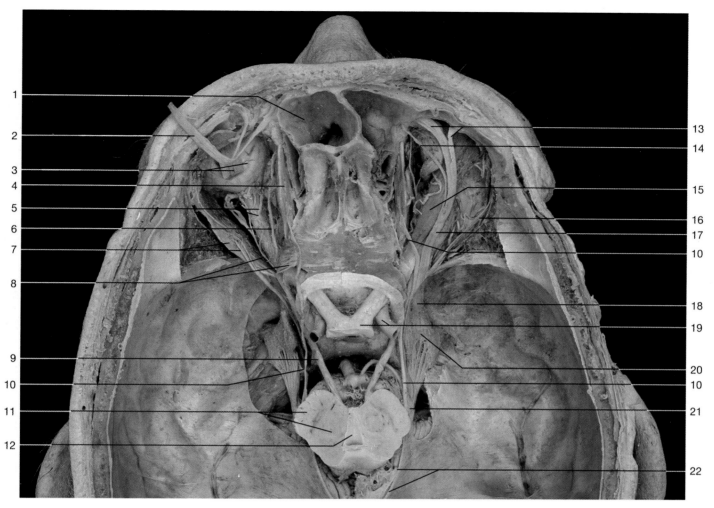

**Cranial nerves of the orbit** (superior aspect). Right side: superficial layer, left side: middle layer of the orbit (superior rectus muscle and frontal nerve divided and reflected). Tentorium and dura mater partly removed.

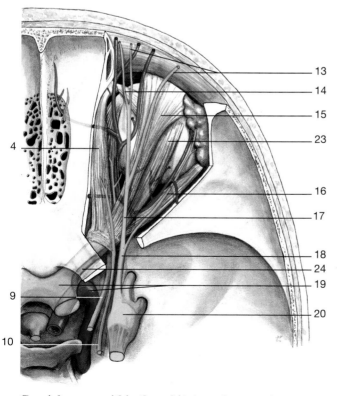

**Cranial nerves within the orbit** (superior aspect).

1  Frontal sinus (enlarged)
2  Frontal nerve (divided and reflected)
3  Superior rectus muscle (divided) and eyeball
4  Superior oblique muscle
5  Short ciliary nerves and optic nerve (n. II)
6  Nasociliary nerve
7  Abducent nerve (n. VI) and lateral rectus muscle
8  Ciliary ganglion and superior rectus muscle (reflected)
9  Oculomotor nerve (n. III)
10  Trochlear nerve (n. IV)
11  Crus cerebri and midbrain
12  Inferior wall of the third ventricle connected with cerebral aqueduct
13  Lateral and medial branches of supra-orbital nerve
14  Supratrochlear nerve
15  Superior levator palpebrae muscle
16  Lacrimal nerve
17  Frontal nerve
18  Ophthalmic nerve (n. V$_1$)
19  Optic chiasma and internal carotid artery
20  Trigeminal ganglion
21  Trigeminal nerve (n. V)
22  Tentorial notch
23  Superior rectus muscle
24  Ophthalmic artery

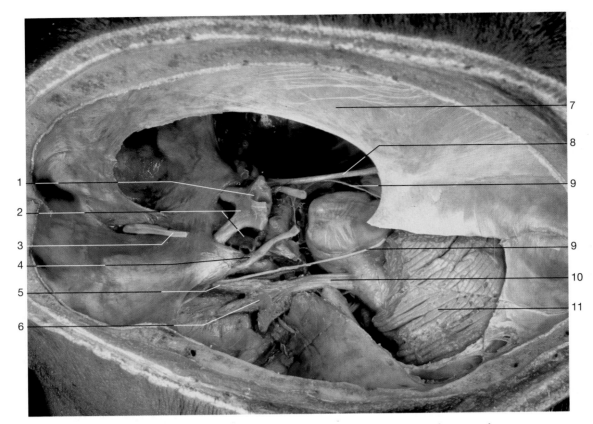

**Cranial nerves at the skull base.** The brain stem was divided and the tentorium fenestrated.
Both hemispheres were removed.

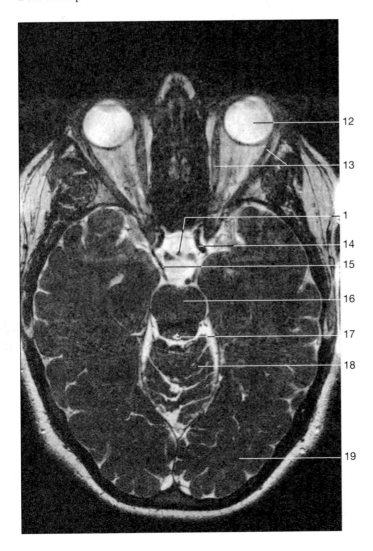

1   Infundibulum
2   Optic chiasma and
    internal carotid artery
3   Olfactory tract
4   Oculomotor nerve (n. III)
5   Ophthalmic nerve (n. V1)
6   Trigeminal ganglion
7   Falx cerebri
8   Tentorial notch
9   Trochlear nerve (n. IV)
10  Trigeminal nerve (n. V)
11  Cerebellum
12  Eyeball
13  Medial and lateral rectus
    muscles
14  Internal carotid artery
15  Oculomotor nerve (n. III)
16  Midbrain
17  Cerebral aqueduct
18  Vermis of cerebellum
19  Occipital lobe of the
    cerebrum
20  Basilar artery

**Four selected sections through the head** taken of a
complete series of MRI scans demonstrating cranial
nerves. (MRI scans of University Erlangen, Dpt. of
Neurosurgery [Head: Prof. R. Fahlbusch].)
**Section 1 at the level of the sella turcica.**

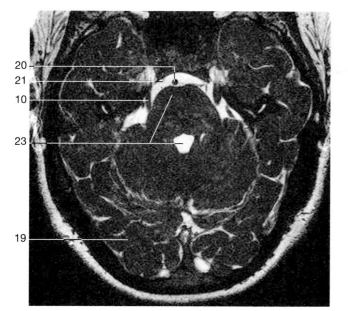

**Section 2 at the level of the pons.**

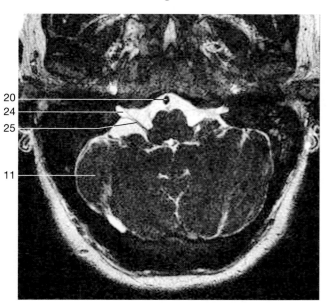

**Section 4 at the level of the medulla oblongata.**

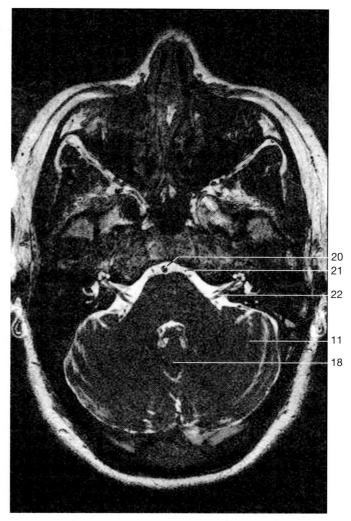

**Section 3 at the level of the skull base and cerebellum.**

21  Abducent nerve (n. VI)
22  Facial nerve (n. VII) and
    vestibulocochlear nerve (n. VIII)
23  Fourth ventricle and pons
24  Jugular foramen
25  Glossopharyngeal nerve (n. IX)
    and vagus nerve (n. X)
26  Optic tract  (n. II)
27  Hypoglossal nerve (n. XII)
28  Accessory nerve (n. XI)
29  Spinal nerves (C$_1$ and C$_2$)

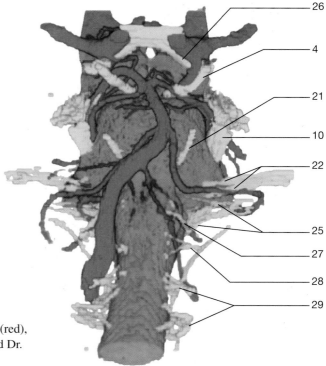

**3-D reconstruction of cranial nerves** (yellow) **and cerebral arteries** (red), based on the MRI scans depicted above (courtesy of Dr. R. Naraghi and Dr. P. Hastreiter, University Erlangen, Dpt. of Neurosurgery).

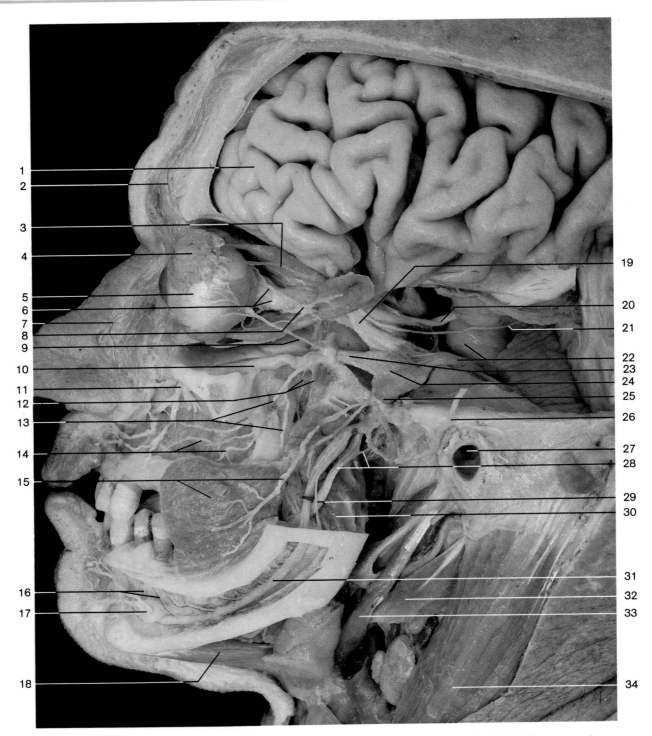

**Dissection of the trigeminal nerve in its entirety.** Lateral wall of cranial cavity, lateral wall of orbit, zygomatic arch, and ramus of the mandible have been removed and the mandibular canal opened.

 1  Frontal lobe of cerebrum
 2  Supra-orbital nerve
 3  Lacrimal nerve
 4  Lacrimal gland
 5  Eyeball
 6  Optic nerve and short ciliary nerves
 7  External nasal branch of
    anterior ethmoidal nerve
 8  Ciliary ganglion
 9  Zygomatic nerve
10  Infra-orbital nerve
11  Infra-orbital foramen and terminal branches
    of infra-orbital nerve

12  Pterygopalatine ganglion and
    pterygopalatine nerves
13  Posterior superior alveolar
    nerves
14  Superior dental plexus
15  Buccinator muscle and buccal nerve
16  Inferior dental plexus
17  Mental foramen and mental nerve
18  Anterior belly of digastric muscle
19  Ophthalmic nerve (n. V$_1$)
20  Oculomotor nerve (n. III)
21  Trochlear nerve (n. IV)
22  Trigeminal nerve and pons

23  Maxillary nerve (n. V$_2$)
24  Trigeminal ganglion
25  Mandibular nerve (n. V$_3$)
26  Auriculotemporal nerve
27  External acoustic meatus (divided)
28  Lingual nerve and chorda tympani
29  Mylohyoid nerve
30  Medial pterygoid muscle
31  Inferior alveolar nerve
32  Posterior belly of digastric muscle
33  Stylohyoid muscle
34  Sternocleidomastoid muscle

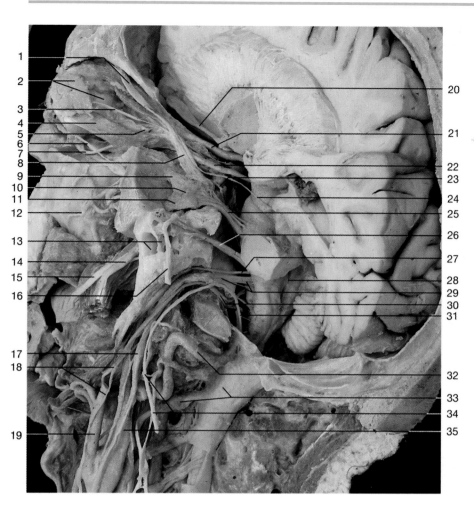

**Cranial nerves in connection with the brain stem.** Left side (lateral superior aspect). Left half of brain and head partly removed. Notice the location of trigeminal ganglion.

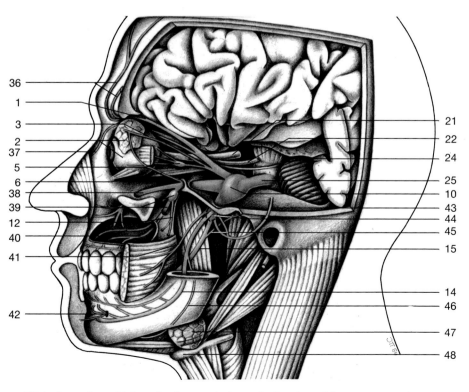

**Main branches of trigeminal nerve** (schematic drawing of figure on opposite page).

1  Frontal nerve
2  Lacrimal gland and eyeball
3  Lacrimal nerve
4  Lateral rectus muscle
5  Ciliary ganglion lateral to optic nerve
6  Zygomatic nerve
7  Inferior branch of oculomotor nerve
8  Ophthalmic nerve (n. V$_1$)
9  Maxillary nerve (n. V$_2$)
10  Trigeminal ganglion
11  Mandibular nerve (n. V$_3$)
12  Posterior superior alveolar nerves
13  Tympanic cavity, external acoustic meatus, and tympanic membrane
14  Inferior alveolar nerve
15  Lingual nerve
16  Facial nerve (n. VII)
17  Vagus nerve (n. X)
18  Hypoglossal nerve (n. XII) and superior root of ansa cervicalis
19  External carotid artery
20  Olfactory tract (n. I)
21  Optic nerve (n. II) (intracranial part)
22  Oculomotor nerve (n. III)
23  Abducent nerve (n. VI)
24  Trochlear nerve (n. IV)
25  Trigeminal nerve (n. V)
26  Vestibulocochlear nerve (n. VIII) and facial nerve (n. VII)
27  Glossopharyngeal nerve (n. IX) (leaving brain stem)
28  Rhomboid fossa
29  Vagus nerve (n. X) (leaving brain stem)
30  Hypoglossal nerve (n. XII) (leaving medulla oblongata)
31  Accessory nerve (n. XI) (ascending from foramen magnum)
32  Vertebral artery
33  Spinal ganglion and dura mater of spinal cord
34  Accessory nerve (n. XI)
35  Internal carotid artery
36  Lateral and medial branch of supra-orbital nerve
37  Infratrochlear nerve
38  Infra-orbital nerve
39  Pterygopalatine ganglion and middle superior alveolar nerve
40  Middle superior alveolar nerves (entering superior dental plexus)
41  Buccal nerve
42  Mental nerve and mental foramen
43  Auriculotemporal nerve
44  Otic ganglion (dotted line)
45  Chorda tympani
46  Mylohyoid nerve
47  Submandibular gland
48  Hyoid bone

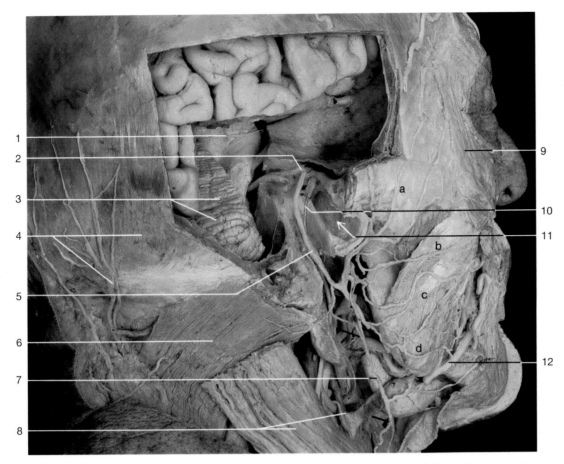

**Dissection of facial nerve in its entirety.** Cranial cavity fenestrated; temporal lobe partly removed. Facial canal and tympanic cavity opened, posterior wall of external acoustic meatus removed.
**Branches of facial nerve:** a = temporal branch; b = zygomatic branches; c = buccal branches; d = marginal mandibular branch.

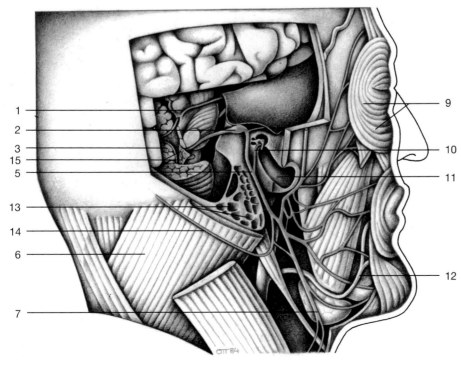

**Facial nerve** (schematic drawing of the dissection above).

1   Trochlear nerve
2   Facial nerve with geniculate ganglion
3   Cerebellum (right hemisphere)
4   Occipital belly of occipitofrontalis and greater occipital nerve
5   Facial nerve at stylomastoid foramen
6   Splenius capitis muscle
7   Cervical branch of facial nerve
8   Sternocleidomastoid muscle and retromandibular vein
9   Orbicularis oculi muscle
10  Chorda tympani
11  External acoustic meatus
12  Facial artery
13  Mastoid air cells
14  Posterior auricular nerve
15  Nucleus and genu of facial nerve

**Cranial nerves in connection with the brain stem** (oblique-lateral aspect). Lateral portion of the skull, brain, neck and facial structures, lateral wall of orbit and oral cavity have been removed. The tympanic cavity has been opened. The mandible has been divided and the muscles of mastication have been removed.

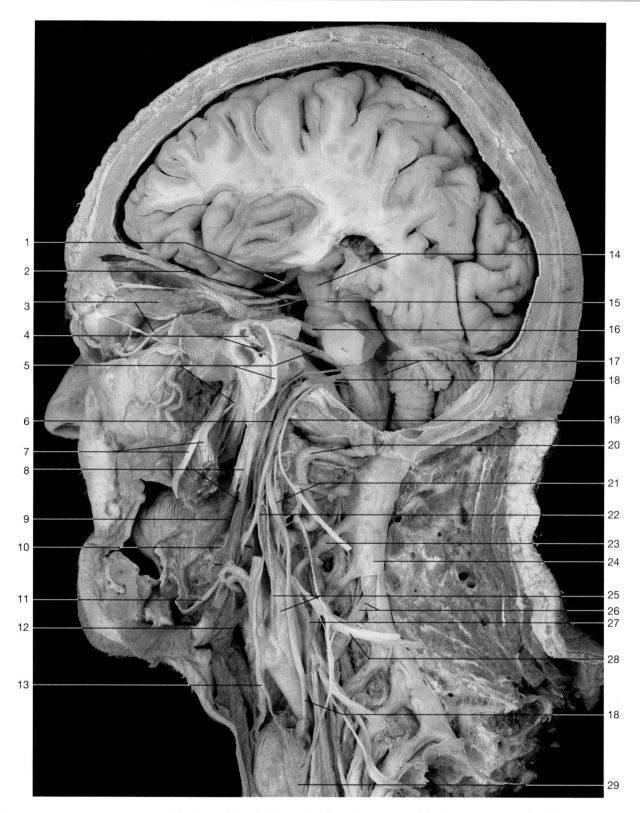

1  Optic tract
2  Oculomotor nerve (n. III)
3  Lateral rectus muscle and inferior branch
   of oculomotor nerve
4  Malleus and chorda tympani
5  Chorda tympani, facial nerve (n. VII), and
   vestibulocochlear nerve (n. VIII)
6  Glossopharyngeal nerve (n. XI)
7  Lingual nerve and inferior alveolar nerve
8  Styloid process and stylohyoid muscle
9  Styloglossus muscle
10 Lingual branches of glossopharyngeal
   nerve

11 Lingual branch of hypoglossal nerve
12 External carotid artery
13 Superior root of ansa cervicalis (branch of
   hypoglossal nerve, derived from $C_1$)
14 Lateral ventricle with choroid plexus and
   cerebral peduncle
15 Trochlear nerve (n. IV)
16 Trigeminal nerve (n. V)
17 Fourth ventricle and rhomboid fossa
18 Vagus nerve (n. X)
19 Accessory nerve (n. XI)
20 Vertebral artery
21 Superior cervical ganglion

22 Hypoglossal nerve (n. XII)
23 Spinal ganglion with dural sheath
24 Dura mater of spinal cord
25 Internal carotid artery and carotid
   sinus branch of glossopharyngeal
   nerve
26 Dorsal roots of spinal nerve
27 Sympathetic trunk
28 Branch of cervical plexus (ventral
   primary ramus of third cervical
   spinal nerve)
29 Ansa cervicalis

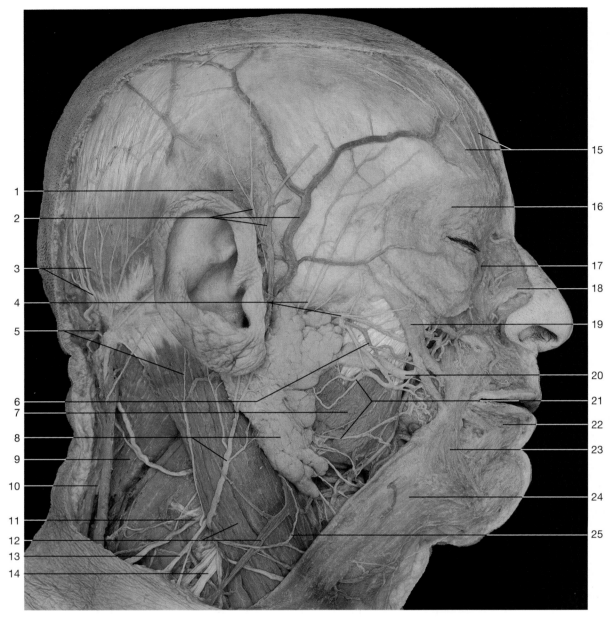

1
2
3
4
5
6
7
8
9
10
11
12
13
14

15
16
17
18
19
20
21
22
23
24
25

Lateral superficial aspect of the face. Peripheral distribution of facial nerve (n. VII).

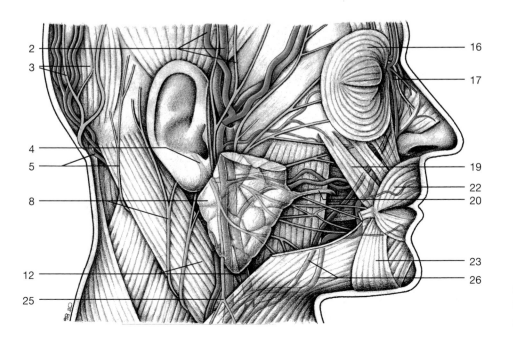

2
3
4
5
8
12
25

16
17
19
22
20
23
26

**Superficial region of the face.** Note the facial plexus within the parotid gland (semischematic drawing).

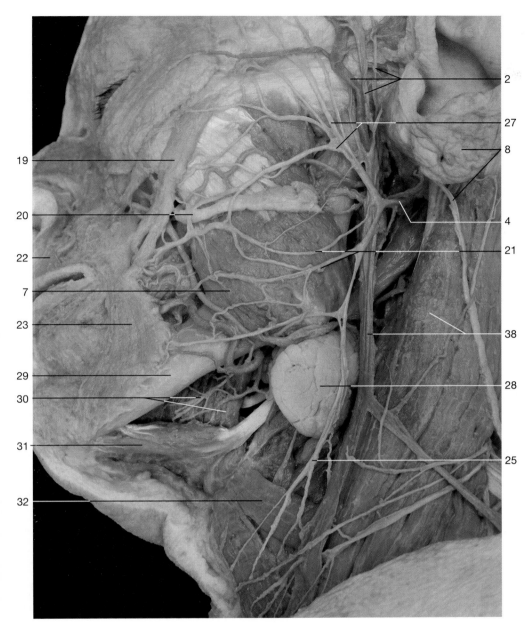

1  Temporoparietalis muscle
2  Superficial temporal artery and vein and auriculotemporal nerve
3  Occipital belly of occipitofrontalis muscle and greater occipital nerve (C₂)
4  Facial nerve (n. VII)
5  Lesser occipital nerve and occipital artery
6  Transverse facial artery
7  Masseter muscle
8  Parotid gland and great auricular nerve
9  Splenius capitis muscle
10  Trapezius muscle
11  Punctum nervosum, point of distribution of cutaneous nerves of cervical plexus
12  Sternocleidomastoid muscle and external jugular vein
13  Supraclavicular nerves
14  Brachial plexus
15  Supra-orbital nerves
16  Orbicularis oculi muscle
17  Angular artery (terminal branch of facial artery)
18  Nasalis muscle
19  Zygomaticus major muscle
20  Parotid duct
21  Zygomatic and buccal branches of facial nerve
22  Orbicularis oris muscle
23  Depressor anguli oris muscle
24  Platysma
25  Cervical branch of facial nerve (anastomosing with transverse cervical nerve of cervical plexus)
26  Facial artery and vein
27  Temporal branches of facial nerve
28  Submandibular gland
29  Mandible
30  Mylohyoideus muscle and nerve
31  Digastricus muscle, anterior belly
32  Omohyoideus muscle
33  Greater petrosal nerve
34  Geniculate ganglion
35  Chorda tympani
36  Posterior auricular nerve
37  Stylomastoid foramen
38  Sternocleidomastoid muscle and retromandibular vein

**Deep dissection of facial nerve. Retromandibular and submandibular region**
(lateral aspect, parotid gland has been removed).

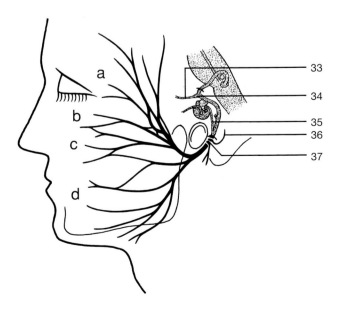

**Main branches of facial nerve** (schematic diagram).
a = temporal branches; b = zygomatic branches;
c = buccal branches; d = marginal mandibular branch.

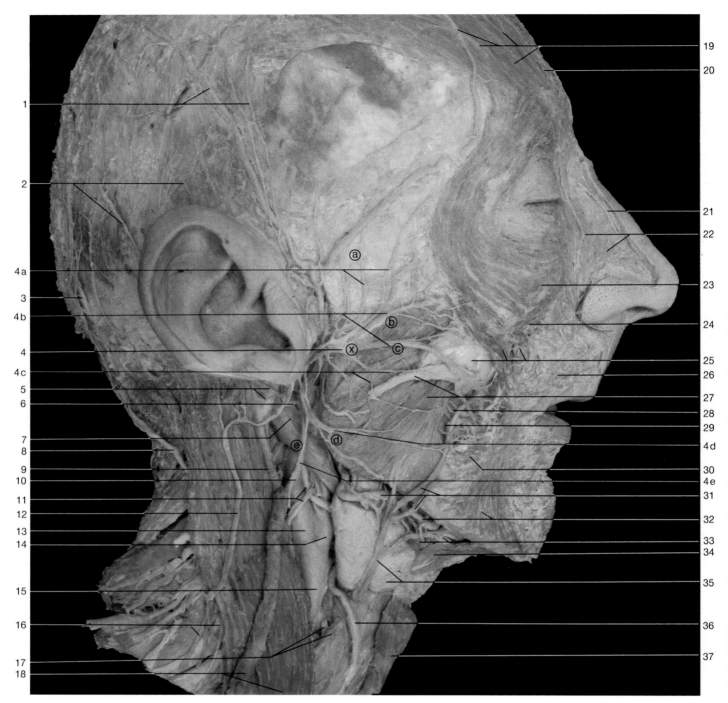

**Lateral superficial aspect of the face.** The parotid gland has been removed to display the parotid plexus of the facial nerve.
a–e = branches of facial nerve: a = temporal branch; b = zygomatic branches; c = buccal branches; d = marginal mandibular branch; e = cervical branch.

1   Superficial temporal artery and
    auriculotemporal nerve
2   Posterior auricular artery and nerve
    and temporoparietalis muscle
3   Occipital artery
4   Facial nerve (n. VII) (parotid plexus [×])
    a   Temporal branches
    b   Zygomatic branches
    c   Buccal branches
    d   Marginal mandibular branch
    e   Cervical branch
5   Posterior auricular nerve
6   Posterior auricular artery
7   Digastric muscle (posterior belly)
8   Lesser occipital nerve
9   Posterior auricular vein

10  Retromandibular vein
11  Hypoglossal nerve
    and sternocleidomastoid artery
12  Great auricular nerve
13  Internal carotid artery
14  External carotid artery
15  Common carotid artery
16  Branches of cervical plexus
17  Superior laryngeal artery and vein
18  External jugular vein and
    sternocleidomastoid muscle
19  Frontal branch of superficial temporal artery,
    lateral branch of supra-orbital nerve, and
    frontal belly of occipitofrontalis muscle
20  Medial branch of supra-orbital nerve
21  Dorsal nasal artery
22  Angular artery and nasalis muscle

23  Orbicularis oculi muscle
24  Zygomaticus minor muscle
25  Buccal fat pad, zygomaticus major
    muscle, and infra-orbital nerve
26  Orbicularis oris muscle
27  Parotid duct and masseter muscle
28  Buccal artery and nerve
29  Buccinator muscle
30  Risorius muscle
31  Facial artery and vein
32  Submental artery and depressor anguli
    oris muscle
33  Mylohyoid nerve and mylohyoid muscle
34  Digastric muscle (anterior belly)
35  Facial vein and submandibular gland
36  Superior thyroid artery
37  Sternohyoid muscle

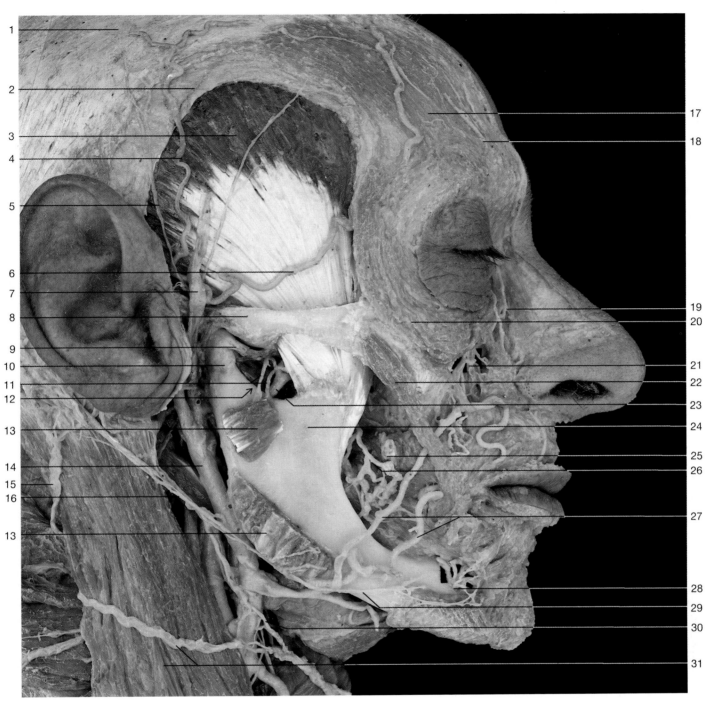

**Lateral superficial aspect of the face.** Masseter muscle and temporal fascia have been partly removed to display the masseteric artery and nerve.

| | | |
|---|---|---|
| 1 Galea aponeurotica | 10 Head of mandible | 22 Zygomaticus major muscle |
| 2 Temporal fascia | 11 Masseteric artery and nerve | 23 Maxillary artery |
| 3 Temporalis muscle | 12 Mandibular notch | 24 Coronoid process |
| 4 Parietal branch of superficial temporal artery | 13 Masseter muscle (divided) | 25 Parotid duct (divided) |
| 5 Auriculotemporal nerve | 14 External carotid artery | 26 Buccal nerve |
| 6 Frontal branch of superficial temporal artery | 15 Great auricular nerve | 27 Facial artery and vein |
| 7 Superficial temporal vein | 16 Facial nerve (reflected) | 28 Mental nerve |
| 8 Zygomatic arch | 17 Frontal belly of occipitofrontalis muscle | 29 Mandibular branch of facial nerve |
| 9 Articular disc of temporomandibular joint | 18 Medial branch of supra-orbital nerve | 30 Cervical branch of facial nerve |
| | 19 Angular artery | 31 Transverse cervical nerve (communicating branch with facial nerve) and sternocleidomastoid muscle |
| | 20 Orbicularis oculi muscle | |
| | 21 Infra-orbital nerve | |

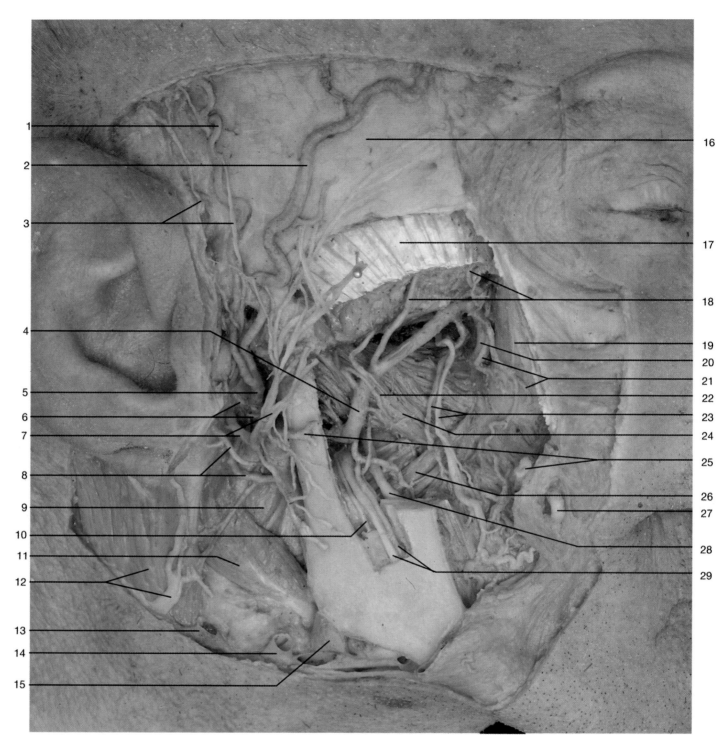

**Deep dissection of facial and retromandibular regions.** The coronoid process together with the insertions of temporalis muscle have been removed to display the maxillary artery. The upper part of the mandibular canal has been opened.

1  Parietal branch of the superficial temporal
   artery
2  Frontal branch of the superficial temporal
   artery
3  Auriculotemporal nerve
4  Maxillary artery
5  Superficial temporal artery
6  Communicating branches between facial
   and auriculotemporal nerves
7  Facial nerve
8  Posterior auricular artery and anterior
   auricular branch of superficial temporal artery
9  Internal jugular vein

10  Mylohyoid nerve
11  Posterior belly of digastric muscle
12  Great auricular nerve and
    sternocleidomastoid muscle
13  External jugular vein
14  Retromandibular vein
15  Submandibular gland
16  Temporal fascia
17  Temporalis tendon
18  Deep temporal arteries
19  Posterior superior alveolar nerve
20  Sphenopalatine artery
21  Posterior superior alveolar arteries

22  Masseteric artery and nerve
23  Buccal nerve and artery
24  Lateral pterygoid
25  Transverse facial artery and
    parotid duct (divided)
26  Medial pterygoid muscle
27  Facial artery
28  Lingual nerve
29  Inferior alveolar artery and nerve
    (mandibular canal opened)

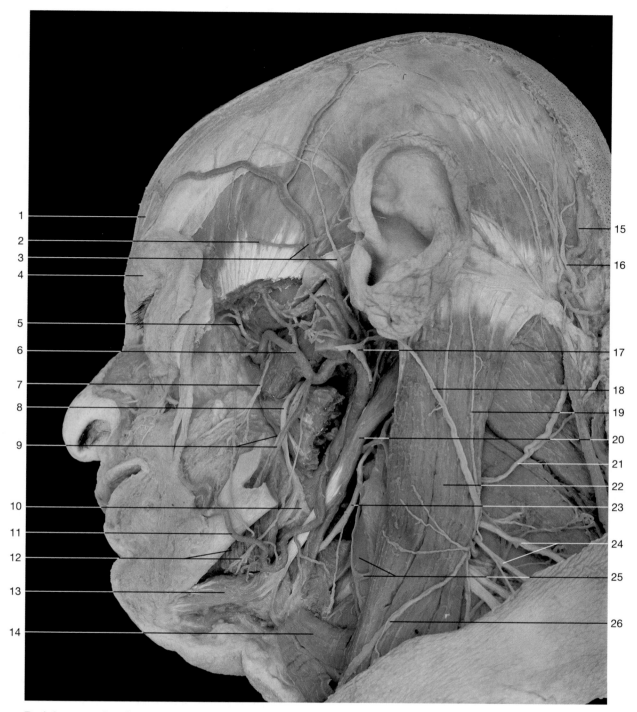

**Peripharyngeal and retromandibular region.** The mandible has been partly removed (oblique lateral aspect).

1  Supra-orbital nerve (medial branch)
2  Temporalis muscle
3  Superficial temporal artery and
   auriculotemporal nerve
4  Orbicularis oculi muscle
5  Anterior deep temporal artery
6  Maxillary artery
7  Buccal nerve
8  Lingual nerve
9  Inferior alveolar nerve and artery

10  Submandibular ganglion
11  Facial artery
12  Mylohyoid muscle and nerve
13  Anterior belly of digastric muscle
14  Omohyoid muscle
15  Occipital artery
16  Greater occipital nerve (C$_2$)
17  Facial nerve (cut) (n. VII)
18  Great auricular nerve
19  Lesser occipital nerve

20  Posterior belly of digastric muscle
21  Accessory nerve (Var.)
22  Sternocleidomastoid muscle
23  Hypoglossus nerve (n. XII)
24  Supraclavicular nerves
   (lateral and intermedial branches)
25  Internal jugular vein and ansa
   cervicalis
26  Anterior supraclavicular nerve

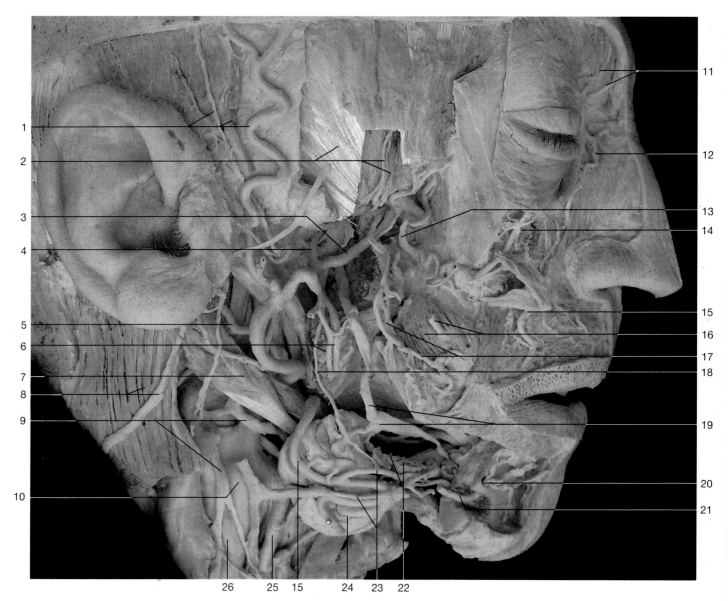

**Dissection of deep facial and retromandibular regions after removal of mandible.** Pterygoid muscles removed, temporalis muscle fenestrated.

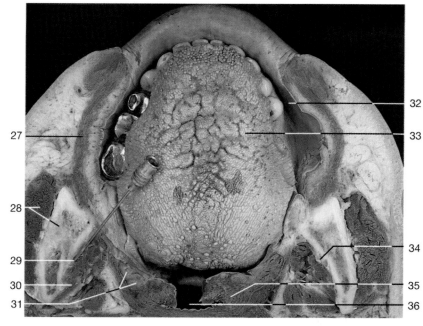

**Transverse section through oral cavity and pharynx.** The location of inferior alveolar nerve and artery is indicated by a needle.

1 Superficial temporal artery and vein and auriculotemporal nerve
2 Temporalis tendon, deep temporal nerves and artery
3 Maxillary artery
4 Middle meningeal artery
5 Occipital artery
6 Inferior alveolar artery and nerve
7 Posterior belly of digastric muscle
8 Great auricular nerve and sternocleidomastoid muscle
9 Hypoglossal nerve and superior root of ansa cervicalis
10 External carotid artery
11 Supratrochlear nerve and medial branch of supra-orbital artery
12 Angular artery
13 Posterior superior alveolar artery
14 Infra-orbital nerve
15 Facial artery
16 Parotid duct (divided) and buccinator muscle
17 Buccal artery and nerve

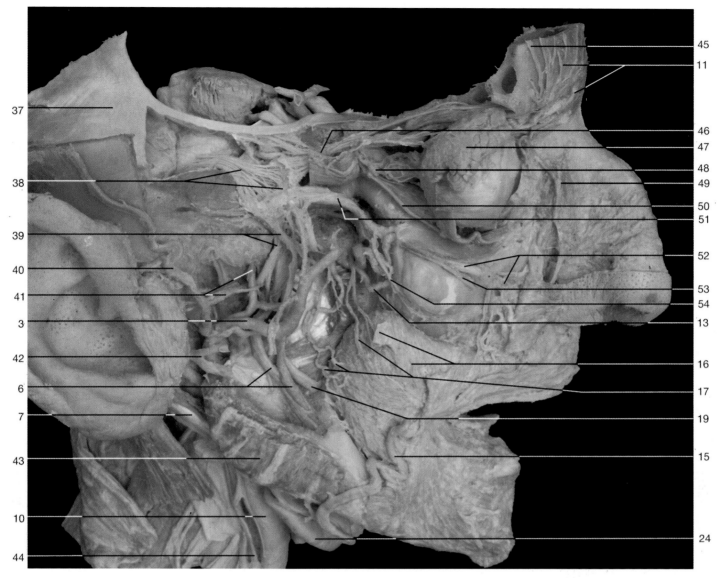

**Para- and retropharyngeal regions.** The mandible and the lateral wall of the orbit have been removed. The main branches of the trigeminal nerve and its ganglion are displayed.

| | | | |
|---|---|---|---|
| 18 | Mylohyoid nerve | 36 | Pharynx |
| 19 | Lingual nerve and submandibular ganglion | 37 | Tentorium of cerebellum |
| 20 | Mental nerve and mental foramen | 38 | Trigeminal nerve and ganglion |
| 21 | Inferior alveolar nerve | 39 | Mandibular nerve |
| 22 | Mylohyoid muscle (divided) and hypoglossal nerve | 40 | Superficial temporal artery |
| 23 | Submental artery and vein | 41 | Auriculotemporal nerve and middle meningeal artery |
| 24 | Submandibular gland | 42 | Facial nerve (divided) |
| 25 | Superior thyroid artery | 43 | Masseter muscle |
| 26 | Common carotid artery | 44 | Superior root of ansa cervicalis |
| 27 | Buccinator muscle | 45 | Lateral branch of supra-orbital nerve |
| 28 | Masseter muscle and mandible | 46 | Ophthalmic nerve |
| 29 | Entrance of mandibular canal | 47 | Lacrimal gland |
| 30 | Medial pterygoid muscle | 48 | Ciliary ganglion and short ciliary nerves |
| 31 | Palatine tonsil | 49 | Angular artery |
| 32 | Oral vestibule | 50 | Inferior branch of oculomotor nerve |
| 33 | Tongue | 51 | Maxillary nerve |
| 34 | Inferior alveolar nerve, artery, and vein | 52 | Infra-orbital nerve |
| 35 | Pharyngeal constrictor muscle | 53 | Anterior superior alveolar nerve |
| | | 54 | Posterior superior alveolar nerve |

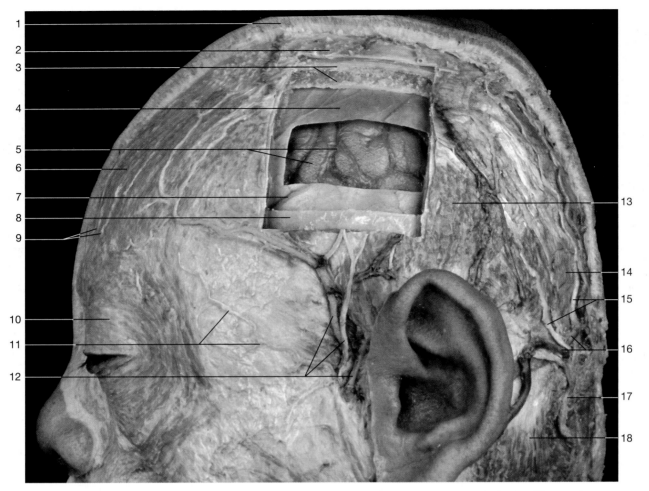

**Nerves and blood vessels of the scalp.** Scalp and meninges are demonstrated by a series of window-like openings.

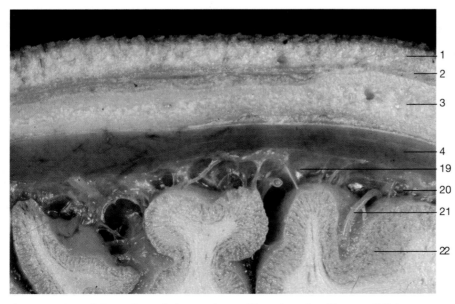

**Cross section of the scalp and the meninges.** The subarachnoid space (20) is shown.

1  Skin
2  Galea aponeurotica
3  Skull diploe
4  Dura mater
5  Arachnoid and pia mater
   with cerebral vessels
6  Frontal belly of occipitofrontalis
   muscle
7  Branch of middle meningeal artery
8  Pericranium (periosteum)
9  Lateral and medial branches of
   supra-orbital nerve
10 Orbicularis oculi muscle
11 Zygomatico-orbital artery
12 Auriculotemporal nerve and
   superficial temporal artery and
   vein
13 Superior auricular muscle
14 Occipital belly of occipitofrontalis
   muscle
15 Occipital nerve
16 Occipital artery and vein
17 Greater occipital nerve

18 Sternocleidomastoid muscle
19 Arachnoid mater
20 Subarachnoid space
21 Pia mater with cerebral vessels
22 Cerebral cortex
23 Arachnoid granulations
24 Confluens sinuum
25 Cerebellum
26 Superior sagittal sinus
27 Inferior sagittal sinus
28 Straight sinus (Sinus rectus)
29 Subdural space
30 Falx cerebri
31 Frontal lobe
32 Chiasmatic cistern
33 Interpeduncular cistern
34 Corpus callosum
35 Cerebellomedullar cistern

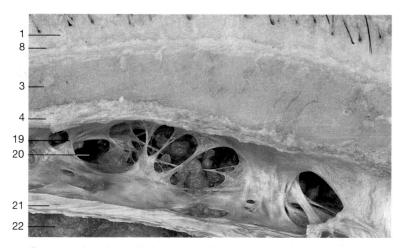

**Cross section through the vertex of the skull** showing the dura, pia, and arachnoid mater. The subarachnoid space (20) appears enlarged.

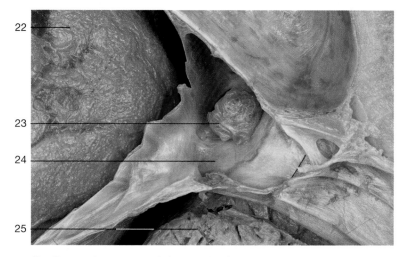

**Confluens sinuum** containing arachnoid granulations of Pacchioni.

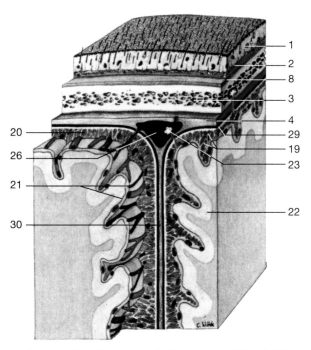

**A coronal section through the vertex of the skull,** showing the arrangement of the meninges.

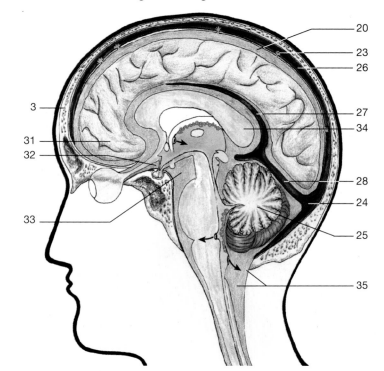

**Subarachnoid cisterns of the brain** (midsagittal section).
Green = cisterns; blue = dural sinus and ventricles;
red = choroid plexus of third and fourth ventricles; arrows = flow of cerebrospinal fluid.

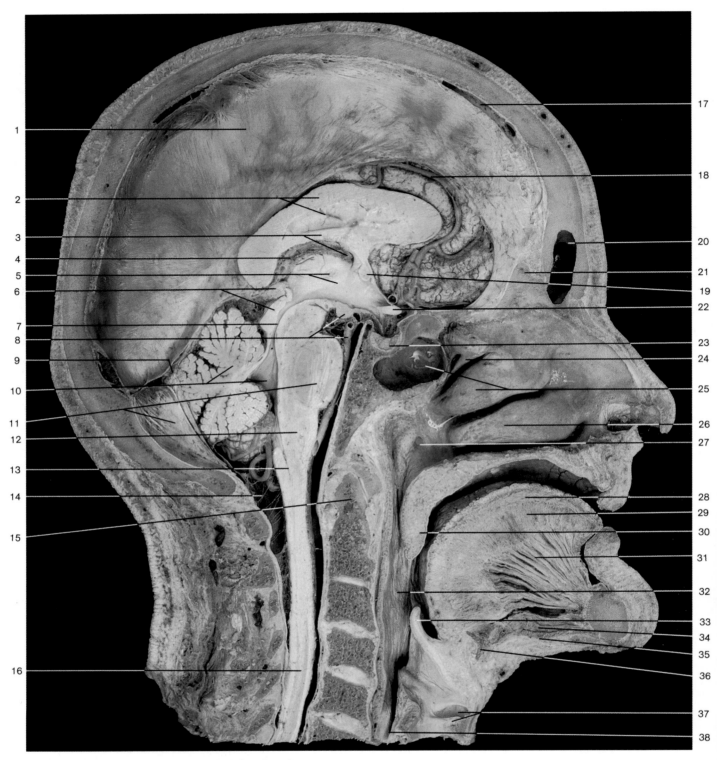

**Median sagittal section through the head and neck.**

1  Falx cerebri
2  Corpus callosum and septum pellucidum
3  Interventricular foramen and fornix
4  Choroid plexus of third ventricle and internal cerebral vein
5  Third ventricle and interthalamic adhesion
6  Pineal body and colliculi of the midbrain
7  Cerebral aqueduct
8  Mamillary body and basilar artery
9  Straight sinus
10  Fourth ventricle and cerebellum
11  Pons and falx cerebelli
12  Medulla oblongata
13  Central canal

14  Cerebellomedullary cistern
15  Dens of the axis (odontoid process)
16  Spinal cord
17  Superior sagittal sinus
18  Anterior cerebral artery
19  Anterior commissure
20  Frontal sinus
21  Crista galli
22  Optic chiasma
23  Pituitary gland (hypophysis)
24  Superior nasal concha
25  Middle nasal concha and sphenoid sinus
26  Inferior nasal concha

27  Pharyngeal opening of auditory tube
28  Superior longitudinal muscle of tongue
29  Vertical muscle of the tongue
30  Uvula
31  Genioglossus muscle
32  Pharynx
33  Epiglottis
34  Geniohyoid muscle
35  Mylohyoid muscle
36  Hyoid bone
37  Vocal fold and sinus of larynx
38  Esophagus

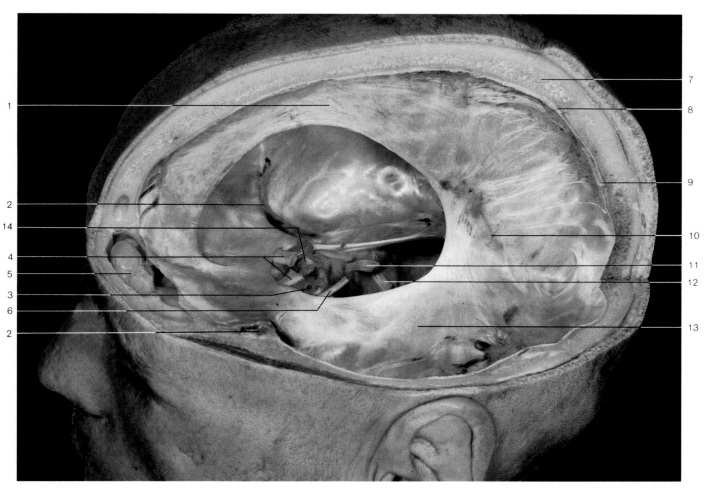

**Dura mater and venous sinuses of the dura mater.** The brain has been removed (oblique lateral aspect).

1  Falx cerebri
2  Position of middle meningeal
   artery and vein
3  Internal carotid artery
4  Optic nerve (n. II)
5  Frontal sinus
6  Oculomotor nerve (n. III)
7  Diploe
8  Dura mater
9  Superior sagittal sinus
10  Straight sinus
11  Trigeminal nerve (n. V)
12  Facial and vestibulocochlear nerve
    (n. VII and n. VIII)
13  Tentorium cerebelli
14  Pituitary gland (hypophysis)
15  Inferior sagittal sinus
16  Sigmoid sinus
17  Confluence of sinuses
18  Inferior petrosal sinus
19  Transverse sinus
20  Superior petrosal sinus
21  Cavernous and intercavernous sinuses

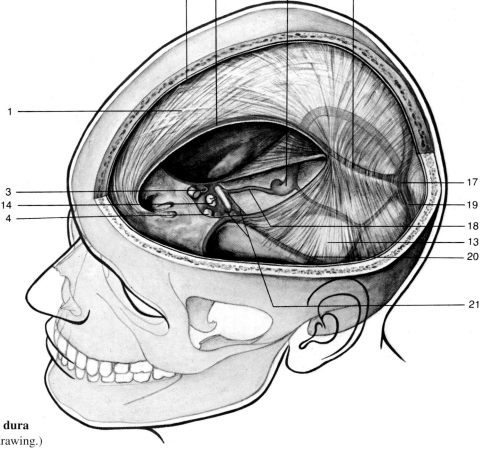

**Dura mater and venous sinuses of the dura mater** (left lateral aspect). (Schematic drawing.)

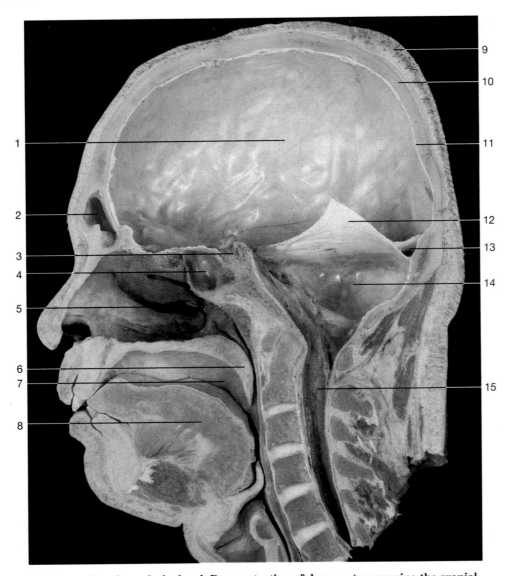

1  Cranial cavity with dura mater
   (right cerebral hemisphere
   has been removed)
2  Frontal sinus
3  Hypophysial fossa with pituitary
   gland
4  Sphenoidal sinus
5  Nasal cavity
6  Soft palate (uvula)
7  Oral cavity
8  Tongue
9  Skin
10  Calvaria
11  Dura mater
12  Tentorium cerebelli
13  Confluence of sinuses
14  Infratentorial space (cerebellum
   and part of the brain stem have
   been removed)
15  Vertebral canal
16  Frontal branch of middle
   meningeal artery and veins
17  Middle meningeal artery
18  Diploe
19  Parietal branch of middle
   meningeal artery and vein
20  Occipital pole of left hemisphere
   covered with dura mater

**Median section through the head. Demonstration of dura mater covering the cranial cavity.** Brain and spinal cord are removed (right half of the head, as seen from medial).

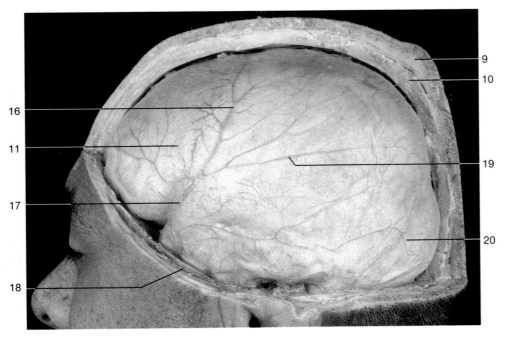

**Dissection of dura mater and meningeal vessels.** Left half of calvaria removed.

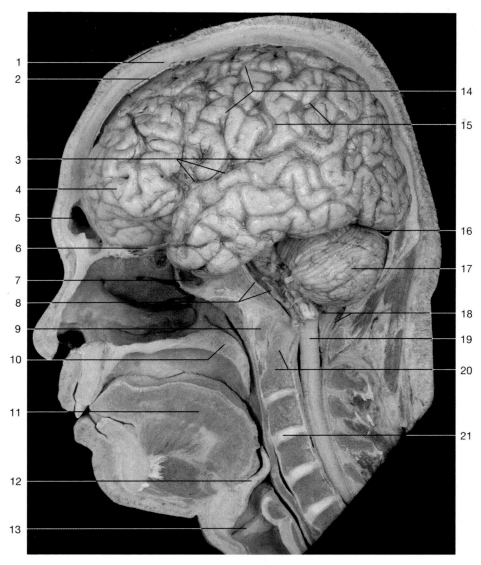

1  Calvaria and skin of the scalp
2  Dura mater (divided)
3  Position of lateral sulcus
4  Frontal lobe covered by arachnoid and pia mater
5  Frontal sinus
6  Olfactory bulb
7  Sphenoidal sinus
8  Dura mater on clivus and basilar artery
9  Atlas (anterior arch, divided)
10 Soft palate
11 Tongue
12 Epiglottis
13 Vocal fold
14 Position of central sulcus
15 Superior cerebral veins
16 Tentorium (divided)
17 Cerebellum
18 Cerebellomedullary cistern
19 Position of foramen magnum and spinal cord
20 Dens of axis
21 Intervertebral disc

**Dissection of the brain with pia mater and arachnoid in situ.** The head is cut in half except for the brain, which is shown in its entirety.

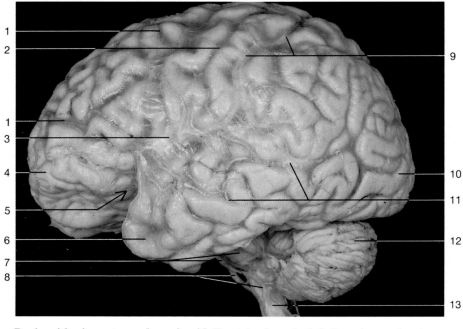

1  Superior cerebral veins
2  Position of central sulcus
3  Position of lateral sulcus and cistern of lateral cerebral fossa
4  Frontal pole
5  Lateral sulcus (arrow)
6  Temporal pole
7  Pons and basilar artery
8  Vertebral arteries
9  Superior anastomotic vein
10 Occipital pole
11 Inferior cerebral veins
12 Hemisphere of cerebellum
13 Medulla oblongata

**Brain with pia mater and arachnoid.** Frontal pole to the left (lateral aspect).

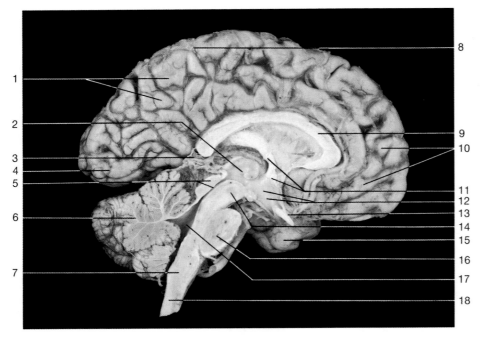

**Brain and brain stem,** median section. Frontal pole to the right.

1  Parietal lobe
2  Thalamus, third ventricle, and intermediate mass
3  Great cerebral vein
4  Occipital lobe
5  Colliculi of the midbrain and cerebral aqueduct
6  Cerebellum
7  Medulla oblongata
8  Central sulcus
9  Corpus callosum
10  Frontal lobe
11  Fornix and anterior commissure
12  Hypothalamus
13  Optic chiasma
14  Midbrain
15  Temporal lobe
16  Pons
17  Fourth ventricle
18  Spinal cord
19  Inferior concha and nasal cavity
20  Alveolar process of maxilla
21  Tongue
22  Dens of axis
23  Oral part of pharynx
24  Alveolar process of mandible
25  Epiglottis

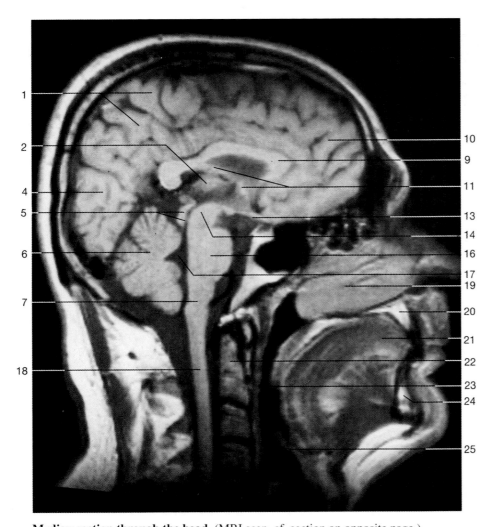

**Median section through the head.** (MRI scan, cf. section on opposite page.)

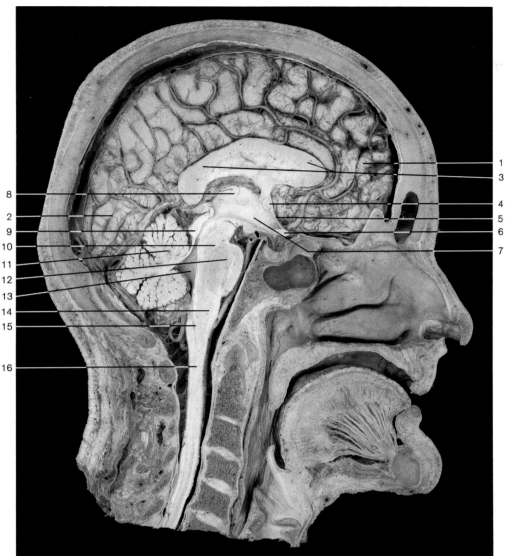

1   Frontal lobe of cerebrum
2   Occipital lobe of cerebrum
3   Corpus callosum
4   Anterior commissure
5   Lamina terminalis
6   Optic chiasma
7   Hypothalamus
8   Thalamus and third
    ventricle
9   Colliculi of the midbrain
10  Midbrain (inferior portion)
11  Cerebellum
12  Pons
13  Fourth ventricle
14  Medulla oblongata
15  Central canal
16  Spinal cord

**Median section through the head.** Regions of the brain. Falx cerebri removed.

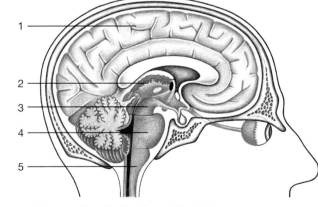

**Scheme of brain divisions** (cf. table).
Red = choroidal plexus. (Schematic drawing.)
1  Telencephalon (yellow) with lateral ventricles
2  Diencephalon (orange) with third ventricle,
   optic nerve, and retina
3  Mesencephalon (blue) with cerebral aqueduct
4  Metencephalon (green) with fourth ventricle
5  Myelencephalon (yellow-green)

| | | |
|---|---|---|
| I.  Prosencephalon (forebrain) | 1.  Telencephalon (cerebral hemispheres, striatum, etc.) | |
| | 2.  Diencephalon (thalamus, metathalamus, hypothalamus, etc.) | |
| II.  Mesencephalon (midbrain) | 3.  Mesencephalon (colliculi, cerebral peduncles, tegmentum) | |
| III.  Rhombencephalon (hindbrain) | 4.  Metencephalon (pons, cerebellum) | |
| | 5.  Myelencephalon (medulla oblongata) | |

**Main divisions of the brain**
I–III = primary brain vesicles; 1–5 = secondary brain vesicles

Diencephalon, midbrain, pons, and medulla oblongata are collectively termed the **brain stem.**

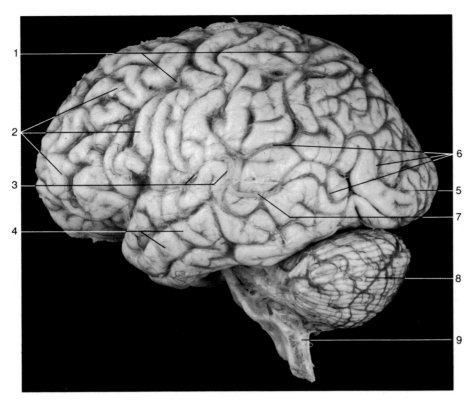

1  Superior cerebral veins and
   parietal lobe
2  Frontal lobe
3  Superficial middle cerebral vein and
   cistern of lateral cerebral fossa
4  Temporal lobe
5  Occipital lobe
6  Inferior cerebral veins and
   transverse occipital sulcus
7  Inferior anastomotic vein
8  Cerebellum
9  Medulla oblongata

**Brain with pia mater. Cerebral veins** (bluish). In the lateral sulcus the cistern of the lateral fossa is recognizable. Frontal lobe to the left.

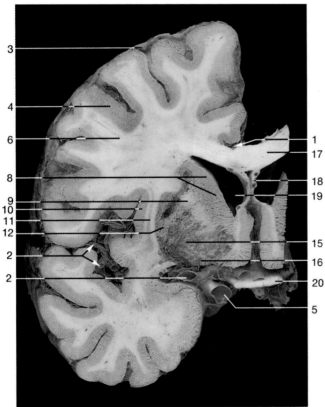

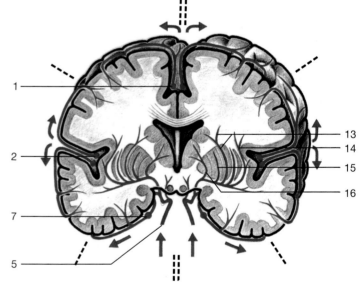

**Arteries of the brain.** Coronal section. Areas supplied by cortical and central arteries. Dotted lines indicate boundaries of arterial supply areas; arrows, direction of blood flow.

◁ **Coronal section through the right hemisphere,** showing arachnoid, pia mater, and the arterial blood supply (anterior aspect).

| | | |
|---|---|---|
| 1  Anterior cerebral artery | 8  Caudate nucleus | 15  Pallidostriate artery |
| 2  Middle cerebral arteries | 9  Internal capsule | 16  Thalamic artery |
| 3  Arachnoid | 10  Insular lobe | 17  Corpus callosum |
| 4  Cortex | 11  Claustrum | 18  Septum pellucidum |
| 5  Internal carotid artery | 12  Putamen | 19  Lateral ventricle |
| 6  Frontal lobe (white matter) | 13  Posterior striate branch | 20  Optic chiasma |
| 7  Posterior cerebral artery | 14  Insular artery | |

1 Olfactory tract
2 Anterior cerebral artery
3 Optic nerve (n. II)
4 Middle cerebral artery
5 Infundibulum
6 Oculomotor nerve (n. III) and posterior communicating artery
7 Posterior cerebral artery
8 Basilar artery and abducent nerve (n. VI)
9 Anterior spinal artery
10 Vertebral artery
11 Cerebellum
12 Anterior communicating artery
13 Internal carotid artery
14 Superior cerebellar artery and pons
15 Labyrinthine arteries
16 Inferior anterior cerebellar artery
17 Inferior posterior cerebellar artery
18 Medulla oblongata
19 Supratrochlear artery
20 Anterior ciliary arteries
21 Lacrimal artery
22 Posterior ciliary arteries
23 Ophthalmic artery with central retinal artery
24 Trigeminal nerve (n. V)
25 Facial nerve (n. VII) and vestibulocochlear nerve (n. VIII)
26 Glossopharyngeal nerve (n. IX), vagus nerve (n. X), and accessory nerve (n. XI)
27 Olfactory bulb
28 Posterior spinal artery

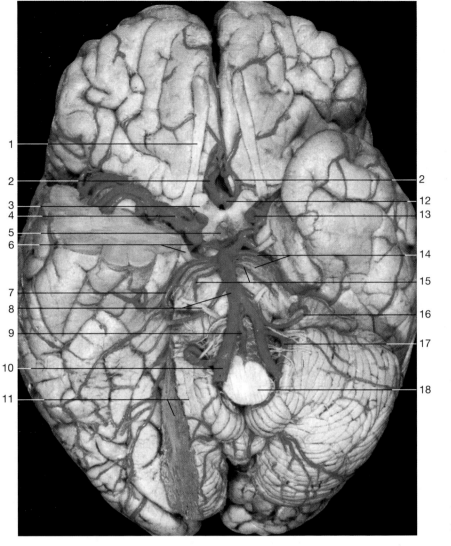

**Arteries of the brain** (inferior aspect, frontal pole above). Right temporal lobe and cerebellum partly removed.

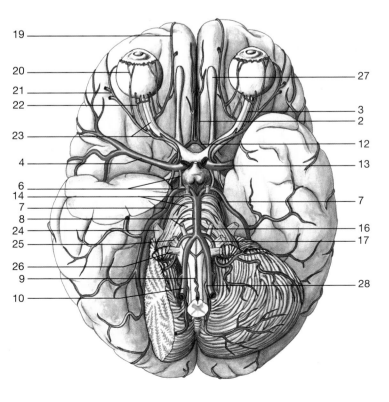

**Arteries of the brain** (inferior aspect). Right temporal lobe and cerebellum partly removed. Note the arterial circle of Willis around the infundibulum.

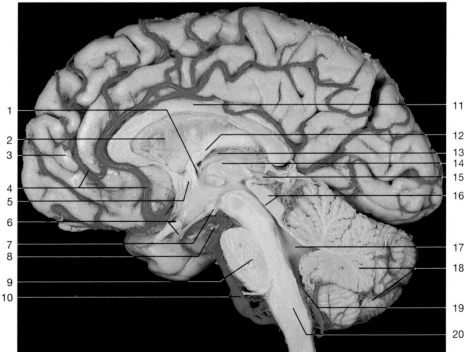

1  Insula
2  Middle cerebral artery (2 branches:
   a Parietal branches,
   b Temporal branches)
3  Basilar artery
4  Vertebral artery
5  Central sulcus
6  Occipital lobe
7  Superior cerebellar artery
8  Cerebellum
9  Anterior cerebral artery
10 Ethmoidal arteries
11 Ophthalmic artery
12 Internal carotid artery
13 Posterior communicating artery
14 Posterior cerebral artery
15 Anterior inferior cerebellar artery
16 Posterior inferior cerebellar artery

**Cerebral arteries.** Lateral aspect of
the left hemisphere. The upper part of
the temporal lobe has been removed to
display the insula and cerebral arteries.

◁ **Arteries of the brain.**

1  Interventricular foramen
2  Septum pellucidum
3  Frontal lobe
4  Anterior cerebral artery
5  Anterior commissure
6  Optic chiasma and infundibulum
7  Mamillary body
8  Oculomotor nerve (n. III)
9  Pons
10 Basilar artery
11 Corpus callosum
12 Fornix
13 Choroid plexus
14 Third ventricle
15 Pineal body
16 Tectum and cerebral aqueduct
17 Fourth ventricle
18 Cerebellum (arbor vitae, vermis)
19 Median aperture of Magendie
20 Medulla oblongata

**Median section through the brain
and brain stem.** Cerebral arteries
injected with red resin.

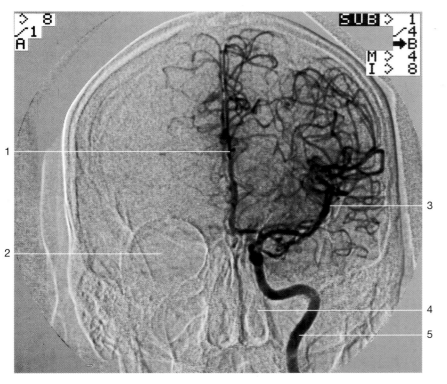

1  Anterior cerebral artery
2  Orbit
3  Middle cerebral artery
4  Nasal cavity
5  Internal carotid artery
6  Arterial circle of Willis
7  Posterior communicating
   artery
8  Posterior cerebral artery
9  Basilar artery
10  Vertebral artery
11  Subclavian artery
12  Aortic arch
13  Common carotid artery

**Arteries of the brain. Angiogram of the left internal carotid artery** (anterior aspect) (courtesy of Prof. Dr. W. Huk, University of Erlangen-Nürnberg).

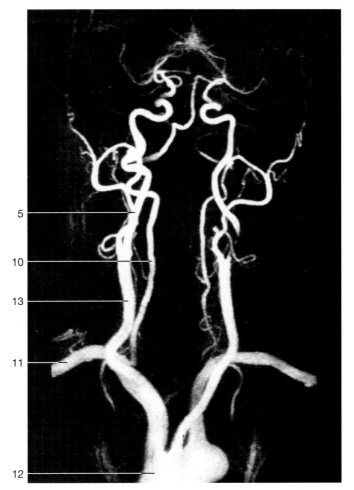

**Cerebral arteries** (schematic drawing).
Left hemisphere and brain stem have been removed.
Note the arterial circle of Willis around the sella turcica.

**Main arteries for brain supply** (MRI angiograph, anterior aspect, courtesy of Prof. Dr. W. Bautz, University of Erlangen-Nürnberg).

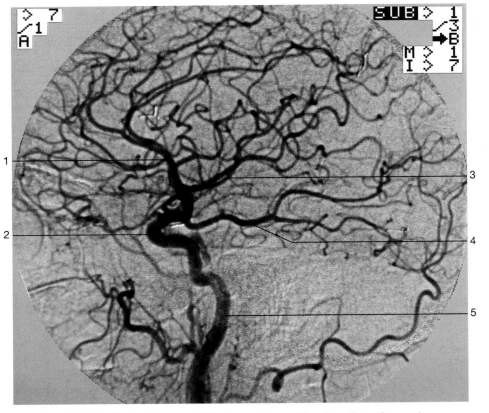

1   Anterior cerebral artery
2   Loop of the internal
    carotid artery
3   Middle cerebral artery
4   Posterior cerebral artery
5   Internal carotid artery
6   Superior cerebellar artery
7   Anterior inferior cerebellar
    artery
8   Posterior inferior cerebellar
    artery
9   Vertebral artery

**Arteries of the brain. Angiogram of the internal carotid artery** (lateral aspect)
(courtesy of Prof. Dr. W. Huk, University of Erlangen-Nürnberg).

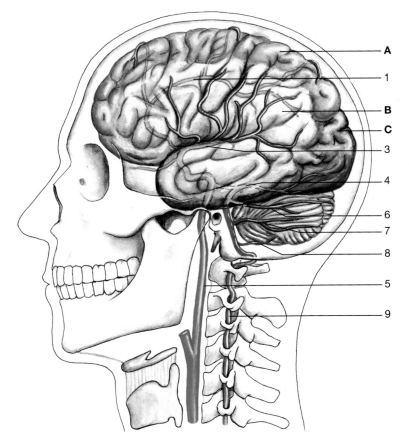

**Cerebral arteries.** The areas supplied by the main arteries are indicated by
different colors (lateral aspect).

**Areas of blood supply of the brain**
(cerebellum = green).
A = Anterior cerebral artery (upper
    and medial parts of the cortex)
    (orange)
B = Middle cerebral artery (lateral
    areas of the frontal, parietal, and
    temporal lobe) (white)
C = Posterior cerebral artery (occipital
    lobe and inferior parts of the
    temporal lobe) (blue)

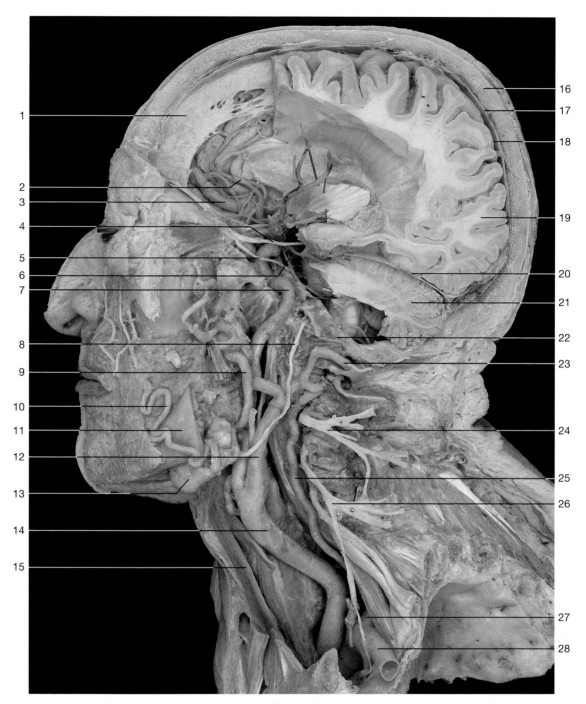

**Dissection of the arteries of the brain and head** (lateral aspect, superficial layers of facial region and left hemisphere and cerebellum partly removed).

| | | | |
|---|---|---|---|
| 1 | Falx cerebri | 16 | Calvaria |
| 2 | Anterior cerebral artery | 17 | Dura mater |
| 3 | Frontal lobe | 18 | Subarachnoidal space |
| 4 | Oculomotor nerve (n. III) | 19 | Occipital lobe |
| 5 | Abducent nerve (n. VI) | 20 | Tentorium of cerebellum |
| 6 | Posterior cerebral artery | 21 | Cerebellum |
| 7 | Internal carotid artery, entering sinus cavernosus | 22 | Base of skull |
| | | 23 | Vertebral artery (on the posterior arch of the atlas) |
| 8 | Hypoglossus nerve (n. XII) | | |
| 9 | Maxillary artery | 24 | Cervical plexus |
| 10 | Facial artery | 25 | Vertebral artery (removed from the cervical vertebrae) |
| 11 | Mandible | | |
| 12 | External carotid artery | 26 | Brachial plexus |
| 13 | Submandibular gland | 27 | Vertebral artery (branching from the subclavian artery) |
| 14 | Common carotid artery | | |
| 15 | Sternohyoid muscle | 28 | Subclavian artery |

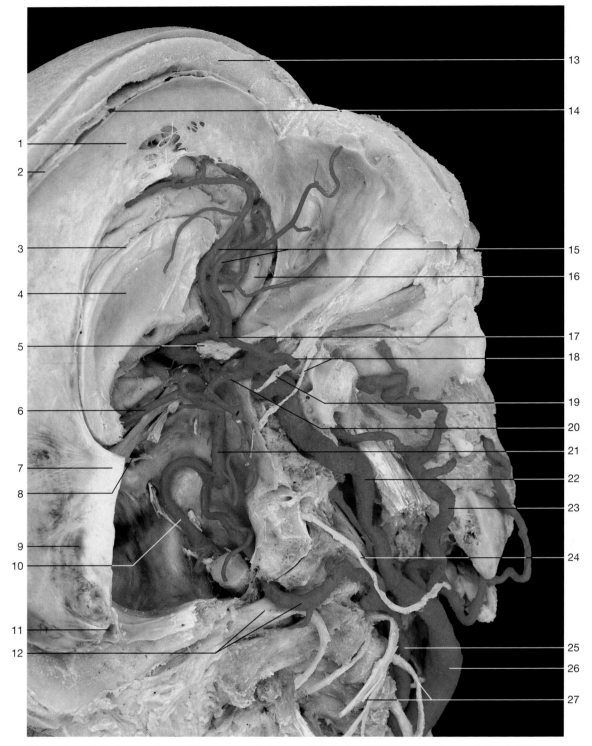

**Dissection of the internal carotid artery and the arterial circle of Willis at the base of the skull** (posterior lateral aspect, right hemisphere, cerebellum, and part of the deep facial regions have been removed).

| | | | | | |
|---|---|---|---|---|---|
| 1 | Falx cerebri | 10 | Left vertebral artery | 19 | Oculomotor nerve (n. III) |
| 2 | Dura mater | 11 | Confluens sinuum (continuing into the transverse sinus) | 20 | Arterial circle of Willis |
| 3 | Corpus callosum | 12 | Atlas (posterior arch) with vertebral artery | 21 | Basilar artery |
| 4 | Septum pellucidum | 13 | Calvaria | 22 | Internal carotid artery |
| 5 | Optic chiasma | 14 | Sinus sagittalis superior | 23 | Maxillary artery |
| 6 | Posterior cerebral artery | 15 | Right and left anterior cerebral artery | 24 | Hypoglossal nerve (n. XII) |
| 7 | Tentorium of cerebellum | 16 | Frontal lobe of the brain | 25 | Vertebral artery |
| 8 | Internal acoustic meatus | 17 | Anterior communicating artery | 26 | Common carotid artery |
| 9 | Sinus sigmoideus | 18 | Medial cerebral artery and abducent nerve (n. VI) | 27 | Cervical plexus |

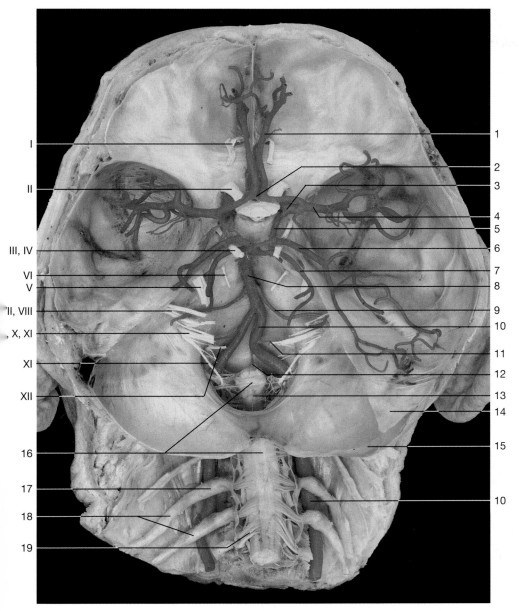

1   Anterior cerebral artery
2   Anterior communicating artery
3   Internal carotid artery
4   Medial cerebral artery
5   Posterior communicating artery
6   Posterior cerebral artery
7   Superior cerebellar artery
8   Basilar artery
9   Anterior inferior cerebellar
    artery with the artery of the
    labyrinth
10  Vertebral artery
11  Posterior inferior cerebellar
    artery
12  Anterior spinal artery
13  Pia mater of spinal cord
14  Tentorium cerebelli
15  Dura mater of the cranial cavity
16  Spinal cord
17  Spinal ganglion
18  Spinal nerves (C$_3$, C$_4$)
19  Posterior root filaments
    (fila radicularia post.)
20  Ophthalmic artery
    (within the orbit)
21  Internal carotid artery
    (within carotid canal)
22  Posterior spinal artery

I     Olfactory tract
II    Optic nerve
III   Oculomotor nerve
IV    Trochlear nerve
V     Trigeminal nerve
VI    Abducent nerve
VII   Facialis nerve
VIII  Vestibulocochlear nerve
IX    Glossopharyngeal nerve
X     Vagus nerve
XI    Accessory nerve
XII   Hypoglossus nerve

**Dissection of the arterial circle of the cerebrum at the base of the skull**
(from above; calvaria and brain have been removed; arteries are colored in red, cranial
nerves [n. I–XII] in yellow).

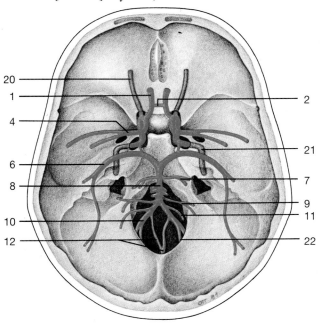

**Arterial circle of Willis** (superior aspect).
(Schematic drawing.)

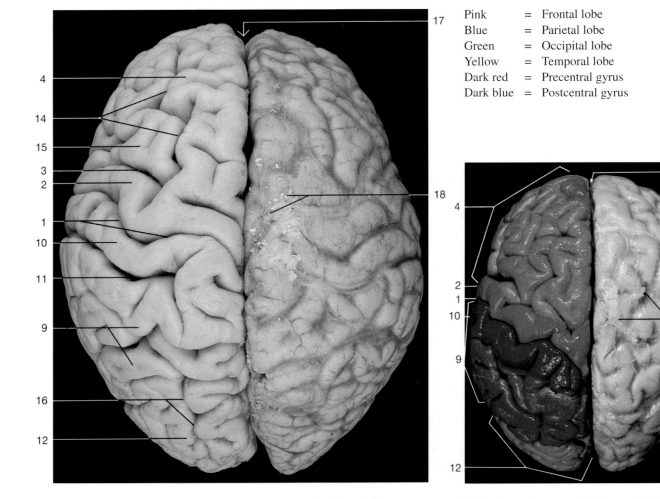

1   Central sulcus
2   Precentral gyrus
3   Precentral sulcus
4   Frontal lobe
5   Anterior ascending ramus of lateral sulcus
6   Anterior horizontal ramus of lateral sulcus
7   Lateral sulcus
8   Temporal lobe
9   Parietal lobe
10  Postcentral gyrus
11  Postcentral sulcus
12  Occipital lobe
13  Cerebellum
14  Superior frontal sulcus
15  Middle frontal gyrus
16  Lunate sulcus
17  Longitudinal fissure
18  Arachnoid granulations

**Brain, left hemisphere** (lateral aspect). Frontal pole to the left.

| Pink | = | Frontal lobe |
| Blue | = | Parietal lobe |
| Green | = | Occipital lobe |
| Yellow | = | Temporal lobe |
| Dark red | = | Precentral gyrus |
| Dark blue | = | Postcentral gyrus |

**Brain** (superior aspect). Right hemisphere with arachnoid and pia mater.

**Brain** (superior aspect). Lobes of the left hemisphere indicated by color; right hemisphere is covered with arachnoid and pia mater.

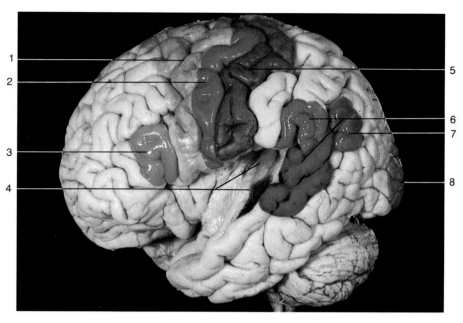

1  Premotor area
2  Somatomotor area
3  Motor speech area of Broca
4  Acoustic area
   (red: high tone, dark green: low tone)
5  Somatosensory area
6  Sensory speech area of Wernicke
7  Reading comprehension area
8  Visuosensory area

**Brain,** left hemisphere (lateral aspect). **Main cortical areas** are colored.
The lateral sulcus has been opened to display the insula and the inner surface of the temporal lobe.

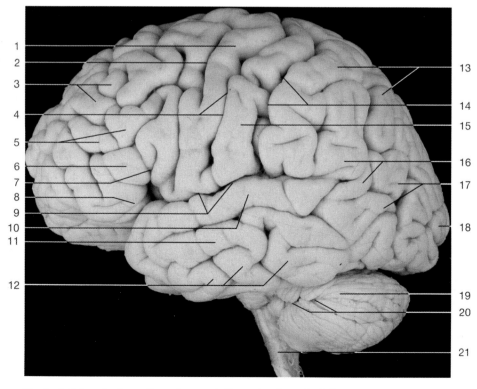

1  Precentral gyrus
2  Precentral sulcus
3  Superior frontal gyrus
4  Central sulcus
5  Middle frontal gyrus
6  Inferior frontal gyrus
7  Ascending ramus ⎫
8  Horizontal ramus ⎬ of lateral
9  Posterior ramus ⎭ sulcus
10 Superior temporal gyrus
11 Middle temporal gyrus
12 Inferior temporal gyrus
13 Parietal lobe
14 Postcentral sulcus
15 Postcentral gyrus
16 Supramarginal gyrus
17 Angular gyrus
18 Occipital lobe
19 Cerebellum
20 Horizontal fissure of cerebellum
21 Medulla oblongata

**Brain, left hemisphere** (lateral aspect). Frontal pole to the left.

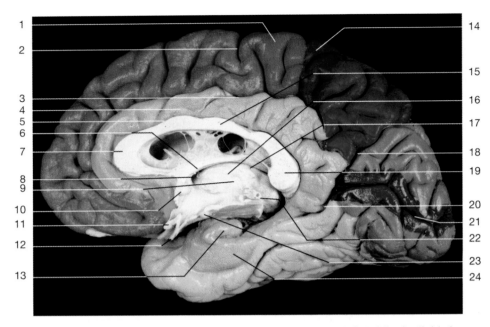

**Brain, right hemisphere** (medial aspect). Frontal pole to the left (midbrain divided, cerebellum and inferior part of brain stem removed).

| | | | | | | |
|---|---|---|---|---|---|---|
| Red | = | Frontal lobe | | Dark blue | = | Postcentral lobe |
| Blue | = | Parietal lobe | | Dark green | = | Calcarine sulcus |
| Green | = | Occipital lobe | | Dark yellow | = | Limbic cortex (cingulate and parahippocampal gyri) |
| Yellow | = | Temporal lobe | | | | |
| Dark red | = | Precentral lobe | | | | |

1  Precentral gyrus
2  Precentral sulcus
3  Cingulate sulcus
4  Cingulate gyrus
5  Sulcus of corpus callosum
6  Fornix
7  Genu of corpus callosum
8  Interventricular foramen
9  Intermediate mass
10 Anterior commissure
11 Optic chiasma
12 Infundibulum
13 Uncus hippocampi
14 Postcentral gyrus
15 Body of corpus callosum
16 Third ventricle and thalamus
17 Stria medullaris
18 Parieto-occipital sulcus
19 Splenium of corpus callosum
20 Communication of calcarine and parieto-occipital sulcus
21 Calcarine sulcus
22 Pineal body
23 Mamillary body
24 Parahippocampal gyrus
25 Olfactory bulb
26 Olfactory tract
27 Gyrus rectus
28 Optic nerve
29 Infundibulum and optic chiasma
30 Optic tract
31 Oculomotor nerve
32 Pedunculus cerebri
33 Red nucleus
34 Cerebral aqueduct
35 Corpus callosum
36 Longitudinal fissure
37 Orbital gyri
38 Lateral root of olfactory tract
39 Medial root of olfactory tract
40 Olfactory tubercle and anterior perforated substance
41 Tuber cinereum
42 Interpeduncular fossa
43 Substantia nigra
44 Colliculi of the midbrain
45 Lateral occipitotemporal gyrus
46 Medial occipitotemporal gyrus

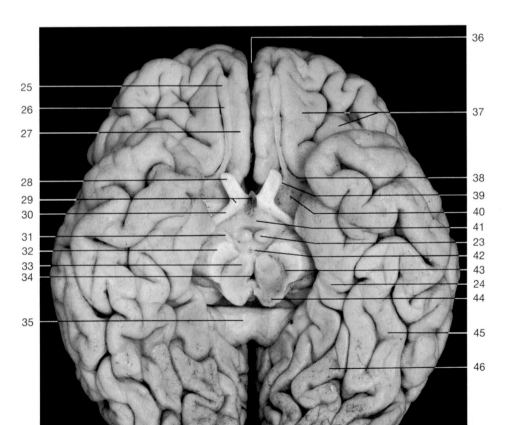

**Brain** (inferior aspect). Midbrain divided. Cerebellum and inferior part of brain stem removed. Frontal pole at the top.

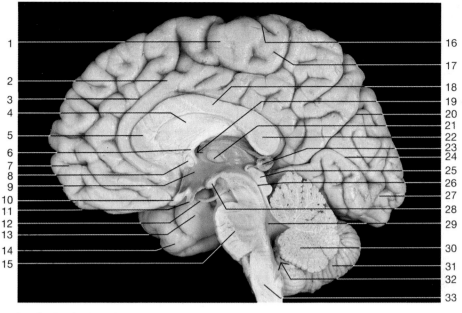

**Brain** (sagittal section). Frontal pole to the left.

1  Precentral gyrus
2  Cingulate gyrus
3  Cingulate sulcus
4  Septum pellucidum
5  Genu of corpus callosum
6  Fornix
7  Frontal lobe
8  Anterior commissure
9  Hypothalamus
10  Optic chiasma
11  Infundibulum
12  Oculomotor nerve
13  Uncus
14  Temporal lobe
15  Pons
16  Central sulcus
17  Postcentral gyrus
18  Body of corpus callosum
19  Interventricular foramen (arrow)
20  Parieto-occipital sulcus
21  Intermediate mass
22  Splenium of corpus callosum
23  Pineal body
24  Calcarine sulcus
25  Colliculi of midbrain
26  Cerebral aqueduct
27  Occipital lobe
28  Mamillary body
29  Fourth ventricle
30  Vermis of cerebellum
31  Right hemisphere of cerebellum
32  Median aperture of Magendie (arrow)
33  Medulla oblongata
34  Olfactory tract
35  Optic nerve
36  Internal carotid artery
37  Interpeduncular cistern
38  Superior cerebellar artery
39  Anterior inferior cerebellar artery
40  Vertebral artery
41  Posterior inferior cerebellar artery
42  Basilar artery
43  Trigeminal nerve (n. V)
44  Facial nerve (n. VII)
45  Accessory nerve (n. XI) and
    hypoglossal nerve (n. XII)
46  Cerebellum

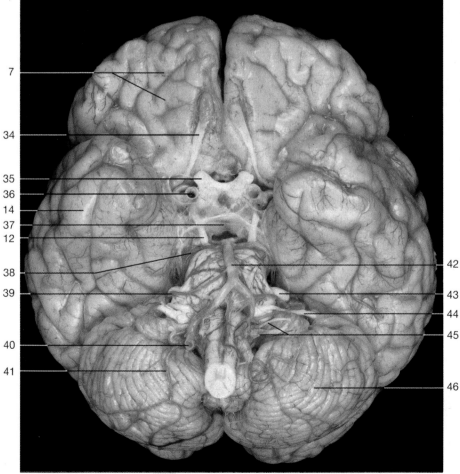

**Brain, with pia mater and blood vessels** (inferior aspect).

1  Superior cerebellar peduncle
2  Middle cerebellar peduncle
3  Cerebellar tonsil
4  Inferior semilunar lobule
5  Vermis
6  Central lobule of vermis
7  Inferior cerebellar peduncle
8  Superior medullary velum
9  Nodule of vermis
10  Flocculus
11  Biventral lobule
12  Left cerebellar hemisphere
13  Inferior semilunar lobule
14  Biventral lobule
15  Vermis of cerebellum
16  Tuber of vermis
17  Pyramid of vermis
18  Uvula of vermis
19  Tonsil of cerebellum
20  Floccule of cerebellum
21  Right cerebellar hemisphere
22  Vermis (central lobule)
23  Cerebellar lingula
24  Ala of central lobule
25  Superior cerebellar peduncle
26  Fastigium
27  Fourth ventricle
28  Middle cerebellar peduncle
29  Nodule of vermis
30  Flocculus of cerebellum
31  Cerebellar tonsil
32  Culmen of vermis
33  Declive of vermis
34  Tuber of vermis
35  Inferior semilunar lobule
36  Pyramid of vermis (cut)
37  Uvula of vermis

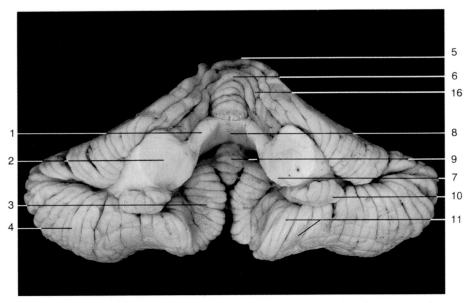

**Cerebellum** (inferior anterior aspect). The cerebellar peduncles have been severed.

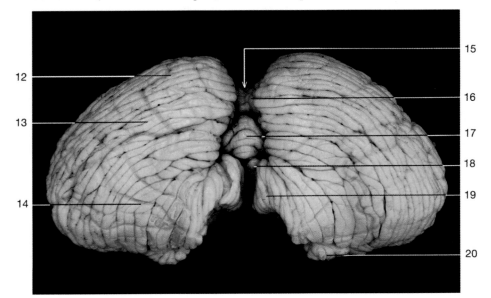

**Cerebellum** (inferior posterior aspect).

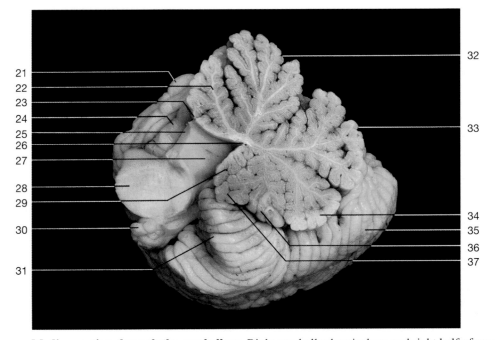

**Median section through the cerebellum.** Right cerebellar hemisphere and right half of vermis.

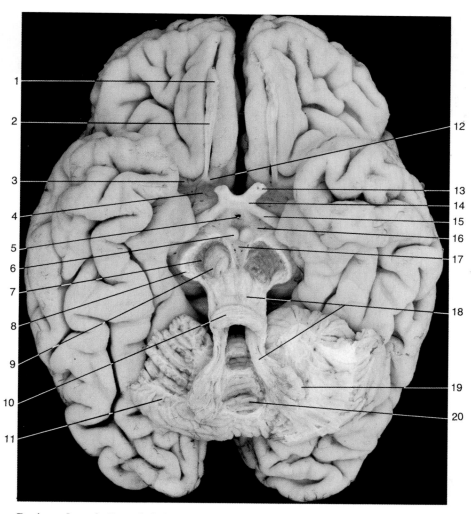

1  Olfactory bulb
2  Olfactory tract
3  Lateral olfactory stria
4  Anterior perforated substance
5  Infundibulum (divided)
6  Mamillary body
7  Substantia nigra
8  Pedunculus cerebri (cut)
9  Red nucleus
10  Decussation of superior cerebellar peduncle
11  Cerebellar hemisphere
12  Medial olfactory stria
13  Optic nerve
14  Optic chiasma
15  Optic tract
16  Posterior perforated substance
17  Interpeduncular fossa
18  Superior cerebellar peduncle and cerebellorubral tract
19  Dentate nucleus
20  Vermis of cerebellum
21  Cingulate gyrus
22  Corpus callosum
23  Stria terminalis
24  Septum pellucidum
25  Columna fornicis
26  Cerebral peduncle at midbrain level
27  Pons
28  Inferior olive
29  Medulla oblongata with lateral pyramidal tract
30  Occipital lobe
31  Calcarine sulcus
32  Thalamus
33  Inferior colliculus with brachium
34  Medial lemniscus
35  Superior cerebellar peduncle
36  Inferior cerebellar peduncle
37  Middle cerebellar peduncle
38  Cerebellar hemisphere

**Brain and cerebellum** (inferior aspect). Parts of the cerebellum have been removed to display the dentate nucleus and the main pathway to the midbrain (cerebellorubral tract).

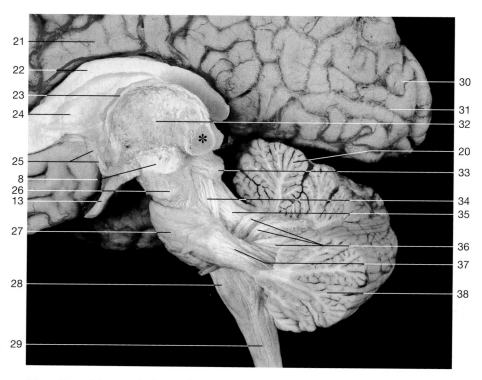

**Dissection of the cerebellar peduncles and their connection with midbrain and diencephalon.** A small part of pulvinar thalami (∗) has been cut to show inferior brachium.

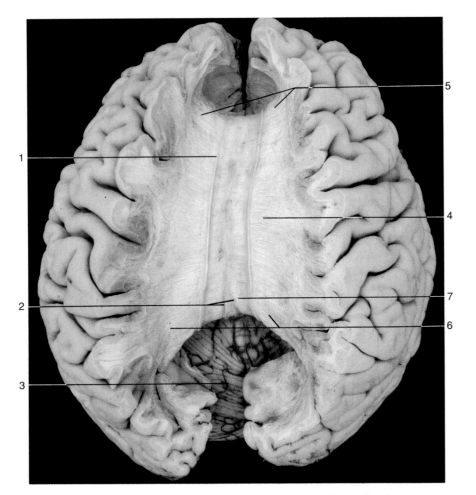

1  Lateral longitudinal stria
   of indusium griseum
2  Medial longitudinal stria
   of indusium griseum
3  Cerebellum
4  Radiating fibers of the corpus callosum
5  Forceps minor of corpus callosum
6  Forceps major of corpus callosum
7  Splenium of corpus callosum

**Dissection of the brain I.** The fiber system of the corpus callosum has been displayed by removing the cortex lying above it. Frontal pole at the top.

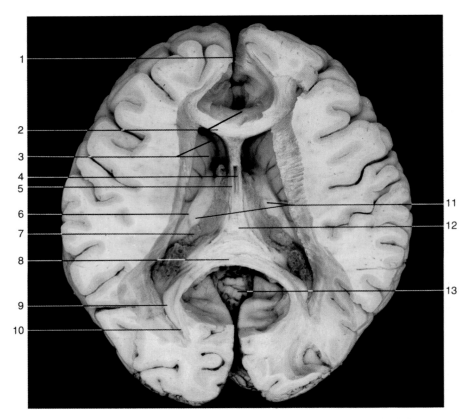

1  Longitudinal cerebral fissure
2  Genu of corpus callosum
3  Head of caudate nucleus and
   anterior horn of lateral ventricle
4  Cavum of septum pellucidum
5  Septum pellucidum
6  Stria terminalis
7  Choroid plexus of lateral ventricle
8  Splenium of corpus callosum
9  Calcar avis
10 Posterior horn of lateral ventricle
11 Thalamus (lamina affixa)
12 Commissure of fornix
13 Vermis of cerebellum

**Dissection of the brain II.** The lateral ventricles and subcortical nuclei of the brain are dissected. The corpus callosum has been partly removed. Frontal pole at the top.

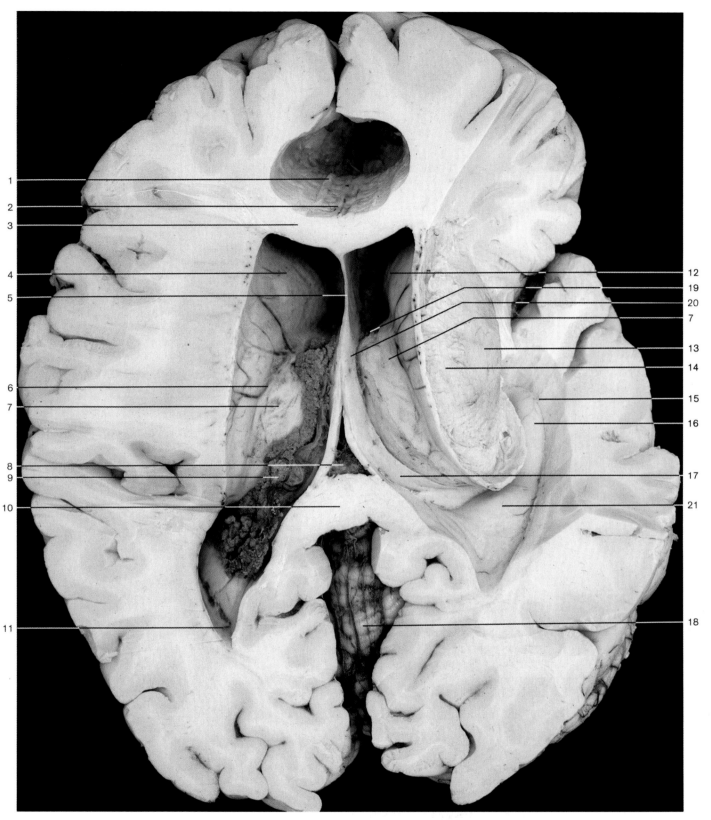

**Dissection of the brain III** (superior view of lateral ventricle and subcortical nuclei of the brain). Corpus callosum partly removed. At right, the entire lateral ventricle has been opened, the insula with claustrum and the extreme and external capsules have been removed, exposing the lentiform nucleus and the internal capsule.

| | | | |
|---|---|---|---|
| 1 | Lateral longitudinal stria | 9 | Choroid plexus of lateral ventricle |
| 2 | Medial longitudinal stria | 10 | Splenium of corpus callosum |
| 3 | Genu of corpus callosum | 11 | Posterior horn of lateral ventricle |
| 4 | Head of caudate nucleus | 12 | Anterior horn of lateral ventricle |
| 5 | Septum pellucidum | | (head of caudate nucleus) |
| 6 | Stria terminalis | 13 | Putamen of lentiform nucleus |
| 7 | Thalamus (lamina affixa) | 14 | Internal capsule |
| 8 | Choroid plexus of third ventricle | 15 | Inferior horn of lateral ventricle |

| | |
|---|---|
| 16 | Pes hippocampi |
| 17 | Crus of fornix |
| 18 | Vermis of cerebellum with arachnoid and pia mater |
| 19 | Interventricular foramen |
| 20 | Right column of fornix |
| 21 | Collateral eminence |

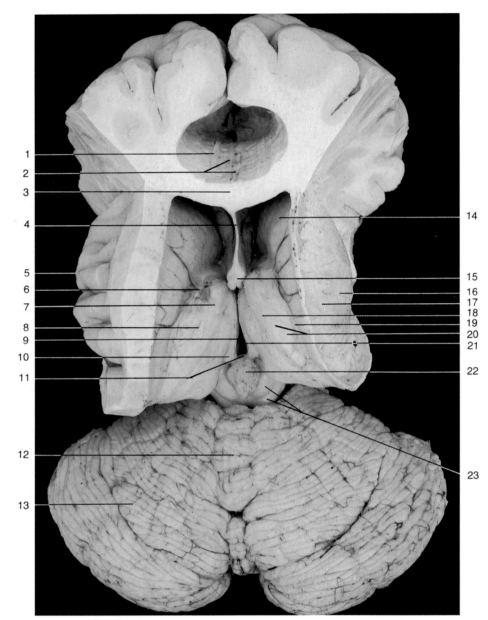

1  Lateral longitudinal stria
2  Medial longitudinal stria
3  Corpus callosum
4  Septum pellucidum
5  Insular gyri
6  Thalamostriate vein
7  Anterior tubercle of thalamus
8  Thalamus
9  Stria medullaris of thalamus
10 Habenular trigone
11 Habenular commissure
12 Vermis of cerebellum
13 Left hemisphere of cerebellum
14 Head of caudate nucleus
15 Columns of fornix
16 Putamen of lentiform nucleus
17 Internal capsule
18 Taenia of choroid plexus
19 Stria terminalis and thalamostriate
   vein
20 Lamina affixa
21 Third ventricle
22 Pineal body
23 Superior and inferior colliculus
   of midbrain

**Dissection of the brain IVa.** Temporal lobe, fornix, and the posterior corpus callosum have been removed (this part of the specimen is depicted below). Frontal pole at top (superior aspect).

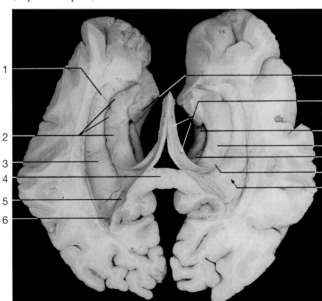

1  Inferior horn of lateral ventricle
2  Hippocampal digitations
3  Collateral eminence
4  Splenium of corpus callosum
5  Calcar avis
6  Posterior horn of lateral ventricle
7  Uncus of parahippocampal gyrus
8  Body and crus of fornix
9  Parahippocampal gyrus
10 Pes hippocampi
11 Dentate gyrus
12 Hippocampal fimbria
13 Lateral ventricle

**Dissection of the brain IVb.** Depicted is the portion of the brain removed from the specimen above. **Temporal lobe and limbic system** (superior aspect). Columns of fornix are cut.

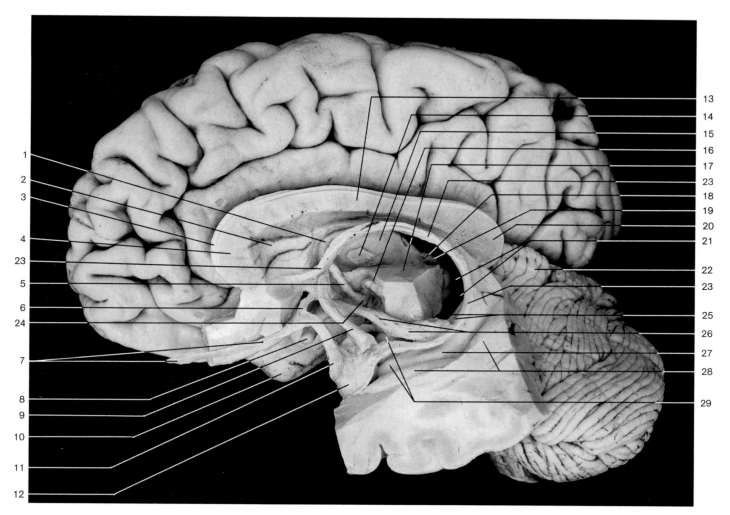

**Dissection of the limbic system.** Left side, lateral aspect. Corpus callosum has been cut in the median plane. The left thalamus and the left hemisphere have been partly removed.

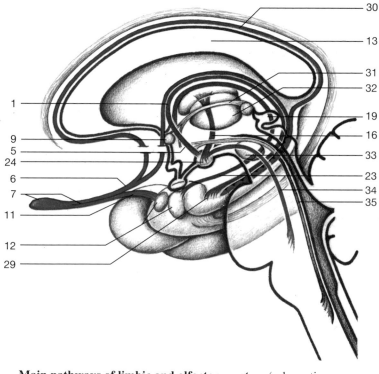

| | | | |
|---|---|---|---|
| 1 | Body of fornix | 20 | Splenium of corpus |
| 2 | Septum pellucidum | | callosum |
| 3 | Lateral longitudinal stria | 21 | Colliculi of midbrain |
| 4 | Genu of corpus callosum | 22 | Vermis of cerebellum |
| 5 | Column of fornix | 23 | Stria terminalis |
| 6 | Medial olfactory stria | 24 | Mamillary body |
| 7 | Olfactory bulb and | 25 | Fimbria of hippocampus |
| | olfactory tract | | and pes hippocampi |
| 8 | Optic nerve | 26 | Left optic tract and |
| 9 | Anterior commissure | | lateral geniculate body |
| | (left half) | 27 | Lateral ventricle and |
| 10 | Right temporal lobe | | parahippocampal gyrus |
| 11 | Lateral olfactory stria | 28 | Collateral eminence |
| 12 | Amygdala | 29 | Hippocampal digitations |
| 13 | Body of corpus callosum | 30 | Supracallosal gyrus |
| 14 | Interthalamic adhesion | | (longitudinal stria) |
| 15 | Third ventricle and right | 31 | Stria medullaris of |
| | thalamus | | thalamus |
| 16 | Mamillothalamic fasciculus | 32 | Thalamus |
| 17 | Part of the thalamus | 33 | Red nucleus |
| 18 | Habenular commissure | 34 | Mamillotegmental |
| 19 | Pineal body | | fasciculus |
| | | 35 | Dorsal longitudinal |
| | | | fasciculus (Schütz) |

**Main pathways of limbic and olfactory system** (schematic drawing). Blue = afferent pathways; red = efferent pathways.

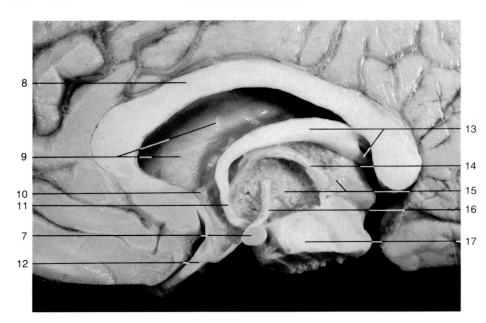

1 Paraventricular nucleus ⎫
2 Pre-optic nucleus            ⎪
3 Ventromedial nucleus    ⎬ Hypothalamic
4 Supra-optic nucleus       ⎪ nuclei
5 Posterior nucleus          ⎪
6 Dorsomedial nucleus    ⎭
7 Mamillary body
8 Corpus callosum
9 Lateral ventricle (showing caudate nucleus)
10 Anterior commissure
11 Column of fornix
12 Optic chiasma
13 Crus of fornix
14 Stria medullaris of thalamus
15 Thalamus and interthalamic adhesion
16 Mamillothalamic fasciculus of Vicq d'Azyr
17 Cerebral peduncle
18 Pineal body
19 Tectum of midbrain
20 Lamina terminalis

**Median section through the diencephalon.** Medial part of the thalamus and septum pellucidum have been removed to show the fornix and mamillothalamic fasciculus.

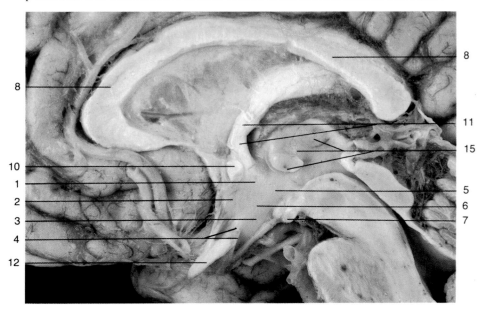

**Median section through the diencephalon and midbrain; location of hypothalamic nuclei.**

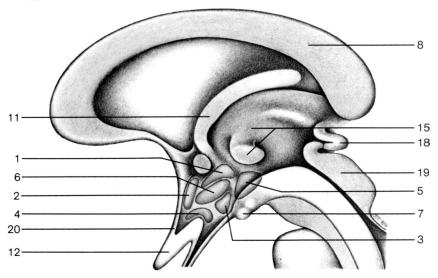

**Position of main hypothalamic nuclei** (schematic diagram).

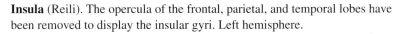

1  Circular sulcus of insula
2  Long gyrus of insula
3  Short gyri of insula
4  Limen insulae
5  Opercula (cut)
   a  Frontal operculum
   b  Frontoparietal operculum
   c  Temporal operculum
6  Corona radiata
7  Lentiform nucleus
8  Anterior commissure
9  Olfactory tract
10  Cerebral arcuate fibers
11  Optic radiation
12  Cerebral peduncle
13  Trigeminal nerve (n. V)
14  Flocculus of cerebellum
15  Pyramidal tract
16  Decussation of pyramidal tract
17  Internal capsule
18  Optic tract
19  Optic nerve (n. II)
20  Infundibulum
21  Temporal lobe (right side)
22  Mamillary bodies
23  Oculomotor nerve (n. III)
24  Transverse fibers of pons

**Insula** (Reili). The opercula of the frontal, parietal, and temporal lobes have been removed to display the insular gyri. Left hemisphere.

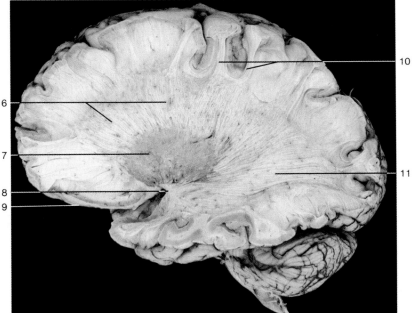

**Dissection of the corona radiata,** left hemisphere. Frontal pole on the left.

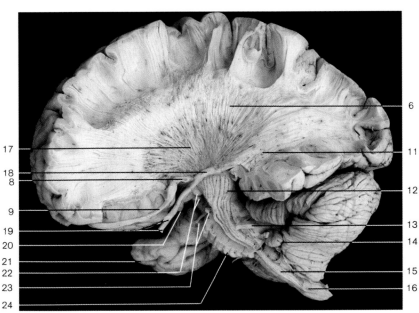

◁ **Corona radiata and internal capsule,** left hemisphere. Lentiform nucleus removed (frontal pole to the left).

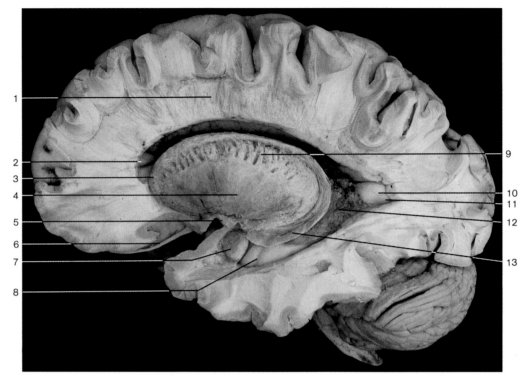

1   Corona radiata
2   Anterior horn of lateral ventricle
3   Head of caudate nucleus
4   Putamen
5   Anterior commissure
6   Olfactory tract
7   Amygdala
8   Hippocampal digitations
9   Internal capsule
10  Calcar avis
11  Posterior horn of lateral ventricle
12  Choroid plexus of lateral ventricle
13  Caudal extremity of caudate nucleus
14  Thalamus
15  Cerebral arcuate fibers
16  Globus pallidus (remnants)

**Dissection of the subcortical nuclei and internal capsule,** left hemisphere (lateral aspect). Frontal pole to the left. The lateral ventricle has been opened, and the insular gyri and claustrum have been removed, revealing the lentiform nucleus and the internal capsule.

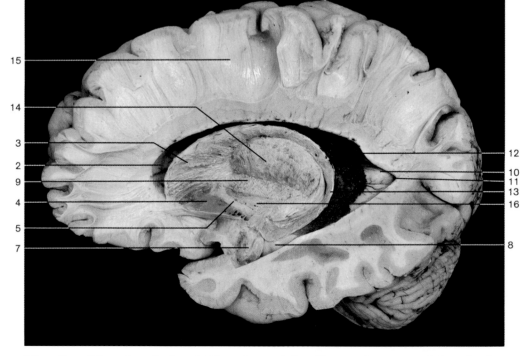

**Dissection of the subcortical nuclei** (lateral aspect). Lentiform nucleus removed, frontal pole to the left.

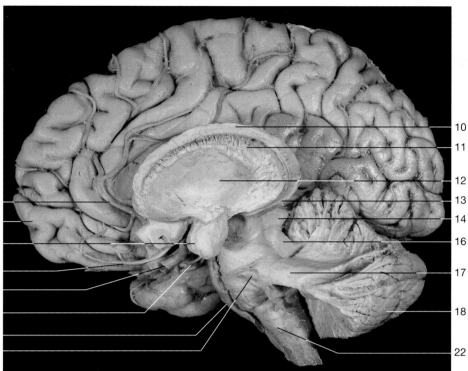

| | |
|---|---|
| 1 | Anterior cerebral artery |
| 2 | Frontal lobe |
| 3 | Amygdala (amygdaloid body) |
| 4 | Olfactory tract |
| 5 | Internal carotid artery |
| 6 | Oculomotor nerve (n. III) |
| 7 | Basilar artery |
| 8 | Trigeminal nerve (n. V) |
| 9 | Hypoglossal nerve (n. XII) |
| 10 | Caudate nucleus |
| 11 | Internal capsule |
| 12 | Lentiform nucleus |
| 13 | Caudal extremity of caudate nucleus |
| 14 | Inferior colliculus of midbrain |
| 15 | Trochlear nerve (n. IV) |
| 16 | Superior cerebellar peduncle |
| 17 | Middle cerebellar peduncle |
| 18 | Cerebellum |
| 19 | Facial nerve (n. VII) and vestibulocochlear nerve (n. VIII) |
| 20 | Abducent nerve (n. VI) |
| 21 | Glossopharyngeal nerve (n. IX), vagus nerve (n. X), and accessory nerve (n. XI) |
| 22 | Inferior olive |

**Right hemisphere together with brain stem and cerebellum.**
The connections of the brain stem with the cerebellum are dissected. The amygdala of the left hemisphere is shown. The corpus callosum has been partly removed.

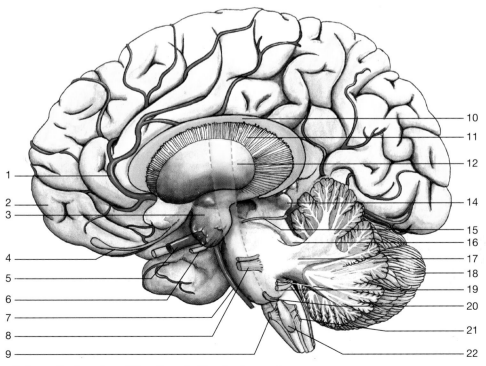

**Schematic drawing of the dissected brain** shown above.
The course of the pyramidal tracts is indicated in red. Cranial nerves yellow.

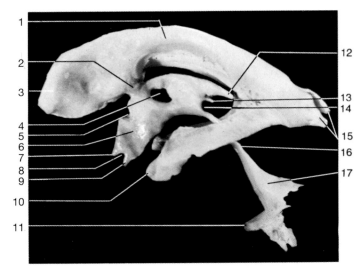

**Cast of ventricular cavities of the brain** (lateral aspect), frontal pole to the left.

1  Central part of the lateral ventricle
2  Interventricular foramen of Monro
3  Anterior horn of the lateral ventricle
4  Site of interthalamic adhesion
5  Notch for anterior commissure
6  Third ventricle
7  Optic recess
8  Notch for optic chiasma
9  Infundibular recess
10  Inferior horn of lateral ventricle with indentation of amygdaloid body
11  Lateral recess and lateral aperture of Luschka
12  Suprapineal recess
13  Pineal recess
14  Notch for posterior commissure
15  Posterior horn of lateral ventricle
16  Cerebral aqueduct

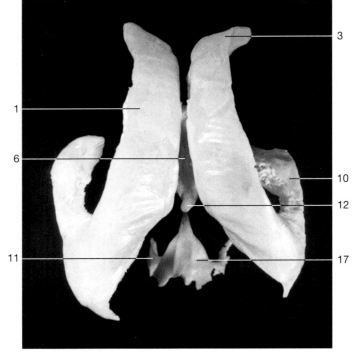

**Cast of ventricular cavities of the brain** (superior aspect, frontal pole at top).

17  Fourth ventricle
18  Median aperture of Magendie
19  Cerebellomedullary cistern
20  Superior sagittal sinus
21  Inferior sagittal sinus
22  Intervaginal space of optic nerve
23  Arachnoid granulations of Pacchioni
24  Straight sinus

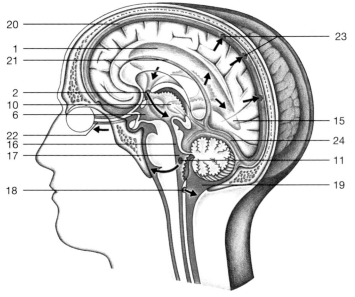

**Position of ventricular cavities** (schematic drawing).
The direction of flow of cerebrospinal fluid is indicated by arrows.
Green = right lateral ventricle; red = choroidal plexus.

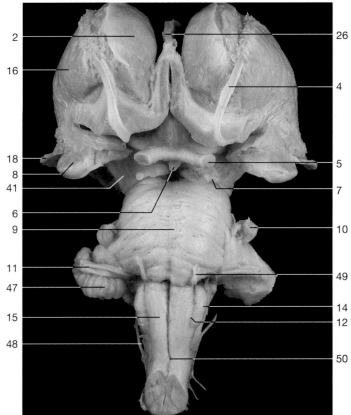

**Brain stem** (ventral aspect). (Numbers see p. 115)

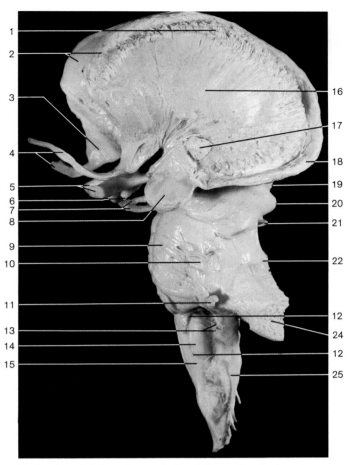

**Brain stem** (left lateral aspect). Cerebellar peduncles have been severed, cerebellum and cerebral cortex have been removed.

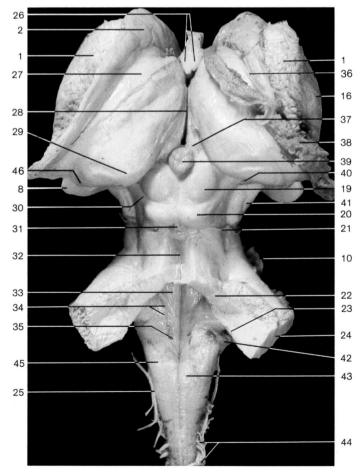

**Brain stem** (dorsal aspect). Cerebellum removed.

1  Internal capsule
2  Head of the caudate nucleus
3  Olfactory trigone
4  Olfactory tracts
5  Optic nerves
6  Infundibulum
7  Oculomotor nerve
8  Amygdaloid body
9  Pons
10  Trigeminal nerve
11  Facial and vestibulocochlear nerves
12  Hypoglossal nerve
13  Glossopharyngeal and vagus nerves
14  Olive (Oliva inf.)
15  Medulla oblongata
16  Lentiform nucleus
17  Anterior commissure
18  Tail of caudate nucleus
19  Superior colliculus
20  Inferior colliculus
21  Trochlear nerve
22  Superior cerebellar peduncle
23  Inferior cerebellar peduncle
24  Middle cerebellar peduncle
25  Accessory nerve (n. XI)
26  Columns of fornix (divided)
27  Lamina affixa
28  Third ventricle
29  Pulvinar of thalamus
30  Inferior brachium
31  Frenulum veli
32  Superior medullary velum
33  Facial colliculus
34  Striae medullares and rhomboid fossa
35  Hypoglossal triangle
36  Stria terminalis and thalamostriate vein
37  Habenular trigone
38  Choroid plexus of lateral ventricle
39  Pineal body
40  Medial geniculate body
41  Cerebral peduncle
42  Choroid plexus of fourth ventricle
43  Clava
44  Dorsal root of cervical nerve
45  Cuneate tubercle
46  Lateral geniculate body
47  Flocculus
48  Accessory nerve (n. XI)
49  Abducent nerve (n. VI)
50  Decussation of the pyramids

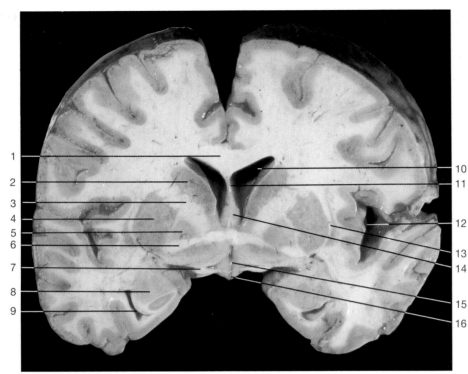

**Coronal section through the brain** at the level of the anterior commissure. Section 1.

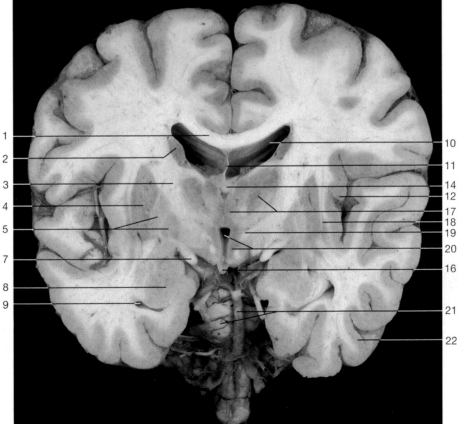

**Coronal section through the brain** at the level of the third ventricle and the interthalamic adhesion. Section 2.

1 Corpus callosum
2 Head of caudate nucleus
3 Internal capsule
4 Putamen
5 Globus pallidus
6 Anterior commissure
7 Optic tract
8 Amygdaloid body
9 Inferior horn of lateral ventricle
10 Lateral ventricle
11 Septum pellucidum
12 Lobus insularis (insula)
13 External capsule
14 Column of fornix
15 Optic recess
16 Infundibulum
17 Thalamus
18 Claustrum
19 Lenticular ansa
20 Third ventricle and hypothalamus
21 Basilar artery and pons
22 Cortex of temporal lobe
23 Inferior colliculus
24 Superior colliculus
25 Cerebral aqueduct
26 Red nucleus
27 Substantia nigra
28 Cerebral peduncle
29 Trochlear nerve (n. IV)
30 Gray matter
31 Nucleus of oculomotor nerve
32 Fibers of oculomotor nerve (n. III)
33 Vermis of cerebellum
34 Fourth ventricle
35 Reticular formation
36 Pons and transverse pontine fibers
37 Emboliform nucleus
38 Dentate nucleus
39 Middle cerebellar peduncle
40 Choroid plexus
41 Hypoglossal nucleus at rhomboid fossa
42 Medial longitudinal fasciculus
43 Trigeminal nerve (n. V.)
44 Inferior olivary nucleus
45 Corticospinal fibers and arcuate fibers
46 Fourth ventricle with choroid plexus
47 Vestibular nuclei
48 Nucleus and tractus solitarius
49 Inferior cerebellar peduncle (restiform body)
50 Reticular formation
51 Medial lemniscus
52 Cuneate nucleus of Burdach
53 Central canal
54 Pyramidal tract
55 Flocculus of cerebellum
56 Cerebellar hemisphere with pia mater
57 "Arbor vitae" of cerebellum
58 Nucleus gracilis of Goll
59 Lateral recess of choroid plexus of fourth ventricle
60 Posterior inferior cerebellar artery
61 Choroid plexus of lateral ventricle

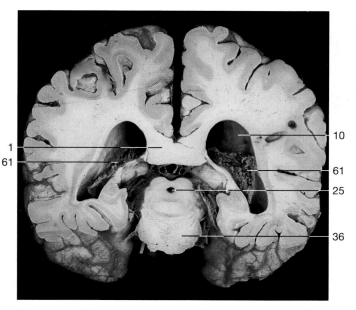

**Coronal section** at the level of **inferior colliculus** (posterior aspect). Section 3.

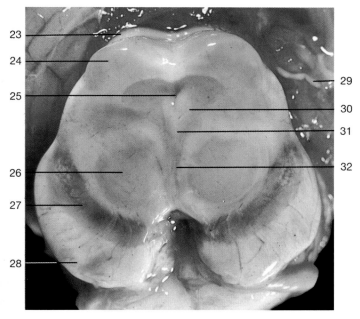

**Cross section of the midbrain** (mesencephalon) at the level of the superior colliculus (superior aspect). Section 4.

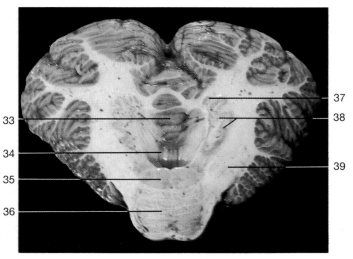

**Cross section through the rhombencephalon** at the level of pons (inferior aspect). Section 5.

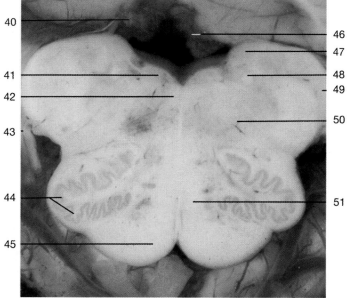

**Cross section of the rhombencephalon** at the level of the olive (inferior aspect). Section 6.

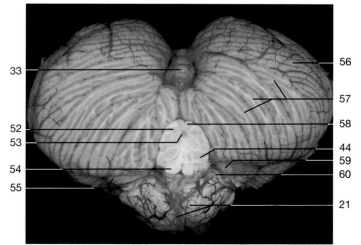

**Cross section through medulla oblongata and cerebellum** (inferior aspect). Section 7.

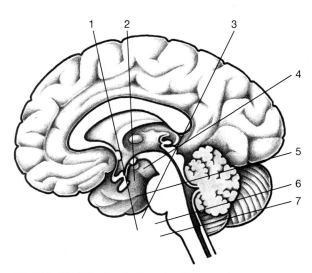

**Right half of the brain.** Levels of the sections are indicated.

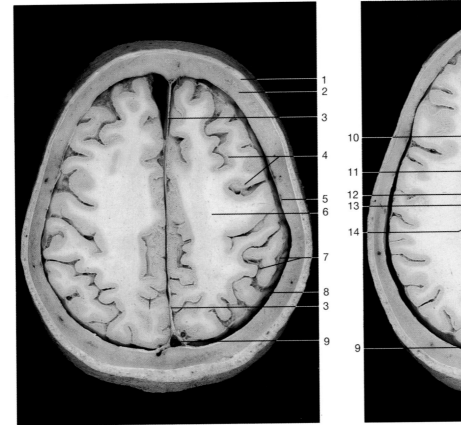

**Horizontal section through the head.**
Section 1.

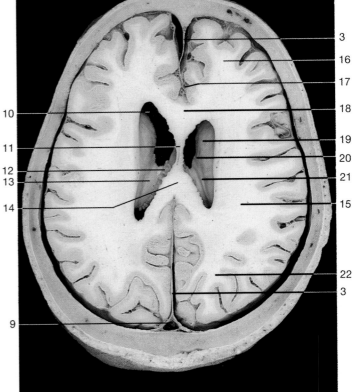

**Horizontal section through the head.**
Section 2.

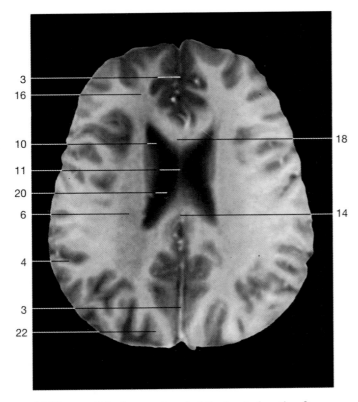

**MRI scan of the human head** at the level of section 2.

1   Skin of scalp
2   Calvaria (diploe of the skull)
3   Falx cerebri
4   Gray matter of brain (cortex)
5   Dura mater
6   White matter of brain
7   Arachnoid and pia mater with vessels
8   Subdural space (slightly expanded due to
    shrinkage of the brain)
9   Superior sagittal sinus
10  Anterior horn of lateral ventricle
11  Septum pellucidum
12  Choroid plexus
13  Thalamus
14  Splenium of corpus callosum
15  Parietal lobe
16  Frontal lobe
17  Anterior cerebral artery
18  Genu of corpus callosum
19  Caudate nucleus
20  Central part of lateral ventricle
21  Stria terminalis
22  Occipital lobe

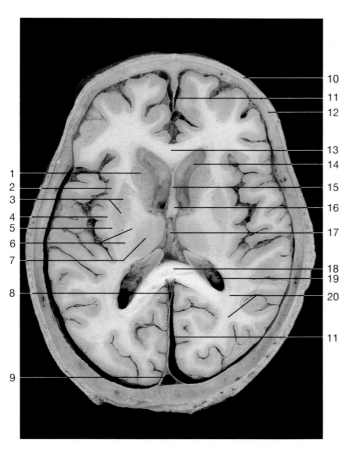

1  Caudate nucleus
2  Lobus insularis (insula)
3  Lentiform nucleus
4  Claustrum
5  External capsule
6  Internal capsule
7  Thalamus
8  Inferior sagittal sinus
9  Superior sagittal sinus
10  Skin of scalp
11  Falx cerebri
12  Calvaria (diploe of skull)
13  Genu of corpus callosum
14  Anterior horn of lateral ventricle
15  Septum pellucidum
16  Column of fornix
17  Choroid plexus of third ventricle
18  Splenium of corpus callosum
19  Entrance to inferior horn of lateral ventricle with choroid plexus
20  Optic radiation
21  Third ventricle

**Horizontal section through the head at the level of third ventricle** of internal capsule and neighboring nuclei. Section 3.

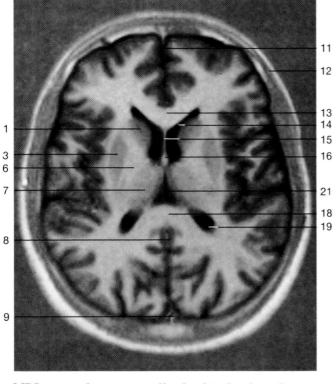

**MRI scan at the corresponding level to the above figure.** Section 3.

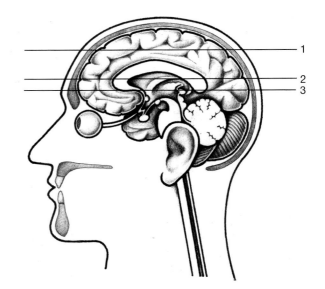

**Sagittal sections through the head.** Levels of the horizontal sections are indicated.

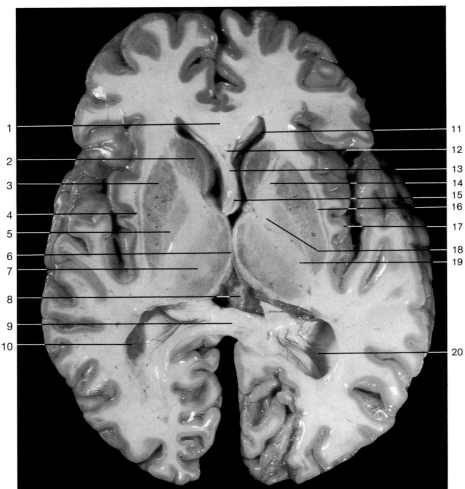

1   Genu of corpus callosum
2   Head of caudate nucleus
3   Putamen
4   Claustrum
5   Globus pallidus
6   Third ventricle
7   Thalamus
8   Pineal body
9   Splenium of corpus callosum
10  Choroid plexus of the lateral
    ventricle
11  Anterior horn of lateral ventricle
12  Cavity of septum pellucidum
13  Septum pellucidum
14  Anterior limb of internal capsule
15  Column of fornix
16  External capsule
17  Lobus insularis (insula)
18  Genu of internal capsule
19  Posterior limb of internal capsule
20  Posterior horn of lateral ventricle
21  Anterior commissure
22  Optic radiation
23  Falx cerebri
24  Maxillary sinus
25  Position of auditory tube
26  Tympanic cavity
27  External acoustic meatus
28  Medulla oblongata
29  Fourth ventricle
30  Cerebellum (left hemisphere)
31  Temporomandibular joint
32  Tympanic membrane
33  Base of cochlea
34  Mastoid air cells
35  Sigmoid sinus
36  Vermis of cerebellum
37  Intermediate mass

**Horizontal section through the brain,** showing the subcortical nuclei and internal capsule. Section 1.

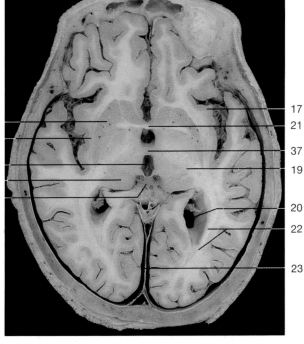

**Horizontal section through the head.** Section 2.

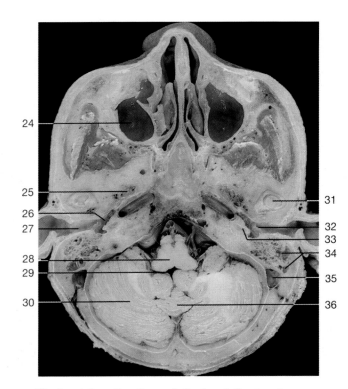

**Horizontal section through the head.** Section 4.

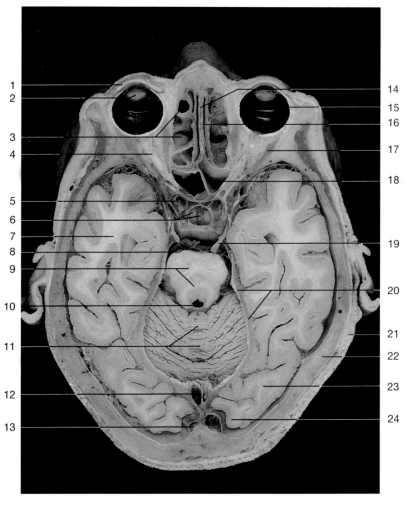

1   Upper lid (tarsal plate)
2   Lens
3   Ethmoidal sinus
4   Optic nerve (n. II)
5   Internal carotid artery
6   Infundibulum and pituitary gland
7   Temporal lobe
8   Basilar artery
9   Pons (cross section of brain stem)
10  Cerebral aqueduct (beginning of fourth ventricle)
11  Vermis of cerebellum
12  Straight sinus
13  Transverse sinus
14  Nasal septum
15  Eyeball (sclera)
16  Nasal cavity
17  Lateral rectus muscle
18  Sphenoidal sinus
19  Oculomotor nerve (n. III)
20  Tentorium of cerebellum
21  Skin of scalp
22  Calvaria
23  Occipital lobe
24  Striate cortex (visual cortex)

**Horizontal section through the head.** Section 3.

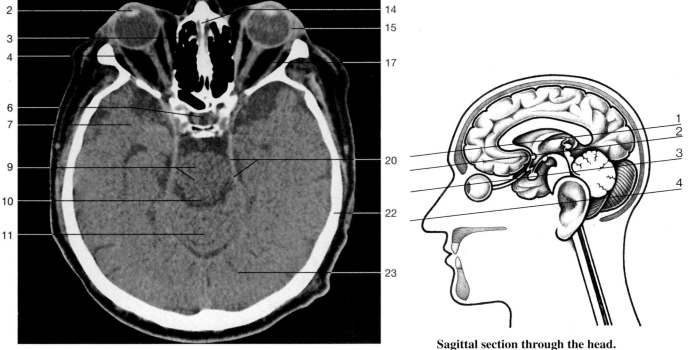

**Horizontal section through the head.** (CT scan.) Section 3.

**Sagittal section through the head.**
Levels of the horizontal sections are indicated.

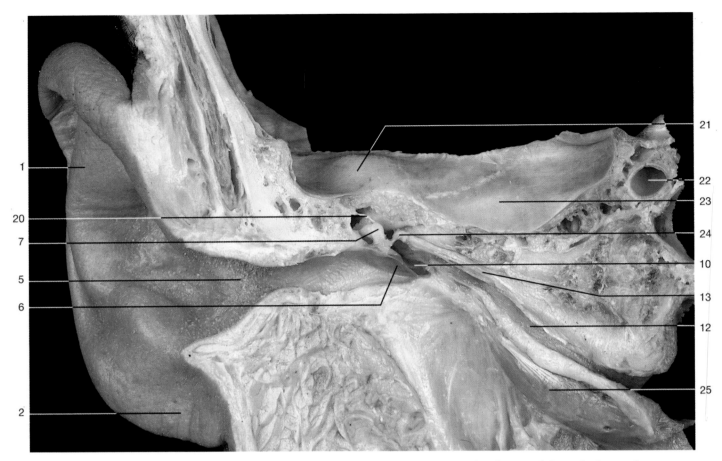

**Longitudinal section through the right temporal bone I.** The outer and middle ear and auditory ossicles and tube are shown (anterior aspect).

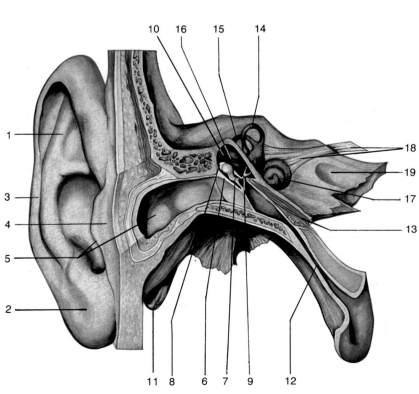

**Right auditory and vestibular apparatus** (anterior aspect).
(Schematic drawing.)

**Outer ear**
1  Auricle
2  Lobule of auricle
3  Helix
4  Tragus
5  External acoustic meatus

**Middle ear**
6  Tympanic membrane
7  Malleus
8  Incus
9  Stapes
10  Tympanic cavity
11  Mastoid process
12  Auditory tube
13  Tensor tympani muscle

**Inner ear**
14  Anterior semicircular duct
15  Posterior semicircular duct
16  Lateral semicircular duct
17  Cochlea
18  Vestibulocochlear nerve
19  Petrous part of the temporal bone

**Additional structures**
20  Superior ligament of malleus
21  Arcuate eminence
22  Internal carotid artery
23  Anterior surface of pyramid with dura mater
24  Stapes
25  Levator veli palatini muscle

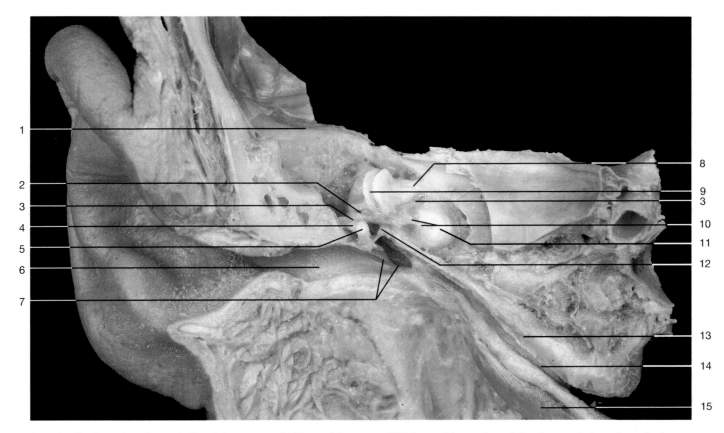

**Longitudinal section through the right outer, middle, and inner ear II.** The cochlea and semicircular canals have been further dissected (anterior aspect).

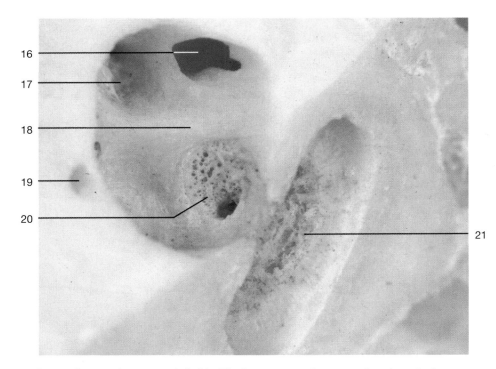

1   Roof of tympanic cavity
2   Lateral osseous semicircular canal
3   Facial nerve
4   Incus
5   Malleus
6   External acoustic meatus
7   Tympanic cavity and tympanic membrane
8   Vestibulocochlear nerve
9   Anterior osseous semicircular canal
10  Geniculate ganglion and greater petrosal nerve
11  Cochlea
12  Stapes
13  Tensor tympani muscle
14  Auditory tube
15  Levator veli palatini muscle
16  Area of facial nerve
17  Superior vestibular area
18  Transverse crest
19  Foramen singulare
20  Foraminous spiral tract (outlet of cochlear part of vestibulocochlear nerve)
21  Base of cochlea

**Internal acoustic meatus,** left side. The bone was partly removed to show the bottom of the meatus.

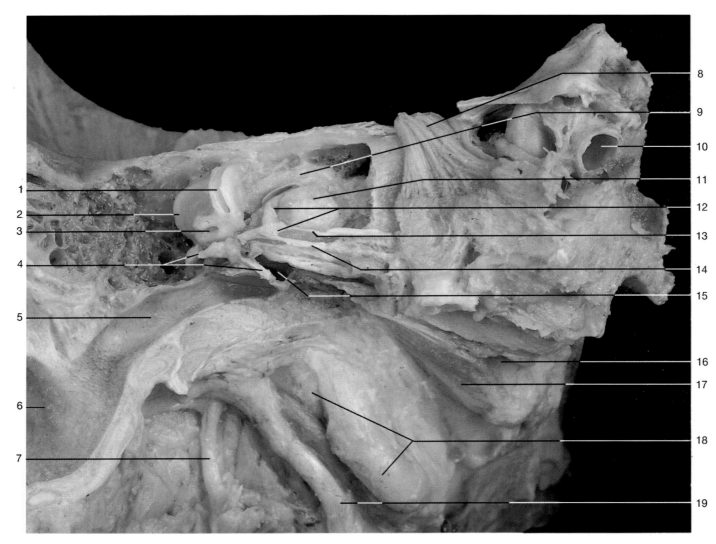

**Longitudinal section through the outer, middle, and inner ear III.** Deeper dissection to display facial nerve and lesser and greater petrosal nerves (anterior aspect).

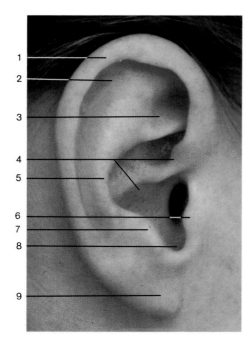

**Right auricle** (lateral aspect).

◁
1  Helix
2  Scaphoid fossa
3  Triangular fossa
4  Concha
5  Antihelix
6  Tragus
7  Antitragus
8  Intertragic notch
9  Lobule

△
1   Anterior osseous semicircular canal (opened)
2   Posterior osseous semicircular canal
3   Lateral osseous semicircular canal (opened)
4   Facial nerve and chorda tympani
5   External acoustic meatus
6   Auricle
7   Facial nerve
8   Trigeminal nerve
9   Bony base of internal acoustic meatus
10  Internal carotid artery within cavernous sinus
11  Cochlea
12  Facial nerve with geniculate ganglion
13  Greater petrosal nerve
14  Lesser petrosal nerve
15  Tympanic cavity
16  Auditory tube
17  Levator veli palatini muscle
18  Internal carotid artery and internal jugular vein
19  Styloid process

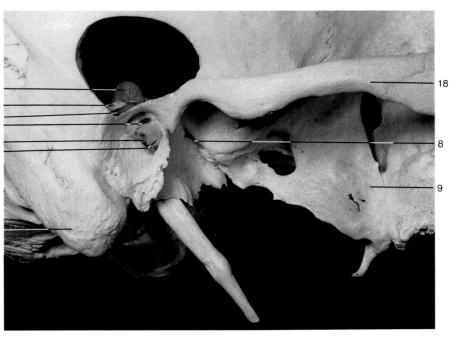

1  Anterior semicircular canal (red)
2  Posterior semicircular canal (yellow)
3  Lateral or horizontal semicircular canal (green)
4  Fenestra vestibuli
5  Fenestra cochleae
6  Tympanic cavity
7  Mastoid process
8  Petrotympanic fissure (red probe: chorda tympani)
9  Lateral pterygoid plate
10  Mastoid air cells
11  Facial canal (blue)
12  Foramen ovale
13  Carotid canal (red)
14  Tympanic ring
15  Petromastoid part of temporal bone
16  Squamous part of temporal bone
17  Squamomastoid suture
18  Zygomatic process of temporal bone
19  Incisure of tympanic ring
20  Promontory
21  Apex of cochlea (cupula)
22  Spiral canal of cochlea at base of cochlea
23  Epitympanic recess
24  Auditory ossicles and tympanic cavity
25  Hypotympanic recess
26  Canaliculus chordae tympani (green probe)
27  Mastoid process
28  Canaliculus for stapedius nerve (red)
29  Cochlea
30  Canaliculus mastoideus (red probe)

**Right temporal bone** (lateral aspect). Petrosquamous portion has been partly removed to display the semicircular canals.

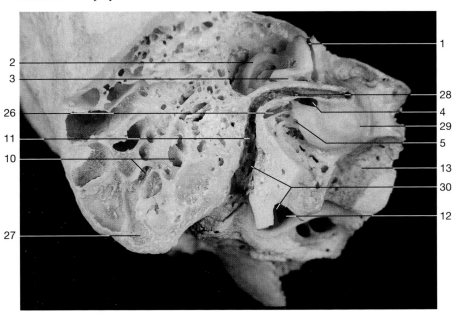

**Right temporal bone** (lateral aspect). Mastoid air cells and facial canal had been opened. The three semicircular canals were dissected.

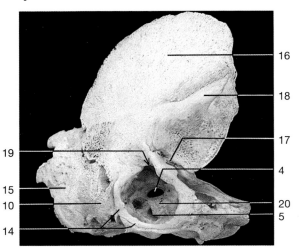

**Right temporal bone of the newborn** (lateral aspect).

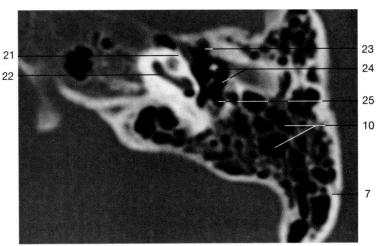

**Frontal section through petrous part.** (CT scan.)

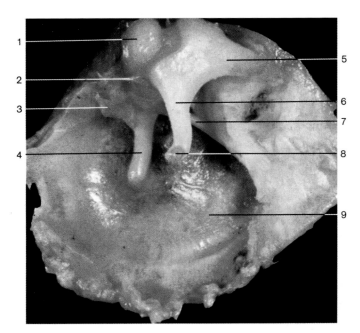

1  Head of malleus
2  Anterior ligament of malleus
3  Tendon of tensor tympani muscle
4  Handle of malleus
5  Short crus of incus
6  Long crus of incus
7  Chorda tympani
8  Lenticular process
9  Tympanic membrane

**Tympanic membrane with malleus and incus** (internal aspect; right side).

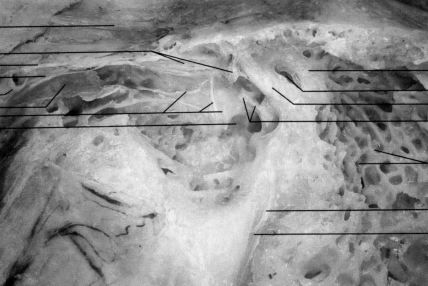

1  Tympanic antrum
2  Lateral semicircular canal (opened)
3  Facial canal
4  Stapes with tendon of stapedius
5  Mastoid air cells
6  Chorda tympani (intracranial part)
7  Greater petrosal nerve
8  Tensor tympani muscle (processus cochleariformis)
9  Lesser petrosal nerve
10  Anterior tympanic artery
11  Middle meningeal artery
12  Auditory tube
13  Promontory with tympanic plexus
14  Fenestra cochleae

**Tympanic cavity, medial wall.** External auditory meatus and lateral wall of tympanic cavity together with incus. Malleus and tympanic membrane have been removed; mastoid air cells are opened (left side).

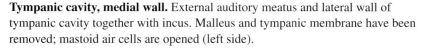
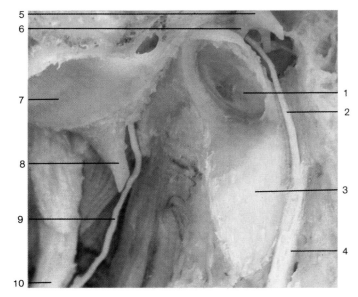

1  Tympanic membrane
2  Chorda tympani (intracranial part)
3  Floor of the external acoustic meatus
4  Facial nerve and facial canal
5  Incus
6  Head of malleus
7  Mandibular fossa
8  Spine of sphenoid
9  Chorda tympani (extracranial part)
10  Styloid process

**Tympanic membrane** (lateral aspect). External acoustic meatus and facial canal have been opened to expose the chorda tympani (magn. ~1.5×) (left side).

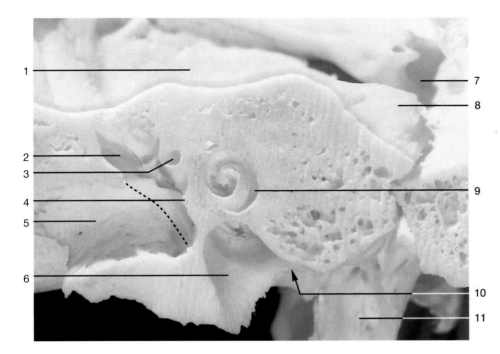

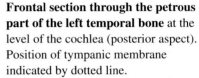

**Frontal section through the petrous part of the left temporal bone** at the level of the cochlea (posterior aspect). Position of tympanic membrane indicated by dotted line.

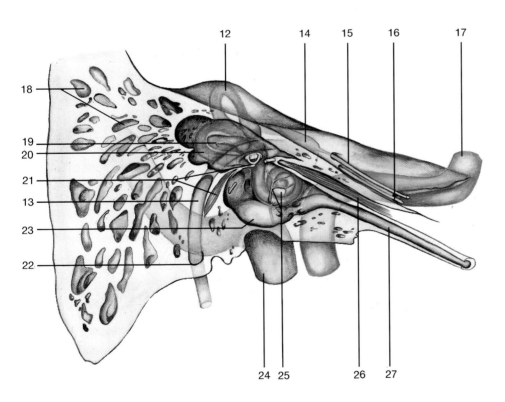

**Medial wall of tympanic cavity** and its relation to neighboring structures of the inner ear, facial nerve, and blood vessels. (Schematic drawing.) Frontal section through the right temporal bone (anterior aspect).

| | | |
|---|---|---|
| 1 Anterior surface of the pyramid | 10 Carotid canal | 20 Posterior semicircular duct |
| 2 Mastoid antrum | 11 Pterygoid process | 21 Stapes with stapedius muscle |
| 3 Lateral semicircular canal | 12 Anterior semicircular duct | 22 Stylomastoid foramen |
| 4 Cochleariform process | 13 Facial nerve | 23 Inferior recess of tympanic cavity |
| 5 External acoustic meatus | 14 Geniculate ganglion | (hypotympanon) |
| 6 Jugular fossa | 15 Greater petrosal nerve | 24 Internal jugular vein |
| 7 Foramen lacerum | 16 Lesser petrosal nerve | 25 Promontory with tympanic plexus |
| 8 Apex of petrous part | 17 Internal carotid artery | (position of cochlea) |
| 9 Position of cochlea (modiolus with | 18 Mastoid air cells | 26 Tensor muscle of tympanum |
| crista spiralis ossea) | 19 Lateral semicircular duct | 27 Auditory tube |

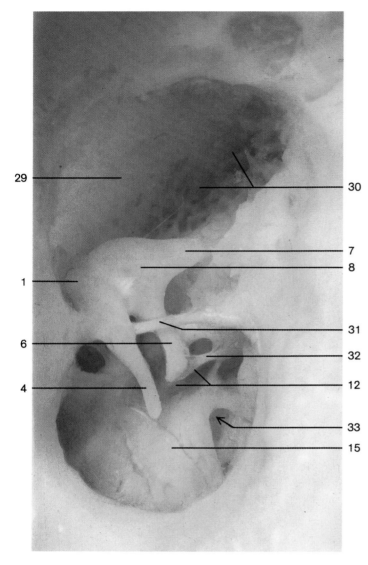

**Tympanic cavity with malleus, incus, and stapes,** left side (lateral aspect). Tympanic membrane removed, mastoid antrum opened.

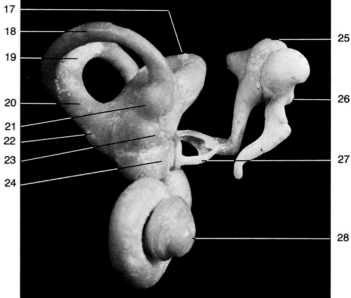

**Chain of auditory ossicles** in connection with the inner ear, left side (anterior-lateral aspect).

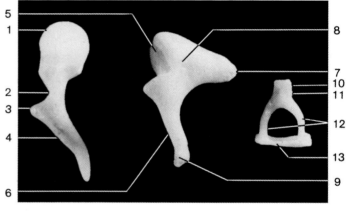

**Auditory ossicles** (isolated).

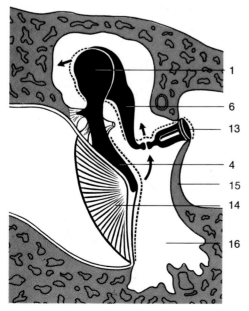

**Position and movements of the auditory ossicles** (schematic diagram).

**Malleus**
1  Head
2  Neck
3  Lateral process
4  Handle

**Incus**
5  Articular facet for malleus
6  Long crus
7  Short crus
8  Body
9  Lenticular process

**Stapes**
10  Head
11  Neck
12  Anterior and posterior crura
13  Base

**Walls of tympanic cavity**
14  Tympanic membrane
15  Promontory
16  Hypotympanic recess of tympanic cavity

**Internal ear (labyrinth)**
17  Lateral semicircular duct
18  Anterior semicircular duct
19  Posterior semicircular duct
20  Common crus
21  Ampulla
22  Beginning of endolymphatic duct
23  Utricular prominence
24  Saccular prominence
25  Incus
26  Malleus
27  Stapes
28  Cochlea

**Tympanic cavity**
29  Epitympanic recess
30  Mastoid antrum
31  Chorda tympani
32  Tendon of stapedius muscle
33  Round window (fenestra cochleae)

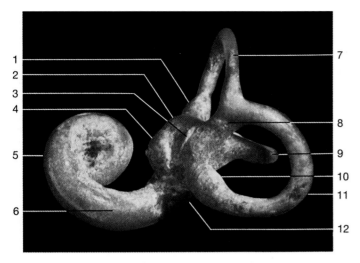

| | |
|---|---|
| 1 Ampulla (anterior semicircular canal) | 16 External acoustic meatus |
| 2 Elliptical recess | 17 Mastoid air cells |
| 3 Aqueduct of the vestibule | 18 Tympanic cavity and fenestra cochleae (probe) |
| 4 Spherical recess | 19 External acoustic meatus |
| 5 Cochlea | 20 Facial canal |
| 6 Base of cochlea | 21 Base of cochlea and canalis musculotubarius |
| 7 Anterior semicircular canal | 22 Malleus and incus |
| 8 Crus commune or common limb | 23 Stapes |
| 9 Lateral semicircular canal | 24 Tympanic membrane |
| 10 Posterior bony ampulla | 25 Tympanic cavity |
| 11 Posterior semicircular canal (posterior canal) | 26 Aqueduct of cochlea |
| 12 Fenestra cochleae | 27 Saccus endolymphaticus |
| 13 Bony ampulla | 28 Ductus endolymphaticus |
| 14 Fenestra vestibuli | 29 Macula of utricle |
| 15 Cupula of cochlea | 30 Macula of saccule |

**Cast of the right labyrinth** (posterior-medial aspect).

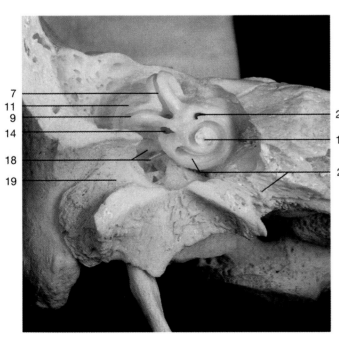

**Cast of the right labyrinth** (lateral aspect).

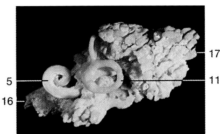

**Cast of the labyrinth and mastoid cells.**
Life size (posterior aspect).

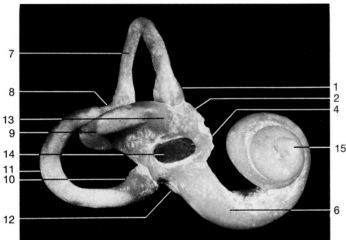

**Dissection of bony labyrinth in situ.** Semicircular canals and cochlear duct opened.

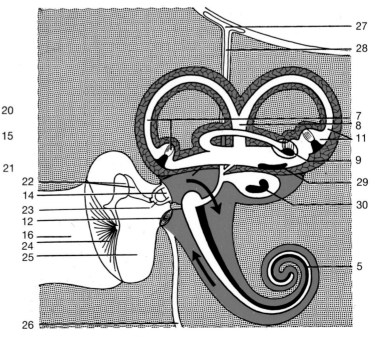

**Auditory and vestibular apparatus.** Arrows: direction of sound waves; blue = perilymphatic ducts. (Schematic diagram.)

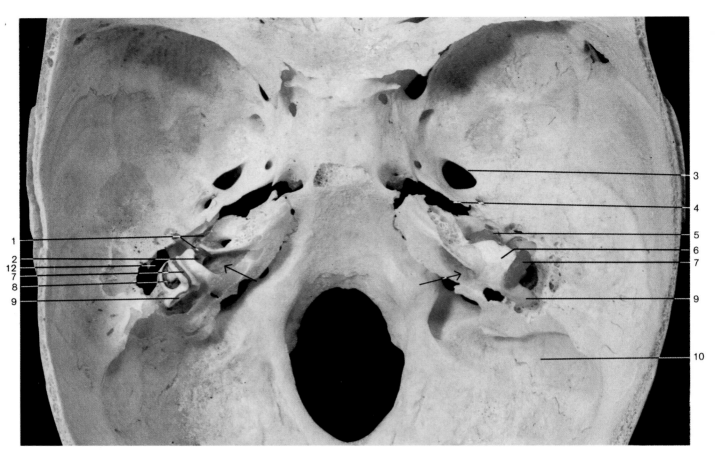

**Bony labyrinth, petrous part of the temporal bone** (from above). At left: semicircular canals opened; at right, closed. Arrows: internal acoustic meatus.

| | | | |
|---|---|---|---|
| 1 | Facial canal and semicanal of auditory tube | 9 | Posterior semicircular canal |
| 2 | Superior vestibular area | 10 | Groove for sigmoid sinus |
| 3 | Foramen ovale | 11 | Sigmoid sinus |
| 4 | Foramen lacerum | 12 | Tympanic cavity |
| 5 | Cochlea | 13 | Auditory tube |
| 6 | Vestibule | 14 | Mastoid air cells |
| 7 | Anterior semicircular canal | 15 | Facial and vestibulocochlear nerves |
| 8 | Lateral semicircular canal | 16 | Temporal fossa |

| | |
|---|---|
| 17 | Fenestra vestibuli |
| 18 | Promontory |
| 19 | Zygomatic process |
| 20 | Fenestra cochleae |
| 21 | Mastoid process |

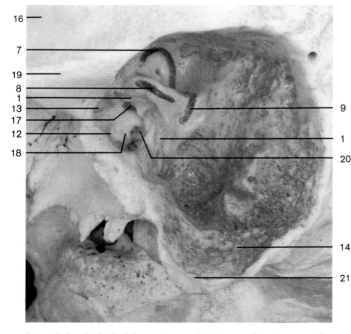

**Bony labyrinth** (left lateral aspect). Temporal and tympanic bone partly removed, semicircular canals opened.

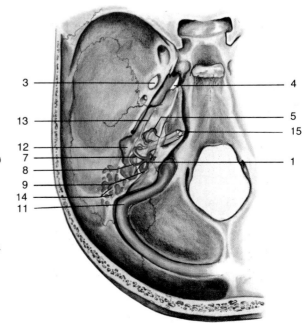

**Internal ear.** Diagram showing the position of the membranous labyrinth and the tympanic cavity.

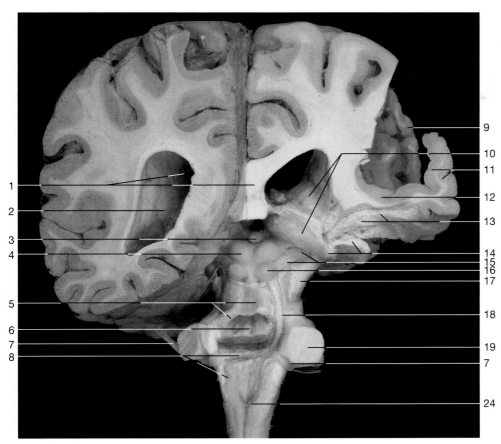

1  Left lateral ventricle
   and corpus callosum
2  Thalamus
3  Pineal gland (epiphysis)
4  Superior colliculus
5  Superior medullary velum and
   superior cerebellar peduncle
6  Rhomboid fossa
7  Vestibulocochlear nerve (n. VIII)
8  Dorsal acoustic striae and
   inferior cerebellar peduncle
9  Insular lobe
10 Caudate nucleus and thalamus
11 Temporal lobe (superior temporal
   gyrus) (area of acoustic centers)
12 Transverse temporal gyri of
   Heschl (area of primary
   acoustic centers)
13 Acoustic radiation of internal
   capsule
14 Lateral geniculate body and
   optic radiation (cut)
15 Medial geniculate body and
   brachium of inferior colliculus
16 Inferior colliculus
17 Cerebral peduncle
18 Lateral lemniscus
19 Middle cerebellar peduncle
20 Dorsal (posterior) cochlear
   nucleus
21 Ventral (anterior) cochlear
   nucleus
22 Inferior olive with olivocochlear tract of Rasmussen (red)
23 Ganglion spirale
24 Obex
25 Frontal lobe
26 Temporal lobe
27 Middle temporal gyrus (area of
   tertiary acoustic centers)
28 Trapezoid body

**Dissection of the brain stem showing the auditory pathway.** Cerebellum and posterior part of the two hemispheres have been removed (dorsal aspect).

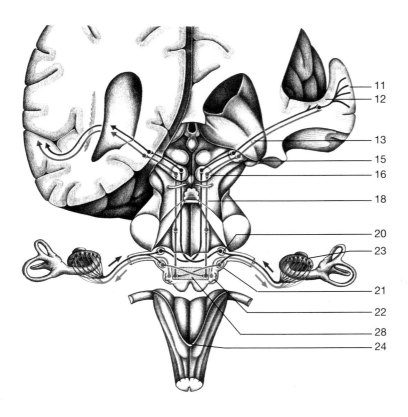

**Auditory pathway** (schematic drawing, compare with figure above). Red = descending (efferent) pathway (olivocochlear tract of Rasmussen); green and blue = ascending (afferent) pathways.

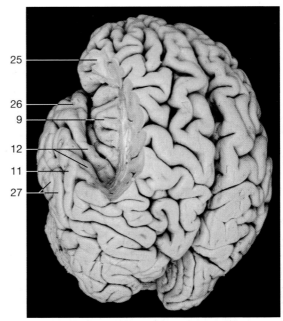

**Auditory areas in the left hemisphere** (superior lateral aspect). Parts of the frontal and parietal lobe have been removed.

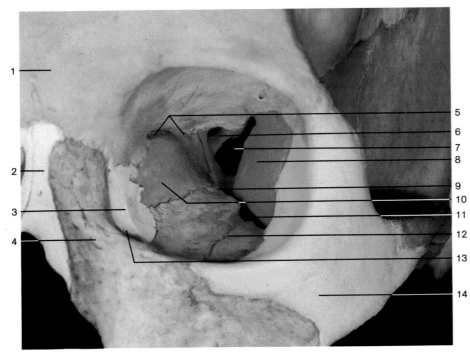

**Bones of the left orbit** (indicated by different colors).

1　Frontal bone
2　Nasal bone
3　Lacrimal bone
4　Maxilla (frontal process)
5　Ethmoidal foramina
6　Lesser wing of sphenoid bone
　　and optic canal
7　Superior orbital fissure
8　Greater wing of sphenoid bone
9　Orbital process of palatine bone
10　Orbital plate of ethmoid bone
11　Inferior orbital fissure
12　Infra-orbital sulcus
13　Nasolacrimal canal
14　Zygomatic bone
15　Frontal sinus
16　Superior rectus muscle
17　Orbital fatty tissue
18　Optic nerve
19　Sclera
20　Inferior rectus muscle
21　Periorbita and maxilla
22　Maxillary sinus
23　Levator palpebrae superioris
　　muscle
24　Superior conjunctival fornix
25　Superior tarsal plate
26　Inferior tarsal plate
27　Inferior conjunctival fornix
28　Inferior oblique muscle
29　Lateral rectus muscle
30　Medial rectus muscle
31　Superior oblique muscle
32　Nasal septum
33　Middle nasal concha
34　Inferior nasal concha
35　Tenon's space
36　Ophthalmic artery
37　Cornea
38　Lens

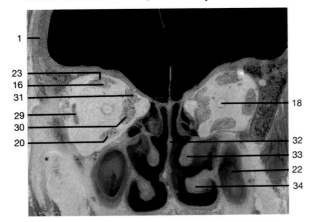

**Frontal section through the posterior part of the orbit.**

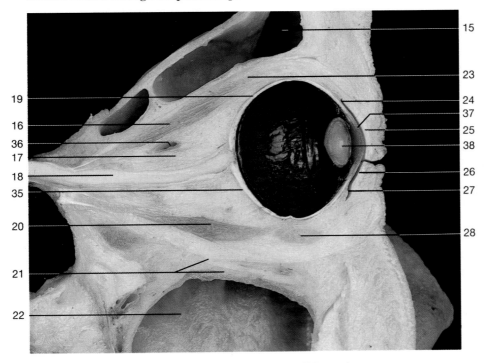

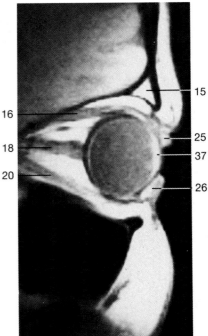

**Sagittal section through orbit and eyeball.** (Right: MRI scan.)

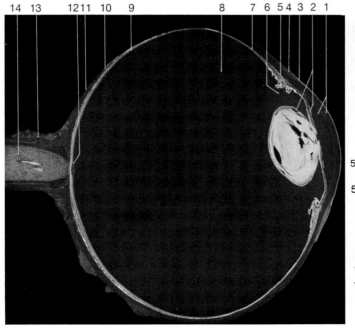

14 13  1211 10   9        8    7 6 54 3 2 1

**Horizontal section through the human eye** (2×).

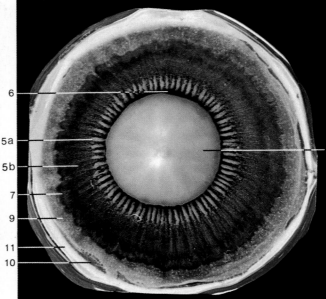

6
5a
5b
7
9
11
10
15

**Anterior segment of the eyeball** (posterior aspect).
The opacity of the lens is an artifact.

◁

**Organization of the eyeball.**
Demonstration of vascular tunic of bulb
(schematic drawing).

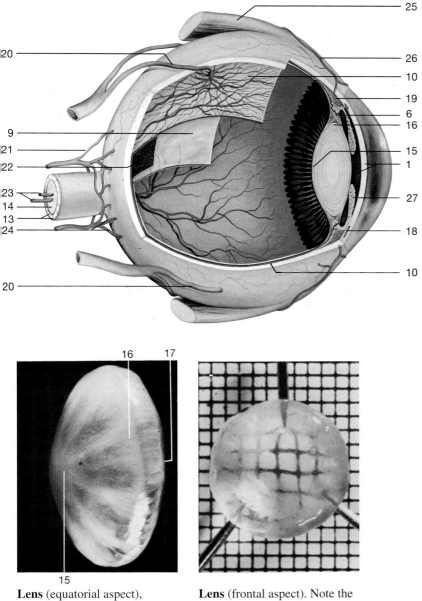

25
20
26
10
19
6
16
9
21
15
22
1
23
14
13
27
24
18
20
10

16   17

15

**Lens** (equatorial aspect),
anterior pole to the right.

**Lens** (frontal aspect). Note the
magnification effect.

1   Cornea and anterior chamber
2   Iris and lens
3   Transitional zone between corneal
    and conjunctival epithelium
4   Conjunctiva of the eyeball
5   Ciliary body
    a  Ciliary processes (pars plicata)
    b  Ciliary ring (pars plana)
6   Zonular fibers
7   Ora serrata
8   Vitreous body
9   Retina
10  Choroid
11  Sclera
12  Optic disc
13  Dura mater and subarachnoid space
14  Optic nerve (n. II)
15  Lens (posterior pole)
16  Equator of lens
17  Lens (anterior pole)
18  Canal of Schlemm
19  Ciliary muscle
20  Vena vorticosa
21  Long posterior ciliary artery
22  Retinal pigmented epithelium
23  Central retinal artery and vein
24  Short posterior ciliary arteries
25  External ocular muscle
26  Anterior ciliary artery
27  Iris

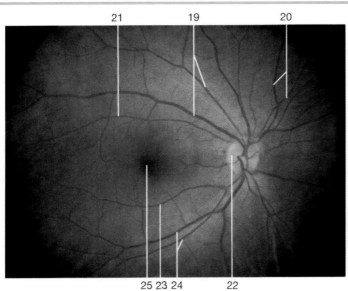

**Fundus of a normal right eye** (courtesy of Prof. Dr. R. Okamura, Univ. Eye Dept., Kumamoto, Japan). Notice, the arteries are smaller and lighter than the veins.

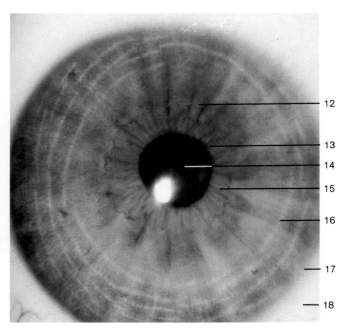

**Anterior segment of the human eye** (courtesy of Prof. Dr. G. O. H. Naumann, Eye Dept., University of Erlangen, Germany). Note the colored iris (16) and the location of the lens behind the iris (14).

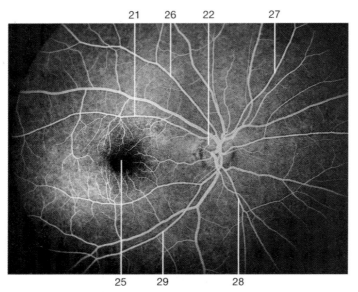

**Fluorescent angiography of the right eye;** retinal vessels. The same eye as above (courtesy of Prof. Dr. R. Okamura, Univ. Eye Dept., Kumamoto, Japan).

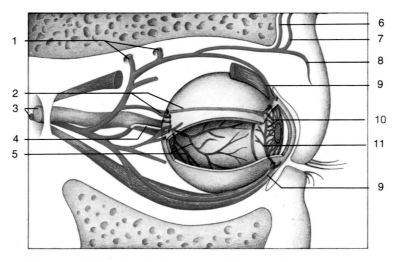

**Diagram of the ophthalmic artery and its branches.**

1  Posterior and anterior ethmoidal arteries
2  Long and short posterior ciliary arteries
3  Optic nerve and ophthalmic artery
4  Central retinal artery
5  Retinal arteries
6  Supratrochlear artery
7  Supra-orbital artery
8  Dorsal nasal artery
9  Anterior ciliary artery
10  Iridial arteries
11  Circulus arteriosus major of iris
12  Iridial fold
13  Pupillary margin of iris
14  Anterior pole of lens
15  Lesser circle of iris
16  Greater circle of iris
17  Margin of cornea or limbus
18  Sclera
19  Superior temporal artery and vein of retina
20  Superior nasal artery and vein of retina
21  Superior macular artery
22  Optic disc
23  Inferior macular artery
24  Inferior temporal artery and vein
25  Fovea centralis and macula lutea
26  Superior temporal artery ⎫
27  Superior nasal artery      ⎬ of retina
28  Inferior nasal artery      ⎪
29  Inferior temporal artery ⎭

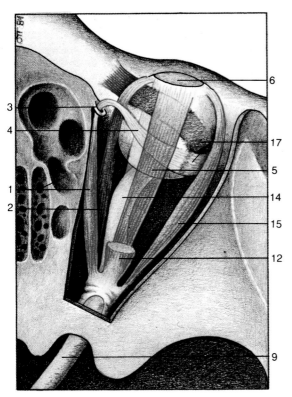

**Schematic diagram of the extra-ocular muscles.**
Right orbit (from above). Levator palpebrae
superioris muscle has been severed.

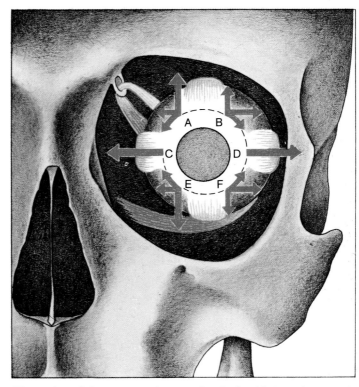

**The action of the extra-ocular muscles.** Left orbit (anterior aspect).

| | | | |
|---|---|---|---|
| A | Superior rectus muscle | D | Lateral rectus muscle |
| B | Inferior oblique muscle | E | Inferior rectus muscle |
| C | Medial rectus muscle | F | Superior oblique muscle |

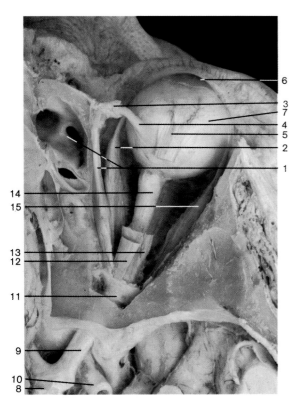

**Right orbit with eyeball and extra-ocular
muscles** (from above). The roof of the orbit has
been removed, the superior rectus muscle and the
levator palpebrae superioris muscle have been
severed.

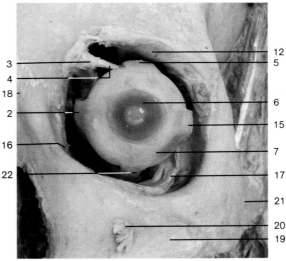

**Left orbit with eyeball and extra-ocular muscles**
(anterior aspect). Lids, conjunctiva, and lacrimal
apparatus have been removed.

| | | | |
|---|---|---|---|
| 1 | Superior oblique muscle and ethmoid air cells | 12 | Levator palpebrae superioris muscle |
| 2 | Medial rectus muscle | 13 | Superior rectus muscle |
| 3 | Trochlea | 14 | Optic nerve (extracranial part) |
| 4 | Tendon of superior oblique muscle | 15 | Lateral rectus muscle |
| 5 | Superior rectus muscle | 16 | Nasolacrimal duct |
| 6 | Cornea | 17 | Inferior oblique muscle |
| 7 | Eyeball | 18 | Nasal bone |
| 8 | Optic chiasma | 19 | Maxilla |
| 9 | Optic nerve (intracranial part) | 20 | Infra-orbital foramen and nerves |
| 10 | Internal carotid artery | 21 | Zygomatic bone |
| 11 | Common annular tendon | 22 | Inferior rectus muscle |

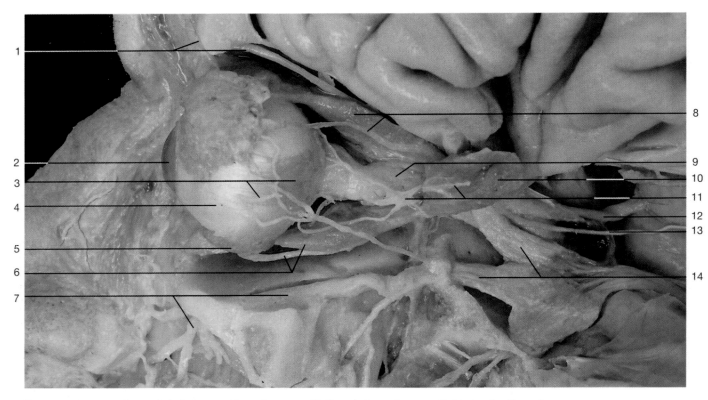

**Extra-ocular muscles and their nerves** (lateral aspect of left eye). Lateral rectus divided and reflected.

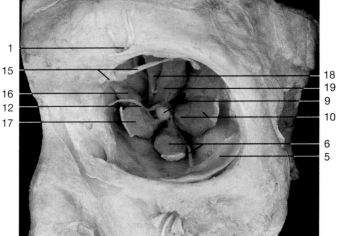

**Left orbit with extra-ocular muscles** (anterior aspect). Eyeball removed.

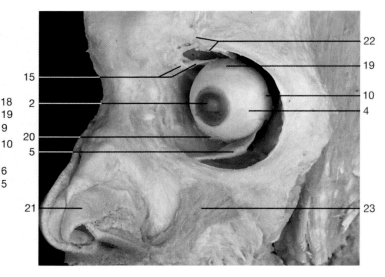

**Extra-ocular eye muscles** (anterior-lateral aspect).

 1  Supra-orbital nerve
 2  Cornea
 3  Insertion of lateral rectus muscle
 4  Eyeball (sclera)
 5  Inferior oblique muscle
 6  Inferior rectus muscle and inferior branch of oculomotor nerve
 7  Infra-orbital nerve
 8  Superior rectus muscle and lacrimal nerve
 9  Optic nerve
10  Lateral rectus muscle
11  Ciliary ganglion and abducens nerve (n. VI)
12  Oculomotor nerve (n. III)

13  Trochlear nerve (n. IV)
14  Ophthalmic nerve (n. V$_1$) and maxillary nerve (n. V$_2$)
15  Trochlea and tendon of superior oblique muscle
16  Superior oblique muscle
17  Medial rectus muscle
18  Levator palpebrae superioris muscle
19  Superior rectus muscle
20  Inferior rectus muscle
21  Greater alar cartilage
22  Supra-orbital nerve and levator palpebrae superioris muscle
23  Levator labii superioris muscle

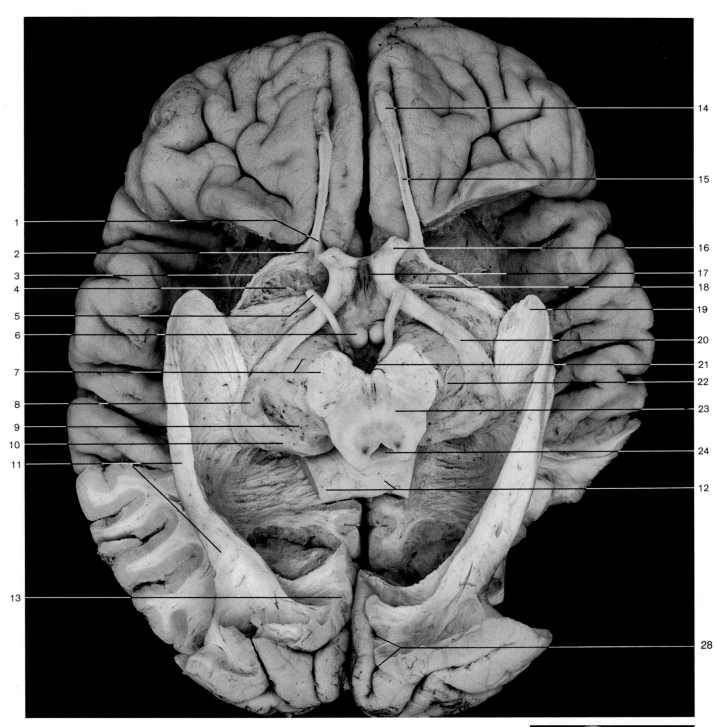

**Dissection of the visual pathway** (inferior aspect). Frontal pole at top, midbrain divided.

1   Medial olfactory stria
2   Olfactory trigone
3   Lateral olfactory stria
4   Anterior perforated substance
5   Oculomotor nerve (n. III)
6   Mamillary body
7   Cerebral peduncle
8   Lateral geniculate body
9   Medial geniculate body
10  Pulvinar of thalamus
11  Optic radiation
12  Splenium of the corpus callosum (commissural fibers)
13  Cuneus
14  Olfactory bulb

15  Olfactory tract
16  Optic nerve (n. II)
17  Infundibulum
18  Anterior commissure
19  Genu of optic radiation
20  Optic tract
21  Interpeduncular fossa and posterior perforated substance
22  Trochlear nerve (n. IV)
23  Substantia nigra
24  Cerebral aqueduct
25  Visual cortex
26  Line of Gennari
27  Gyrus of striate cortex
28  Calcarine sulcus

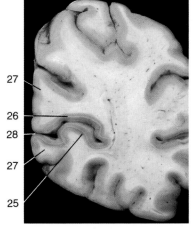

**Frontal section of the striate cortex** at the level of the striate area in the occipital lobe.

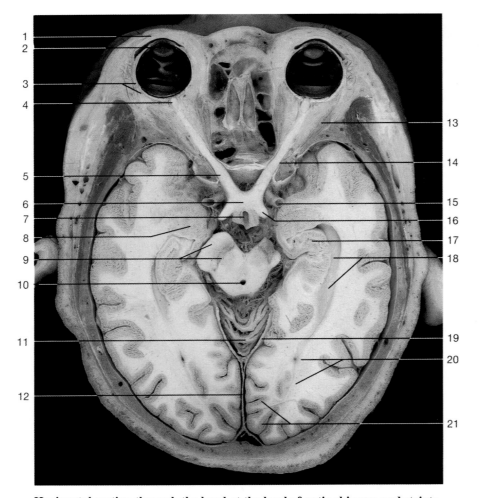

1   Upper lid
2   Cornea
3   Eyeball (sclera, retina)
4   Head of optic nerve
5   Optic nerve
6   Optic chiasma
7   Infundibular recess of hypothalamus
8   Amygdaloid body
9   Substantia nigra and crus cerebri
10  Cerebral aqueduct
11  Vermis of cerebellum
12  Falx cerebri
13  Lateral rectus muscle
14  Optic canal
15  Internal carotid artery
16  Optic tract
17  Hippocampus
18  Inferior horn of lateral ventricle
19  Tentorium cerebelli
20  Optic radiation of Gratiolet
21  Visual cortex (area calcarina,
    striate cortex)
22  Lens
23  Eyeball
24  Ethmoidal cells
25  Optic nerve with dura sheath
26  Cerebral peduncle
27  Aqueduct of mesencephalon
28  Vermis of cerebellum

**Horizontal section through the head at the level of optic chiasma and striate cortex** (superior aspect). Note the relationship of hypothalamic infundibulum to optic chiasma.

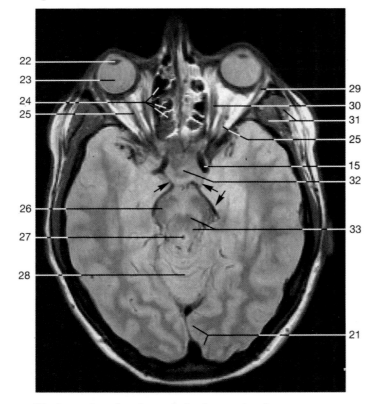

**Horizontal section through the human head**
(MRI scan, courtesy of Prof. W. J. Huk, Erlangen, Germany).
Arrows = branches of arterial circle of Willis.

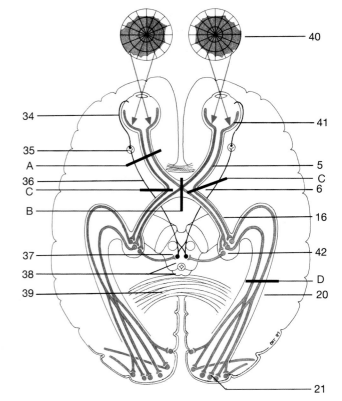

**Diagram of the visual pathway** and path of the light reflex.

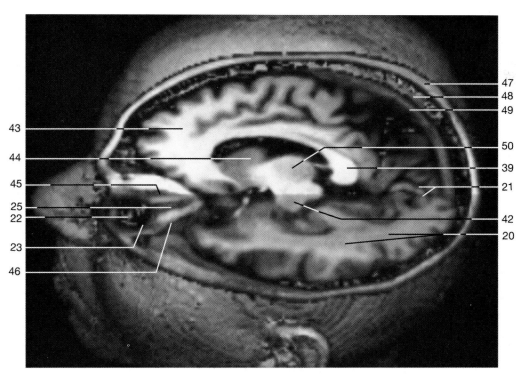

| | |
|---|---|
| 29 | Lateral rectus muscle |
| 30 | Medial rectus muscle |
| 31 | Temporalis muscle |
| 32 | Hypophysis (pituitary gland) |
| 33 | Midbrain |
| 34 | Ciliary nerves (long and short) |
| 35 | Ciliary ganglion |
| 36 | Oculomotor nerve |
| 37 | Accessory oculomotor nucleus |
| 38 | Colliculi of midbrain |
| 39 | Corpus callosum |
| 40 | Visual field |
| 41 | Retina |
| 42 | Lateral geniculate body |
| 43 | Frontal lobe |
| 44 | Caudate nucleus |
| 45 | Medial rectus muscle |
| 46 | Lateral rectus muscle |
| 47 | Skin |
| 48 | Diploe (skull) |
| 49 | Dura mater |
| 50 | Thalamus |
| 51 | Anterior cerebral artery |
| 52 | Caudate nucleus |
| 53 | Frontal sinus |
| 54 | Internal capsule |
| 55 | Lentiform nucleus (putamen) |
| 56 | Hippocampus |
| 57 | Temporal lobe of left hemisphere |

**3-D reconstruction of the human visual system** (MRI scan flash 40°, courtesy of Prof. W. J. Huk, University of Erlangen, Germany).

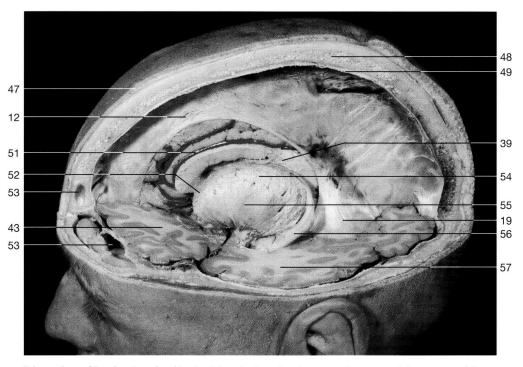

**Dissection of brain stem in situ.** Left hemisphere has been partly removed (compare with MRI scan above).

In **binocular vision** the visual field (40) is projected upon portions of both retinae (blue and red in the drawing). In the chiasma the fibers from the two retinal portions are combined to form the left optic tract. The fibers of the two eyes remain separated from each other throughout the entire visual pathway up to their final termination in the calcarine cortex (21). **Injuries** on the optic pathway produce visual defects whose nature depends on the location of the injury. Destruction of one optic nerve (A) produces blindness in the corresponding eye with loss of pupillary light reflex. If lesions of the **chiasma** destroy the crossing fibers of the nasal portions of the retina (B), both temporal fields of vision are lost (bitemporal hemianopsia). If both lateral angles of the chiasma are compressed (C), the nondecussating fibers from the temporal retinae are affected, resulting in loss of nasal visual fields (binasal hemianopsia). Lesions posterior to the chiasma (D) (i.e., optic tract, lateral geniculate body, optic radiation, or visual cortex) result in a loss of the entire opposite field of vision (homonymous hemianopsia).

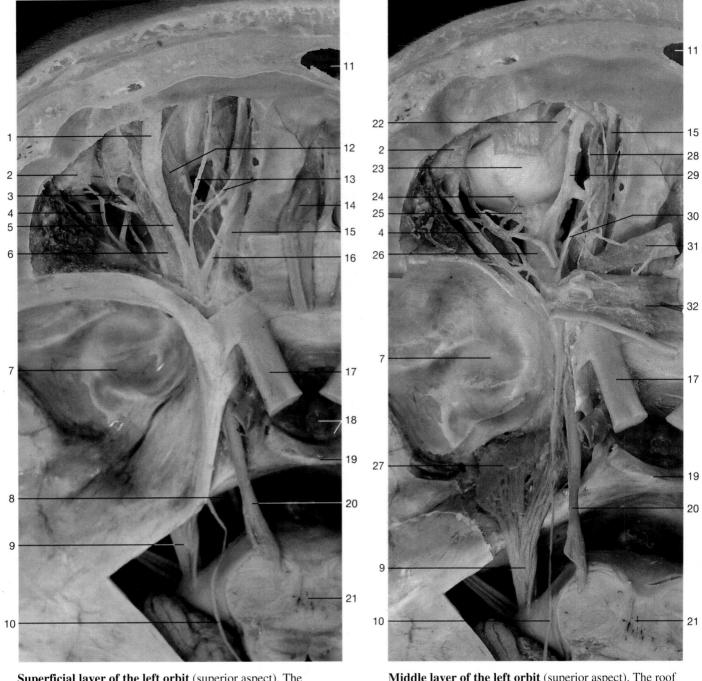

**Superficial layer of the left orbit** (superior aspect). The roof of the orbit and a portion of the left tentorium have been removed.

**Middle layer of the left orbit** (superior aspect). The roof of the orbit has been removed and the superior extra-ocular muscles have been divided and reflected.

| | | | |
|---|---|---|---|
| 1 | Lateral branch of frontal nerve | 10 | Trochlear nerve (intracranial part) (n. IV) |
| 2 | Lacrimal gland | 11 | Frontal sinus |
| 3 | Lacrimal vein | 12 | Levator palpebrae superioris muscle |
| 4 | Lacrimal nerve | 13 | Branches of supratrochlear nerve |
| 5 | Frontal nerve | 14 | Olfactory bulb |
| 6 | Superior rectus | 15 | Superior oblique muscle |
| 7 | Middle cranial fossa | 16 | Trochlear nerve (intra-orbital part) (n. IV) |
| 8 | Abducent nerve (n. VI) | 17 | Optic nerve (intracranial part) |
| 9 | Trigeminal nerve (n. V) | 18 | Pituitary gland and infundibulum |

| | |
|---|---|
| 19 | Dorsum sellae |
| 20 | Oculomotor nerve (n. III) |
| 21 | Midbrain |
| 22 | Tendon of superior oblique muscle |
| 23 | Eyeball |
| 24 | Vena vorticosa |
| 25 | Short ciliary nerves |
| 26 | Optic nerve (extracranial part) |
| 27 | Trigeminal ganglion |

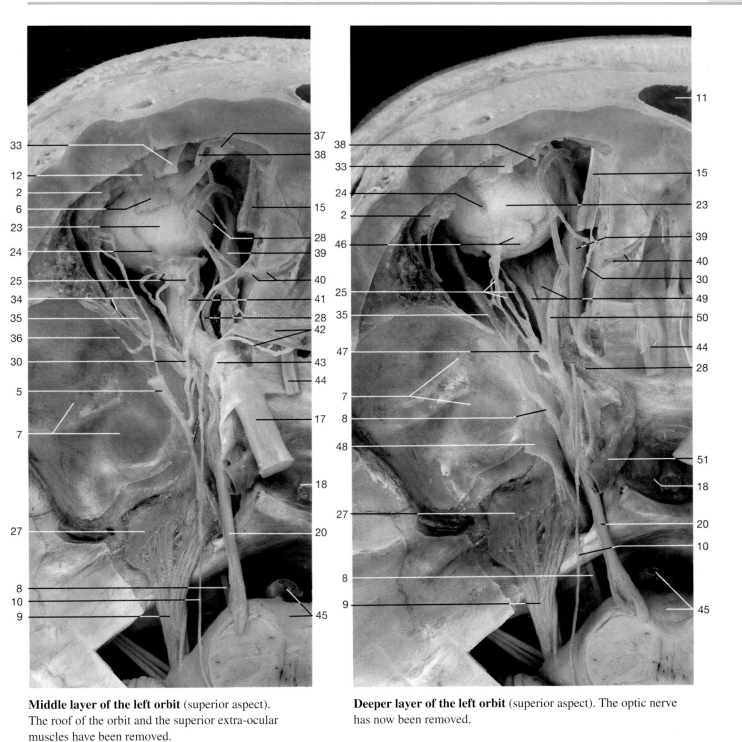

**Middle layer of the left orbit** (superior aspect). The roof of the orbit and the superior extra-ocular muscles have been removed.

**Deeper layer of the left orbit** (superior aspect). The optic nerve has now been removed.

28  Ophthalmic artery
29  Superior ophthalmic vein
30  Nasociliary nerve
31  Levator palpebrae superioris muscle (reflected)
32  Superior rectus muscle (reflected)
33  Lateral branch of supra-orbital nerve
34  Lacrimal nerve and artery
35  Lateral rectus muscle
36  Meningolacrimal artery (anastomosing with middle meningeal artery)

37  Trochlea
38  Medial branch of supra-orbital nerve
39  Medial rectus muscle
40  Anterior ethmoidal artery and nerve
41  Long ciliary nerve
42  Superior oblique muscle and trochlear nerve
43  Common tendinous ring
44  Olfactory tract

45  Basilar artery and pons
46  Optic nerve (external sheath of optic nerve, divided)
47  Ciliary ganglion
48  Ophthalmic nerve (divided, reflected)
49  Inferior branch of oculomotor nerve and inferior rectus muscle
50  Superior branch of oculomotor nerve
51  Internal carotid artery

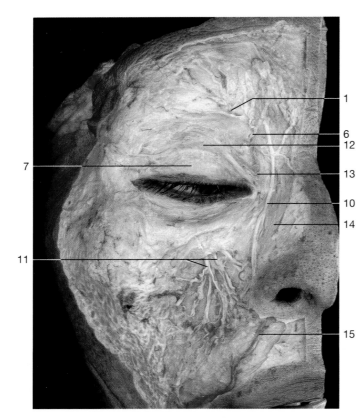

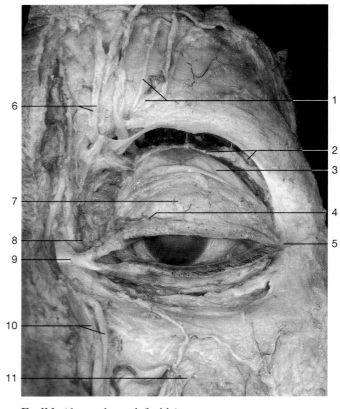

**Eyelids** (superficial layer, right side).

**Eyelids** (deeper layer, left side).

1   Supra-orbital artery, supra-orbital nerve, lateral branch
2   Lacrimal gland
3   Aponeurosis of levator palpebrae superioris muscle
4   Arterial arch of upper eyelid
5   Lateral palpebral ligament
6   Supratrochlear artery, supratrochlear nerve
7   Upper eyelid, superior tarsal plate (tarsus)
8   Lacrimal sac
9   Medial palpebral ligament
10  Angular artery and vein
11  Infra-orbital artery, vein, and nerve
12  Orbital septum

13  Infratrochlear nerve
14  Levator labii superioris alaeque nasi muscle
15  Facial artery and vein
16  Superior lacrimal canaliculus
17  Inferior lacrimal canaliculus
18  Lacrimal papilla and punctum
19  Lacrimal bone
20  Nasolacrimal duct
21  Mucous membrane of nasal cavity
22  Palpebral conjunctiva of lower eyelid
23  Lacrimal sac and superior lacrimal canaliculus
24  Lateral fixation of levator aponeurosis
25  Infra-orbital foramen

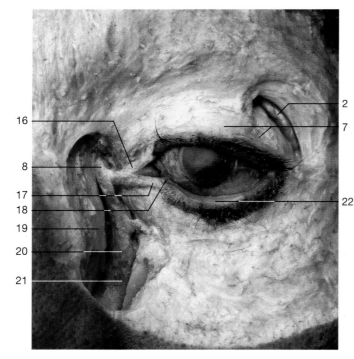

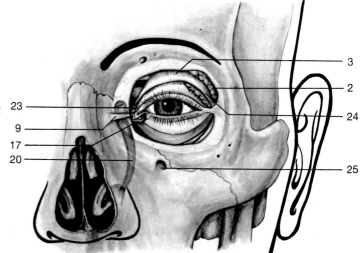

**Lacrimal apparatus of left eye** (anterior aspect).

**Lacrimal apparatus of left eye** (anterior aspect).

1    Crista galli
2    Pituitary gland and
      sella turcica
3    Sphenoidal sinus
      (relatively large)
4    Tubal elevation
5    Pharyngeal opening
      of the auditory tube
6    Pharyngeal recess
7    Atlas (anterior arch)
8    Soft palate
9    Frontal sinus
10   Perpendicular plate of
      ethmoid
11   Cartilage of nasal septum
12   Vomer
13   Hard palate
14   Nasal branch of anterior
      ethmoidal artery and
      anterior ethmoidal nerve
15   Nasopharynx
16   Nasal septum
17   Olfactory nerves
18   Septal artery
19   Crest of nasal septum
20   Incisive canal
21   Anterior ethmoidal artery
22   Olfactory bulb
23   Olfactory tract
24   Internal carotid artery
25   Posterior nasal and septal
      arteries
26   Nasopalatine nerve
27   Choana (arrow)
28   Tongue

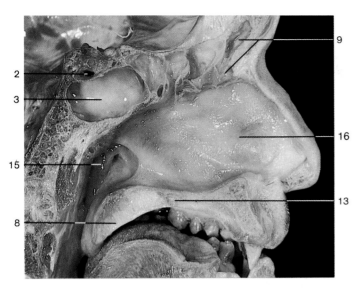

**Nasal septum,** covered by a mucous membrane.

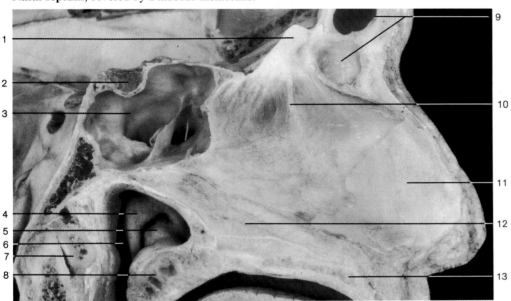

**Nasal septum,** mucous membrane removed.

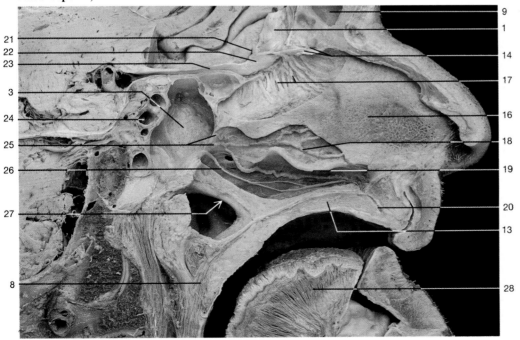

**Nasal septum.** Dissection of nerves and vessels.

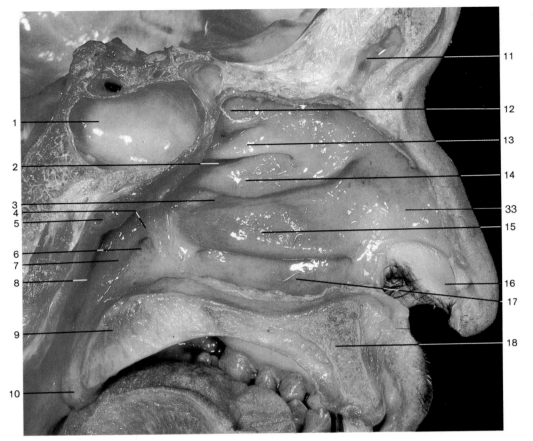

**Lateral wall of the nasal cavity.** Septum removed.

1  Sphenoidal sinus
2  Superior meatus
3  Middle meatus
4  Tubal elevation
5  Pharyngeal tonsil
6  Pharyngeal orifice of
   auditory tube
7  Salpingopharyngeal fold
8  Pharyngeal recess
9  Soft palate
10 Uvula
11 Frontal sinus
12 Spheno-ethmoidal recess
13 Superior nasal concha
14 Middle nasal concha
15 Inferior nasal concha
16 Vestibule
17 Inferior meatus
18 Hard palate
19 Grooves for the middle
   meningeal artery and
   parietal bone (yellow)
20 Maxillary hiatus
21 Perpendicular process of
   palatine bone
22 Openings of ethmoidal air
   cells
23 Opening of frontal sinus
24 Medial pterygoid plate (red)
25 Horizontal plate of palatine
   process
26 Ethmoidal air cells
27 Maxillary sinus
28 Nasal septum
29 Pterygoid hamulus
30 Nasal bone (white)
31 Frontal process of maxilla
   (violet)
32 Palatine process of maxilla
   (violet)
33 Nasal atrium

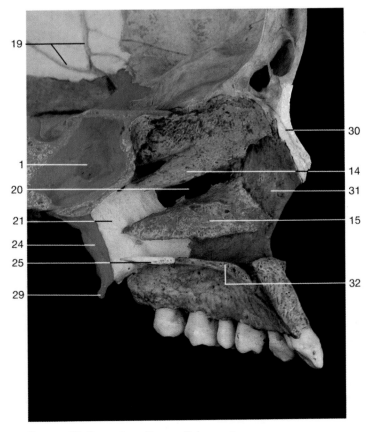

**Bones of left nasal cavity,** medial aspect.

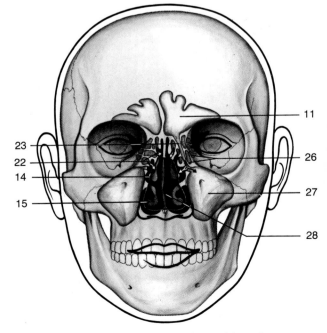

**Schematic diagram showing the position of
paranasal sinuses.** Openings indicated by arrows.

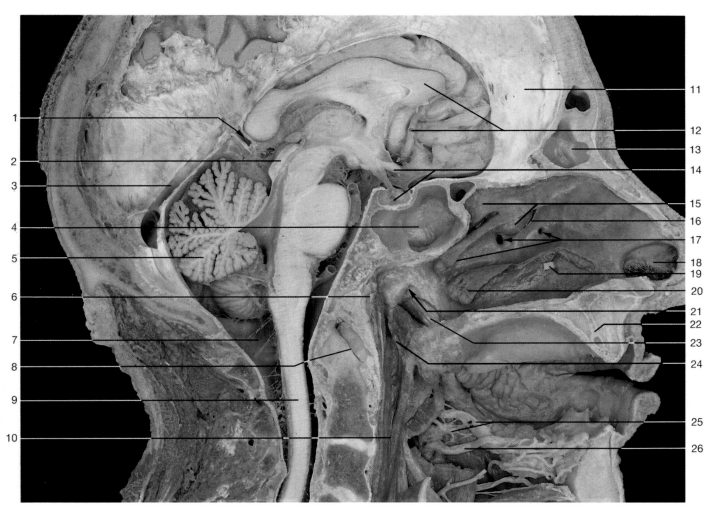

**Median section through the head with nasal and oral cavity.** The middle and inferior nasal conchae have been partly removed to show the openings of paranasal sinuses.

1  Great cerebral vein (Galen's vein)
2  Tectum of midbrain
3  Straight sinus
4  Sphenoidal sinus
5  Cerebellum
6  Pharyngeal tonsil
7  Cerebellomedullary cistern
8  Median atlanto-axial joint
9  Spinal cord
10  Oral part of pharynx
11  Falx cerebri
12  Corpus callosum and anterior cerebral artery
13  Frontal sinus
14  Optic chiasm and pituitary gland
15  Superior nasal concha and ethmoidal bulla
16  Semilunar hiatus
17  Accessory openings to maxillary sinus and cut edge of middle nasal concha
18  Vestibule
19  Opening of nasolacrimal duct
20  Inferior nasal concha (cut)
21  Opening of auditory tube
22  Incisive canal
23  Levator veli palatini muscle
24  Salpingopharyngeal fold
25  Lingual nerve and submandibular ganglion
26  Submandibular duct
27  Nasofrontal duct
28  Nasolacrimal duct
29  Spheno-ethmoidal recess (of Rosenmüller)
30  Salpingopalatine fold

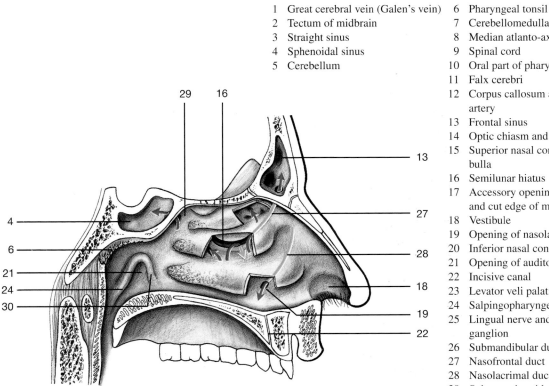

**Lateral wall of nasal cavity.** Openings indicated by red arrows (schematic drawing).

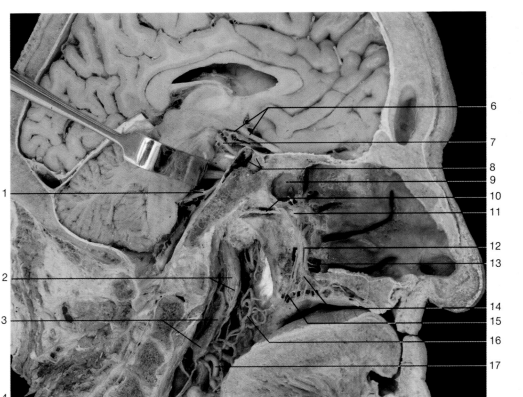

**Nerves of the lateral wall of nasal cavity I.** Sagittal section through the head. Mucous membranes partly removed, pterygoid canal opened.

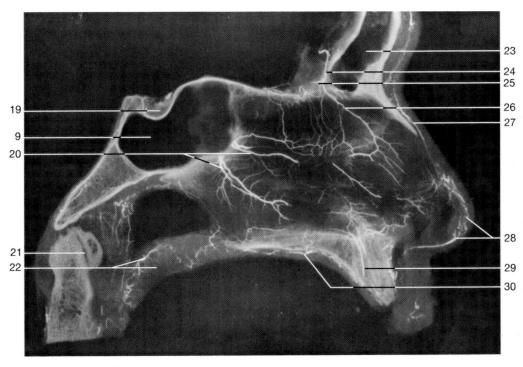

**Arteriogram of the nasal septum,** left side (lateral aspect).

1   Facial nerve
2   Internal carotid artery and internal carotid plexus
3   Superior cervical ganglion
4   Vagus nerve
5   Sympathetic trunk
6   Optic nerve and ophthalmic artery
7   Oculomotor nerve
8   Internal carotid artery and cavernous sinus
9   Sphenoidal sinus
10  Nerve of the pterygoid canal
11  Pterygopalatine ganglion
12  Descending palatine artery
13  Lateral inferior posterior nasal branches and lateral posterior nasal and septal arteries
14  Greater palatine nerves and artery
15  Lesser palatine nerves and arteries
16  Branches of ascending pharyngeal artery
17  Lingual artery
18  Epiglottis
19  Sella turcica
20  Posterior lateral nasal and septal arteries (branches of sphenopalatine artery)
21  Median atlanto-axial joint
22  Soft palate and lesser palatine arteries (branches of descending palatine artery)
23  Frontal sinus
24  Anterior meningeal artery
25  Anterior ethmoidal artery (branch of ophthalmic artery)
26  Septal branch of anterior ethmoidal artery
27  Dorsal nasal artery
28  Nasal branches of anterior ethmoidal artery
29  Incisive canal with nasopalatine artery
30  Hard palate and greater palatine artery (branch of descending palatine artery)
31  Tentorium cerebelli
32  Trochlear nerve
33  Trigeminal nerve with motor root
34  Internal carotid plexus
35  Lingual nerve with chorda tympani
36  Medial pterygoid muscle and medial pterygoid plate
37  Inferior alveolar nerve
38  Sympathetic trunk
39  Oculomotor nerve
40  Palatine nerves
41  Tongue
42  Trigeminal ganglion
43  Trigeminal nerve (n. V)
44  Facial nerve (n. VII)
45  Geniculate ganglion
46  Stylomastoid foramen
47  Medial pterygoid muscle

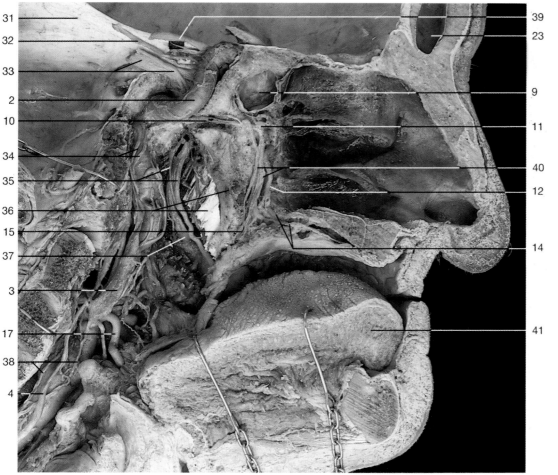

48  Greater petrosal nerve
49  Maxillary nerve
50  Olfactory bulb
51  Olfactory nerves
52  Internal nasal branches
    of anterior ethmoidal
    nerve
53  Lateral superior
    posterior nasal
    branches
54  Lateral inferior
    posterior nasal
    branches
55  Incisive canal with
    nasopalatine nerve
56  Greater palatine nerve
57  Deep petrosal nerve
58  Mandibular nerve
59  Nasal cavity and
    inferior nasal concha
60  Opening of auditory
    tube
61  Tensor veli palatini
    muscle
62  Levator veli palatini
    muscle
63  Pharyngeal recess
    in the nasopharynx
64  Uvula
65  Palatoglossal arch
66  Tonsillar branch of
    ascending palatine
    artery
67  Palatine tonsil
68  Palatopharyngeal arch

**Nerves of the lateral wall of nasal cavity II.** Carotid canal opened, mucous membranes of pharynx and nasal cavity partly removed.

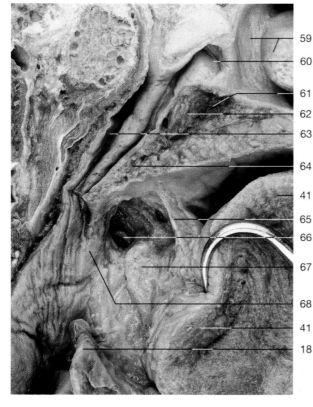

**Dissection of palatine tonsil** located in the lateral wall of the nasopharynx (left side). Root of tongue reflected.

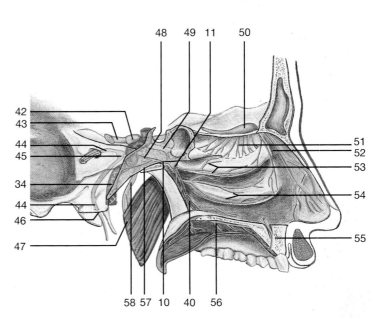

**Nerves of the lateral wall of nasal cavity.** Body of sphenoid bone appears transparent (schematic drawing).

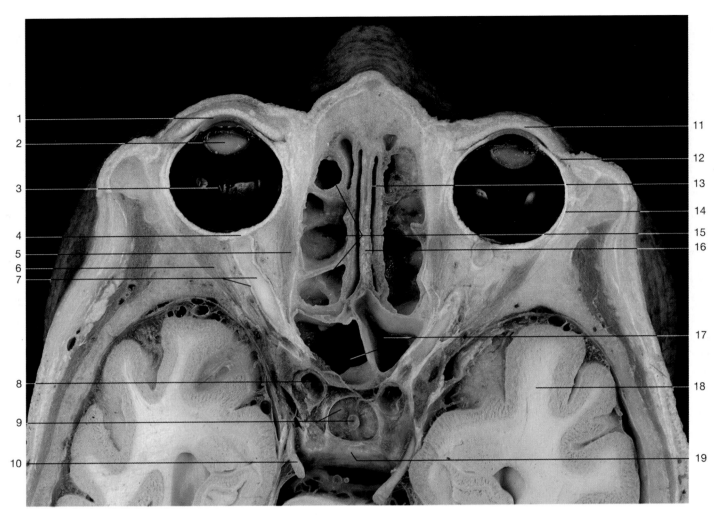

**Horizontal section through the nasal cavity, the orbits, and temporal lobes of the brain at the level of pituitary gland.**

| | | |
|---|---|---|
| 1 Cornea | 4 Head of optic nerve | 7 Optic nerve with dural sheath |
| 2 Lens | 5 Medial rectus muscle | 8 Internal carotid artery |
| 3 Vitreous body (eyeball) | 6 Lateral rectus muscle | 9 Pituitary gland and infundibulum |

10 Oculomotor nerve
11 Superior tarsal plate of eyelid
12 Fornix of conjunctiva
13 Nasal cavity
14 Sclera
15 Ethmoidal sinus
16 Nasal septum
17 Sphenoidal sinus
18 Temporal lobe
19 Clivus
20 Middle cranial fossa
21 External acoustic meatus
22 Superior sagittal sinus
23 Falx cerebri
24 Superior rectus and levator
   palpebrae superioris muscles
25 Eyeball and lacrimal gland
26 Inferior rectus and inferior oblique muscle
27 Zygomatic bone
28 Maxillary sinus
29 Inferior nasal concha
30 Hard palate
31 Superior longitudinal muscle of tongue
32 Lingual septum
33 Inferior longitudinal muscle of tongue
34 Sublingual gland
35 Mandible
36 Calvaria

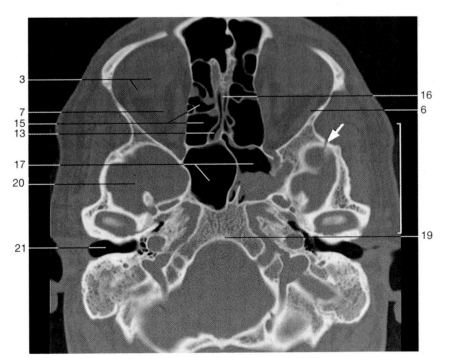

**Horizontal section through the head.** CT scan. Bar = 2 cm.
Arrow: fracture.

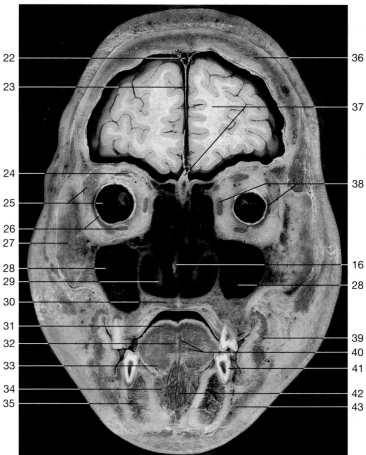

**Coronal section through the head** at the level of the second premolar of the mandible.

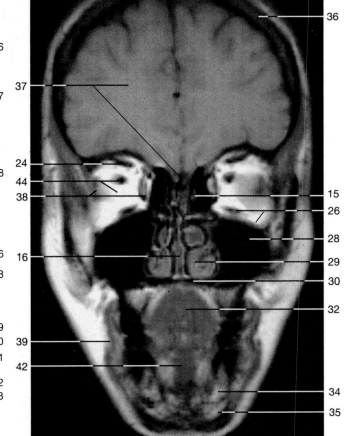

**Coronal section through the head** (MRI scan, courtesy of Prof. Dr. A. Heuck, Munich, Germany). Note the situation of the head cavities.

37 Frontal lobe of brain and crista galli
38 Lateral and medial rectus muscles
39 Buccinator muscle
40 Vertical and transverse muscles of tongue
41 Second premolar of mandible
42 Genioglossus muscle
43 Platysma muscle
44 Orbit and optic nerve
45 Filiform papillae
46 Foramen cecum
47 Root of tongue (lingual tonsil)
48 Palatine tonsil
49 Vallecula of epiglottis
50 Vestibule of larynx
51 Median sulcus of tongue
52 Fungiform papillae
53 Foliate papillae
54 Circumvallate papilla
55 Sulcus terminalis
56 Epiglottis
57 Greater cornu of hyoid bone

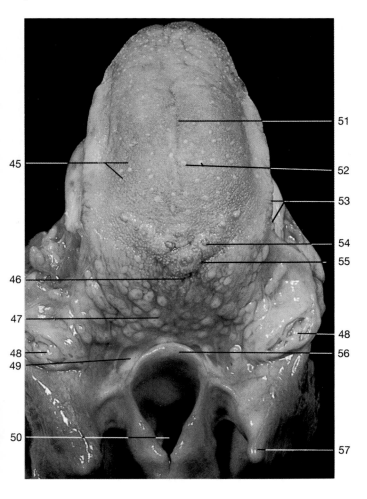

◁ **Dorsal surface of the tongue and laryngeal inlet.**

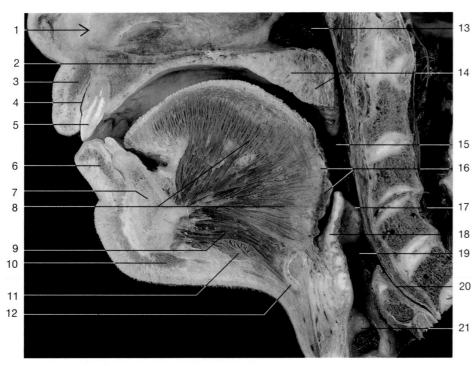

1   Nasal cavity
2   Hard palate
3   Upper lip and orbicularis oris
     muscle
4   Vestibule of oral cavity
5   First incisor
6   Lower lip and orbicularis oris
     muscle
7   Mandible
8   Genioglossus muscle
9   Geniohyoid muscle
10  Anterior belly of diagastric muscle
11  Mylohyoid muscle
12  Hyoid bone
13  Nasopharynx
14  Soft palate and uvula
15  Oropharynx
16  Root of tongue and lingual tonsil
17  Laryngopharynx
18  Epiglottis
19  Ary-epiglottic fold
20  Laryngopharynx continuous with
     esophagus
21  Larynx

**Median sagittal section through the oral cavity and pharynx.**

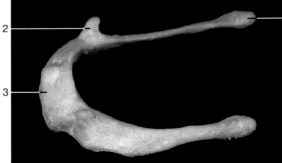

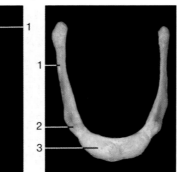

1   Greater cornu ⎫
2   Lesser cornu  ⎬ of hyoid bone
3   Body          ⎭

**Hyoid bone** (oblique lateral aspect).          **Hyoid bone** (anterior aspect).

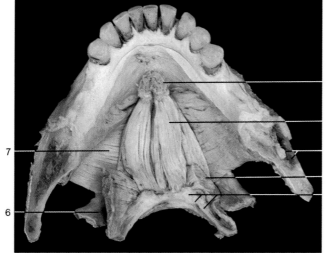

**Muscles of the floor of the oral cavity** (superior aspect).          **Oral diaphragm, muscles** (inferior aspect). Cut on the base.

1   Lesser cornu and body of hyoid bone          7   Mylohyoid muscle
2   Hyoglossus muscle (divided)                  8   Anterior belly of digastric muscle
3   Ramus of mandible and inferior alveolar nerve 9   Hyoid bone
4   Geniohyoid muscle                            10  Mandible
5   Genioglossus muscle (divided)                11  Intermediate tendon of digastric muscle
6   Stylohyoid muscle (divided)

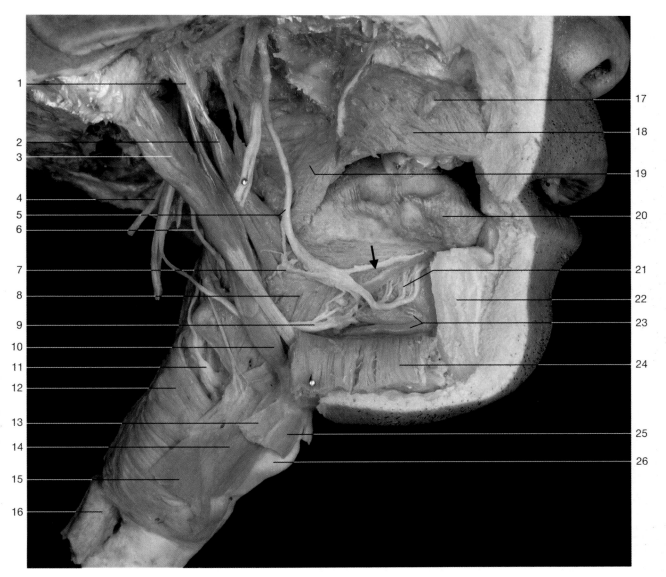

**Parapharyngeal and sublingual regions.** Innervation of the tongue. Lateral part of face and mandible removed, oral cavity opened. Arrow: submandibular duct.

1  Styloid process
2  Styloglossus muscle
3  Digastric muscle (posterior belly)
4  Vagus nerve (n. X)
5  Lingual nerve (n. V₃)
6  Glossopharyngeal nerve (n. IX)
7  Submandibular ganglion
8  Hyoglossus muscle
9  Hypoglossal nerve (n. XII)
10  Stylohyoid muscle
11  Internal branch of superior laryngeal nerve (branch of vagus nerve, not visible)
12  Middle constrictor muscle of pharynx
13  Omohyoid muscle (divided)
14  Thyrohyoid muscle
15  Sternothyroid muscle
16  Esophagus
17  Parotid duct (divided)
18  Buccinator
19  Superior constrictor muscle of pharynx
20  Tongue
21  Terminal branches of lingual nerve
22  Mandible (divided)
23  Genioglossus and geniohyoid muscles
24  Mylohyoid muscle (divided and reflected)
25  Sternohyoid muscle (divided)
26  Thyroid cartilage
27  Anterior belly of digastric muscle
28  Hyoid bone

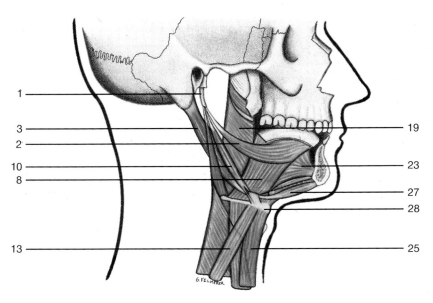

**Supra- and infrahyoid muscles and pharynx** (schematic drawing).

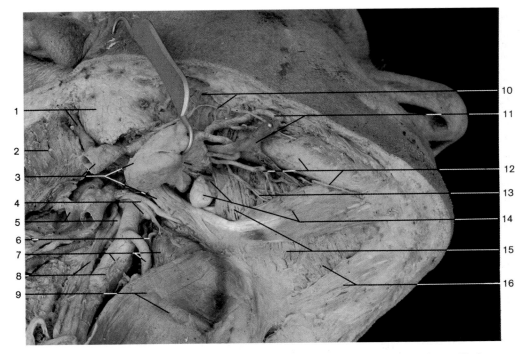

**Submandibular triangle,** superficial dissection. Right side (inferior aspect). Submandibular gland has been reflected.

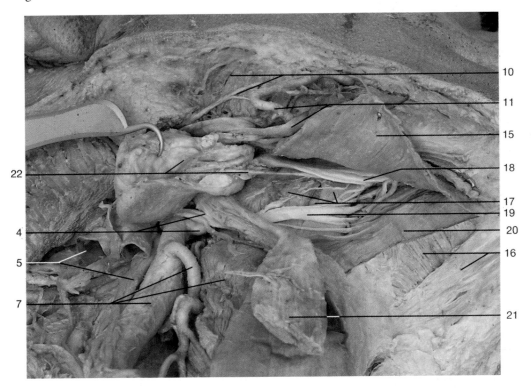

**Submandibular triangle,** deep dissection. Right side. Mylohyoid muscle has been severed and reflected to display the lingual and hypoglossal nerves.

1  Parotid gland and retromandibular vein
2  Sternocleidomastoid muscle
3  Retromandibular vein, submandibular gland, and stylohyoid muscle
4  Hypoglossal nerve and lingual artery
5  Vagus nerve and internal jugular vein
6  Superior laryngeal artery
7  External carotid artery, thyrohyoid muscle, and superior thyroid artery
8  Common carotid artery and superior root of ansa cervicalis
9  Omohyoid and sternohyoid
10  Masseter and marginal mandibular branch of facial nerve
11  Facial artery and vein

12  Mandible and submental artery and vein
13  Mylohyoid nerve
14  Submandibular duct, sublingual gland, and anterior belly of digastric muscle
15  Mylohyoid (right side)
16  Left mylohyoid and anterior belly of left digastric muscle
17  Hyoglossus muscle and lingual artery
18  Lingual nerve
19  Hypoglossal nerve
20  Geniohyoid muscle
21  Anterior belly of right digastric muscle
22  Submandibular gland and duct

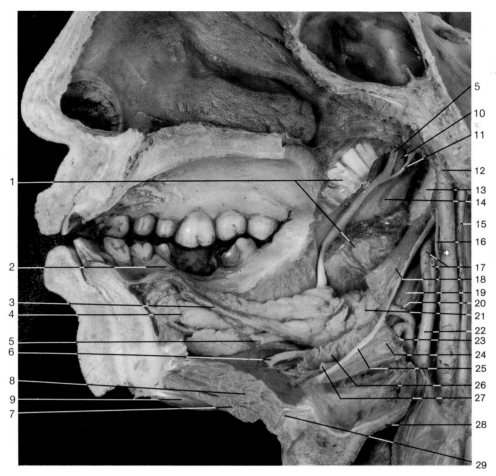

1   Medial pterygoid muscle
2   Sublingual papilla
3   Submandibular duct
4   Sublingual gland
5   Lingual nerve
6   Hypoglossal nerve
7   Mylohyoid muscle
8   Geniohyoid muscle
9   Anterior belly of digastric muscle
10  Inferior alveolar nerve
11  Chorda tympani
12  Internal carotid artery
13  Parotid gland
14  Sphenomandibular ligament
15  Vagus nerve
16  Glossopharyngeal nerve
17  Superficial temporal artery and ascending pharyngeal artery
18  Styloglossus muscle
19  Posterior belly of digastric muscle
20  Facial artery
21  Submandibular gland
22  External carotid artery
23  Lingual artery
24  Middle pharyngeal constrictor muscle
25  Stylohyoid ligament
26  Hyoglossus muscle
27  Deep lingual artery
28  Epiglottis
29  Hyoid bone
30  Buccinator muscle
31  Tongue
32  Mandible (divided)
33  Parotid duct
34  Masseter muscle
35  Right and left sublingual papillae

**Oral cavity** (internal aspect). Tongue and pharyngeal wall removed.

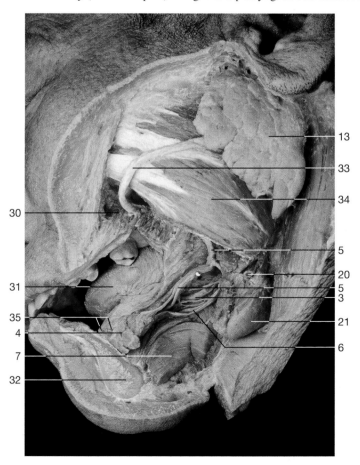

**Dissection of major salivary glands.** Left mandible and buccinator muscle partly removed to view the oral cavity (inferior lateral aspect).

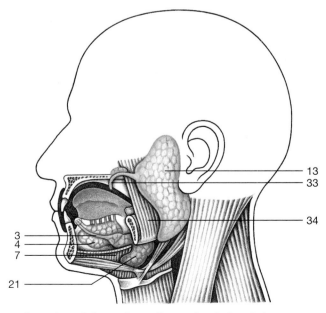

**Location of the major salivary glands** in relation to the oral cavity.

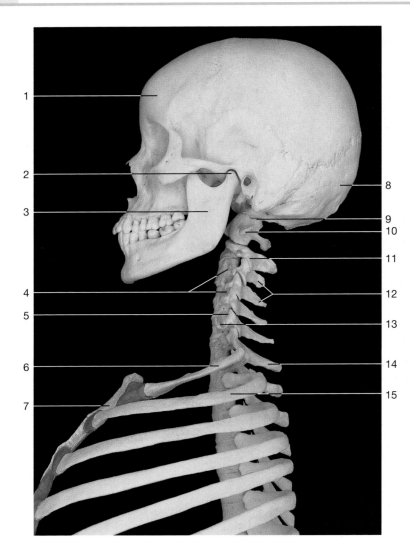

**Cervical spine** between skull and upper thorax (lateral aspect).

1   Frontal bone
2   Temporomandibular joint
3   Mandible
4   Bodies of the third and fourth cervical vertebrae (C₃, C₄)
5   Intervertebral foramen
6   First rib
7   Manubrium of the sternum
8   Occipital bone
9   Atlanto-occipital joint
10  Atlas
11  Axis
12  Spinous processes of the third and fourth cervical vertebrae
13  Transverse process with groove for spinal nerve
14  Vertebra prominens (seventh cervical vertebra)
15  Second rib

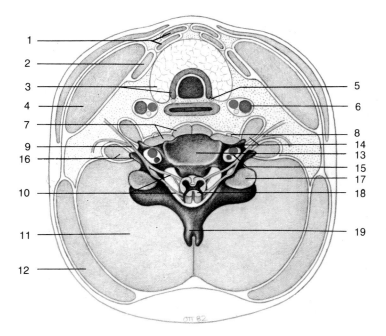

**Cervical vertebra** and the **organization of the neck** (schematic drawing).

1   Sternohyoid and sternothyroid muscles
2   Omohyoid muscle
3   Thyroid gland and trachea
4   Sternocleidomastoid muscle
5   Recurrent laryngeal nerve
6   Internal jugular vein, common carotid artery, and vagus nerve
7   Longus colli and longus capitis muscles
8   Sympathetic trunk
9   Spinal nerve
10  Ventral and dorsal root of spinal nerve
11  True muscles of the neck
12  Trapezius muscle
13  Body of cervical vertebra
14  Anterior tubercle of transverse process and origin of scalenus anterior muscle
15  Vertebral artery and foramen transversarium
16  Posterior tubercle of transverse process and origin of scalenus medius and posterior muscles
17  Superior facet of articular process
18  Spinal cord
19  Spinous process

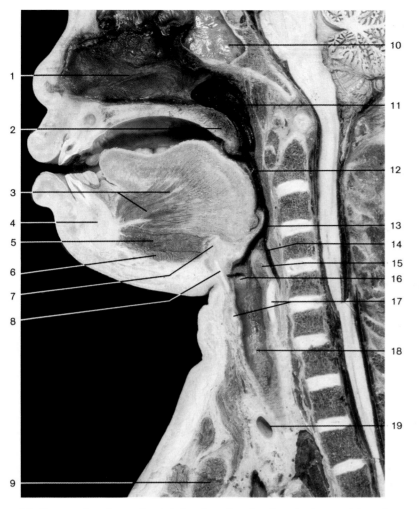

1. Nasal septum
2. Uvula
3. Genioglossus muscle
4. Mandible
5. Geniohyoid muscle
6. Mylohyoid muscle
7. Hyoid bone
8. Thyroid cartilage
9. Manubrium sterni
10. Sphenoidal sinus
11. Nasopharynx
12. Oropharynx
13. Epiglottis
14. Laryngopharynx
15. Arytenoid muscle
16. Vocal fold
17. Cricoid cartilage
18. Trachea
19. Left brachiocephalic vein
20. Thymus
21. Esophagus
22. Occipital lobe
23. Cerebellum and fourth ventricle
24. Medulla oblongata
25. Dens of axis
26. Intervertebral discs
    of cervical vertebral column

**Median section through adult head and neck.** Note the low position of the adult larynx when compared with that of the neonate (cf. with the figure below).

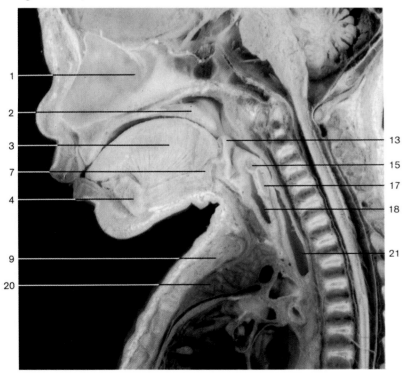

**Median section through neonate head and neck.** Note the high position of the larynx permitting the epiglottis nearly to reach the uvula (cf. with the figure above).

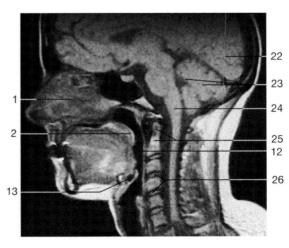

**Sagittal section through the head.** (MRI scan.)

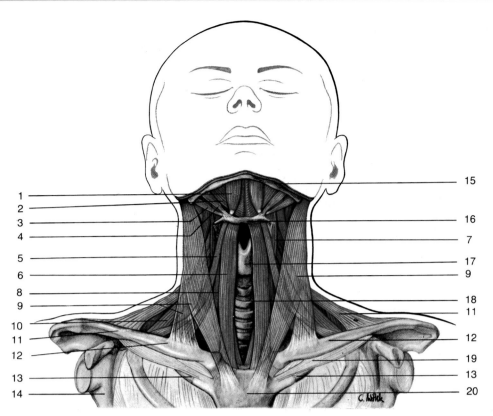

**Muscles of the neck** (anterior aspect).

**Suprahyoid muscles**
1　Anterior belly of digastric muscle
2　Mylohyoid muscle
3　Posterior belly of digastric muscle
4　Stylohyoid muscle

**Infrahyoid muscles**
5　Omohyoid muscle
6　Sternohyoid muscle
7　Thyrohyoid muscle
8　Sternothyroid muscle

**Other structures**
9　Sternocleidomastoid muscle
10　Scalenus muscles
11　Trapezius muscle
12　Clavicle
13　First rib
14　Scapula
15　Mandible
16　Hyoid bone
17　Larynx (thyroid cartilage)
18　Trachea
19　Subclavius muscle
20　Manubrium sterni
21　Mucous membrane of larynx
　　(conus elasticus)
22　Cricoid cartilage
23　Inferior horn of thyroid cartilage
24　Esophagus
25　Body of cervical vertebra
26　Posterior root ganglion
27　Spinal cord
28　Spinous process
29　Internal jugular vein, common
　　carotid artery, and vagus nerve
30　True muscles of the neck (semi-
　　spinalis cervicis and capitis muscles)

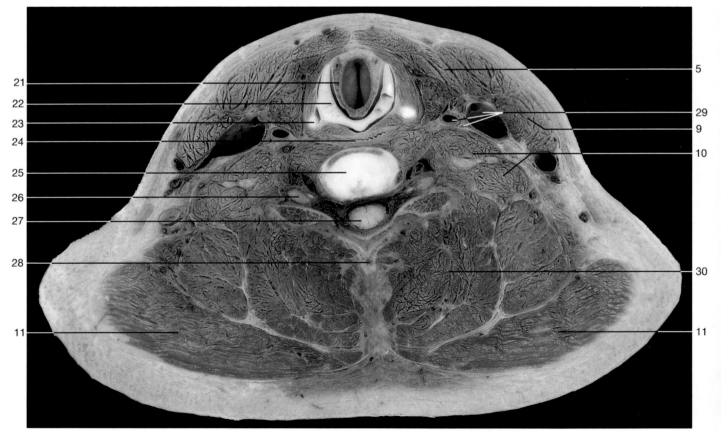

**Cross section of the neck** at the level of the intervertebral disc between the 5th and 6th cervical vertebra (inferior aspect).

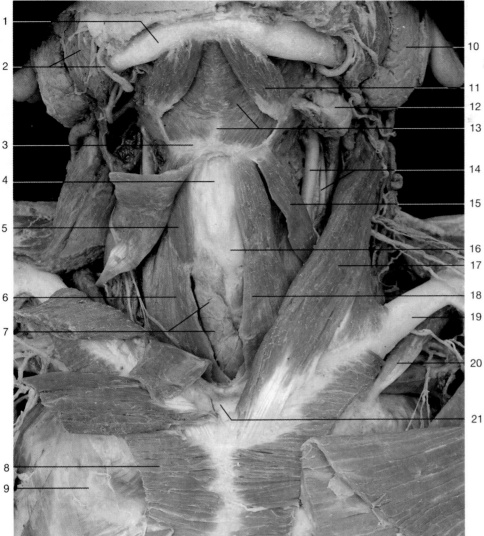

1   Mandible
2   Masseter muscle and facial artery
3   Hyoid bone
4   Median thyrohyoid ligament
5   Thyrohyoid muscle
6   Sternothyroid muscle
7   Thyroid gland (pyramidal lobe)
8   Pectoralis major muscle
9   Second rib
10  Parotid gland
11  Anterior belly of digastric muscle
12  Submandibular gland (divided)
13  Mylohyoid muscle and mylohyoid raphe
14  External carotid artery and vagus nerve
15  Omohyoid muscle
16  Thyroid cartilage
17  Sternocleidomastoid muscle
18  Sternohyoid muscle
19  Clavicle
20  Subclavius muscle
21  Jugular fossa and interclavicular ligament

**Muscles of the neck** (anterior aspect). Sternocleidomastoid and sternohyoid muscles on the right have been divided and reflected.

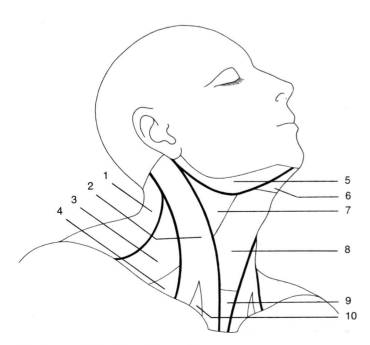

**Regions and triangles of the neck.**

1   Trapezius muscle
2   Sternocleidomastoid muscle
3   Lateral cervical triangle  ⎤ Posterior triangle
4   Supraclavicular triangle   ⎦
5   Submandibular triangle  ⎤
6   Submental triangle      ⎬ Anterior triangle
7   Carotid triangle        ⎦
8   Muscular triangle
9   Jugular fossa
10  Lesser supraclavicular fossa

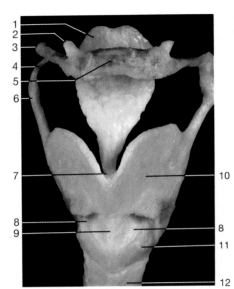

1 Epiglottis
2 Lesser cornu of hyoid bone
3 Greater cornu of hyoid bone
4 Lateral thyrohyoid ligament
5 Body of hyoid bone
6 Superior cornu of thyroid
  cartilage
7 Thyro-epiglottic ligament
8 Conus elasticus
9 Cricothyroid ligament
10 Thyroid cartilage
11 Cricoid cartilage
12 Trachea
13 Corniculate cartilage
14 Arytenoid cartilage
15 Posterior crico-arytenoid
   ligament
16 Cricothyroid joint
17 Crico-arytenoid joint

**Cartilages of the larynx and the hyoid bone** (anterior aspect).

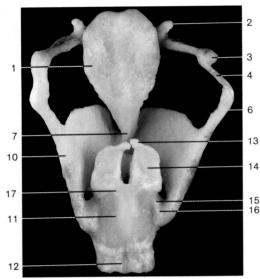

**Cartilages of the larynx and the hyoid bone** (posterior aspect).

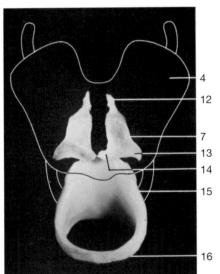

**Cartilages of the larynx** (anterior aspect). Thyroid cartilage is indicated by the outline.

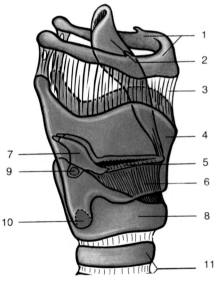

1 Hyoid bone
2 Epiglottis
3 Thyrohyoid membrane
4 Thyroid cartilage
5 Vocal ligament
6 Conus elasticus
7 Arytenoid cartilage
8 Cricoid cartilage
9 Crico-arytenoid joint
10 Cricothyroid joint
11 Tracheal cartilages
12 Corniculate cartilage
13 Muscular process of arytenoid
   cartilage
14 Vocal process of arytenoid
   cartilage
15 Lamina of cricoid cartilage
16 Arch of cricoid cartilage

**Cartilages and ligaments of the larynx** (lateral aspect). (Schematic drawing.)

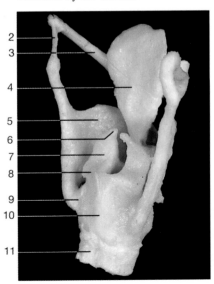

**Cartilages of the larynx** (oblique-posterior aspect).

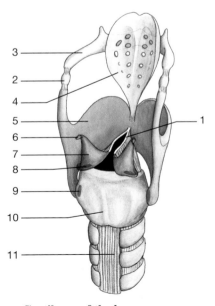

1 Vocal ligament
2 Lateral thyrohyoid ligament
3 Greater cornu of hyoid bone
4 Epiglottis
5 Thyroid cartilage
6 Corniculate cartilage
7 Arytenoid cartilage
8 Crico-arytenoid joint
9 Cricothyroid joint
10 Cricoid cartilage
11 Trachea

**Cartilages of the larynx** (oblique-posterior aspect).

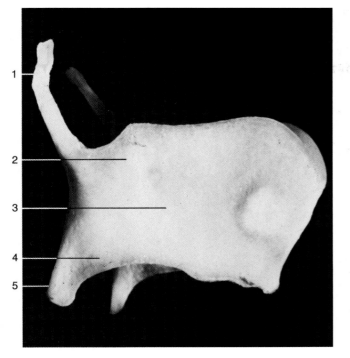

**Thyroid cartilage** (lateral aspect).

1  Superior cornu
2  Superior thyroid tubercle
3  Lamina of thyroid cartilage

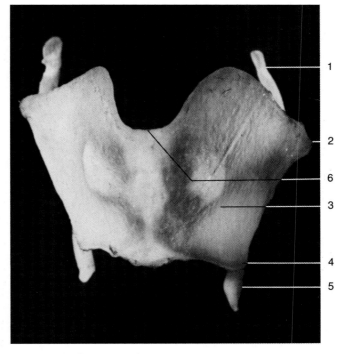

**Thyroid cartilage** (anterior aspect).

4  Inferior thyroid tubercle
5  Inferior cornu
6  Superior thyroid notch

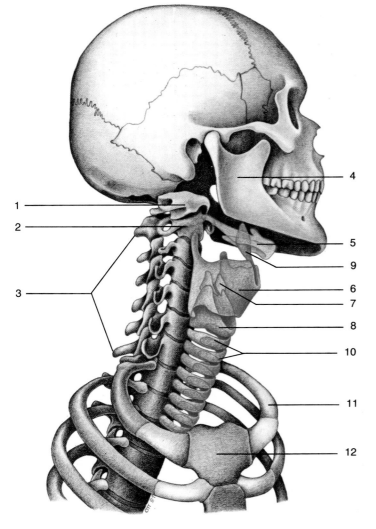

1  Atlas
2  Axis
3  Cervical vertebrae ($C_2$–$C_7$)
4  Mandible
5  Hyoid bone
6  Thyroid cartilage
7  Arytenoid cartilage
8  Cricoid cartilage
9  Epiglottis
10  Tracheal cartilages
11  First rib
12  Manubrium sterni

**Position of the larynx** in the neck (oblique-lateral aspect).
(Schematic drawing.)

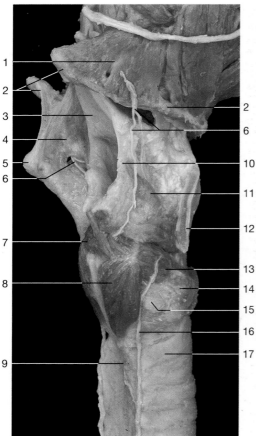

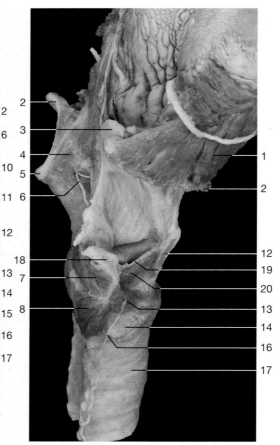

1   Hyoglossus muscle
2   Hyoid bone
3   Epiglottis
4   Thyrohyoid membrane
5   Superior cornu of thyroid
    cartilage
6   Superior laryngeal nerve
7   Transverse arytenoid
    muscle
8   Posterior crico-arytenoid
    muscle
9   Transverse muscle of
    trachea
10  Ary-epiglottic fold
11  Thyro-epiglottic muscle
12  Thyroid cartilage
13  Lateral crico-arytenoid
    muscle
14  Cricoid cartilage
15  Articular facet for thyroid
    cartilage
16  Inferior laryngeal nerve
    (branch of recurrent nerve)
17  Trachea
18  Arytenoid cartilage
19  Vocal ligament
20  Vocalis muscle (part of
    thyro-arytenoid muscle)
21  Thyrohyoideus muscle
22  Cricothyroideus muscle
23  Root of tongue
24  Cuneiform tubercle
25  Corniculate tubercle
26  Ary-epiglottic muscle

**Laryngeal muscles I** (lateral aspect).
Thyroid cartilage (12) and thyro-arytenoid
muscle have been partly removed.

**Laryngeal muscles II** (lateral aspect).
Half of the thyroid cartilage (12) has been removed. Dissection of the vocal ligament (19).

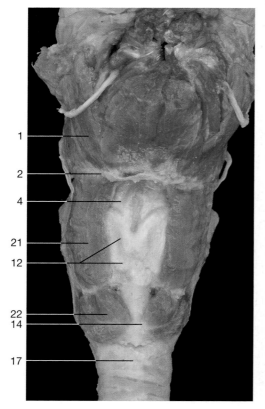

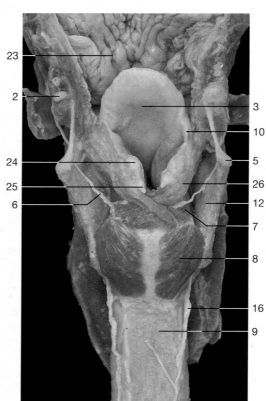

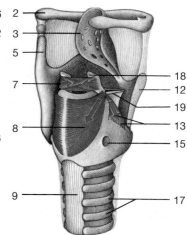

**Laryngeal muscles and larynx**
(anterior aspect).

**Laryngeal muscles and larynx**
(posterior aspect).

**Action of internal muscles of
the larynx** (schematic drawing).

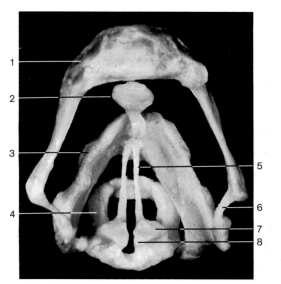

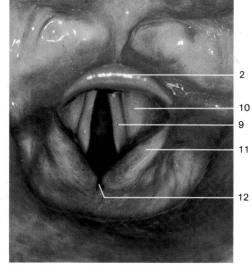

1. Hyoid bone
2. Epiglottis
3. Thyroid cartilage
4. Cricoid cartilage
5. Vocal ligament
6. Thyrohyoid ligament
7. Arytenoid cartilage
8. Corniculate cartilage
9. Vocal fold
10. Vestibular fold
11. Ary-epiglottic fold
12. Interarytenoid notch
13. Mandible
14. Anterior belly of digastric muscle
15. Mylohyoid muscle
16. Pyramidal lobe of thyroid gland
17. Sternohyoid and sternothyroid muscles
18. Common carotid artery
19. Internal jugular vein
20. Rima glottidis
21. Sternocleidomastoid muscle
22. Transverse arytenoid muscle
23. Pharynx and inferior constrictor muscle
24. Ventricle of larynx
25. Vocalis muscle
26. Trachea
27. Superior cornu of thyroid cartilage
28. Root of tongue (lingual tonsil)
29. Piriform recess
30. Vocalis muscle
31. Lateral crico-arytenoid muscle
32. Thyroid gland

**Laryngeal cartilages** (superior aspect).

**Glottis in vivo** (superior aspect).

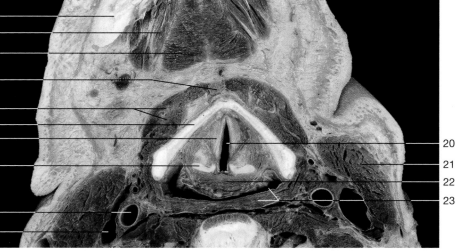

**Horizontal section through the larynx** at the level of the vocal folds (superior aspect).

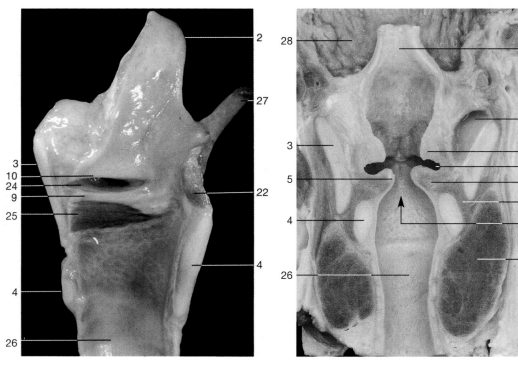

**Sagittal section through the larynx.**

**Coronal section through larynx and trachea.**

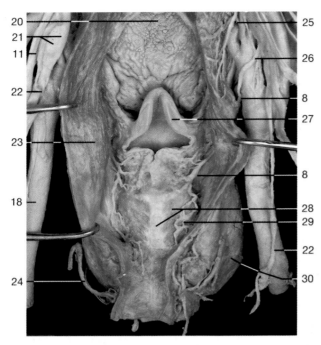

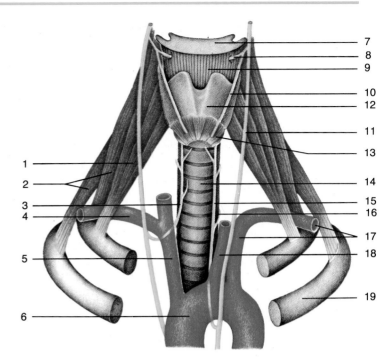

**Larynx and its innervation** (posterior aspect).
Dissection of superior and inferior laryngeal nerves.
Pharynx has been opened.

**Innervation of the larynx** (schematic diagram).

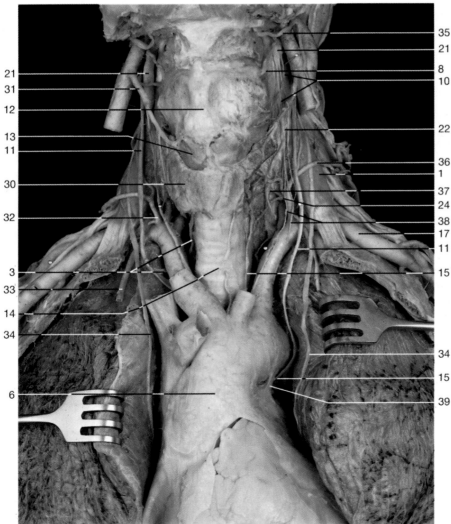

**Larynx and thoracic organs** (anterior aspect). Dissection of vagus and recurrent laryngeal nerves.

1  Scalenus anterior muscle
2  Scalenus medius and posterior muscles
3  Right recurrent laryngeal nerve
4  Right subclavian artery
5  Brachiocephalic trunk
6  Aortic arch
7  Hyoid bone
8  Internal branch of superior laryngeal nerve
9  Thyrohyoid membrane
10 External branch of superior laryngeal nerve
11 Vagus nerve
12 Thyroid cartilage
13 Cricothyroid muscle
14 Trachea
15 Left recurrent laryngeal nerve
16 Esophagus
17 Left subclavian artery
18 Left common carotid artery
19 Second rib
20 Tongue
21 Superior cervical ganglion
22 Sympathetic trunk
23 Inferior constrictor muscle of pharynx
24 Inferior thyroid artery
25 Glossopharyngeal nerve
26 Superior laryngeal nerve
27 Epiglottis
28 Posterior crico-arytenoid muscle and cricoid cartilage
29 Inferior laryngeal branch of recurrent laryngeal nerve
30 Thyroid gland
31 Superior thyroid artery
32 Thyrocervical trunk
33 Internal thoracic artery
34 Phrenic nerve
35 Hypoglossal nerve
36 Transverse cervical artery
37 Middle cervical ganglion
38 Middle cervical cardiac nerves (branches of sympathetic trunk)
39 Ligamentum arteriosum

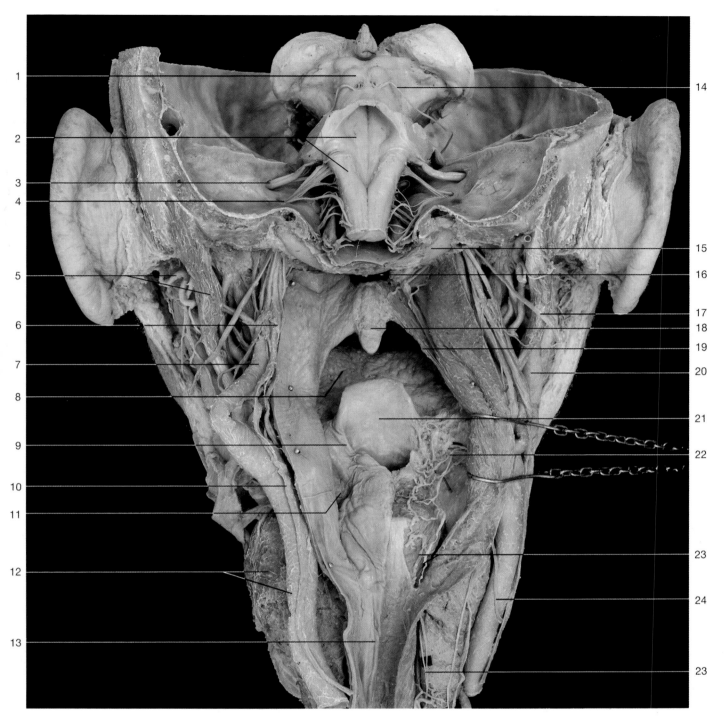

**Larynx and oral cavity** (posterior aspect). Mucous membrane on the right half of pharynx has been removed.

1   Midbrain (inferior colliculus)
2   Rhomboid fossa and medulla oblongata
3   Vestibulocochlear and facial nerve
4   Glossopharyngeal, vagus, and accessory nerves
5   Occipital artery and posterior belly of digastric muscle
6   Superior cervical ganglion
7   Internal carotid artery
8   Oral cavity (tongue)
9   Ary-epiglottic fold
10  Vagus nerve
11  Piriform recess
12  Thyroid gland and common carotid artery
13  Esophagus
14  Trochlear nerve
15  Occipital condyle
16  Nasal cavity (choana)
17  Accessory nerve
18  Uvula and soft palate
19  Palatopharyngeus muscle
20  External carotid artery
21  Epiglottis
22  Internal branch of superior laryngeal nerve
23  Inferior laryngeal nerve
24  Ansa cervicalis

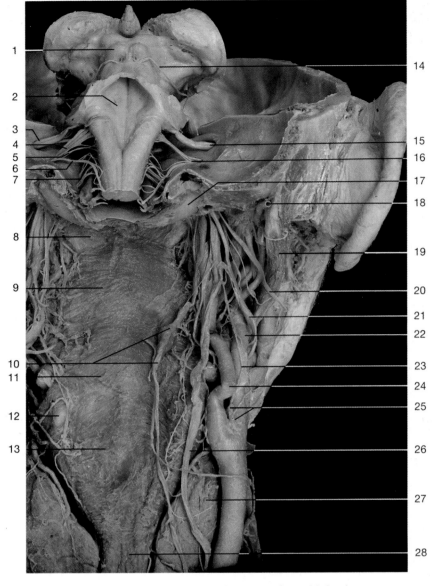

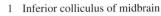

1   Inferior colliculus of midbrain
2   Facial colliculus in floor of rhomboid fossa
3   Vestibulocochlear and facial nerves
4   Glossopharyngeal nerve
5   Vagus nerve
6   Accessory nerve
7   Hypoglossal nerve
8   Pharyngobasilar fascia
9   Superior constrictor muscle of pharynx
10  Sympathetic trunk and superior cervical
    ganglion (medially displaced)
11  Middle constrictor muscle of pharynx
12  Greater cornu of hyoid bone
13  Inferior constrictor muscle of pharynx
14  Trochlear nerve
15  Internal acoustic meatus with facial and
    vestibulocochlear nerves
16  Jugular foramen with glossopharyngeal,
    vagus, and assessory nerves
17  Occipital condyle
18  Occipital artery
19  Posterior belly of digastric muscle
20  Accessory nerve (extracranial part)
21  Hypoglossal nerve (extracranial part)
22  External carotid artery
23  Carotid sinus nerve
24  Internal carotid artery
25  Carotid sinus and carotid body
26  Vagus nerve
27  Thyroid gland
28  Esophagus
29  Choanae
30  Medial pterygoid plate
31  Foramen lacerum
32  Pharyngeal tubercle
33  Hard palate
34  Greater and lesser palatine foramen
35  Pterygoid hamulus
36  Lateral pterygoid plate
37  Pterygoid canal
38  Foramen ovale
39  Mandibular fossa
40  Carotid canal
41  Styloid process and stylomastoid
    foramen

**Pharynx and parapharyngeal nerves in connection with brain stem**
(posterior aspect).

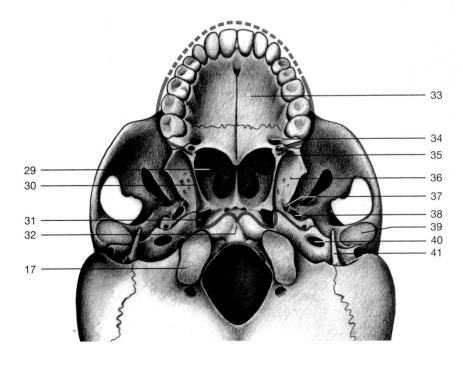

**Inferior aspect of the skull.**

Red line = outline of superior constrictor
muscle in continuation with buccinator
muscle and orbicularis oris muscle.
(Semischematic drawing.)

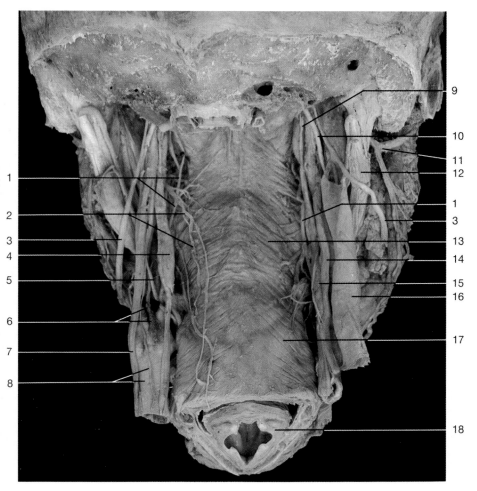

1 Ascending pharyngeal artery
2 Pharyngeal plexus
3 Accessory nerve
4 Superior cervical ganglion of
  sympathetic trunk
5 Superior laryngeal nerve
6 Carotid body and carotid sinus
  nerve
7 Left vagus nerve
8 Common carotid artery and cardiac
  branch of vagus nerve
9 Glossopharyngeal nerve
10 Hypoglossal nerve
11 Facial nerve
12 Posterior belly of digastric muscle
13 Middle constrictor muscle
   of pharynx
14 Right vagus nerve
15 Sympathetic trunk
16 Internal jugular vein
17 Inferior constrictor muscle
   of pharynx
18 Larynx
19 Buccinator muscle
20 Soft palate and palatine glands
21 Palatine tonsil
22 Uvula of palate
23 Pharynx (oral part)
24 Parotid gland
25 Longus capitis muscle
26 Median atlanto-axial joint and
   anterior arch of atlas
27 Dens of axis
28 Spinal cord
29 Dura mater
30 Incisive papilla
31 Oral vestibule
32 Masseter muscle
33 Mandible
34 Mandibular canal with vessels and
   nerve
35 Medial pterygoid muscle
36 External carotid artery
37 Internal carotid artery
38 Atlas
39 Vertebral artery
40 Splenius capitis muscle
41 Semispinalis capitis muscle

**Parapharyngeal nerves and vessels.** Dorsal aspect of the pharynx.

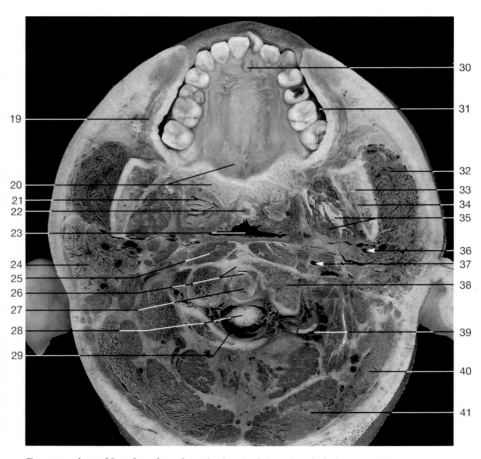

**Cross section of head and neck** at the level of the atlas (inferior aspect).

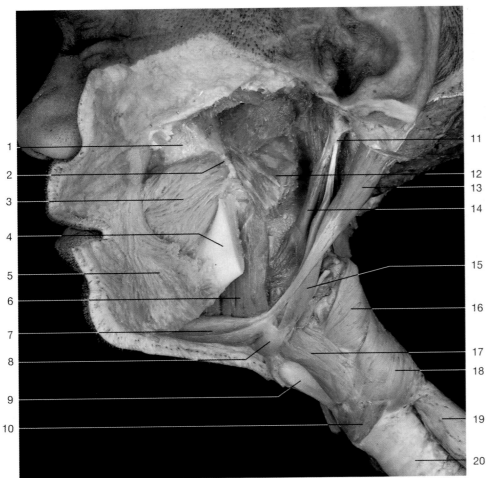

**Dissection of pharynx, supra-, and infrahyoid muscles I.** Mandible partly removed (lateral aspect).

1   Maxilla
2   Pterygomandibular raphe
3   Buccinator muscle
4   Mandible (divided)
5   Depressor anguli oris muscle
6   Mylohyoid muscle
7   Anterior belly of digastric muscle
8   Hyoid bone
9   Thyroid cartilage
10  Cricothyroid muscle
11  Styloid process
12  Medial pterygoid muscle (divided)
13  Posterior belly of digastric muscle
14  Styloglossus muscle
15  Stylohyoid muscle
16  Thyropharyngeal part of inferior constrictor muscle of pharynx
17  Thyrohyoid muscle
18  Cricopharyngeal part of inferior constrictor muscle of pharynx
19  Esophagus
20  Trachea
21  First molar of maxilla
22  Tongue
23  Inferior longitudinal muscle of tongue
24  Genioglossus muscle
25  Superior constrictor muscle of pharynx
26  Hypoglossal nerve
27  Hyoglossus muscle
28  Superior laryngeal nerve and superior laryngeal artery

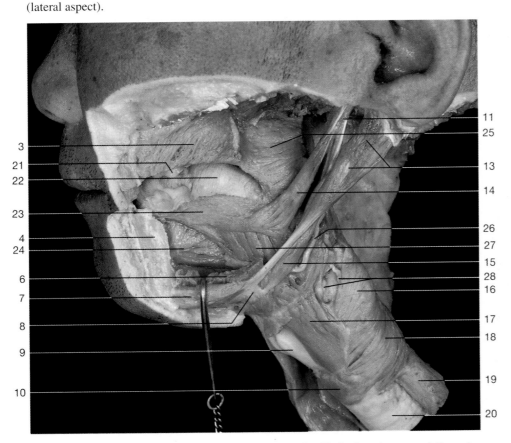

**Dissection of pharynx, supra-, and infrahyoid muscles II.** Oral cavity opened (lateral aspect).

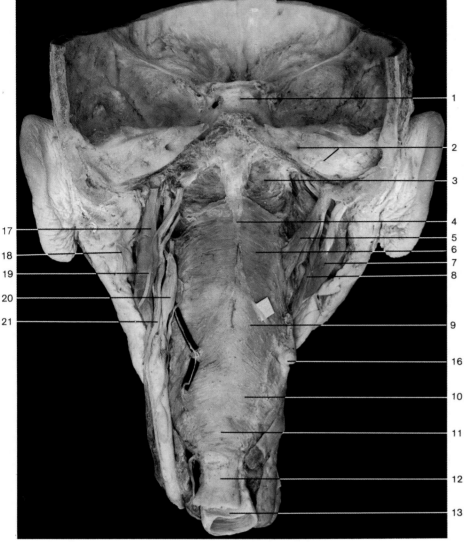

1   Sella turcica
2   Internal acoustic meatus and petrous part of temporal bone
3   Pharyngobasilar fascia
4   Fibrous raphe of pharynx
5   Stylopharyngeal muscle
6   Superior constrictor muscle of pharynx
7   Posterior belly of digastric muscle
8   Stylohyoid muscle
9   Middle constrictor muscle of pharynx
10  Inferior constrictor muscle of pharynx
11  Muscle-free area (Killian's triangle)
12  Esophagus
13  Trachea
14  Thyroid and parathyroid glands
15  Medial pterygoid muscle
16  Greater horn of hyoid bone
17  Internal jugular vein
18  Parotid gland
19  Accessory nerve
20  Superior cervical ganglion of sympathetic trunk
21  Vagus nerve
22  Laimer's triangle (area prone to developing diverticula)
23  Orbicularis oculi muscle
24  Nasal muscle
25  Levator labii superioris and levator labii alaeque nasi muscles
26  Levator anguli oris muscle
27  Orbicularis oris muscle
28  Buccinator muscle
29  Depressor labii inferioris muscle
30  Hyoglossus muscle
31  Thyrohyoid muscle
32  Thyroid cartilage
33  Cricothyroid muscle
34  Pterygomandibular raphe
35  Tensor veli palatini muscle
36  Levator veli palatini muscle
37  Depressor anguli oris muscle
38  Mentalis muscle
39  Styloglossus muscle

**Muscles of the pharynx** (posterior aspect).

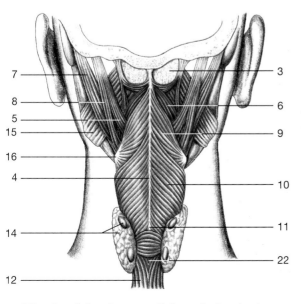

**Muscles of the pharynx.** (Schematic drawing.)

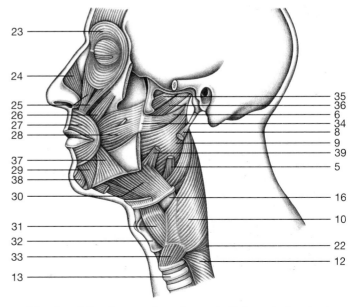

**Muscles of the pharynx** (lateral aspect). (Schematic drawing.)

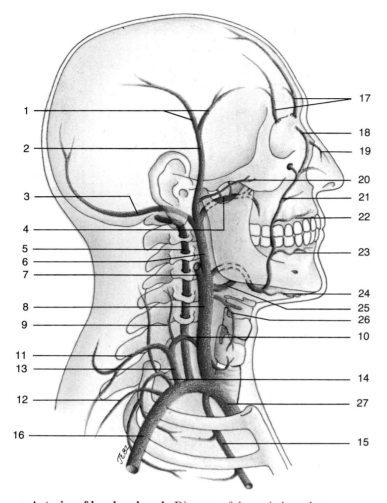

1   Frontal and parietal branches of superficial
    temporal artery
2   Superficial temporal artery
3   Occipital artery
4   Maxillary artery
5   Vertebral artery
6   External carotid artery
7   Internal carotid artery
8   Common carotid artery (divided)
9   Ascending cervical artery
10  Inferior thyroid artery
11  Transverse cervical artery with two branches
    (superficial cervical artery and descending
    scapular artery)
12  Suprascapular artery
13  Thyrocervical trunk
14  Costocervical trunk with two branches
    (deep cervical artery and superior intercostal artery)
15  Internal thoracic artery
16  Axillary artery
17  Supra-orbital and supratrochlear arteries
18  Angular artery
19  Dorsal nasal artery
20  Transverse facial artery
21  Facial artery
22  Superior labial artery
23  Inferior labial artery
24  Submental artery
25  Lingual artery
26  Superior thyroid artery
27  Brachiocephalic trunk

**Arteries of head and neck.** Diagram of the main branches
of external carotid and subclavian artery.

▷   **To page 169:**

1   Galea aponeurotica
2   Frontal branch  ⎫  of superficial
3   Parietal branch ⎭  temporal artery
4   Superior auricular muscle
5   Superficial temporal artery and vein
6   Middle temporal artery
7   Auriculotemporal nerve
8   Branches of facial nerve
9   Facial nerve
10  External carotid artery within the retromandibular fossa
11  Posterior belly of digastric muscle
12  Sternocleidomastoid artery
13  Sympathetic trunk and superior cervical ganglion
14  Sternocleidomastoid muscle (divided and reflected)
15  Clavicle (divided)
16  Transverse cervical artery
17  Ascending cervical artery and phrenic nerve
18  Scalenus anterior muscle
19  Suprascapular artery
20  Dorsal scapular artery

21  Brachial plexus and axillary artery
22  Thoraco-acromial artery
23  Lateral thoracic artery
24  Median nerve (displaced) and
    pectoralis minor muscle (reflected)
25  Frontal belly of occipitofrontalis muscle
26  Orbital part of orbicularis oculi muscle
27  Angular artery and vein
28  Facial artery
29  Superior labial artery
30  Zygomaticus major muscle
31  Inferior labial artery
32  Parotid duct
33  Buccal fat pad
34  Maxillary artery
35  Masseter muscle
36  Facial artery and mandible
37  Submental artery
38  Anterior belly of
    digastric muscle

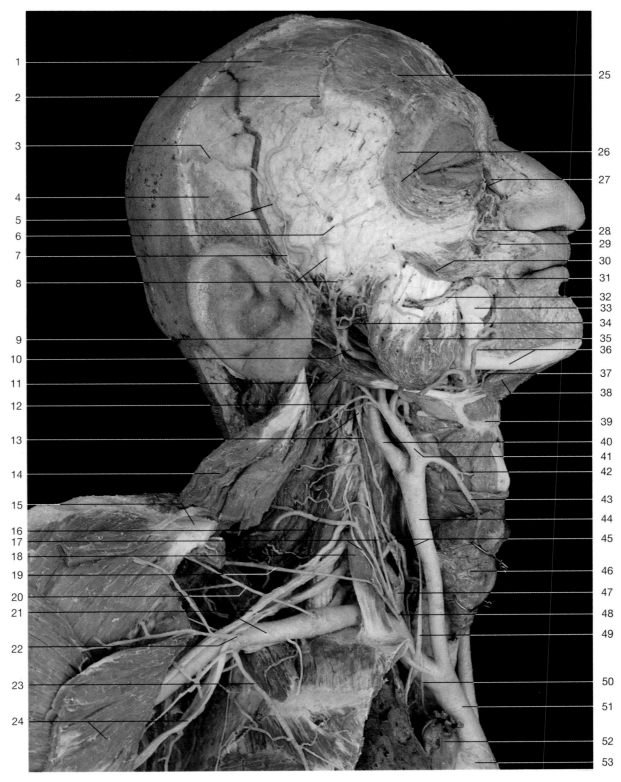

**Main branches of head and neck arteries** (lateral aspect). Anterior thoracic wall and clavicle partly removed; pectoralis muscles have been reflected to display the subclavian and axillary arteries.

39  Hyoid bone
40  Internal carotid artery
41  External carotid artery
42  Superior laryngeal artery
43  Superior thyroid artery
44  Common carotid artery
45  Thyroid ansa of sympathetic
    trunk and inferior thyroid artery

46  Thyroid gland (right lobe)
47  Vertebral artery
48  Thyrocervical trunk
49  Vagus nerve
50  Ansa subclavia of sympathetic trunk
51  Brachiocephalic trunk
52  Superior vena cava (divided)
53  Aortic arch

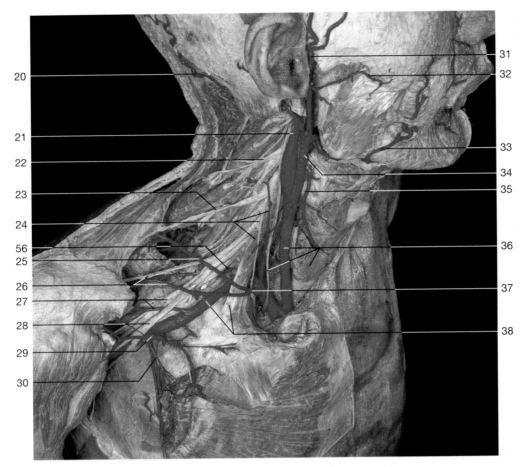

**Arteries of head and neck** (anterior-lateral aspect). Clavicle, sternocleidomastoid muscle and veins have been partly removed; the arteries were colored.

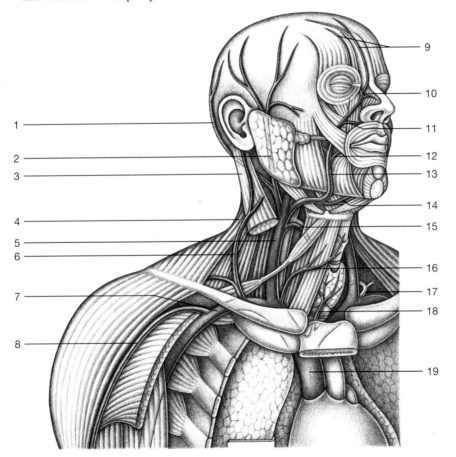

**Veins of head and neck.** Sternocleidomastoid muscle and anterior thoracic wall partly removed. Note the venous connection with the superior vena cava.

1　Occipital vein
2　Superficial temporal vein
3　Sternocleidomastoid muscle
4　Trapezius muscle
5　Internal jugular vein
6　External jugular vein
7　Subclavian vein
8　Cephalic vein
9　Supra-orbital veins
10　Angular vein
11　Superior labial vein
12　Inferior labial vein
13　Facial vein
14　Submental vein
15　Superior thyroid vein
16　Anterior jugular vein
17　Thoracic duct
18　Inferior thyroid vein
19　Superior vena cava
20　Occipital branch of occipital artery
21　Internal carotid artery
22　Cervical plexus
23　Supraclavicular nerve
24　Phrenic nerve and ascending cervical artery on scalenus anterior muscle
25　Superficial cervical artery
26　Suprascapular artery and nerve
27　Brachial plexus and anterior circumflex humeral artery
28　Lateral cord of brachial plexus
29　Thoraco-acromial artery
30　Lateral thoracic artery
31　Superficial temporal artery
32　Transverse facial artery
33　Facial artery
34　External carotid artery
35　Superior thyroid artery
36　Common carotid artery, vagus nerve, and thyroid gland
37　Thyrocervical trunk
38　Subclavian artery and scalenus anterior muscle
39　Parotid gland and facial nerve
40　Great auricular nerve
41　External jugular vein
42　Brachial plexus
43　Cephalic vein in deltopectoral groove
44　Axillary vein and artery
45　Right brachiocephalic vein
46　Superior vena cava
47　Right lung (reflected)
48　Superficial temporal artery and vein
49　Facial artery and vein
50　Cervical branch of facial nerve and submandibular gland
51　Internal jugular vein, common carotid artery, and omohyoid muscle
52　Anterior jugular vein and thyroid gland
53　Jugular venous arch
54　Left brachiocephalic vein
55　Pericardium of heart (location of right atrium)
56　Transverse cervical artery

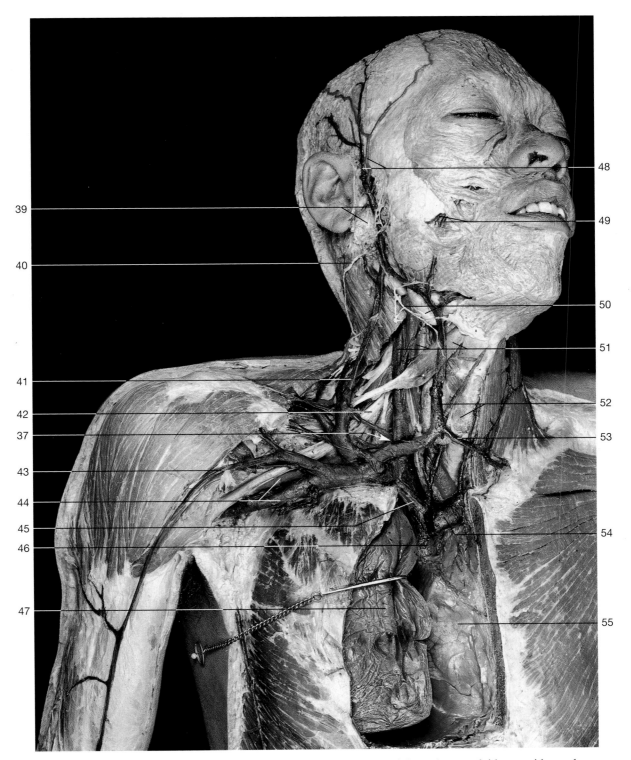

**Veins of head and neck** (anterior aspect). Part of the thoracic wall, clavicle, and sternocleidomastoid muscle have been removed. Veins were colored blue; arteries, red.

The **internal jugular vein** is the continuation of the sigmoid sinus, which drains most of the venous blood from the brain together with the external cerebrospinal fluid. By joining the subclavian vein it forms the right brachiocephalic vein, which continues on the right side directly into the superior vena cava. The common way to introduce the lead from a pacemaker device into the heart is by way of the cephalic vein. On the left side the thoracic duct joins the internal jugular vein at that point where the subclavian vein and the internal jugular vein form the left brachiocephalic vein. Note that the subclavian vein lies in front of the scalenus anterior muscle, whereas the subclavian artery together with the plexus brachialis lie posterior to that muscle. The cephalic vein joins the axillary vein by passing into the deltopectoral triangle. The subclavian vein is strongly fixed to the first rib, so that it can be punctured with a needle at that point (underneath the sternal end of the clavicle) to introduce a catheter (subclavian line).

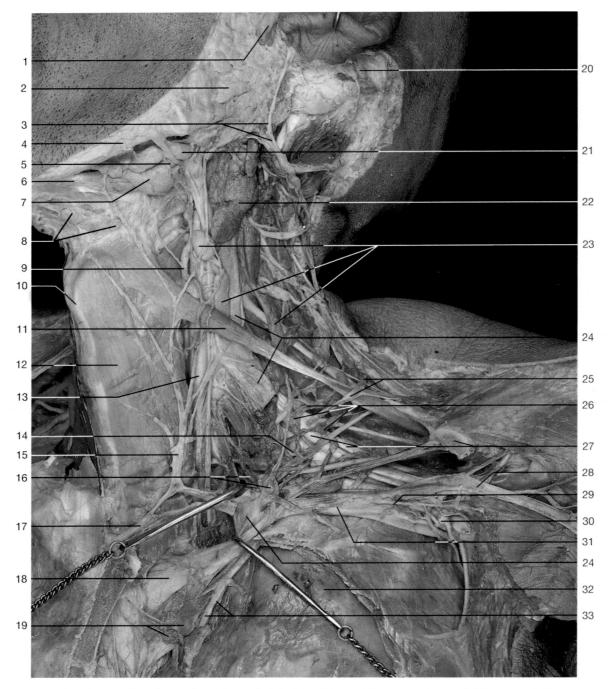

**Lymph nodes and lymph vessels of the neck,** left side oblique (oblique-lateral aspect). The sternocleido-mastoid muscle and the left half of the thoracic wall have been removed. Lower part of the internal jugular vein has been cut and laterally displaced to show the thoracic duct.

1 Superficial parotid lymph node
2 Parotid gland
3 Great auricular nerve
4 Mandible
5 Facial vein
6 Anterior belly of digastric muscle
7 Submandibular gland
8 Submental lymph nodes
9 Superior thyroid artery
10 Thyroid cartilage
11 Omohyoid muscle
12 Sternohyoid muscle

13 Common carotid artery
14 Supraclavicular lymph nodes
15 Anterior jugular vein
16 Thoracic duct and internal jugular vein
17 Jugular venous arch
18 Left brachiocephalic vein
19 Superior mediastinal lymph nodes
20 Retro-auricular lymph nodes
21 Submandibular nodes
22 Superficial cervical lymph nodes
23 Jugulodigastric lymph nodes and jugular
   trunk

24 Internal jugular vein
25 External jugular vein
26 Jugulo-omohyoid lymph nodes
27 Brachial plexus
28 Cephalic vein
29 Subclavian trunk
30 Infraclavicular lymph nodes
31 Subclavian vein
32 Lung
33 Internal thoracic artery and vein

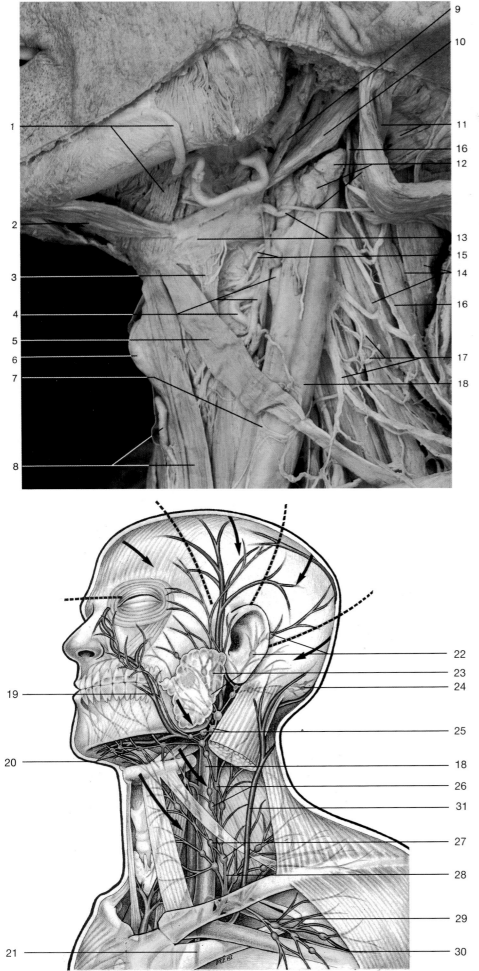

**Carotid triangle,** left side (lateral aspect). Sternocleidomastoid muscle reflected.

1  Mylohyoid muscle and facial artery
2  Anterior belly of digastric muscle
3  Thyrohyoid
4  External carotid artery, superior thyroid artery, and vein
5  Omohyoid muscle
6  Thyroid cartilage
7  Ansa cervicalis
8  Sternohyoid muscle and superior thyroid artery
9  Stylohyoid muscle
10  Posterior belly of digastric muscle
11  Sternocleidomastoid muscle (reflected)
12  Superior cervical lymph nodes and sternocleidomastoid artery
13  Hyoid bone and hypoglossal nerve (n. XII)
14  Splenius capitis and levator scapulae muscles
15  Superior laryngeal artery and internal branch of superior laryngeal nerve
16  Accessory nerve
17  Cervical plexus
18  Internal jugular vein
19  Facial vein
20  Submental nodes
21  Thoracic duct
22  Retro-auricular nodes
23  Parotid nodes
24  Occipital nodes
25  Submandibular nodes
26  Jugulodigastric nodes    ⎤ deep cervical
27  Jugulo-omohyoid nodes    ⎦ nodes
28  Jugular trunk
29  Subclavian trunk
30  Infraclavicular nodes
31  External jugular vein

**Lymph nodes and veins of head and neck.** Dotted lines = border between irrigation areas; arrows: direction of lymph flow.

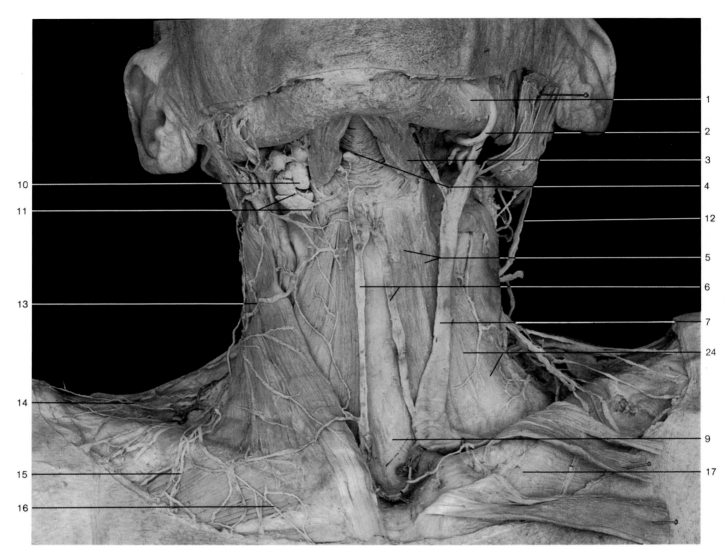

**Neck** (anterior aspect). The superficial fascia has been removed.

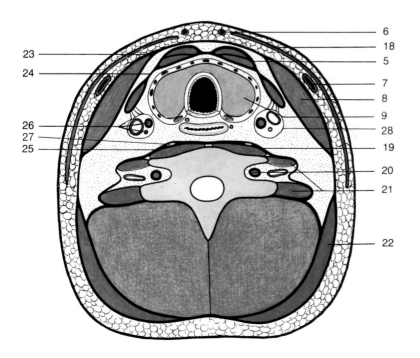

| | |
|---|---|
| 1 | Mandible |
| 2 | Facial artery and vein |
| 3 | Anterior belly of digastric muscle |
| 4 | Mylohyoid muscle |
| 5 | Infrahyoid muscles (sternohyoid, sternothyroid, and omohyoid) |
| 6 | Anterior jugular veins |
| 7 | External jugular vein |
| 8 | Sternocleidomastoid muscle |
| 9 | Thyroid gland |
| 10 | Submandibular gland |
| 11 | Cervical branch of facial nerve |
| 12 | Great auricular nerve |
| 13 | Transverse cervical nerves |
| 14 | Lateral supraclavicular nerves |
| 15 | Middle supraclavicular nerves |
| 16 | Medial supraclavicular nerves |
| 17 | Clavicle |
| 18 | Platysma muscle |
| 19 | Prevertebral lamina of cervical fascia, covering longus colli muscle |
| 20 | Vertebral artery and vein |
| 21 | Scalenus muscles |
| 22 | Trapezius muscle |
| 23 | Superficial lamina of cervical fascia |
| 24 | Pretracheal lamina of cervical fascia |
| 25 | Prevertebral lamina of cervical fascia |
| 26 | Carotid sheath with common carotid artery, internal jugular vein, and vagus nerve |
| 27 | Cervical part of sympathetic trunk |
| 28 | Carotid sheath |

Cutaneous branches of cervical plexus (12, 13, 14, 15, 16)

◁ **Cross section of the neck** at the level of the thyroid gland. Notice the position of the three laminae of cervical fascia (23, 24, 25).

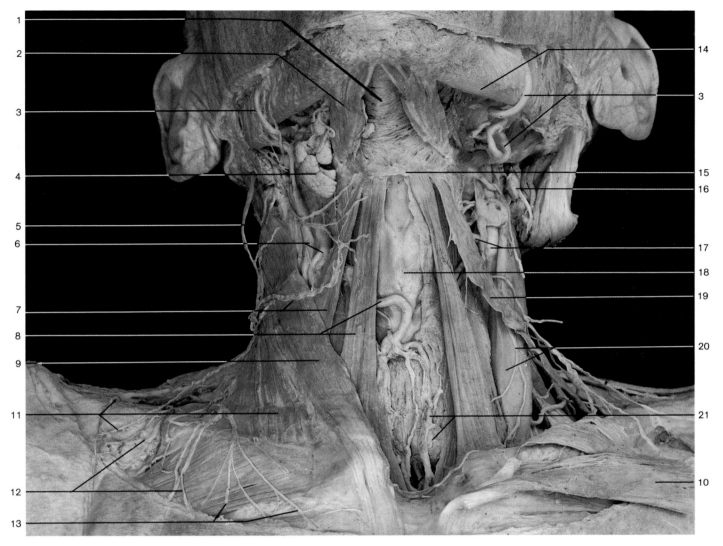

**Anterior triangle** (anterior aspect). The pretracheal lamina of cervical fascia and left sternocleidomastoid muscle have been removed.

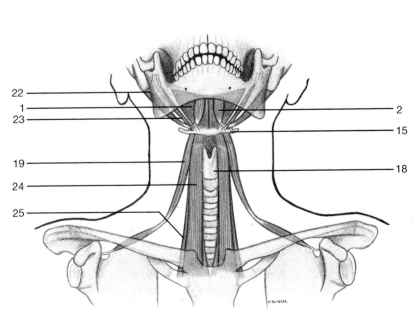

**Supra- and infrahyoid muscles** (schematic drawing).

1  Mylohyoid muscle
2  Anterior belly of digastric muscle
3  Facial artery
4  Submandibular gland
5  Great auricular nerve
6  Internal jugular vein and common carotid artery
7  Transverse cervical nerve and omohyoid muscle
8  Sternohyoid muscle and superior thyroid artery
9  Sternocleidomastoid muscle (sternal head)
10  Left sternocleidomastoid muscle (reflected)
11  Sternocleidomastoid muscle (clavicular head)
     and lateral supraclavicular nerves
12  Middle supraclavicular nerves
13  Medial supraclavicular nerves
14  Mandible
15  Hyoid bone
16  Superficial cervical lymph nodes
17  Left superior thyroid artery and external carotid
     artery
18  Thyroid cartilage
19  Omohyoid muscle (superior belly)
20  Internal jugular vein and branches of ansa
     cervicalis
21  Thyroid gland and unpaired inferior thyroid vein
22  Posterior belly of digastric muscle
23  Stylohyoid muscle
24  Sternohyoid muscle
25  Sternothyroid muscle

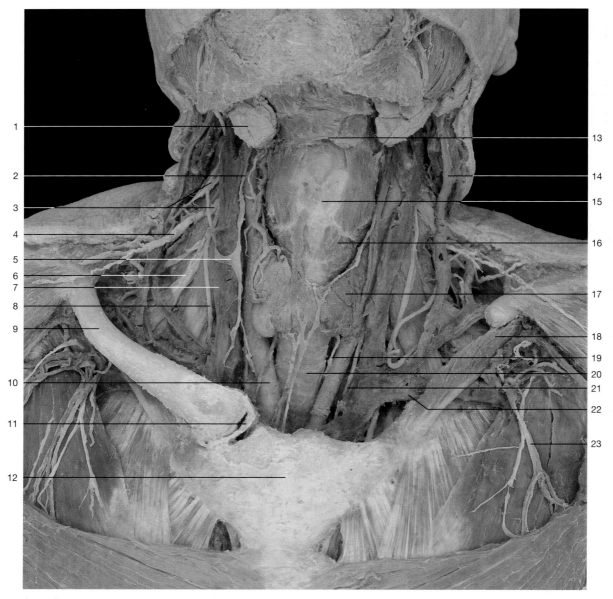

| | | | | |
|---|---|---|---|---|
| 1 | | | 13 |
| 2 | | | 14 |
| 3 | | | 15 |
| 4 | | | 16 |
| 5 | | | |
| 6 | | | 17 |
| 7 | | | |
| 8 | | | |
| 9 | | | 18 |
| | | | 19 |
| | | | 20 |
| 10 | | | 21 |
| | | | 22 |
| 11 | | | 23 |
| 12 | | | |

**Anterior region of the neck.** Sternocleidomastoid muscles and left clavicle have been removed. Thyroid gland in relation to trachea, larynx, and vessels of the neck is shown.

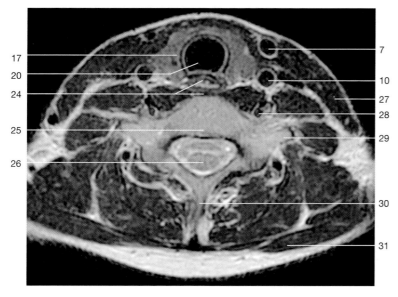

| | | |
|---|---|---|
| 17 | | 7 |
| 20 | | 10 |
| 24 | | 27 |
| | | 28 |
| 25 | | 29 |
| 26 | | |
| | | 30 |
| | | 31 |

**Cross section of the neck** at the level of the thyroid gland (MRI scan, courtesy of Prof. Dr. A. Heuck, Munich).

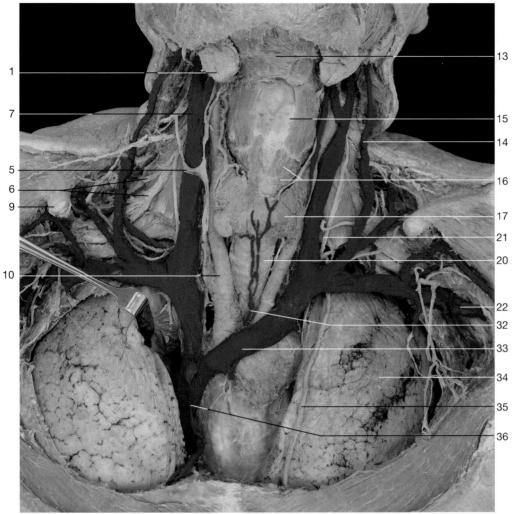

1  Submandibular gland
2  Cervical branch of facial nerve (n. VII)
3  Cervical plexus
4  Middle supraclavicular nerves
5  Ansa cervicalis
6  Brachial plexus
7  Internal jugular vein
8  Phrenic nerve
9  Clavicle
10  Common carotid artery
11  Sternoclavicular articulation with articular disc
12  Manubrium of sternum
13  Hyoid bone
14  External jugular vein
15  Thyroid cartilage
16  Cricothyroid muscle
17  Thyroid gland
18  Subclavius muscle
19  Recurrent laryngeal nerve
20  Trachea
21  Vagus nerve (n. X)
22  Subclavian vein
23  Middle pectoral nerve
24  Esophagus
25  Body of cervical vertebra
26  Spinal cord
27  Sternocleidomastoid muscle
28  Vertebral artery
29  Transverse process of cervical vertebra
30  Spinous process of cervical vertebra
31  Trapezius muscle
32  Inferior thyroid veins
33  Left brachiocephalic vein
34  Superior lobe of left lung
35  Internal thoracic artery
36  Superior vena cava
37  Superior thyroid artery
38  Inferior thyroid artery
39  Thyrocervical trunk
40  Subclavian artery
41  Aortic arch

**Anterior region of neck and thoracic cavity.** Both clavicles, sternum, and ribs have been removed. Main veins are colored in blue.

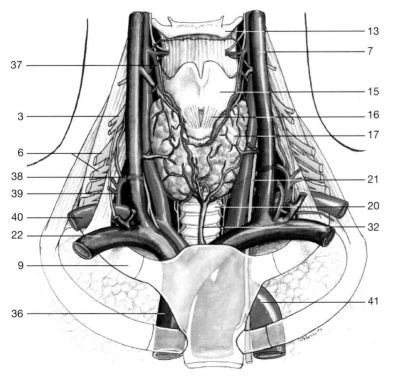

**Anterior region of the neck** (schematic drawing). Regional anatomy of the thyroid gland with related blood vessels.

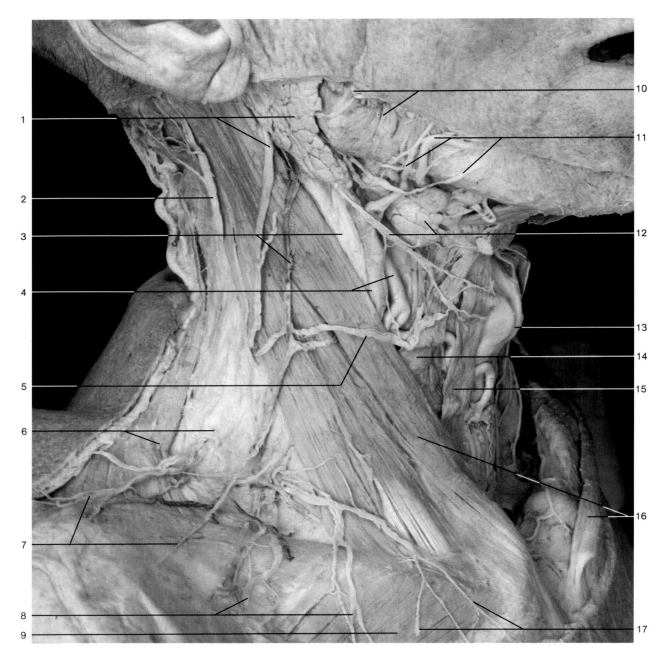

**Posterior and carotid triangles** (lateral aspect). Superficial dissection.

1  Parotid gland and great auricular nerve
2  Lesser occipital nerve
3  Internal and external jugular veins
4  Retromandibular vein and external carotid artery
5  Transverse cervical nerve with communicating branch to cervical branch of facial nerve
6  Trapezius muscle and superficial lamina of cervical fascia
7  Lateral supraclavicular nerves
8  Middle supraclavicular nerves
9  Pectoralis major muscle
10  Buccal branch of facial nerve and masseter muscle
11  Facial artery and vein and mandibular branch of facial nerve
12  Cervical branch of facial nerve and submandibular gland
13  Thyroid cartilage
14  Omohyoid muscle
15  Sternohyoid muscle
16  Sternocleidomastoid muscle
17  Medial supraclavicular nerves
18  Mandibular branch of facial nerve
19  Cervical branch of facial nerve with communicating branch to transverse cervical nerve

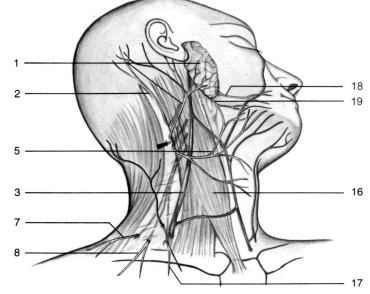

**Cutaneous branches of cervical plexus.** Erb's point is indicated by an arrowhead (schematic diagram).

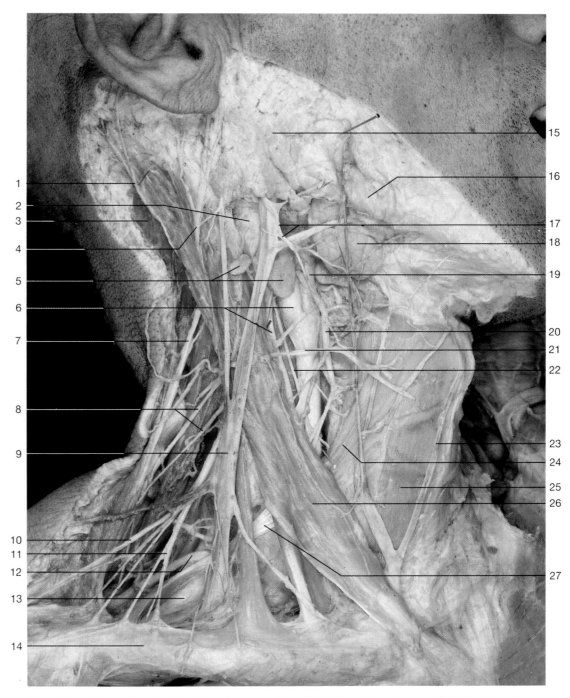

**Posterior and carotid triangles** (lateral aspect). Superficial dissection. The superficial lamina of cervical fascia has been removed to display the cutaneous branches of the cervical plexus and subcutaneous veins.

| | |
|---|---|
| 1 Lesser occipital nerve | 15 Parotid gland |
| 2 Internal jugular vein | 16 Mandible |
| 3 Splenius capitis muscle | 17 Cervical branch of facial nerve |
| 4 Great auricular nerve | 18 Submandibular gland |
| 5 Submandibular nodes | 19 External carotid artery |
| 6 Internal carotid artery and vagus nerve | 20 Superior thyroid artery |
| 7 Accessory nerve | 21 Transverse cervical nerve |
| 8 Muscular branches of cervical plexus | 22 Superior root of ansa cervicalis |
| 9 External jugular vein | 23 Anterior jugular vein |
| 10 Posterior supraclavicular nerves | 24 Omohyoid muscle |
| 11 Middle supraclavicular nerves | 25 Sternohyoid muscle |
| 12 Suprascapular artery | 26 Sternocleidomastoid muscle |
| 13 Pretracheal lamina of fascia of neck | 27 Intermediate tendon of omohyoid muscle |
| 14 Clavicle | |

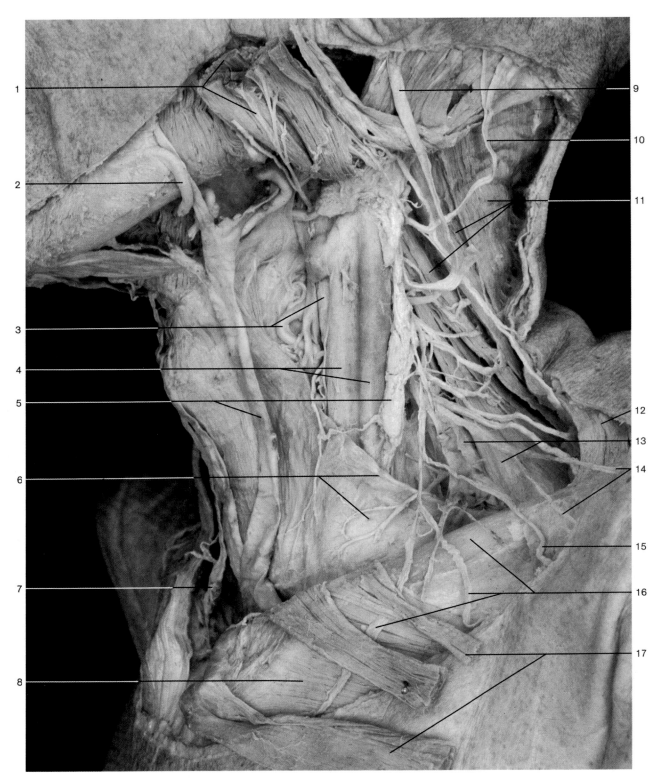

**Neck,** superficial dissection (lateral aspect). Sternocleidomastoid muscle has been cut and reflected to display the pretracheal lamina of the cervical fascia.

1 Sternocleidomastoid muscle (reflected) and
   branch of accessory nerve
2 Facial artery
3 External carotid artery and superior thyroid artery
4 Internal jugular vein
5 Deep cervical lymph nodes and external jugular vein
6 Omohyoid muscle and pretracheal lamina of cervical fascia
7 Anterior jugular vein
8 Pectoralis major muscle

9 Great auricular nerve
10 Lesser occipital nerve
11 Splenius capitis and levator scapulae muscles
12 Trapezius muscle
13 Scalenus medius muscle and brachial plexus
14 Posterior supraclavicular nerves
15 Middle supraclavicular nerve
16 Clavicle and anterior supraclavicular nerves
17 Sternocleidomastoid muscle (reflected)

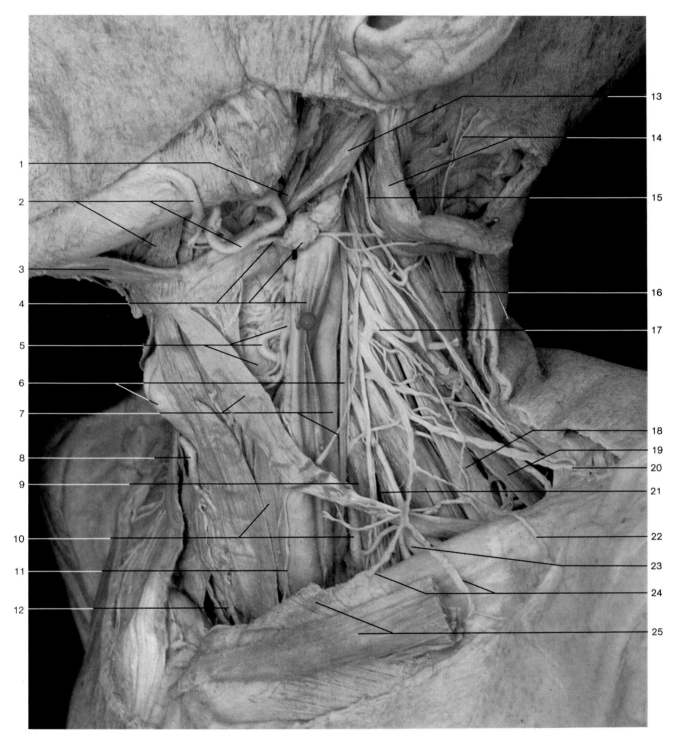

**Neck,** deep dissection (lateral aspect). The internal jugular vein has been reflected to expose the carotid artery and vagus nerve.

| | |
|---|---|
| 1 Stylohyoid muscle | 13 Posterior belly of digastric muscle |
| 2 Facial artery and mylohyoid muscle | 14 Sternocleidomastoid muscle and lesser occipital nerve |
| 3 Anterior belly of digastric muscle | 15 Accessory nerve |
| 4 Internal jugular vein, hypoglossal nerve, and superficial cervical lymph nodes | 16 Splenius capitis muscle |
| 5 Superior thyroid artery and vein and inferior pharyngeal constrictor muscle | 17 Cervical plexus |
| 6 Thyroid cartilage and vagus nerve | 18 Scalenus posterior muscle |
| 7 Ansa cervicalis, omohyoid muscle, and common carotid artery | 19 Levator scapulae muscle |
| 8 Right superior thyroid artery | 20 Posterior supraclavicular nerves |
| 9 Scalenus anterior muscle | 21 Phrenic nerve |
| 10 Sternothyroid muscle and inferior thyroid artery | 22 Middle supraclavicular nerve |
| 11 Muscular branches of ansa cervicalis to the infrahyoid muscles | 23 Brachial plexus |
| 12 Inferior thyroid vein | 24 Anterior supraclavicular nerves |
| | 25 Sternocleidomastoid muscle |

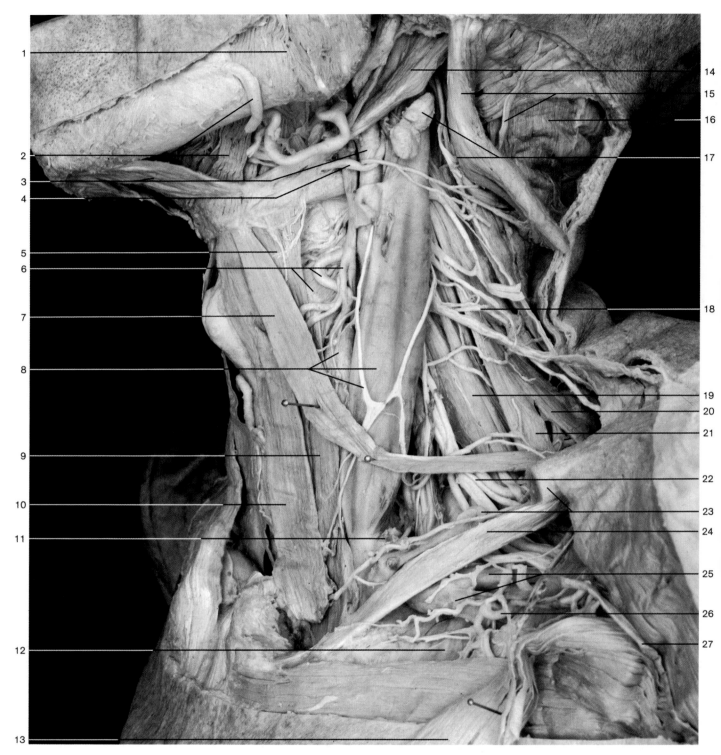

**Neck,** deeper dissection (lateral aspect). **Ansa cervicalis.** The cervical fascia and the clavicle are partly removed. Ansa cervicalis and infrahyoid muscles are displayed.

| | | |
|---|---|---|
| 1 | Masseter muscle | 9 Sternothyroid muscle |
| 2 | Mylohyoid muscle and facial artery | 10 Sternohyoid muscle |
| 3 | External carotid artery and anterior belly of digastric muscle | 11 Thoracic duct |
| 4 | Hypoglossal nerve | 12 Pectoralis minor muscle |
| 5 | Thyrohyoid muscle | 13 Pectoralis major muscle |
| 6 | Superior thyroid artery and vein and inferior pharyngeal constrictor muscle | 14 Posterior belly of digastric muscle |
| 7 | Omohyoid muscle (superior belly) | 15 Sternocleidomastoid muscle and lesser occipital nerve |
| 8 | Ansa cervicalis, thyroid gland, and internal jugular vein | 16 Splenius capitis muscle |

1 Masseter muscle
2 Mylohyoid muscle and facial artery
3 External carotid artery and
anterior belly of digastric muscle
4 Hypoglossal nerve
5 Thyrohyoid muscle
6 Superior thyroid artery and vein and
inferior pharyngeal constrictor muscle
7 Omohyoid muscle (superior belly)
8 Ansa cervicalis, thyroid gland, and
internal jugular vein

9 Sternothyroid muscle
10 Sternohyoid muscle
11 Thoracic duct
12 Pectoralis minor muscle
13 Pectoralis major muscle
14 Posterior belly of digastric muscle
15 Sternocleidomastoid muscle and lesser
occipital nerve
16 Splenius capitis muscle
17 Superficial cervical lymph nodes and
accessory nerve

18 Cervical plexus
19 Scalenus medius muscle
20 Levator scapulae muscle
21 Scalenus posterior muscle
22 Brachial plexus
23 Transverse cervical artery and
clavicle
24 Subclavius muscle
25 Subclavian artery and vein
26 Thoraco-acromial artery
27 Cephalic vein

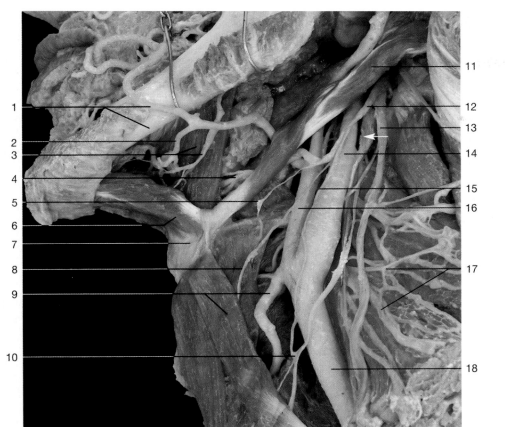

1  Facial artery and mandible
2  Submental artery
3  Mylohyoid muscle and nerve
4  Hypoglossal nerve
   (lingual branches)
5  Thyrohyoid branch of hypoglossal
   nerve (n. XII)
6  Anterior belly of digastric muscle
7  Hyoid bone
8  Omohyoid branch of hypoglossal
   nerve (n. XII)
9  Omohyoid muscle and superior
   thyroid artery
10 Ansa cervicalis
11 Posterior belly of digastric muscle
12 Hypoglossal nerve (n. XII)
13 Vagus nerve (n. X)
14 Internal carotid artery
15 Superior root of ansa cervicalis
16 External carotid artery
17 Cervical plexus
18 Common carotid artery

**Neck, submandibular region** (lateral aspect). **Hypoglossal nerve** (n. XII). Mandible slightly elevated. Arrow = superior cervical ganglion.

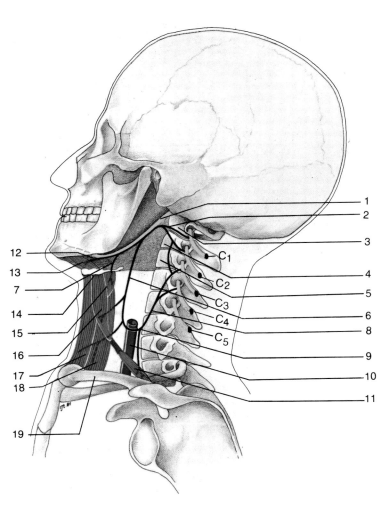

1  Hypoglossal nerve (n. XII)
2  Communication from the ventral ramus
   of the first cervical spinal nerve
3  Atlas
4  Axis
5  Third cervical vertebra
6  Superior root of ansa cervicalis
7  Thyrohyoid branch of hypoglossal nerve
8  Inferior root of ansa cervicalis
9  Ansa cervicalis
10 Internal jugular vein
11 Inferior belly of omohyoid muscle
12 Geniohyoid branch of hypoglossal nerve
13 Geniohyoid muscle
14 Hyoid bone
15 Thyrohyoid muscle
16 Superior belly of omohyoid muscle
17 Sternohyoid muscle
18 Sternothyroid muscle
19 Clavicle

**Ansa cervicalis. Innervation of infrahyoid muscles.**
Cervical plexus and its communication with the hypoglossal nerve.
$C_1$–$C_4$ = ventral rami of cervical spinal nerves of the first four segments.

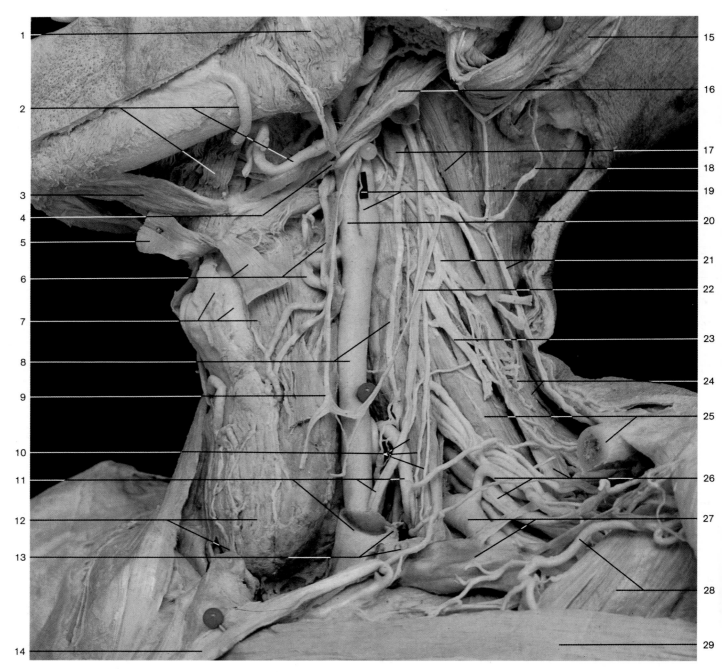

**Neck,** deep dissection (lateral aspect). Clavicle partly removed to show the slit between the scalenus muscles. Internal jugular vein removed.

| | | |
|---|---|---|
| 1 Masseter muscle | 11 Inferior thyroid artery, vagus nerve, and internal jugular vein (cut) | 21 Cervical plexus and accessory nerve |
| 2 Mylohyoid muscle and facial artery | | 22 Inferior root of ansa cervicalis |
| 3 Anterior belly of digastric muscle | 12 Thyroid gland and unpaired inferior thyroid venous plexus | 23 Supraclavicular nerve |
| 4 Hypoglossal nerve | | 24 Levator scapulae muscle |
| 5 Sternohyoid muscle | 13 Thoracic duct and left subclavian trunk | 25 Scalenus medius muscle and clavicle |
| 6 Omohyoid muscle, superior thyroid artery and vein | 14 Subclavius muscle (reflected) | 26 Transverse cervical artery, brachial plexus, and scalenus posterior muscle |
| 7 Sternothyroid muscle, thyroid cartilage, and pyramidal lobe of thyroid gland | 15 Sternocleidomastoid muscle (reflected) | |
| | 16 Posterior belly of digastric muscle | 27 Subclavian artery and vein |
| 8 Common carotid artery and sympathetic trunk | 17 Superior cervical ganglion and splenius muscle | 28 Thoraco-acromial artery and pectoralis minor muscle |
| 9 Ansa cervicalis | 18 Lesser occipital nerve | 29 Pectoralis major muscle |
| 10 Phrenic nerve, ascending cervical artery, and anterior scalenus muscle | 19 Internal carotid artery and branch of the glossopharyngeal nerve to the carotid body | |
| | 20 External carotid artery | |

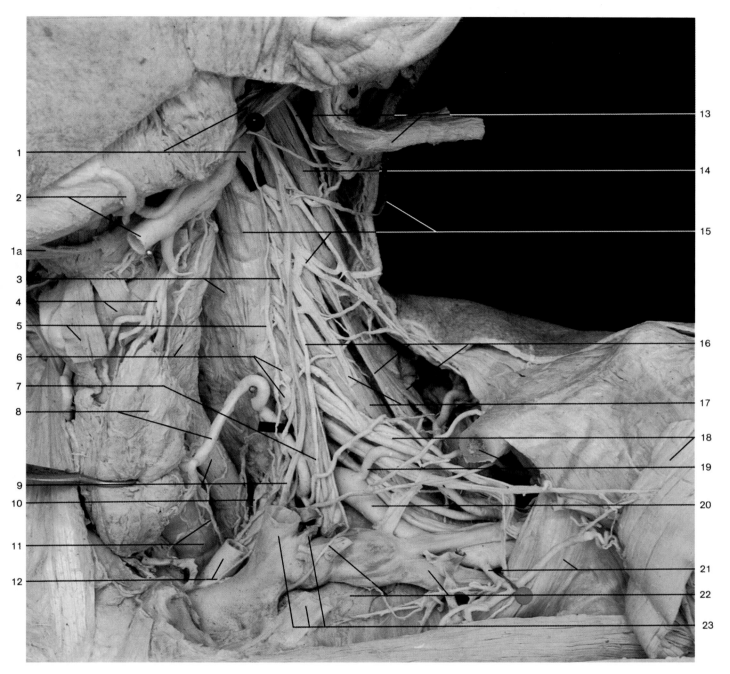

**Neck,** deepest dissection (anterolateral aspect). Thyroid gland reflected to expose the esophagus and the recurrent laryngeal nerve.

1  Superior cervical ganglion of sympathetic trunk and posterior belly of digastric muscle
1a Anterior belly of digastric muscle
2  Facial artery and common carotid artery (reflected anteriorly)
3  Ascending cervical artery and longus colli muscle
4  Omohyoid muscle and superior thyroid artery
5  Sympathetic trunk and sternohyoid muscle
6  Middle cervical ganglion and inferior pharyngeal constrictor muscle
7  Scalenus anterior muscle and phrenic nerve
8  Thyroid gland and inferior thyroid artery
9  Vagus nerve and esophagus
10 Stellate ganglion
11 Recurrent laryngeal nerve and trachea

12 Common carotid artery and cervical cardiac branch of vagus nerve
13 Sternocleidomastoid muscle and accessory nerve
14 Splenius capitis muscle
15 Lesser occipital nerve, longus capitis muscle, and cervical plexus
16 Phrenic nerve, scalenus posterior muscle, and levator scapulae muscle
17 Supraclavicular nerves and scalenus medius muscle
18 Brachial plexus and pectoralis major muscle (clavicular head)
19 Transverse cervical artery and clavicle
20 Subclavian artery
21 Thoraco-acromial artery and pectoralis minor muscle
22 First rib, accessory phrenic nerve, and subclavian vein
23 Internal jugular vein, thoracic duct, and subclavius muscle

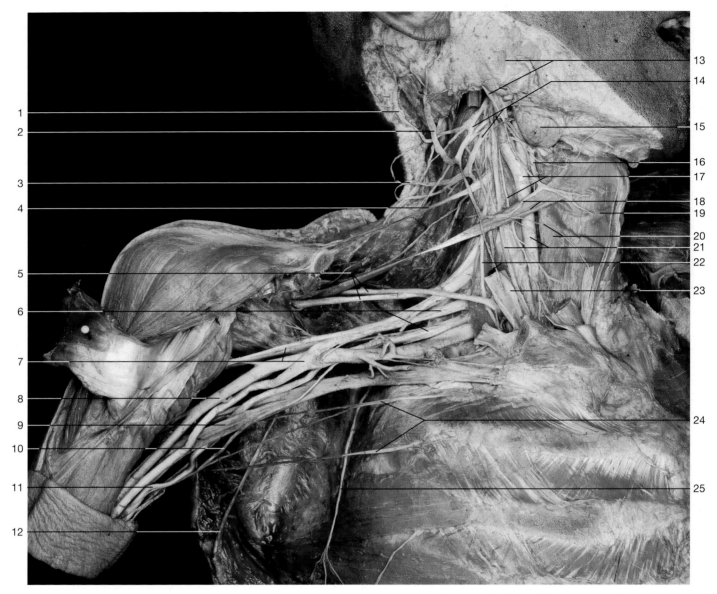

**Neck and arm,** deepest dissection (anterior-lateral aspect). Cervical and brachial plexus and their relation to the blood vessels are shown. Note the location and content of scalene triangle. Sternocleidomastoid muscle and clavicle have been removed; the internal jugular vein was divided to display the roots of cervical and brachial plexus.

| | |
|---|---|
| 1 Lesser occipital nerve | 15 Submandibular gland |
| 2 Great auricular nerve | 16 Superior thyroid artery |
| 3 Cutaneous branches of cervical plexus | 17 Common carotid artery dividing in internal and external |
| 4 Supraclavicular nerve | carotid artery and superior root of ansa cervicalis |
| 5 Suprascapular nerve and artery | 18 Omohyoid muscle and cervical branch of facial nerve |
| 6 Brachial plexus | joining the transverse cervical nerve (C$_2$, C$_3$) |
| 7 Median nerve (with two roots) and musculocutaneous nerve | 19 Sternohyoid muscle |
| 8 Axillary artery | 20 Transverse cervical nerve and sternothyroid muscle |
| 9 Axillary vein | 21 Common carotid artery and vagus nerve |
| 10 Medial brachial cutaneous nerve | 22 Phrenic nerve and scalenus anterior muscle |
| 11 Ulnar nerve | 23 Internal jugular vein |
| 12 Thoracodorsal nerve | 24 Intercostobrachial nerves |
| 13 Parotid gland and facial nerve (cervical branch) | 25 Long thoracic nerve |
| 14 Cervical plexus | |

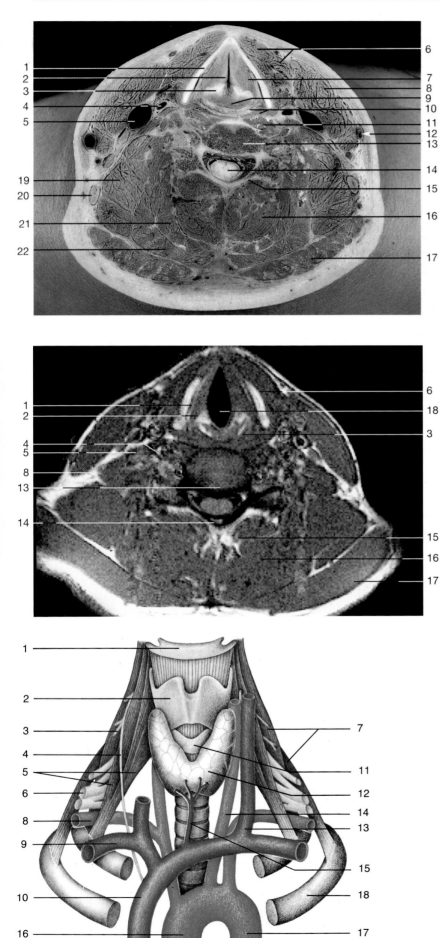

◁ **Horizontal section through the neck** at the level of the fissure of glottis, viewed from above.

1   Thyroid cartilage
2   Vocal fold and glottis (rima glottidis)
3   Arytenoid cartilage
4   Common carotid artery
5   Internal jugular vein
6   Infrahyoid muscles
7   Lateral thyro-arytenoid muscle
8   Sternocleidomastoid muscle
9   Transverse arytenoid muscle
10  Laryngopharynx and inferior constrictor muscle of pharynx
11  Longus colli muscle
12  External jugular vein
13  Body of cervical vertebra ($C_5$)
14  Spinal cord
15  Vertebra arch
16  Deep muscles of neck (semispinalis cervicis muscle)
17  Trapezius muscle
18  Rima glottidis
19  Levator scapulae muscle
20  Lymph node
21  Semispinalis capitis muscle
22  Splenius capitis muscle

◁ **Section through the neck at the level of larynx.** (MRI scan.)

**Scalene triangle, arrangements of blood vessels, and brachial plexus at the lower part of the neck** (schematic diagram).

1   Hyoid bone
2   Thyroid cartilage
3   Cervical plexus ($C_1$–$C_4$)
4   Phrenic nerve ($C_4$)
5   Scalenus anterior muscle
6   Brachial plexus ($C_5$–$T_1$)
7   Scalenus medius and posterior muscles
8   Subclavian artery
9   Subclavian vein
10  Superior vena cava
11  Cricoid cartilage
12  Thyroid gland
13  Internal jugular vein
14  Common carotid artery
15  Inferior thyroid vein
16  Ascending aorta
17  Descending aorta
18  Second rib

# 3 Trunk

**Median sagittal section through the vertebral column, head, and thorax of the adult.**

**Skeleton of the trunk,** vertebral column, thorax, and pelvis (posterior aspect).

| | | | |
|---|---|---|---|
| 1 | Atlas | 14 | Twelfth rib |
| 2 | Axis | 15 | Lumbar vertebrae |
| 3 | Seventh cervical vertebra (vertebra prominens) | 16 | Sacral promontory |
| 4 | Vertebral canal | 17 | Hip bone |
| 5 | First rib | 18 | Pubic symphysis |
| 6 | Clavicle | 19 | Sacrum |
| 7 | Manubrium sterni | 20 | Obturator foramen |
| 8 | Body of sternum | 21 | Acetabulum |
| 9 | Costal arch | 22 | Scapula with coracoid process |
| 10 | Acromion | 23 | Posterior superior iliac spine |
| 11 | Spine of scapula | 24 | Posterior inferior iliac spine |
| 12 | Glenoid cavity (lateral angle of scapula) | 25 | Ischial spine |
| 13 | Eleventh rib | 26 | Ischial tuberosity |

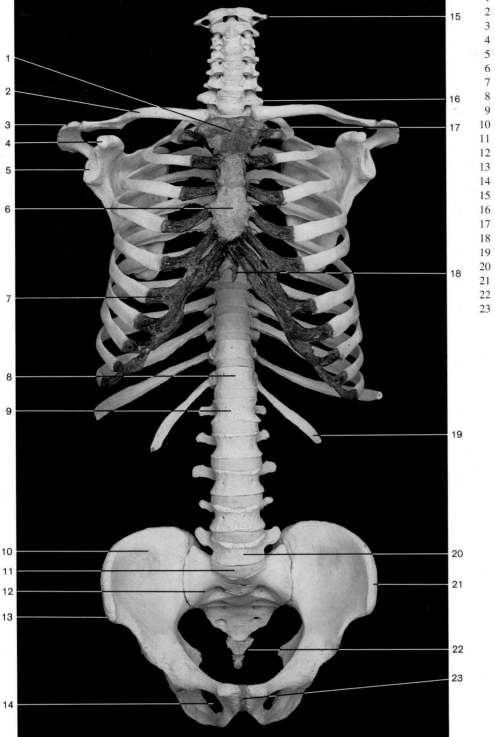

1 Manubrium sterni
2 Clavicle
3 Acromion
4 Coracoid process
5 Glenoid cavity
6 Body of sternum
7 Costal cartilage
8 Body of the twelfth thoracic vertebra
9 Body of the first lumbar vertebra
10 Hip bone
11 Sacral promontory
12 Sacrum
13 Anterior superior iliac spine
14 Obturator foramen
15 Atlas
16 Seventh cervical vertebra
17 First rib
18 Xiphoid process
19 Twelfth rib
20 Body of the fifth lumbar vertebra
21 Iliac crest
22 Coccyx
23 Pubic symphysis

**Skeleton of the trunk,** vertebral column, pelvis, thorax, and shoulder girdle (anterior aspect).

The trunk is divided into segments best visible in the thoracic region, where each segment consists of a pair of ribs connected anteriorly by the sternum and posteriorly by a thoracic vertebra. In the lumbar part of the vertebral column, only vestiges of ribs are present, they form what appear to be the transverse processes. In cervical vertebrae, remnants of ribs are part of the transverse processes. Each segment also comprises muscles (e.g., intercostal muscles), nerves, and vessels. However, in the cervical and lumbar region the muscular segments fuse with each other, forming large muscle plates, for example, the oblique muscles of the abdomen, while vessels and nerves still retain their segmental pattern.

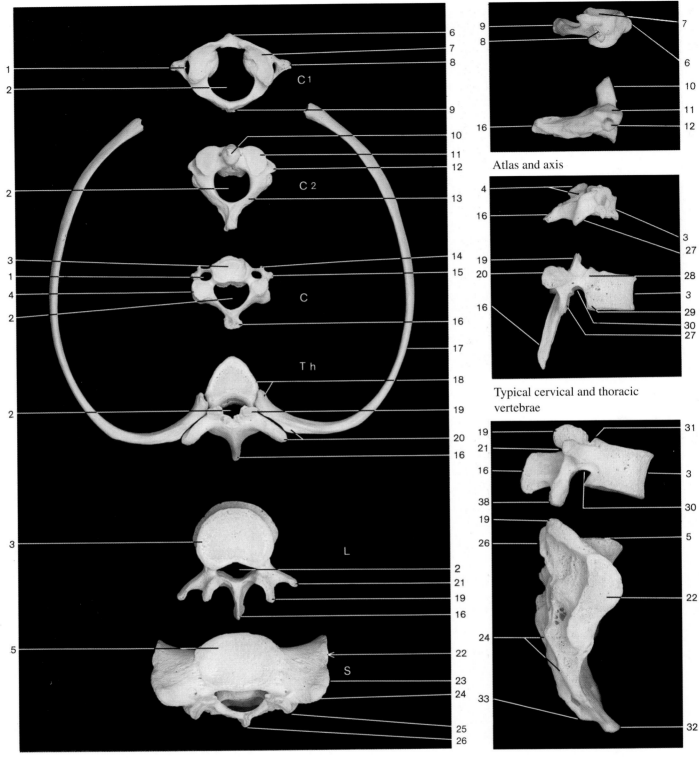

**Representative vertebrae from each region of the vertebral column** (superior aspect).
From top to bottom: atlas (C₁), axis (C₂), cervical vertebra (C),
thoracic vertebra (Th), lumbar vertebra (L), and sacrum (S).

Atlas and axis

Typical cervical and thoracic vertebrae

Typical lumbar vertebra and sacrum

**Representative vertebrae from each region of the vertebral column** (lateral aspect, ventral surface on the right).

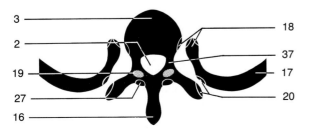

**General organization of ribs and vertebrae** (schematic diagram).

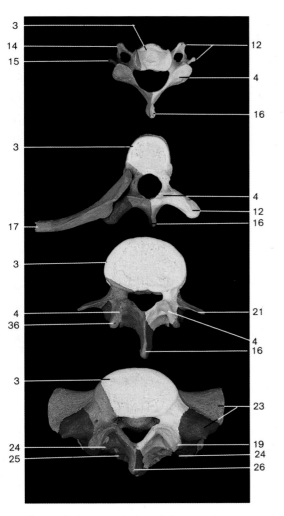

**General characteristics of the vertebrae.**
Typical cervical, thoracic, and lumbar vertebrae and sacrum.

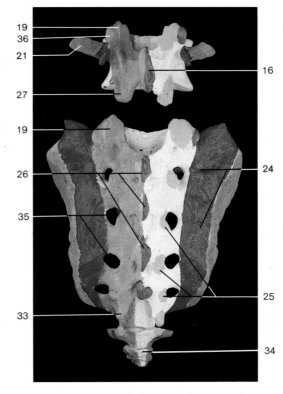

**General characteristics of lumbar vertebrae and sacrum** (posterior aspect).

| | | |
|---|---|---|
| Green | = | Ribs or homologous processes |
| Red | = | Muscular processes (transverse and spinous processes) |
| Orange | = | Laminae and articular processes |
| Yellow and blue | = | Articular facets |

1  Foramen transversarium
2  Vertebral foramen
3  Body of vertebra
4  Superior articular facet
5  Base of sacrum
6  Anterior tubercle of atlas
7  Superior articular facet of atlas
8  Transverse process
9  Posterior tubercle of atlas
10  Dens of axis
11  Superior articular surface
12  Transverse process
13  Arch of vertebra
14  Anterior tubercle of transverse process
15  Posterior tubercle of transverse process
16  Spinous process
17  Shaft of rib
18  Body of vertebra and head of rib articulating with each other (costovertebral joint)
19  Superior articular process

20  Transverse process and tubercle of rib articulating with each other (costotransverse joint)
21  Costal process
22  Auricular surface
23  Lateral part of sacrum
24  Lateral sacral crest
25  Intermediate sacral crest
26  Median sacral crest
27  Inferior articular facet
28  Superior demifacet for head of rib
29  Inferior demifacet for head of rib
30  Inferior vertebral notch
31  Superior vertebral notch
32  Apex of the sacrum
33  Sacral cornu
34  Coccyx
35  Dorsal sacral foramina
36  Mamillary process
37  Pedicle
38  Inferior articular process

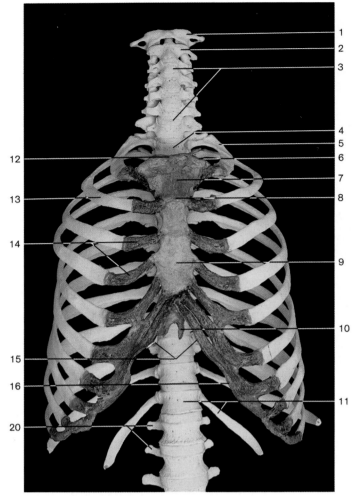

**Skeleton of the thorax** (anterior aspect).

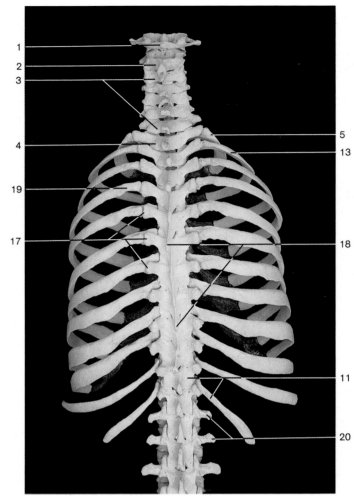

**Skeleton of the thorax** (posterior aspect).

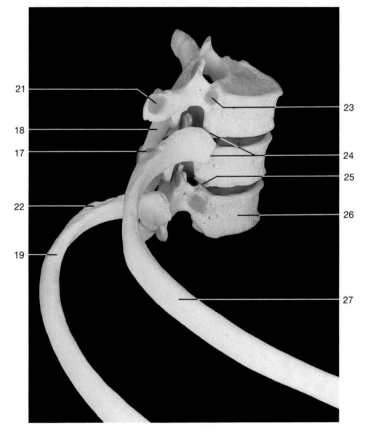

**Costovertebral articulation** (right lateral aspect).

1   Atlas
2   Axis
3   Cervical vertebrae
4   First thoracic vertebra
5   First rib
6   Facet for clavicle and clavicular notch
7   Manubrium sterni
8   Sternal angle
9   Body of sternum
10  Xiphoid process
11  Twelfth thoracic vertebra and rib
12  Jugular notch
13  Second rib
14  Costal cartilages
15  Infrasternal angle
16  Costal arch
17  Costotransverse joints between the transverse processes
    of thoracic vertebra and the tubercles of the ribs
18  Spinous processes
19  Costal angle
20  Costal processes of lumbar vertebrae
21  Facet for articulation with rib
22  Tubercle of rib
23  Superior facet for articulation with head of rib
24  Articulation of head of rib with two vertebrae
25  Inferior facet for articulation with head of rib
26  Body of thoracic vertebra
27  Body or shaft of rib

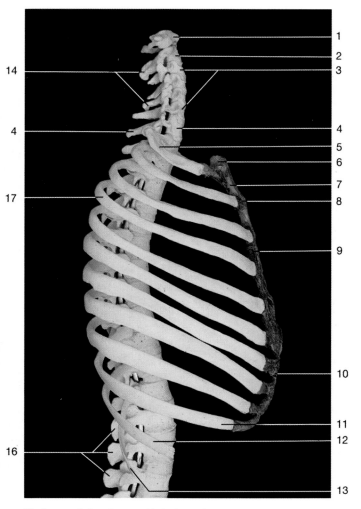

**Skeleton of the thorax** (right lateral aspect).

1   Atlas
2   Axis
3   Cervical vertebrae
4   Seventh cervical vertebra (vertebra prominens)
5   First rib
6   Facet for clavicle
7   Manubrium sterni
8   Sternal angle
9   Body of sternum
10  Costal arch
11  Tenth rib
12  Eleventh rib
13  Twelfth rib
14  Spinous processes of cervical vertebrae
15  Spinous processes of thoracic vertebrae
16  Spinous processes of lumbar vertebrae
17  Costal angle
18  Intervertebral foramina
19  Intervertebral discs
20  Cervical curvature
21  Thoracic curvature
22  Lumbar curvature
23  Sacrum
24  Coccyx

**Vertebral column**
(right lateral aspect).

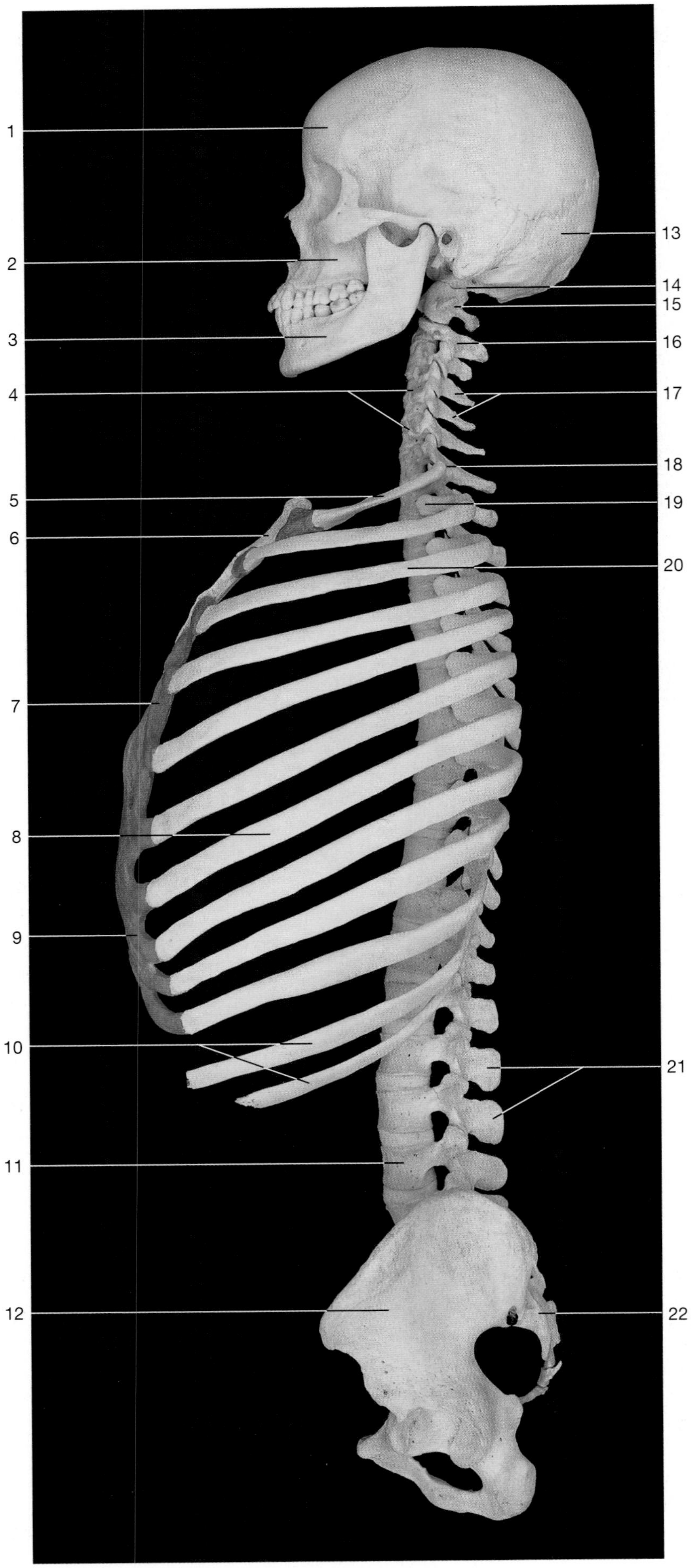

1   Frontal bone
2   Maxilla
3   Mandible
4   Bodies of cervical vertebrae
5   First rib
6   Manubrium of sternum
7   Sternum (corpus sterni)
8   Seventh rib (last of the true ribs)
9   Costal arch (arcus costalis)
10  Floating ribs (costae fluctuantes)
11  Body of fourth lumbar vertebra
12  Pelvis
13  Occipital bone
14  Atlanto-occipital joint
15  Atlas
16  Axis
17  Spinous processes of cervical vertebrae ($C_4$, $C_5$)
18  Costotransverse joint of first rib
19  Head of second rib
20  Third rib
21  Spinous processes of lumbar vertebrae ($L_2$, $L_3$)
22  Sacrum

**Vertebral column and thorax** in connection with head and pelvis (lateral aspect).

1  Atlas
2  Dens of axis
3  Axis
4  Body of cervical vertebra
5  Intervertebral discs
6  Sternocleidomastoid muscle
7  Scalenus muscles
8  Body of vertebra
9  Superior articular facet
10  Vertebral arch
11  Transverse process of vertebra
12  Zygapophysial joint
13  Spinous process
14  Articular facet
     of costovertebral joint
15  Transverse process
     with articular facet
     of costotransverse joint
16  Costal process of lumbar
     vertebra
17  Sacrum
18  Median sacral crest
19  Dorsal sacral foramina
20  Coccyx

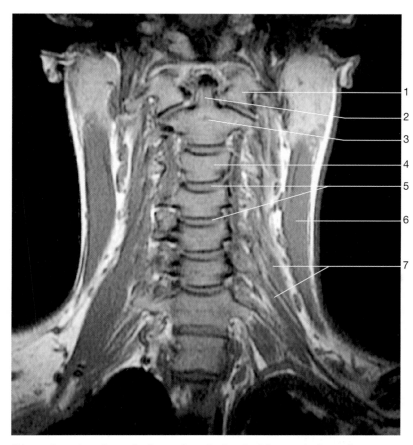

**Coronal section through the neck** at the level of the cervical vertebrae (MRI scan, courtesy of Prof. Dr. A. Heuck, Munich).

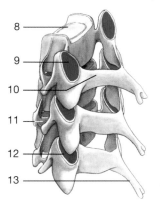

**Cervical vertebrae** (lateral aspect, articular facets blue).

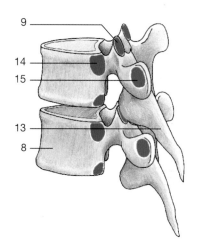

**Thoracic vertebrae** (lateral aspect, articular facets blue).

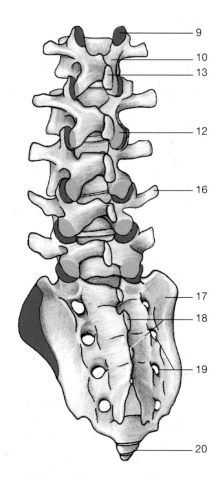

**Lumbar vertebrae with sacrum and coccyx** (posterior aspect, articular facets blue).

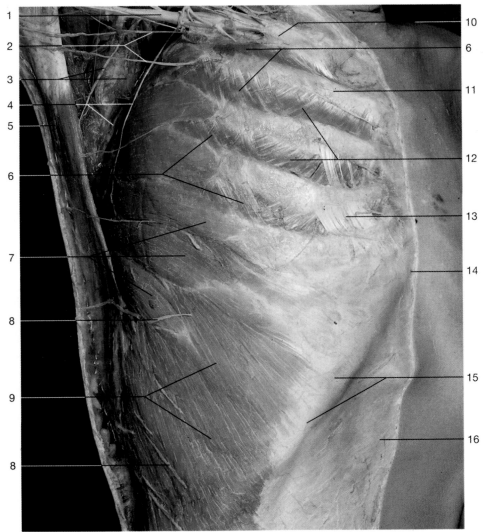

1   Axillary vein
2   Intercostobrachial nerves
3   Subscapularis muscle and
    thoracodorsal nerve
4   Long thoracic nerve, lateral
    thoracic artery and vein
5   Latissimus dorsi muscle
6   External intercostal muscles
7   Serratus anterior muscle
8   Lateral cutaneous branches of
    intercostal nerves
9   External abdominal oblique muscle
10  Clavicle (divided)
11  Second rib (costochondral
    junction)
12  Internal intercostal muscles
13  External intercostal membrane
14  Position of xiphoid process
15  Costal arch or margin
16  Anterior layer of rectus sheath

**Muscles of the thorax,** superficial layer (lateral aspect). Upper limb elevated.
Pectoralis major and minor muscles have been removed.

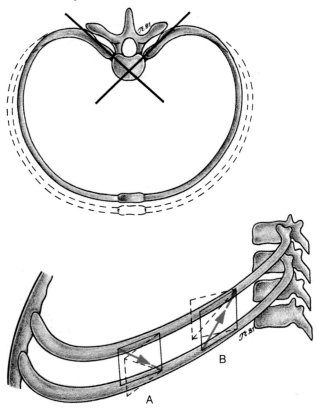

**Effect of intercostal muscles on the costovertebral and
costotransverse joints.** Axes of movement indicated by lines;
direction of movements indicated by red arrows.
A = Action of internal intercostal muscles (expiration);
B = Action of external intercostal muscles (inspiration).

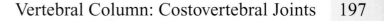

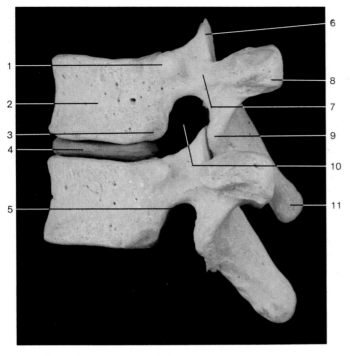

**Two thoracic vertebrae** (left lateral aspect).

| | | | |
|---|---|---|---|
| 1 | Superior demifacet for head of rib | 8 | Transverse process and facet for tubercle of rib |
| 2 | Body of vertebra | 9 | Inferior articular process |
| 3 | Inferior demifacet for head of rib | 10 | Intervertebral foramen |
| 4 | Intervertebral disc | 11 | Spinous process |
| 5 | Inferior vertebral notch | 12 | Anterior longitudinal ligament |
| 6 | Superior articular facet and superior articular process | 13 | Intra-articular ligament |
| 7 | Pedicle | 14 | Radiate ligament |

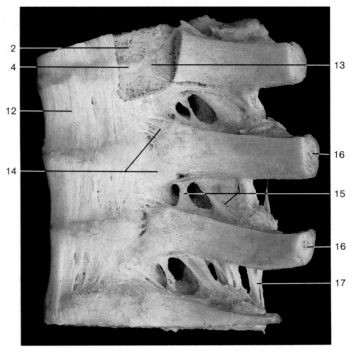

**Ligaments of thoracic vertebrae and costovertebral joints** (left anterolateral aspect). In the upper joint, most of the radiate ligament and the anterior part of the head of the rib have been removed to expose the two joint cavities and the interposed intra-articular ligament.

| | |
|---|---|
| 15 | Superior costotransverse ligament |
| 16 | Body of rib |
| 17 | Intertransverse ligament |

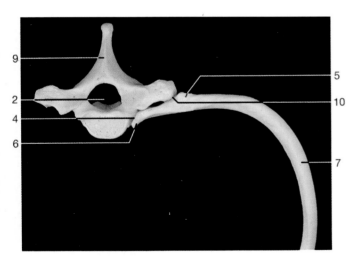

**Location of costovertebral joints** (superior aspect).

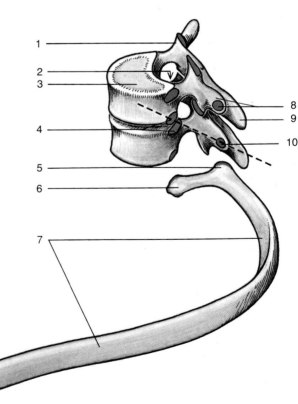

**Costovertebral joints.** Two thoracic vertebrae with an articulating rib (separated). Axis of movement indicated by dotted line. Blue = articular facets. (Schematic diagram.)

| | | | |
|---|---|---|---|
| 1 | Superior articular process | 7 | Shaft or body of rib |
| 2 | Vertebral canal | 8 | Transverse process with articular facet |
| 3 | Body of thoracic vertebra | 9 | Spinous process |
| 4 | Costovertebral joint (articular facets) | 10 | Costotransverse joint (articular facets) |
| 5 | Tubercle of rib | | |
| 6 | Head of rib | | |

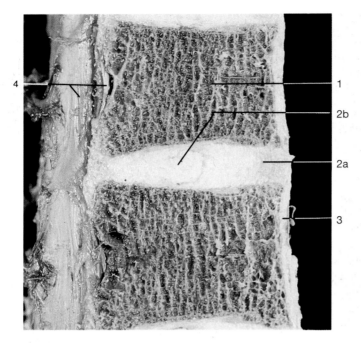

**Median-sagittal section of the bodies of the vertebrae,** showing the **intervertebral discs,** each of which consists of an outer laminated portion and an inner core.

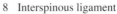

**Ligaments of the vertebral column** (dorsal aspect).

1   Body of vertebra
2   Intervertebral disc
  a  Outer portion (anulus fibrosus)
  b  Inner core (nucleus pulposus)
3   Anterior longitudinal ligament
4   Posterior longitudinal ligament and spinal dura mater
5   Costal process of lumbar vertebra
6   Sacrum
7   Supraspinous ligament

8   Interspinous ligament
9   Intertransverse ligament
10  Superior costotransverse ligament
11  Transverse process of thoracic vertebra
12  Rib
13  Ligamentum flavum
14  Spinous process
15  Intervertebral foramen

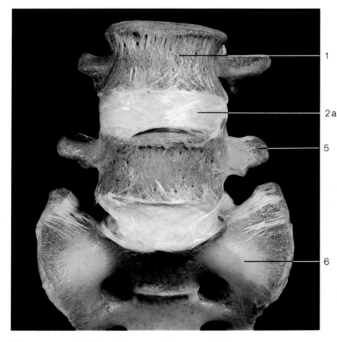

**The two caudal lumbar vertebrae and the sacrum with their intervertebral discs** (anterior aspect). Anterior longitudinal ligament removed.

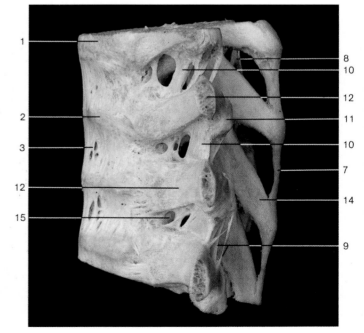

**Ligaments of the vertebral column,** thoracic part (left lateral aspect).

**Disarticulated thorax skeleton.**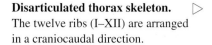
The twelve ribs (I–XII) are arranged
in a craniocaudal direction.

1   Anterior longitudinal ligament
2   Body of vertebra
3   Intervertebral disc
4   Intra-articular ligament
5   Radiate ligament
6   Posterior longitudinal ligament
7   Superior articular facet
8   Articular facets of
     costovertebral joints
9   Superior costotransverse ligament
10  Costovertebral joint
11  Rib
12  Interspinal ligament
13  Costotransverse joint
14  Lateral costotransverse ligament
15  Spinous process
16  Supraspinal ligament
17  Nucleus pulposus
18  Costal process
19  Vertebral arch
20  Intervertebral foramen
21  Intertransverse ligament

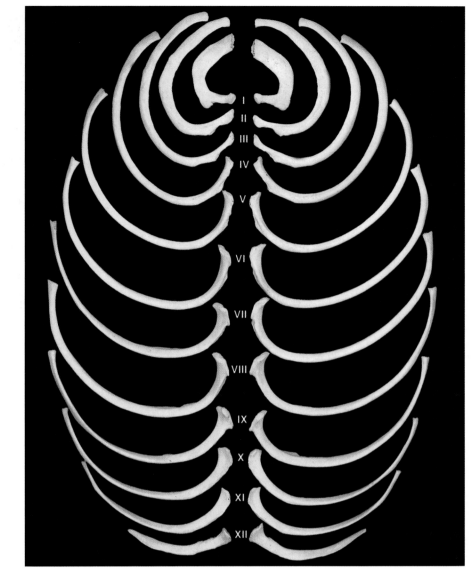

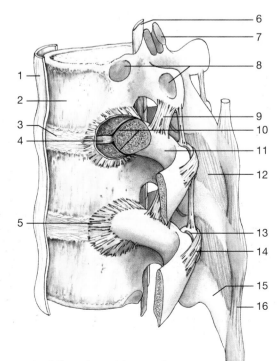

**Ligaments of thoracic vertebrae and
costovertebral joints** (lateral aspect).

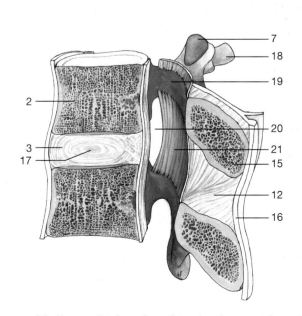

**Median-sagittal section of two lumbar vertebrae** showing
ligaments and vertebral discs.

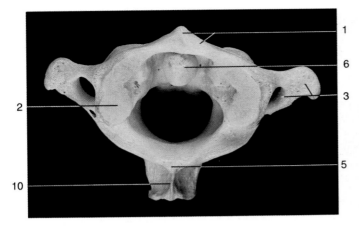

**Atlas and axis** (from above).

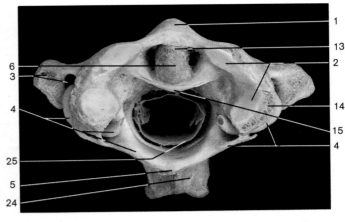

**Median atlanto-axial joint and transverse ligament of atlas** (from above). Dens of axis partly severed.

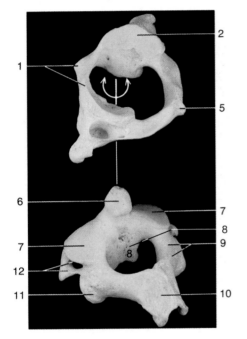

| | |
|---|---|
| 1 | Anterior arch of atlas with anterior tubercle |
| 2 | Superior articular facet of atlas |
| 3 | Foramen transversarium and transverse process |
| 4 | Posterior arch of atlas and vertebral artery |
| 5 | Posterior tubercle of atlas |
| 6 | Dens of axis |
| 7 | Superior articular surface of axis |
| 8 | Body of axis |
| 9 | Pedicle and lamina of axis |
| 10 | Spinous process |
| 11 | Inferior articular process |
| 12 | Transverse process and foramen transversarium of axis |
| 13 | Median atlanto-axial joint (anterior part) |
| 14 | Articular capsule of atlanto-occipital joint |
| 15 | Transverse ligament of atlas |
| 16 | Occipital bone |
| 17 | Atlanto-occipital joint |
| 18 | Lateral atlanto-axial joint |
| 19 | Third cervical vertebra |
| 20 | Superior longitudinal band of cruciform ligament |
| 21 | Alar ligaments |
| 22 | Transverse ligament of atlas |
| 23 | Inferior longitudinal band of cruciform ligament |
| 24 | Spinous process of axis |
| 25 | Dura mater |
| 26 | Occipital bone |

**Atlas and axis.** Left oblique posterolateral aspect, demonstrating the articulation of the dens of axis with atlas (cf. arrows).

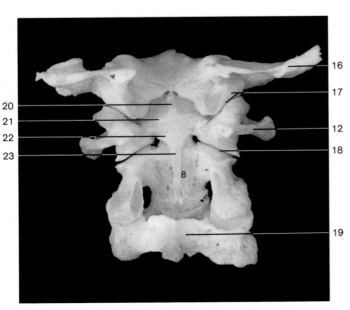

**Atlanto-occipital and atlanto-axial joints** (posterior aspect). Posterior part of occipital bone, posterior arch of atlas, and axis have been removed to show the cruciform ligament.

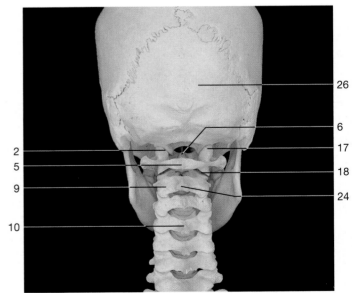

**Head and cervical spine** (posterior aspect). Bones of atlanto-occipital and atlanto-axial joints.

1  Cerebellum
2  Occipital condyle
3  Atlanto-occipital joint
4  Atlas
5  Lateral atlanto-axial joint
6  Intervertebral disc
7  Cistern of pons
8  Head of mandible
9  Dens of axis
10  Axis
11  Body of cervical vertebra (C$_3$)
12  External occipital protuberance
13  Foramen magnum
14  Transverse process of atlas
15  Posterior longitudinal ligament
16  Spinous process of cervical vertebra
17  Occipital bone
18  Membrana tectoria
19  Dorsum sellae
20  Clivus
21  Sella turcica
22  Superior orbital fissure
23  Internal acoustic meatus
24  Jugular foramen
25  Hypoglossal canal
26  Superior longitudinal
   band of cruciform ligament
27  Alar ligaments
28  Transverse ligament of atlas
29  Inferior longitudinal band of
   cruciform ligament

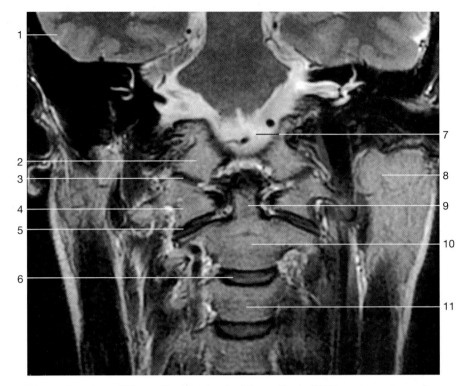

**Coronal section of the neck** at the level of dens of axis (MRI scan, courtesy of Prof. Dr. A. Heuck, Munich).

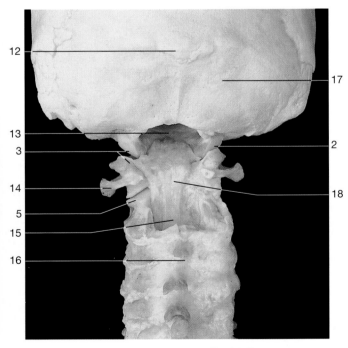

**Cervical vertebral column and skull with ligaments**
(posterior aspect). Posterior arches of atlas and axis removed to show the membrana tectoria.

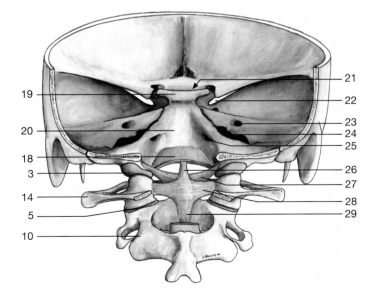

**Atlanto-occipital and atlanto-axial joints with ligaments**
(posterior aspect). Posterior part of occipital bone and posterior arch of atlas have been removed to show the cruciform ligament.

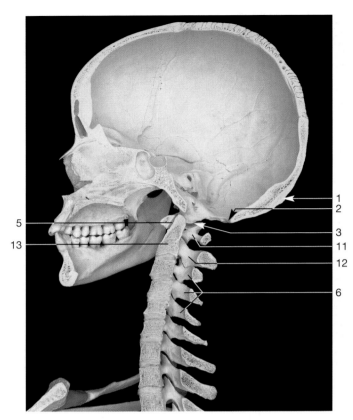

**Cervical vertebral column in relation to the head** (midsagittal section) (medial aspect).

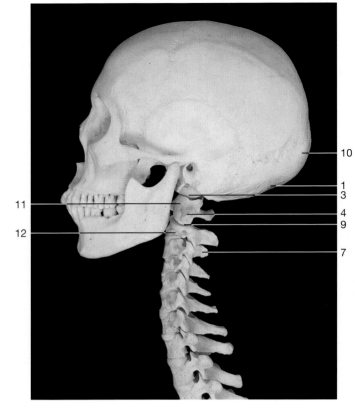

**Atlas and axis in relation to the head** (lateral aspect).

1   External occipital protuberance
2   Foramen magnum
3   Atlanto-occipital joint
4   Transverse process of atlas
5   Median atlanto-axial joint
6   Vertebral canal
7   Spinous process of third cervical vertebra
8   Occipital condyle

9   Lateral atlanto-axial joint
10  Occipital bone
11  Atlas
12  Axis
13  Dens of axis
14  Hypoglossal canal
15  Spinous process of axis

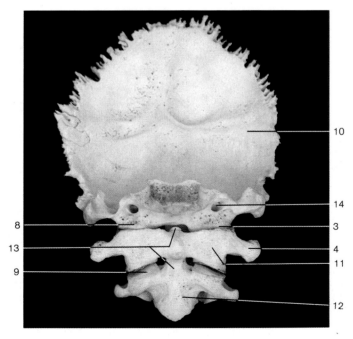

**Occipital bone, atlas, and axis** (anterior aspect).

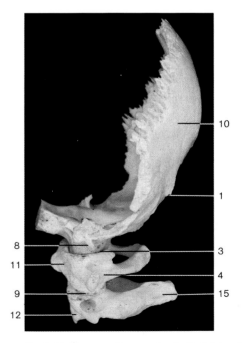

**Occipital bone, atlas, and axis** (left lateral aspect).

1   Pons
2   Base of skull (clivus)
3   Medulla oblongata
4   Atlas (anterior arch)
5   Dens of axis
6   Intervertebral disc
7   Body of cervical vertebra (C$_4$)
8   Site of larynx
9   Trachea
10  Cerebellum
11  Cerebellomedullary cistern
12  Spinal cord
13  Trapezius muscle
14  Muscles of the neck
15  Spinous process of cervical
    vertebra (C$_7$)
16  Internal jugular vein
17  Common carotid artery
18  Vagus nerve (n. X)
19  Larynx
20  Body of cervical vertebra
21  Vertebral artery
22  Spinal nerve with spinal ganglion
23  Transverse process of cervical vertebra
24  Spinous process of cervical vertebra

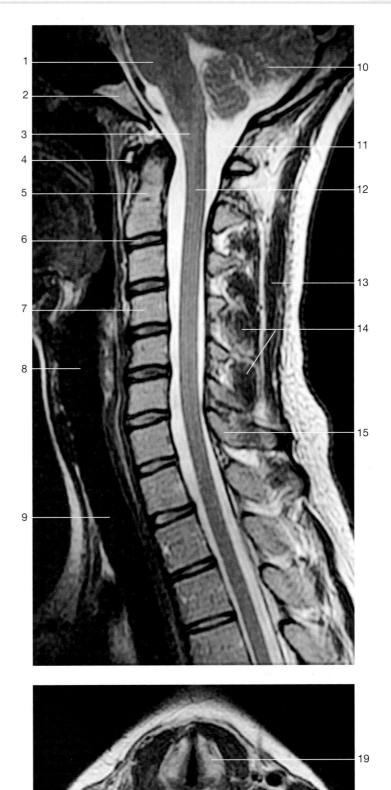

**Median-sagittal section of the neck** showing the spinal cord in connection with medulla oblongata (MRI scan, courtesy of Prof. Dr. A. Heuck, Munich).

**Horizontal section of the neck** at the level of the larynx (MRI scan, courtesy of Prof. Dr. A. Heuck, Munich).

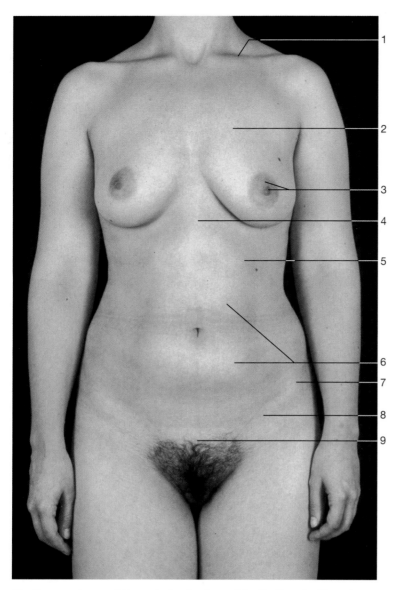

1  Clavicle
2  Pectoralis major muscle
3  Areola and nipple
4  Infrasternal angle
5  Costal arch
6  Rectus abdominis muscle
7  Anterior superior iliac spine
8  Inguinal ligament
9  Mons pubis
10 Epidermis
11 Subcutaneous layer
12 Muscles of the back
13 Kidney
14 Body of lumbar vertebra
15 External abdominal oblique
   muscle
16 Small intestine
17 Deltoid muscle
18 Anterior serratus muscle
19 External intercostal muscle
20 Internal abdominal oblique
   muscle
21 Transverse abdominal muscle
22 Rectus sheath
23 Spermatic cord
24 Pectoralis minor muscle
25 Linea alba

**Surface anatomy of the anterior body wall in the female.** Note the differences in thickness and structure of skin and hairs (compare with the section below).

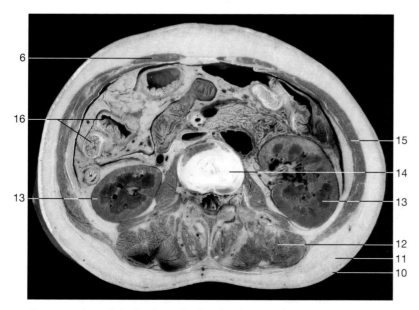

**Cross section of the body** at the first lumbar vertebra. Note the differences in thickness of the subcutaneous layers.

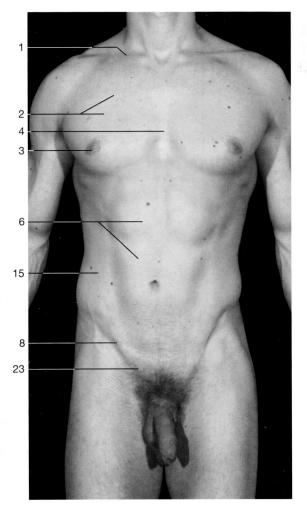

**Surface anatomy of the anterior body wall in the male.** Localization and structure of the muscles can be identified.

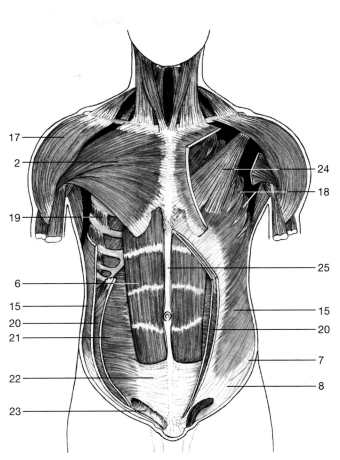

**Muscles of the anterior body wall** (schematic drawing).

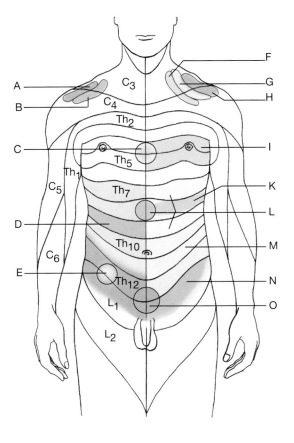

**Head's areas**

A = Duodenum
B = Gallbladder, liver ($C_3$–$C_4$)
C = Esophagus ($Th_4$, $Th_5$)
D = Liver, gallbladder ($Th_6$–$Th_{11}$)
E = Colon, vermiform appendix
    ($Th_{11–12}$, $L_1$)
F = Heart
G = Pancreas
H = Stomach ($C_3$, $C_4$)
I = Heart ($Th_3$, $Th_4$)
K = Pancreas ($Th_8$)
L = Stomach ($Th_6$–$Th_9$)
M = Small intestine ($Th_{10}$–$L_1$)
N = Kidney, ureter, testis ($Th_{10}$–$L_1$)
O = Urinary bladder ($Th_{11}$–$L_1$)

◁ **Segments of anterior body wall.**
Head's areas are indicated.

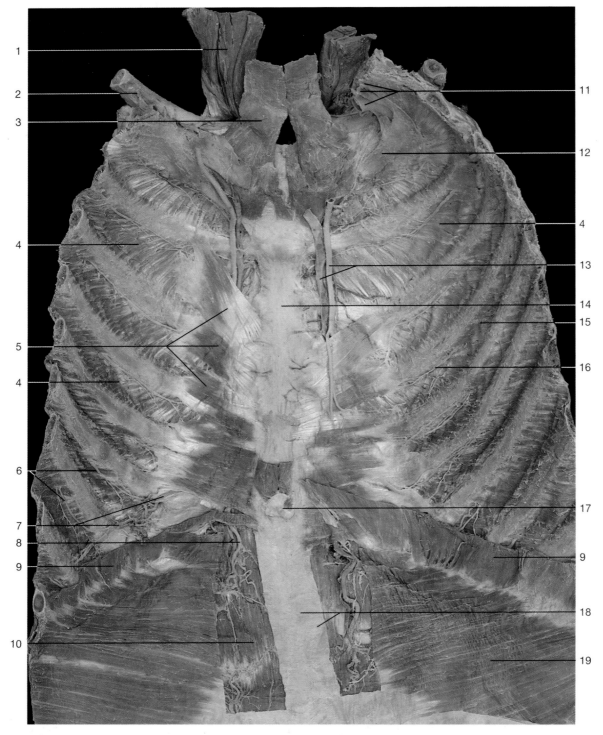

**Anterior thoracic wall** (posterior aspect). Diaphragm partly removed, posterior layer of rectus sheath fenestrated on both sides.

1  Sternocleidomastoid muscle (divided)
2  Clavicle
3  Sternothyroid muscle
4  Internal intercostal muscle
5  Transversus thoracic muscle
6  Intercostal arteries and nerves
7  Musculophrenic artery
8  Superior epigastric artery and vein
9  Diaphragm (divided)
10  Rectus abdominis muscle

11  Subclavian artery and brachial plexus
12  First rib
13  Internal thoracic artery and vein
14  Sternum
15  Innermost intercostal muscle
16  Intercostal artery and vein
17  Xiphoid process
18  Linea alba and posterior layer of rectus sheath
19  Transversus abdominis muscle

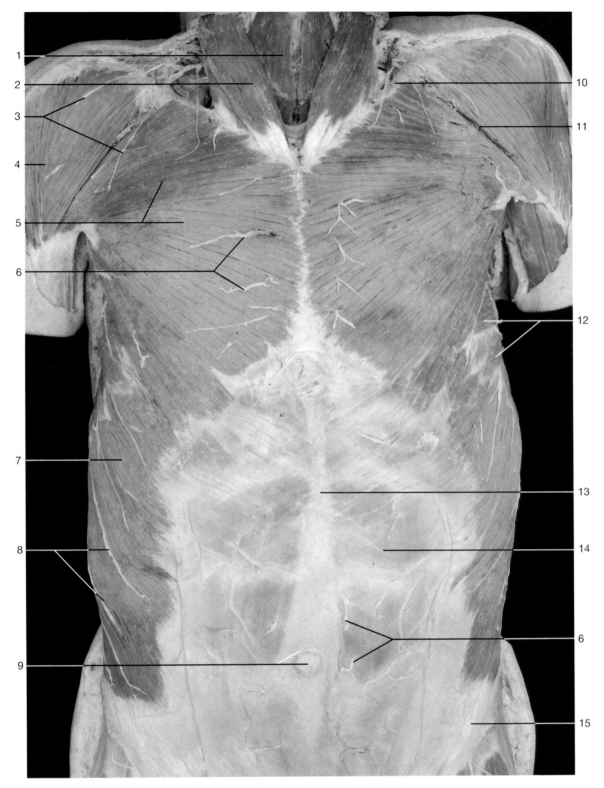

**Superficial muscles of the anterior thoracic and abdominal wall.** The fascia of pectoralis major muscle and the abdominal wall have been removed; the anterior layer of the sheath of the rectus abdominis muscle is displayed.

| | |
|---|---|
| 1  Sternohyoid muscle | 9  Umbilicus and umbilical ring |
| 2  Sternocleidomastoid muscle | 10  Clavicle |
| 3  Supraclavicular nerves (branches of cervical plexus) | 11  Cephalic vein |
| 4  Deltoid muscle | 12  Serratus anterior muscle |
| 5  Pectoralis major muscle | 13  Linea alba |
| 6  Anterior cutaneous branches of intercostal nerves | 14  Sheath of rectus abdominis muscle (anterior layer) |
| 7  External abdominal oblique muscle | 15  Inguinal ligament |
| 8  Lateral cutaneous branches of intercostal nerves | |

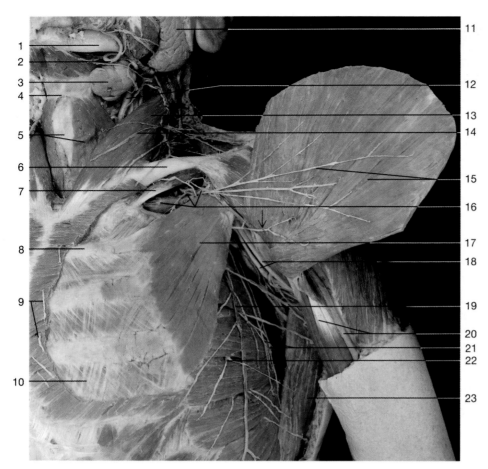

**Thoracic wall I** (anterior aspect). Left pectoralis major muscle has been divided and reflected. Note the connection of the cephalic vein with the subclavian vein. Arrow: medial pectoral nerve.

1   Mandible
2   Facial artery
3   Submandibular gland
4   Hyoid bone
5   Thyroid cartilage and sternohyoid muscle
6   Clavicle
7   Subclavius muscle
8   Second rib
9   Anterior cutaneous branches of intercostal nerves
10  External intercostal membrane
11  Parotid gland
12  External carotid artery
13  Sternocleidomastoid muscle and cutaneous branches of cervical plexus
14  Supraclavicular nerves
15  Pectoralis major muscle and lateral pectoral nerves
16  Thoraco-acromial artery and subclavian vein
17  Pectoralis minor muscle
18  Median and ulnar nerve
19  Thoraco-epigastric vein
20  Cephalic vein and long head of biceps brachii muscle
21  Lateral thoracic artery and long thoracic nerve
22  Lateral cutaneous branches of intercostal nerve
23  Latissimus dorsi muscle
24  Median nerve
25  Axillary artery
26  Intercostobrachial nerves
27  Thoracodorsal nerve
28  Long thoracic nerve
29  Latissimus dorsi muscle
30  Serratus anterior muscle
31  Thoraco-acromial artery
32  Clavicle
33  External intercostal muscle
34  Third rib
35  Internal intercostal muscle
36  Anterior intercostal artery and vein, and intercostal nerve
37  Costal arch or margin

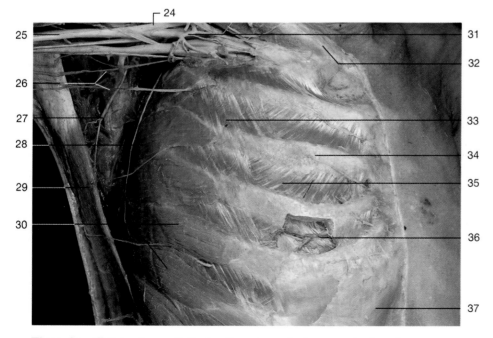

**Thoracic wall** (lateral aspect). Pectoralis major and minor muscles have been removed. A section of the fourth rib has been cut and removed to display the intercostal vessels and nerve.

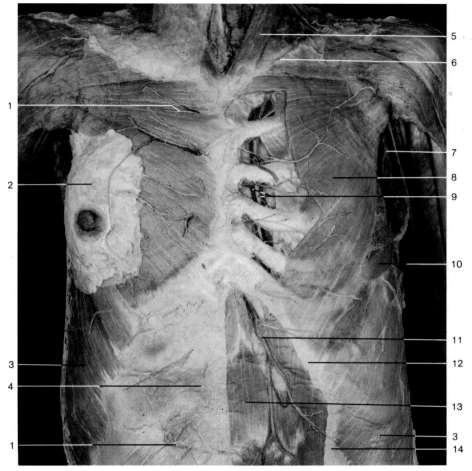

1   Anterior perforating branches
    of intercostal nerve
2   Mammary gland
3   External abdominal oblique muscle
4   Rectus sheath (anterior layer)
5   Sternocleidomastoid muscle
6   Clavicle
7   Lateral thoracic artery
    and vein
8   Pectoralis major muscle
9   Internal thoracic artery
    and vein
10  Serratus anterior muscle
11  Superior epigastric artery
    and vein
12  Costal margin
13  Rectus abdominis muscle
14  Cut edge of the anterior layer
    of the rectus sheath
15  Subclavian artery
16  Highest intercostal artery
17  Internal thoracic artery
18  Musculophrenic artery
19  Superficial epigastric artery
20  Deep circumflex iliac artery
21  Superior epigastric artery
22  Inferior epigastric artery
23  Superficial circumflex iliac artery

**Thoracic wall II** (anterior aspect). Dissection of the **internal thoracic artery and vein.** Left pectoralis major muscle partly removed. Anterior lamina of the rectus sheath on the left side has been removed.

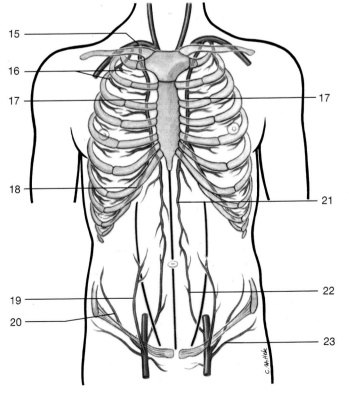

**Main arteries of thoracic and abdominal wall.**

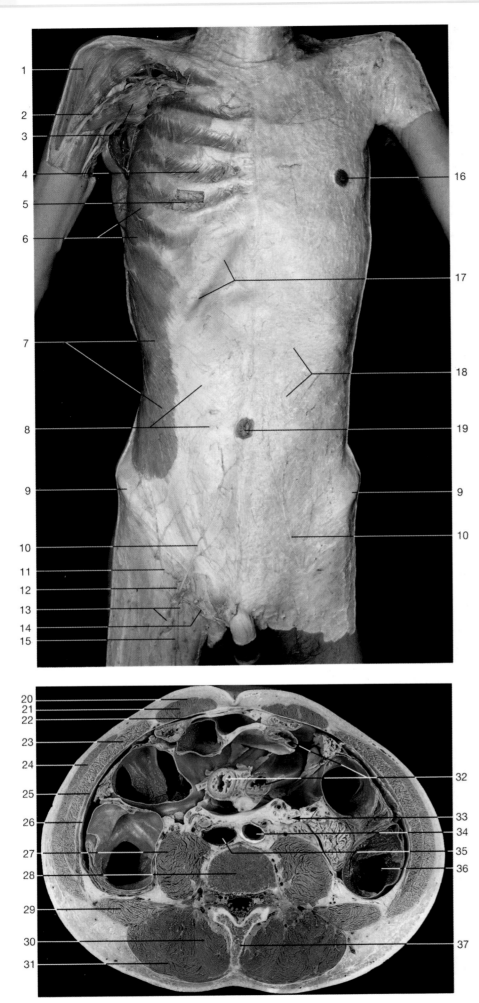

1   Deltoid muscle
2   Cephalic vein
3   Pectoralis major muscle (divided)
4   Internal intercostal muscle
5   Intercostal artery and vein (intercostal
    space, fenestrated)
6   Serratus anterior muscle
7   External abdominal oblique muscle
8   Anterior layer of rectus sheath
9   Iliac crest
10  Superficial epigastric vein
11  Superficial circumflex iliac vein
12  Saphenous opening
13  Superficial inguinal lymph nodes
14  Superficial external pudendal veins
15  Great saphenous vein
16  Nipple
17  Costal margin
18  Subcutaneous fatty tissue
19  Umbilicus
20  Anterior layer of rectus sheath
21  Rectus abdominis muscle
22  Posterior layer of rectus sheath
23  Internal abdominal oblique muscle
24  External abdominal oblique muscle (cut)
25  Transversus abdominis muscle
26  Transversal fascia and peritoneum
27  Psoas major muscle
28  Body of lumbar vertebra (L$_4$)
29  Quadratus lumborum muscle
30  Medial tract of erector spinae muscle
31  Lateral tract of erector spinae muscle
    (longissimus and iliocostalis muscles)
32  Small intestine
33  Left ureter
34  Abdominal aorta
35  Inferior vena cava
36  Descending colon
37  Spinous process

**Thoracic and abdominal wall I.** Right
pectoralis major and minor muscles
are divided. Muscles of thoracic
and abdominal wall on right side are
displayed.

**Horizontal section of the trunk at the
level of the umbilicus,** superior to
arcuate line (inferior aspect).

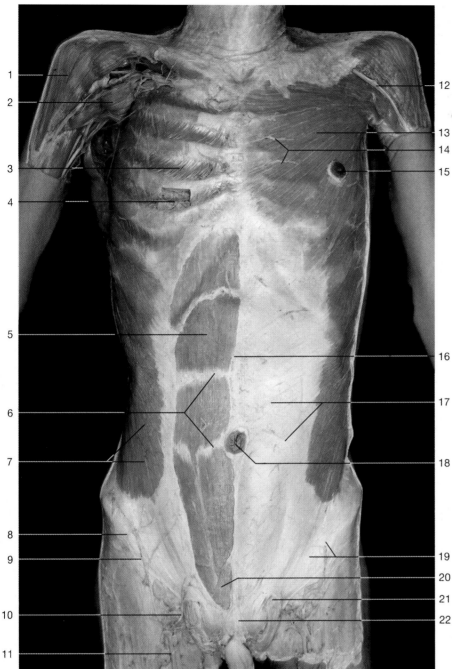

1 Deltoid muscle
2 Pectoralis major muscle (divided)
3 Internal intercostal muscle
4 Intercostal artery and vein
5 Rectus abdominis muscle
6 Tendinous intersections
7 External abdominal oblique muscle
8 Anterior superior iliac spine
9 Superficial circumflex iliac vein
10 Superficial epigastric vein
11 Great saphenous vein
12 Cephalic vein
13 Pectoralis major muscle
14 Anterior cutaneous branches of intercostal nerves
15 Nipple
16 Linea alba
17 Anterior layer of rectus sheath
18 Umbilicus
19 Inguinal ligament
20 Pyramidal muscle
21 Superficial inguinal ring and spermatic cord
22 Suspensory ligament of penis
23 Longissimus and iliocostalis muscles
24 Multifidus muscle
25 Quadratus lumborum muscle
26 Latissimus dorsi muscle
27 Psoas major muscle
28 Spinous process
29 Body of first lumbar vertebra
30 Transversus abdominis muscle
31 Internal abdominal oblique muscle

**Thoracic and abdominal wall II.**
Right pectoralis major and minor muscles and anterior layer of rectus sheath have been removed on the right side.

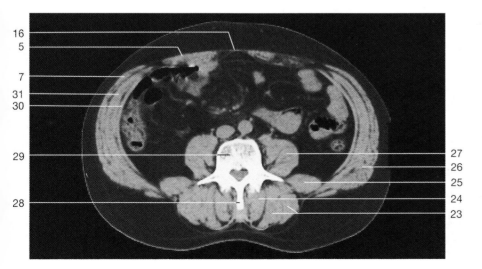

**Horizontal section through the body**
at the level of fourth lumbar vertebra; seen from below. (CT scan.)

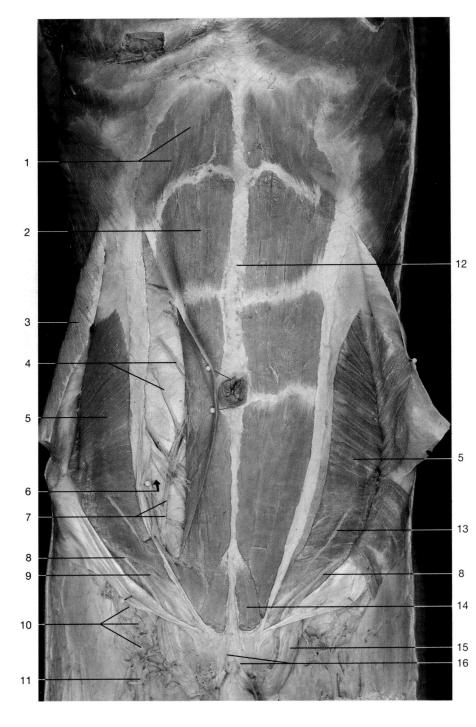

1   Costal margin
2   Rectus abdominis muscle
3   External abdominal oblique muscle
    (reflected)
4   Thoraco-abdominal (intercostal) nerves
    with accompanying vessels
5   Internal abdominal oblique muscle
6   Arcuate line (arrow)
7   Inferior epigastric artery and vein
8   Ilio-inguinal nerve
9   Position of deep inguinal ring
10  Superficial inguinal lymph nodes
11  Great saphenous vein
12  Linea alba
13  Iliohypogastric nerve
14  Pyramidal muscle
15  Spermatic cord
16  Fundiform ligament of penis

**Thoracic and abdominal wall III.**
External abdominal oblique muscle has
been divided and reflected on both sides.
The right rectus muscle has been reflected
medially to display the posterior layer of rectus sheath. Arrow: location of arcuate line.

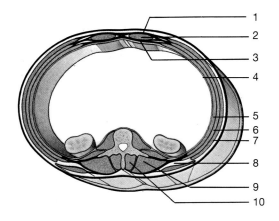

1   Anterior layer of rectus sheath
2   Rectus abdominis muscle
3   Posterior layer of rectus sheath
4   Transversalis fascia
5   Transversus abdominis muscle
6   Internal oblique muscle
7   External oblique muscle
8   Thoracolumbar fascia with
    superficial and deep layer
9   Lateral column of erector spinae muscle
10  Medial column of intrinsic muscles
    of the back

**Horizontal section of the trunk** superior
to arcuate line (schematic drawing).

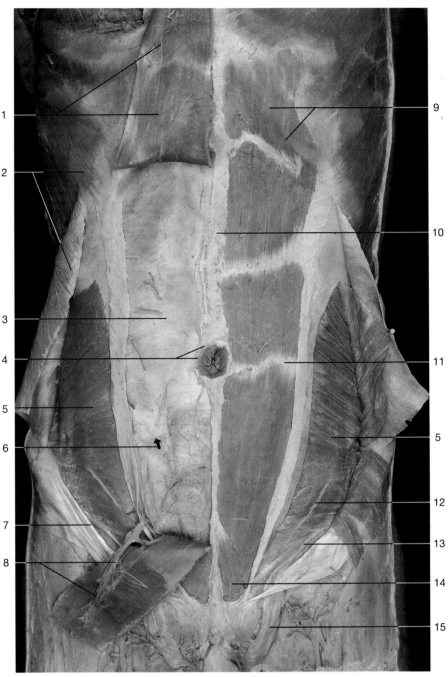

1   Rectus abdominis muscle (reflected)
2   External abdominal oblique muscle
    (divided)
3   Posterior layer of rectus sheath
4   Umbilical ring
5   Internal abdominal oblique muscle
6   Arcuate line (arrow)
7   Inguinal ligament
8   Inferior epigastric artery and vein
    and rectus abdominis muscle
    (divided and reflected)
9   Costal margin
10  Linea alba
11  Tendinous intersection
12  Iliohypogastric nerve
13  Ilio-inguinal nerve
14  Pyramidal muscle
15  Spermatic cord

**Thoracic and abdominal wall IV.**
External abdominal oblique muscle has
been divided and reflected on both sides.
The right rectus muscle has been cut and
reflected to display the posterior layer of
rectus sheath. Arrow: location of arcuate line.

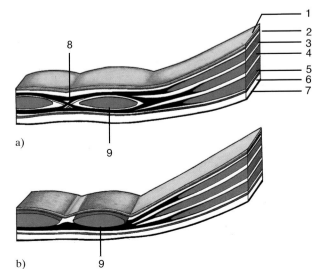

1   Peritoneum
2   Transversalis fascia (green)
3   Transversus abdominis muscle
4   Internal abdominal oblique muscle
5   External abdominal oblique muscle
6   Fascia of external abdominal oblique
    muscle (green)
7   Skin
8   Linea alba
9   Rectus abdominis muscle

**Transverse sections through the
abdominal wall** superior (a) and inferior (b)
to arcuate line.

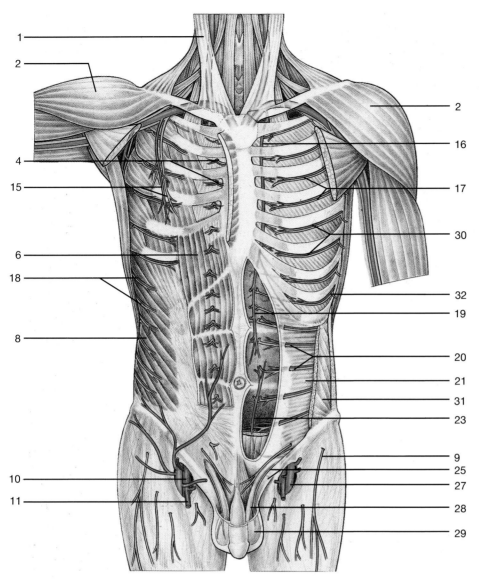

1 Sternocleidomastoid muscle
2 Deltoid muscle
3 Pectoralis major muscle
4 Anterior cutaneous branches of
  intercostal nerves
5 Cut edge of anterior layer of rectus
  sheath
6 Rectus abdominis muscle
7 Tendinous intersection
8 External abdominal oblique muscle
9 Lateral femoral cutaneous nerve
10 Femoral vein
11 Great saphenous vein
12 Medial supraclavicular nerves
13 Pectoralis minor muscle (reflected)
   and medial pectoral nerves
14 Axillary vein
15 Long thoracic nerve and lateral
   thoracic artery
16 Internal thoracic artery
17 Intercostal nerves
18 Lateral cutaneous branches of
   intercostal nerves
19 Superior epigastric artery
20 Thoraco-abdominal (intercostal)
   nerves
21 Transversus abdominis muscle
22 Posterior layer of rectus sheath
23 Inferior epigastric artery
24 Lateral femoral cutaneous nerve
25 Inguinal ligament and ilio-inguinal
   nerve
26 Femoral nerve
27 Femoral artery
28 Spermatic cord
29 Testis
30 Posterior intercostal arteries
31 Internal abdominal oblique muscle
32 Lateral cutaneous branch of
   intercostal nerve
33 Dorsal branch of spinal nerve
34 Latissimus dorsi muscle
35 Deep muscles of the back (medial
   and lateral tract)
36 Anterior layer of rectus sheath
37 Posterior layer of rectus sheath
38 Thoracolumbar fascia
39 Spinal cord
40 Aorta
41 Ventral root ⎫ of spinal
42 Dorsal root ⎭ nerve

**Thoracic and abdominal wall** (schematic drawing). Note the segmental organization of the blood vessels and nerves. Right side: superficial layers; left side: deeper layers.

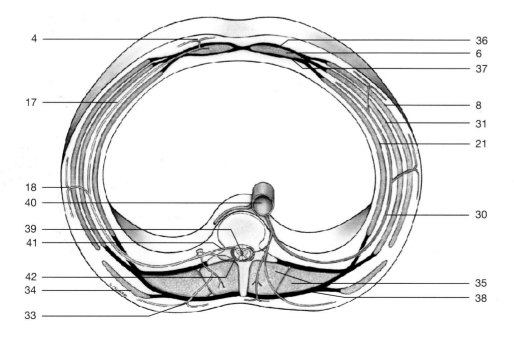

**Horizontal section of the abdominal wall** (from below) showing the location of the intercostal arteries (left side) and nerves (right side).

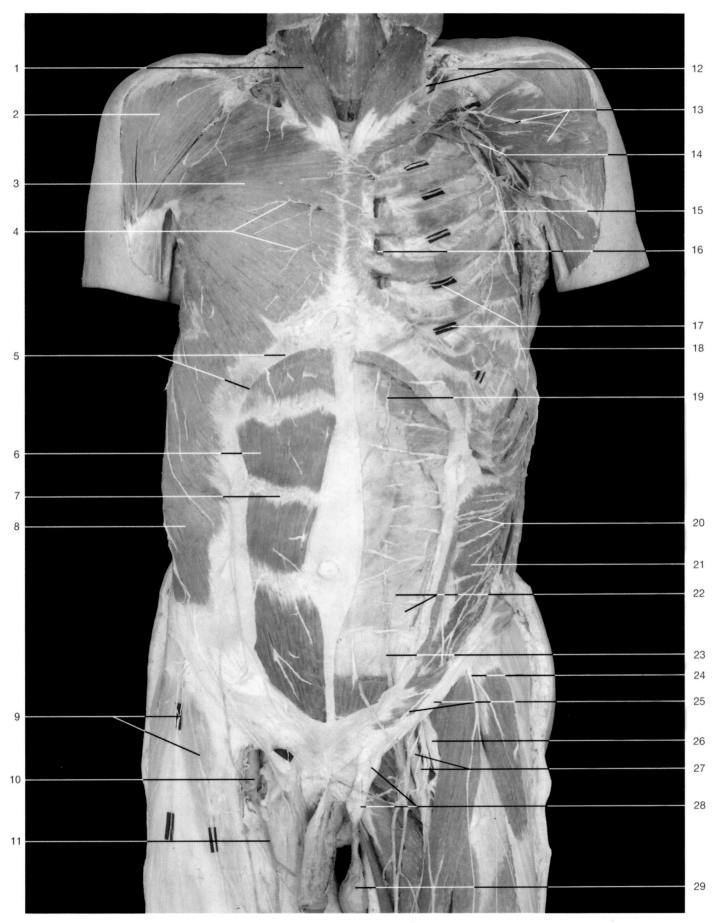

**Thoracic wall and abdominal wall V.** Right side: superficial layers; left side: deeper layers (anterior aspect). Pectoralis major and minor muscles, the external and internal intercostal muscles on the left side have been removed to display the intercostal nerves. The anterior layer of rectus sheath, the left rectus abdominis muscle, and the external and internal abdominal oblique muscles have been removed to show the thoraco-abdominal nerves within the abdominal wall.

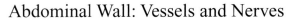

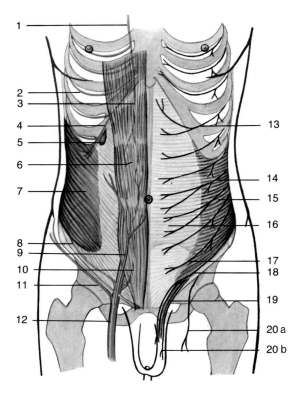

1   Rectus abdominis muscle
2   Tendinous intersection
3   Internal abdominal oblique muscle
4   External abdominal oblique muscle
    (reflected)
5   Anterior superior iliac spine
6   Ilio-inguinal nerve
7   Spermatic cord
8   Costal margin
9   Superior epigastric artery
10  Thoraco-abdominal (intercostal)
    nerves
11  Posterior layer of rectus sheath
12  Transversus abdominis muscle
13  Semilunar line
14  Arcuate line
15  Inferior epigastric artery
16  Inguinal ligament

**Abdominal wall with vessels and nerves.** The left rectus abdominis muscle has
been divided and reflected to display the inferior epigastric vessels. The left internal
abdominal oblique muscle has been removed to show the thoraco-abdominal nerves.

1   Internal thoracic artery
2   Intercostal artery
3   Superior epigastric artery
4   Musculophrenic artery
5   Gallbladder
6   Rectus abdominis muscle
7   External abdominal oblique muscle
8   Deep circumflex iliac artery
9   Superficial epigastric artery
10  Inferior epigastric artery
11  Superficial circumflex iliac artery
12  Femoral artery
13  Intercostal nerve
14  Thoraco-abdominal nerve (T$_{10}$)
15  Transversus abdominis muscle
16  Posterior layer of the rectus sheath
17  Iliohypogastric nerve (L$_1$)
18  Ilio-inguinal nerve (L$_1$)
19  Spermatic cord
20  Genitofemoral nerve (L$_1$, L$_2$)
    a  Femoral branch
    b  Genital branch

**Arteries and nerves that supply the thoracic and abdominal wall.** Note their
segmental arrangement (schematic drawing).

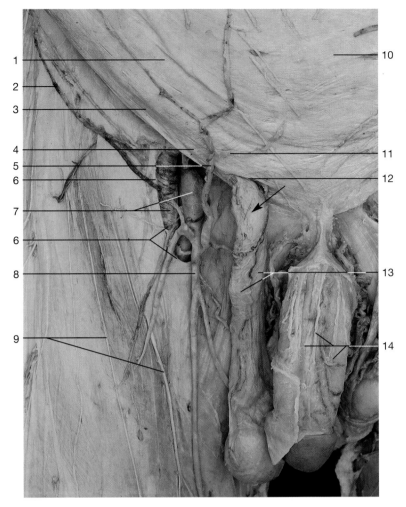

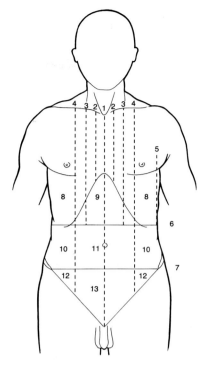

**Inguinal canal in the male I** (superficial layer, anterior aspect).
There is a small inguinal hernia (arrow).

**Regions and reference lines**
for delineating surface projections.

**Reference lines and regions**
1 Median line
2 Lateral sternal line
3 Parasternal line
4 Midclavicular line
5 Axillary line
6 Transpyloric plane
7 Transtubercular plane
8 Hypochondriac region
9 Epigastric region
10 Lumbar region
11 Umbilical region
12 Iliac region
13 Hypogastric region

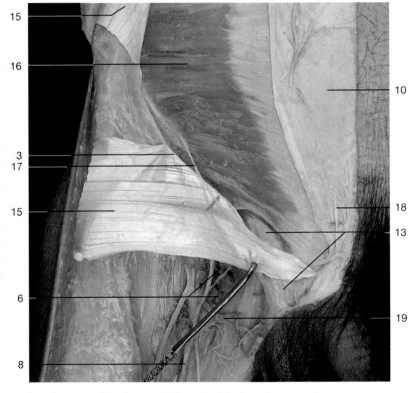

**Inguinal canal in the male II,** right side (anterior aspect).
The external abdominal oblique muscle has been divided to display
the inguinal canal.

1 Aponeurosis of external abdominal oblique muscle
2 Superficial circumflex iliac vein
3 Inguinal ligament
4 Lateral crus of inguinal ring
5 Superficial epigastric vein
6 Saphenous opening
7 Femoral artery and vein
8 Great saphenous vein
9 Anterior cutaneous branches of femoral nerve
10 Anterior layer of rectus sheath
11 Intercrural fibers
12 Superficial inguinal ring
13 Spermatic cord and genital branch
   of genitofemoral nerve
14 Penis with dorsal nerves and deep dorsal vein
   of penis
15 Aponeurosis of external abdominal oblique
   muscle (divided and reflected)
16 Internal abdominal oblique muscle
17 Ilio-inguinal nerve
18 Anterior cutaneous branches of iliohypogastric
   nerve
19 Superficial external pudendal veins

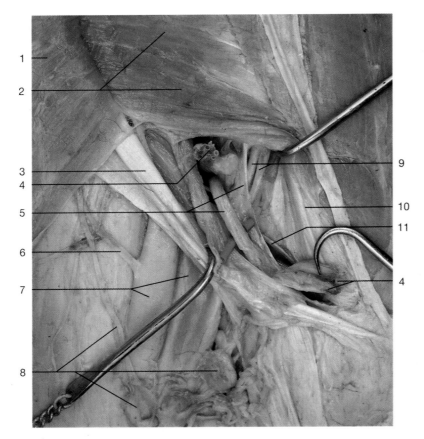

**Inguinal canal in the male III.** Deep dissection (anterior aspect, right side). Spermatic cord with exception of ductus deferens (probe) has been divided and reflected.

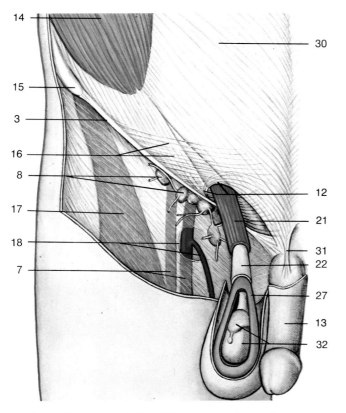

**General characteristics of lower part of anterior abdominal wall and inguinal canal** (schematic drawing).

1   Internal abdominal oblique muscle (reflected)
2   Transversus abdominis muscle
3   Inguinal ligament
4   Spermatic cord with the exception of the ductus deferens (divided and reflected)
5   Ductus deferens and interfoveolar ligament
6   Superficial circumflex iliac artery
7   Femoral artery and vein
8   Superficial inguinal lymph nodes and inguinal lymph vessel
9   Inferior epigastric artery and vein
10  Falx inguinalis or conjoint tendon (cut)
11  Pubic branch of inferior epigastric artery
12  Superficial inguinal ring
13  Penis
14  External abdominal oblique muscle
15  Anterior superior iliac spine
16  Intercrural fibers
17  Fascia lata and sartorius muscle
18  Saphenous opening and great saphenous vein
19  Deep inguinal ring
20  Skin of scrotum and dartos muscle
21  Cremaster muscle
22  Internal spermatic fascia
23  Ductus deferens
24  Epididymis
25  Peritoneum (blue)
26  Remnant of processus vaginalis
27  Tunica vaginalis testis
28  Rectus abdominis muscle
29  Spermatic cord with ductus deferens covered by external spermatic fascia
30  Anterior layer of rectus sheath
31  Suspensory ligament of penis
32  Testis and epididymis
33  Ductus deferens
34  Pampiniform venous plexus and testicular artery
35  Inferior epigastric artery
36  Lateral femoral cutaneous nerve
37  Ilio-inguinal nerve
38  Femoral nerve
39  Sartorius muscle
40  Deep dorsal vein of penis

**Inguinal hernias** may either pass through the inguinal canal lateral to the inferior epigastric artery (indirect or lateral inguinal hernias, A and C) or directly penetrate the abdominal wall through the inguinal triangle located medial to the inferior epigastric artery (direct or medial inguinal hernias, B). The lateral hernias can be congenital if the vaginal process remains open (C) or acquired (A) if the hernia develops independently of a patent processus vaginalis.

**Femoral hernias** generally protrude through the femoral ring below the inguinal ligament. Proper assessment of the site of herniation requires the identification of both the inguinal ligament and the epigastric artery.

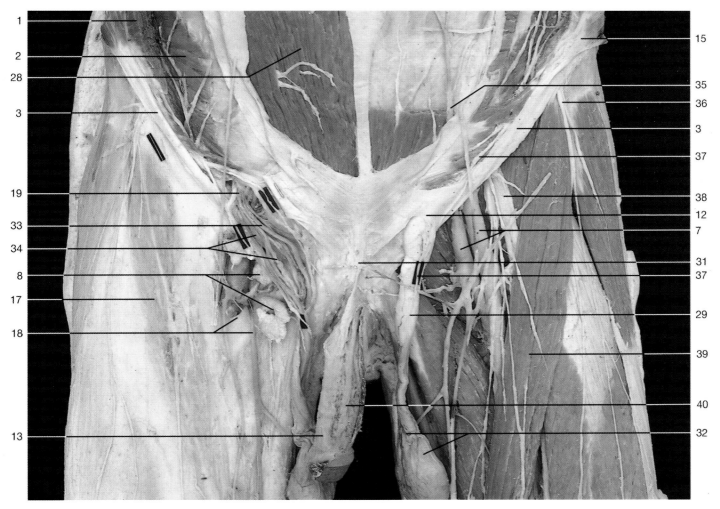

**Inguinal and femoral region in the male** (anterior aspect). On the right, the spermatic cord was dissected to display the ductus deferens and the accompanying vessels and nerves. The fascia lata on the left side has been removed.

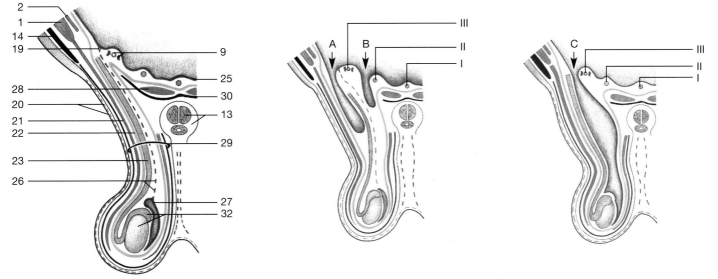

**Layers of spermatic cord and types of hernias.** Left: normal situation; middle: location of acquired inguinal hernias; A = indirect; B = direct inguinal hernia. Right: congenital indirect inguinal hernia (C); the vaginal process remained open.

I    = Median umbilical fold containing urachus chord.
II   = Medial umbilical fold with remnants of umbilical artery.
III  = Lateral umbilical fold with inferior epigastric artery and vein.

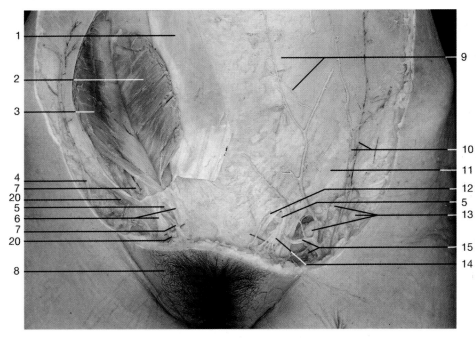

1  Aponeurosis of external abdominal oblique muscle
2  Internal abdominal oblique muscle (divided and reflected)
3  Transversus abdominis muscle
4  Superficial circumflex iliac artery and vein
5  Superficial inguinal ring with fat pad
6  Medial and lateral crural fibers
7  Round ligament (ligamentum teres uteri)
8  Labium majus pudendi
9  Anterior layer of rectus sheath
10  Superficial epigastric artery and vein
11  Inguinal ligament
12  Cutaneous branch of ilio-inguinal nerve
13  Superficial inguinal lymph nodes
14  Entrance of round ligament into the labium majus
15  External pudendal artery and vein
16  Position of deep inguinal ring
17  Ilio-inguinal nerve
18  Internal abdominal oblique muscle
19  Pubic branch of inferior epigastric artery
20  Genital branch of genitofemoral nerve
21  Fat pad of inguinal canal
22  Ilio-inguinal nerve
23  Sheath of round ligament (inguinal canal)
24  Transversalis fascia

**Inguinal region in the female** (anterior aspect). Left side: superficial layer; right side: external and internal abdominal oblique muscle divided and reflected.

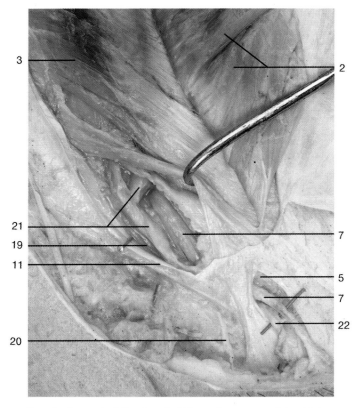

**Inguinal canal of the female I** (anterior aspect, right side). The external abdominal oblique muscle has been divided and reflected, to display the ilio-inguinal nerve and the round ligament.

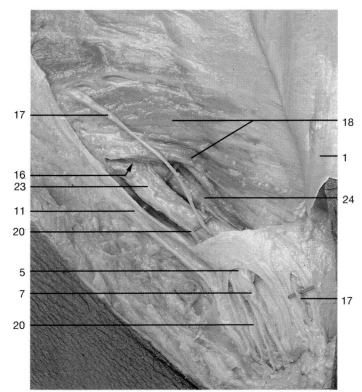

**Inguinal canal of the female II** (anterior aspect, right side). The external and internal abdominal oblique muscle have been divided and reflected to show the content of the inguinal canal.

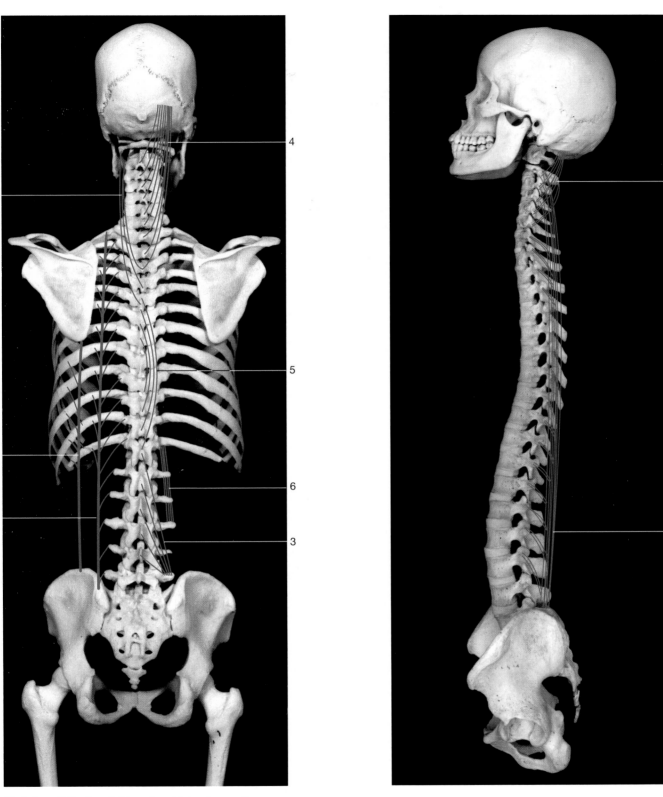

**Skeleton of the trunk** (dorsal and lateral aspect).
The long muscles of the back [longissimus (1) and iliocostalis (2) muscle] originate at the sacrum and pelvis and insert at the spinous or transverse processes of the vertebrae or at the ribs. There are also muscles that insert at the occipital bone. The long muscles form the lateral tract, whereas muscles of the medial tract are situated within the groove between the spinous and transverse processes of the vertebrae [transversospinal (3) and spinotransversal (4) muscles] or between the spinous processes [spinalis muscles (5)] or between the transverse processes [intertransversarii muscles (6)] of the vertebrae.

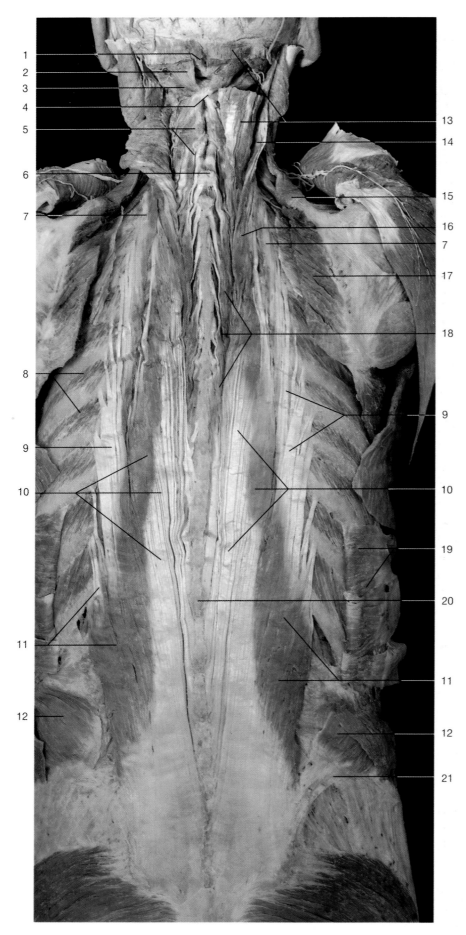

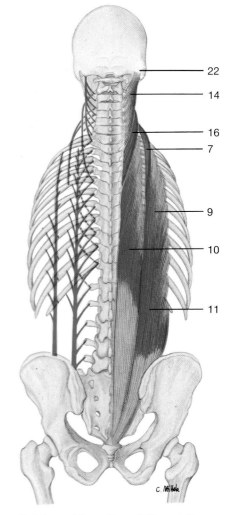

**Origin and insertion of iliocostalis and longissimus muscles** (schematic drawing).

**Muscles of the back I.** Dissection of the erector spinae muscle (lateral column of the intrinsic back muscles).

1   Rectus capitis posterior minor muscle
2   Rectus capitis posterior major muscle
3   Obliquus capitis inferior muscle
4   Spinous process of axis
5   Semispinalis cervicis muscle
6   Spinous process of seventh vertebra
7   Iliocostalis cervicis muscle
8   External intercostal muscles
9   Iliocostalis thoracis muscle
10  Longissimus thoracis muscle
11  Iliocostalis lumborum muscle
12  Internal abdominal oblique muscle
13  Semispinalis capitis muscle (divided)
14  Longissimus capitis muscle
15  Levator scapulae muscle
16  Longissimus cervicis muscle
17  Rhomboid major muscle
18  Spinalis thoracis muscle
19  Serratus posterior inferior muscle (reflected)
20  Spinous process of second lumbar vertebra
21  Iliac crest
22  Mastoid process

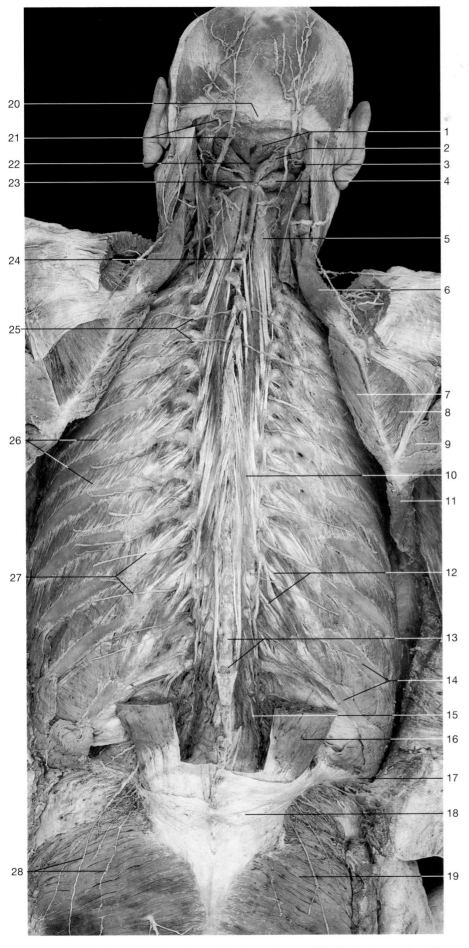

1   Rectus capitis posterior minor muscle
2   Rectus capitis posterior major muscle
3   Obliquus capitis superior muscle
4   Obliquus capitis inferior muscle
5   Semispinalis cervicis muscle
6   Levator scapulae muscle
7   Rhomboideus major muscle
8   Scapula with infraspinatus muscle
9   Teres major muscle
10  Spinalis muscle
11  Latissimus dorsi muscle
12  Levatores costarum muscles
13  Spinous processes of lumbar vertebrae
14  Ribs (Th$_{11}$, Th$_{12}$)
15  Multifidus muscle
16  Longissimus and iliocostalis
    muscles (cut)
17  Iliac crest (lumbar triangle)
18  Thoracolumbar fascia
19  Gluteus maximus muscle
20  Protuberantia occipitalis externa
21  Occipital artery and greater occipital
    nerve (C$_2$)
22  Spinous process of atlas
23  Spinous process of axis
24  Spinous process of seventh cervical
    vertebra (vertebra prominens)
25  Medial branches of dorsal branches
    of spinal nerves
26  External intercostal muscles
27  Lateral branches of dorsal branches
    of spinal nerves
28  Superior cluneal nerves

**Muscles of the back II.** Dissection of the deeper layer of the intrinsic muscles of the back (longissimus and iliocostalis muscles are cut).

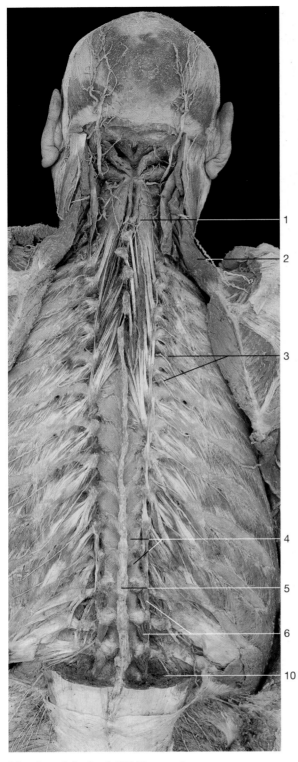

**Muscles of the back III.** Deepest layer.

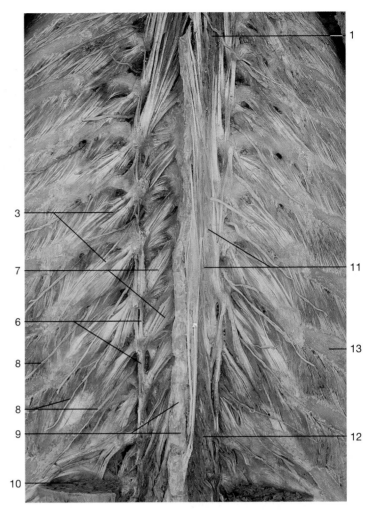

**Muscles of the back III.** Deepest layer. Lumbar region (higher magnification).

1   Semispinalis cervicis muscle
2   Levator scapulae muscle
3   Levatores costarum muscles
4   Vertebral arches of lumbar vertebrae
5   Supraspinal ligaments
6   Intertransverse lumbar muscles
7   Lumbar rotator muscles
8   Cutaneous branches of spinal nerves
9   Lumbar interspinal muscles
10  Longissimus and iliocostalis muscle (cut)
11  Spinal muscle of the back
12  Multifidus muscle
13  Tenth rib ($T_{10}$)

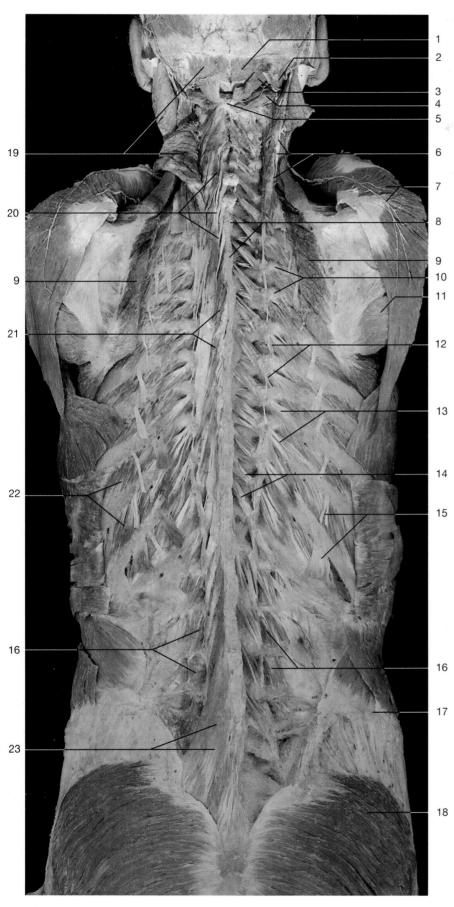

**Muscles of the back IV.** Transversospinal muscles, deepest layer on the right, where all parts of semispinalis and multifidus muscles have been removed.

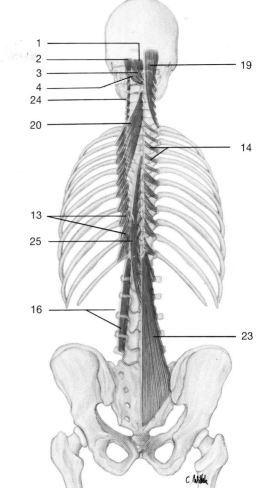

**Medial column of intrinsic muscles of the back.** Transversospinal and intertransversal system (schematic drawing).

1  Rectus capitis posterior minor muscle
2  Obliquus capitis superior muscle
3  Rectus capitis posterior major muscle
4  Obliquus capitis inferior muscle
5  Spinous process of axis
6  Longissimus capitis muscle
7  Trapezius muscle (reflected) and
   accessory nerve (n. XI)
8  Spinous processes
9  Rhomboid major muscle
10  Transverse processes of thoracic
   vertebrae
11  Teres major muscle
12  Intertransverse ligaments
13  Levatores costarum muscles
14  Rotatores muscles
15  Tendons of iliocostalis muscle
16  Intertransversarii lumborum muscles (lateral)
17  Iliac crest
18  Gluteus maximus muscle
19  Semispinalis capitis muscle
20  Semispinalis cervicis muscle
21  Semispinalis thoracis muscle
22  External intercostal muscles
23  Multifidus muscle
24  Posterior cervical intertransversarii muscles
25  Spinalis thoracis muscle

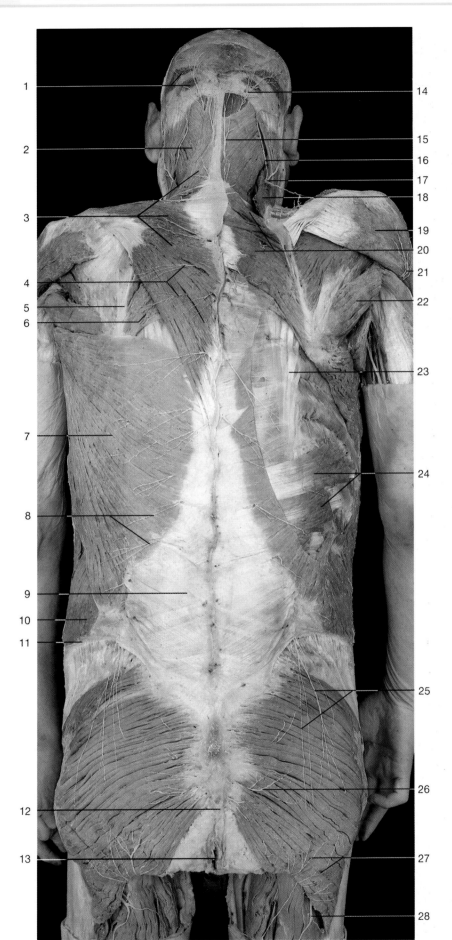

1   Occipital belly of occipitofrontalis muscle
2   Splenius capitis muscle
3   Trapezius muscle
4   Medial cutaneous branches of dorsal rami
    of spinal nerves
5   Medial margin of scapula
6   Rhomboid major muscle
7   Latissimus dorsi muscle
8   Lateral cutaneous branches of dorsal rami
    of spinal nerves
9   Thoracolumbar fascia
10  External abdominal oblique muscle
11  Iliac crest
12  Last coccygeal vertebra
13  Anus
14  Greater occipital nerve
15  Third occipital nerve
16  Lesser occipital nerve
17  Cutaneous branches of cervical plexus
18  Levator scapulae muscle
19  Deltoid muscle
20  Rhomboid major and minor muscles
21  Upper lateral cutaneous nerve of arm
    (branch of axillary nerve)
22  Teres major muscle
23  Iliocostalis thoracis muscle
24  Serratus posterior inferior muscle
25  Superior cluneal nerves
26  Middle cluneal nerves
27  Inferior cluneal nerves
28  Posterior femoral cutaneous nerve

▷  **To page 227**

1   Trapezius muscle
2   Infraspinatus muscle
3   Left latissimus dorsi muscle
4   Thoracolumbar fascia
5   Splenius cervicis muscle
6   Serratus posterior superior muscle
7   Medial branches of dorsal rami
    of thoracic spinal nerves
8   Lateral branches of dorsal rami
    of thoracic spinal nerves
9   Iliocostalis muscle
10  Serratus posterior inferior muscle
11  Latissimus dorsi muscle (reflected)

**Innervation of the back I.** Superficial (left) and deeper (right) layers.
Right trapezius and latissimus dorsi muscles removed.

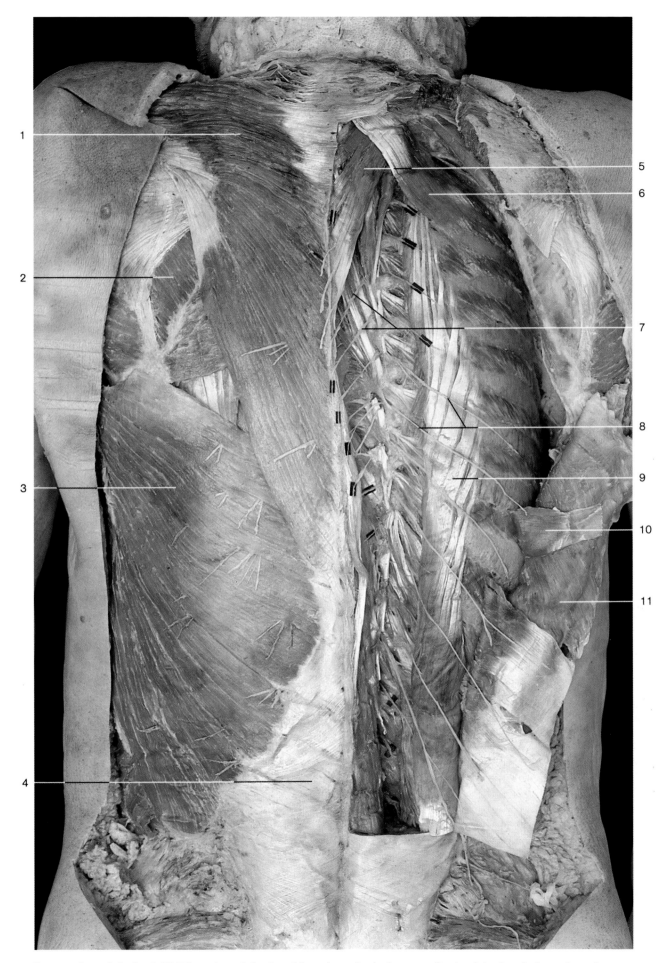

**Innervation of the back II.** Dissection of the dorsal branches of spinal nerves. On the right, longissimus thoracis muscle has been removed and iliocostalis muscle laterally reflected.

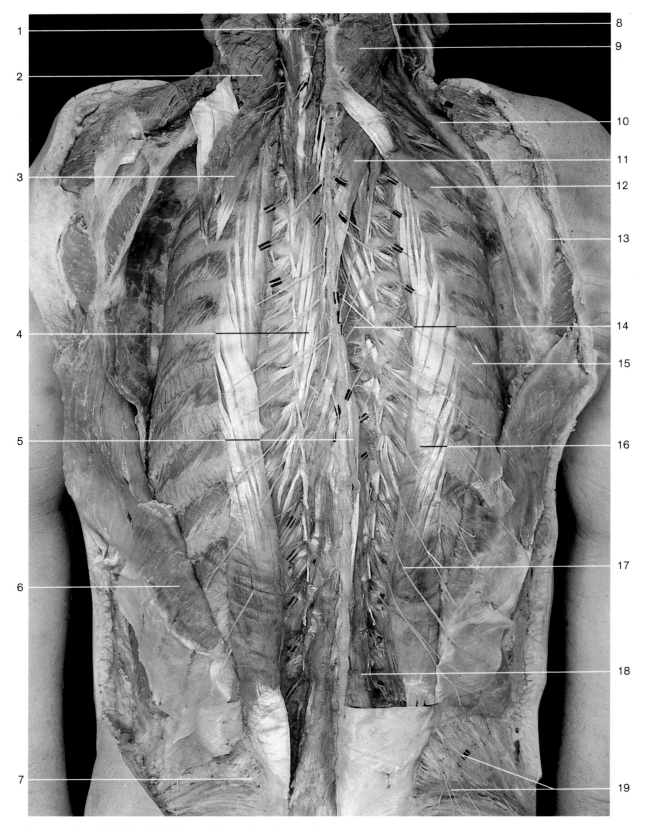

**Innervation of the back III.** Deeper layer (dorsal aspect).

| | | |
|---|---|---|
| 1  Semispinalis capitis muscle | 7  Iliac crest | 14  Medial branches of dorsal rami |
| 2  Left splenius capitis muscle | 8  Lesser occipital nerve | of spinal nerves |
| (cut and reflected) | 9  Splenius capitis muscle | 15  Rib and external intercostal muscle |
| 3  Left splenius cervicis muscle | 10  Levator scapulae muscle | 16  Iliocostalis thoracis muscle |
| (cut and reflected) | 11  Splenius cervicis muscle | 17  Lateral branches of dorsal rami |
| 4  Semispinalis thoracis muscle | 12  Serratus posterior superior muscle | of spinal nerves |
| 5  Spinalis thoracis muscle | 13  Scapula | 18  Multifidus muscle |
| 6  Latissimus dorsi muscle (reflected) | | 19  Superior cluneal nerves |

1 Greater occipital nerve ($C_2$)
2 Suboccipital nerve ($C_1$)
3 Medial branches of dorsal rami of spinal nerves
4 Lateral branches of dorsal rami of spinal nerves
5 Superior cluneal nerves ($L_1$–$L_3$)
6 Middle cluneal nerves ($S_1$–$S_3$)
7 Inferior cluneal nerves (derived from branches of the sacral plexus, ventral rami)
8 Lesser occipital nerve
9 Great auricular nerve
10 Trapezius muscle
11 Deltoid muscle
12 Latissimus dorsi muscle
13 Gluteus maximus muscle
14 External intercostal muscle
15 Internal intercostal muscle
16 Innermost intercostal muscle
17 Dorsal ramus of spinal nerve
18 Spinal nerve and spinal ganglion
19 Sympathetic trunk with ganglion
20 Intercostal nerve
21 Lateral cutaneous branch ⎫
22 Anterior cutaneous branch ⎬ of intercostal nerve

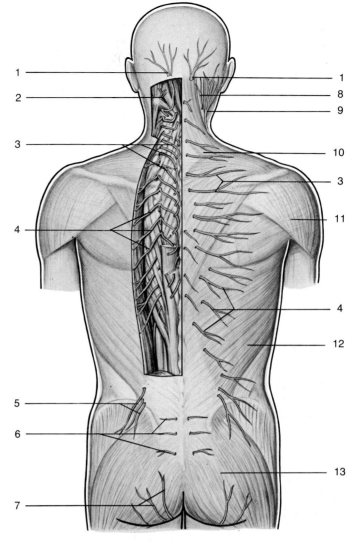

**General characteristics of the innervation of the back.**
Distribution of dorsal branches of spinal nerves. Note the segmental arrangement of the innervation of the dorsal part of the trunk (schematic drawing).

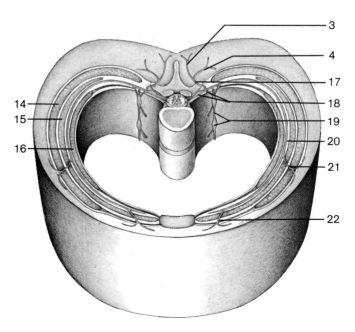

**Position and branches of spinal nerves in one segment of thoracic wall** (schematic drawing).

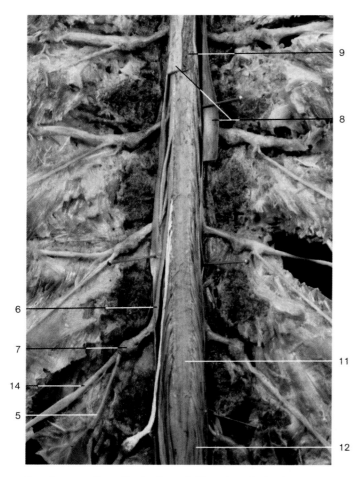

**Lumbar portion of spinal cord.** Note the relation between the nervous and muscular segments.

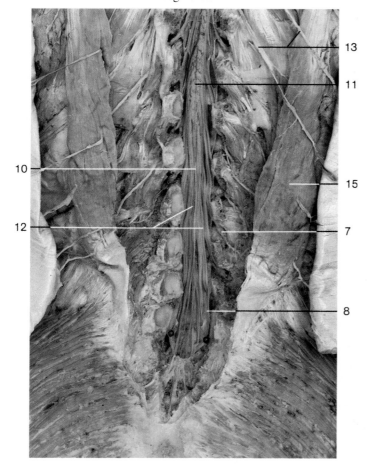

**Terminal part of spinal cord.** Dura removed.

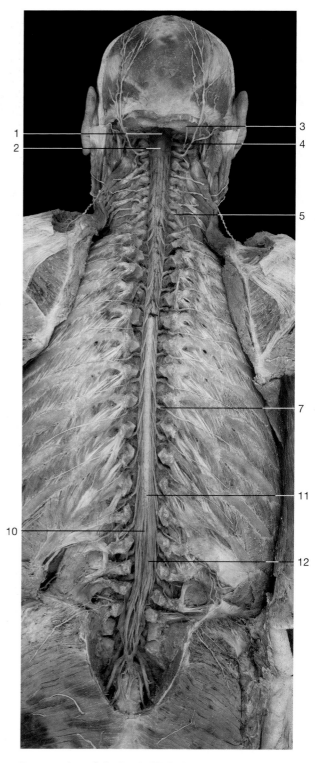

**Innervation of the back IV. Spinal cord in the vertebral canal** (opened). Longissimus dorsi and iliocostal muscles have been removed.

| | | | |
|---|---|---|---|
| 1 | Cerebellomedullary cistern | 9 | Spinal arachnoid mater |
| 2 | Medulla oblongata | 10 | Filum terminale |
| 3 | Third cervical nerve (C$_3$) | 11 | Conus medullaris |
| 4 | Greater occipital nerve (C$_2$) | 12 | Cauda equina |
| 5 | Dorsal primary ramus | 13 | Lateral branches of dorsal rami of spinal nerves |
| 6 | Dorsal roots | 14 | Ventral ramus of spinal nerve (intercostal nerve) |
| 7 | Spinal ganglion | 15 | Iliocostalis muscle |
| 8 | Spinal dura mater | | |

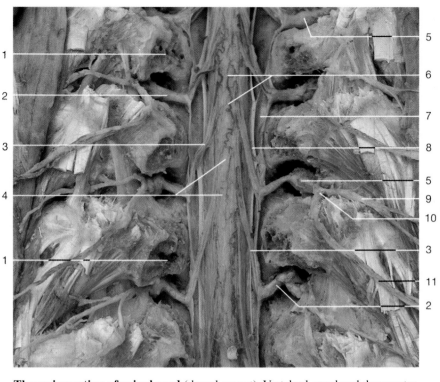

1    Arch of vertebra (divided)
2    Spinal nerve with meningeal coverings
3    Dorsal roots of thoracic spinal nerves
4    Spinal cord (thoracic portion)
5    Spinal ganglia with meningeal coverings
6    Pia mater with blood vessels
7    Dura mater (opened)
8    Denticulate ligament
9    Lateral branch of dorsal ramus
10   Dorsal ramus of spinal nerve
     (dividing into a medial and lateral branch)
11   Medial branch of dorsal ramus
     of spinal nerve
12   Spinal dura mater
13   Spinal nerves of sacral segments
14   Filum terminale

**Thoracic portion of spinal cord** (dorsal aspect). Vertebral canal and dura mater opened.

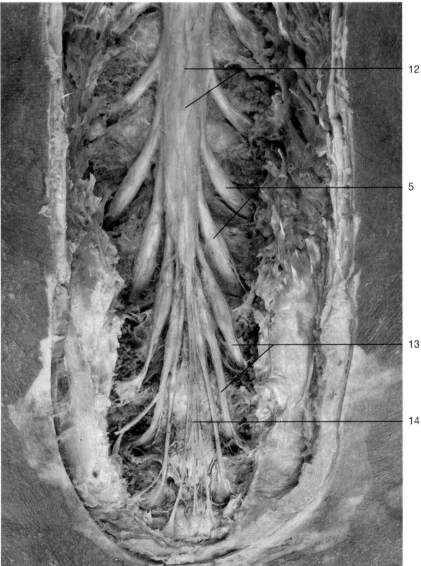

**Terminal part of spinal cord with dura mater** (dorsal aspect). Dorsal part of sacrum removed.

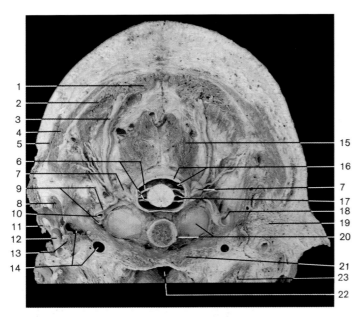

**Horizontal section of the neck.** Dissection of the second cervical spinal nerve. Posterior surface at top of figure.

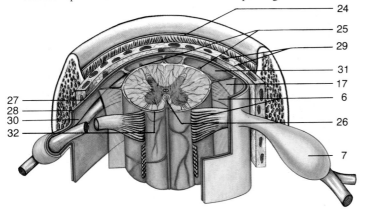

**Meningeal coverings of the spinal cord** (anterior aspect). (Schematic drawing.)

1   Trapezius muscle
2   Semispinalis capitis muscle
3   Dorsal ramus of spinal nerve
4   Sternocleidomastoid muscle
5   Platysma muscle
6   Dorsal and ventral roots of spinal nerves
7   Spinal ganglion
8   Posterior belly of digastric muscle
9   Ventral ramus of spinal nerve
10  Vertebral artery
11  Great auricular nerve
12  Superficial temporal artery
13  Styloid process
14  Internal jugular vein and internal carotid artery
15  Rectus capitis posterior major muscle
16  Dura mater and subarachnoid space
17  Denticulate ligament
18  Vertebral artery
19  Parotid gland
20  Dens of axis (divided) and inferior articular facet of atlas
21  Longus capitis muscle
22  Pharyngeal cavity
23  Medial pterygoid muscle
24  Periosteum of vertebral canal
25  Posterior spinal arteries
26  Anterior spinal artery

**Meningeal coverings**
27  Dura mater
28  Subdural space
29  Extradural or epidural space with venous plexus and fatty tissue
30  Arachnoid (green)
31  Subarachnoid space
32  Pia mater (pink)
33  Nucleus pulposus
34  Crus of diaphragm
35  Intervertebral disc
36  Body of first lumbar vertebra
37  Spinal cord
38  Conus medullaris
39  Cauda equina
40  Filum terminale
41  Spinous process

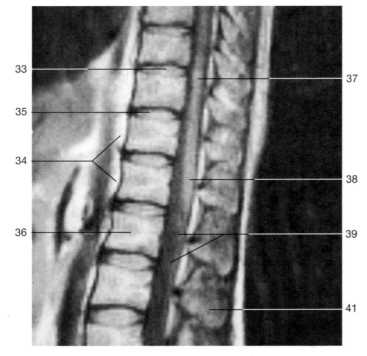

**Sagittal section through the vertebral canal,** $T_9$–$L_2$. (MRI scan.)

**Sagittal section through the vertebral canal,** $T_{12}$–$L_2$. Notice red bone marrow (unfixed).

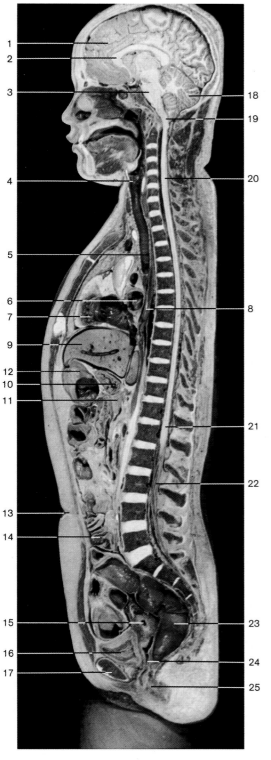

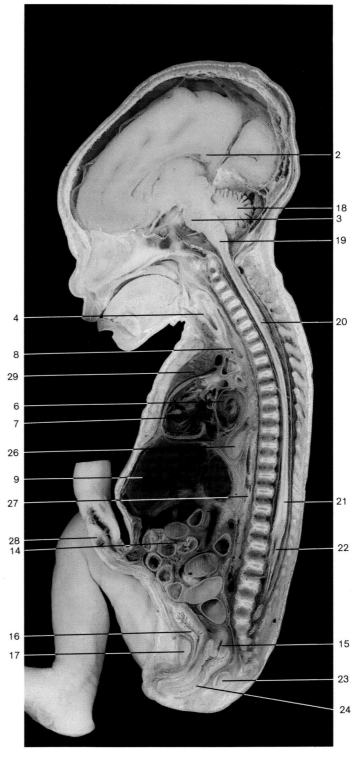

**Median section of the head and trunk in the adult** (female). The conus medullaris of the spinal cord is located at the level of $L_1$.

**Median section of the head and trunk in the neonate.** Note that in the neonate the conus medullaris of the spinal cord extends far more caudally than in the adult.

| 1 | Cerebrum | 11 | Pancreas | 21 | Conus medullaris |
|---|----------|----|----------|----|------------------|
| 2 | Corpus callosum | 12 | Transverse colon | 22 | Cauda equina |
| 3 | Pons | 13 | Umbilicus | 23 | Rectum |
| 4 | Larynx | 14 | Small intestine | 24 | Vagina |
| 5 | Trachea | 15 | Uterus | 25 | Anus |
| 6 | Left atrium | 16 | Urinary bladder | 26 | Inferior vena cava |
| 7 | Right ventricle | 17 | Pubic symphysis | 27 | Aorta |
| 8 | Esophagus | 18 | Cerebellum | 28 | Umbilical cord |
| 9 | Liver | 19 | Medulla oblongata | 29 | Thymus |
| 10 | Stomach | 20 | Spinal cord | | |

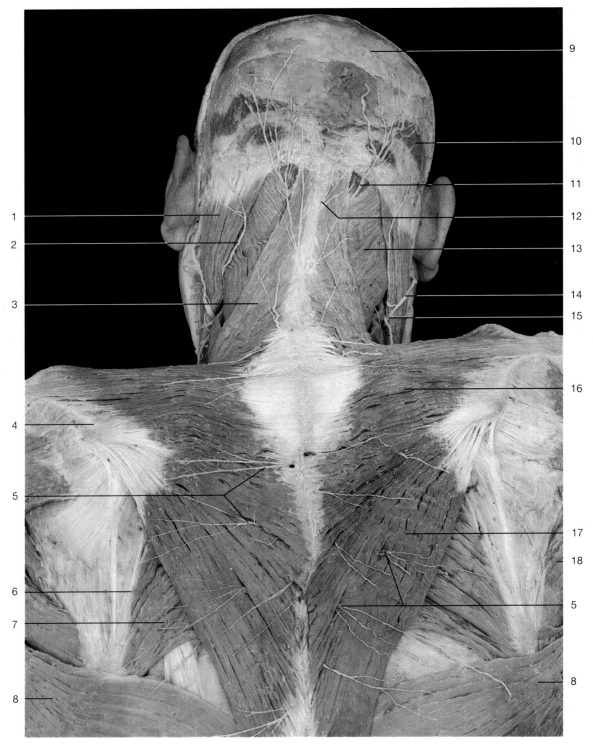

**Dorsal aspect of the neck I. Superficial layer.** Nuchal region and shoulder.

1   Sternocleidomastoid muscle
2   Lesser occipital nerve
3   Descending fibers of trapezius muscle
4   Spine of scapula
5   Medial cutaneous branches of dorsal rami of spinal nerves
6   Medial margin of scapula
7   Rhomboid major muscle
8   Latissimus dorsi muscle
9   Galea aponeurotica

10   Occipital belly of occipitofrontalis muscle
11   Greater occipital nerve
12   Third occipital nerve
13   Splenius capitis muscle
14   Great auricular nerve
15   Cutaneous nerves of cervical plexus
16   Transverse fibers of trapezius muscle
17   Ascending fibers of trapezius muscle
18   Teres major muscle

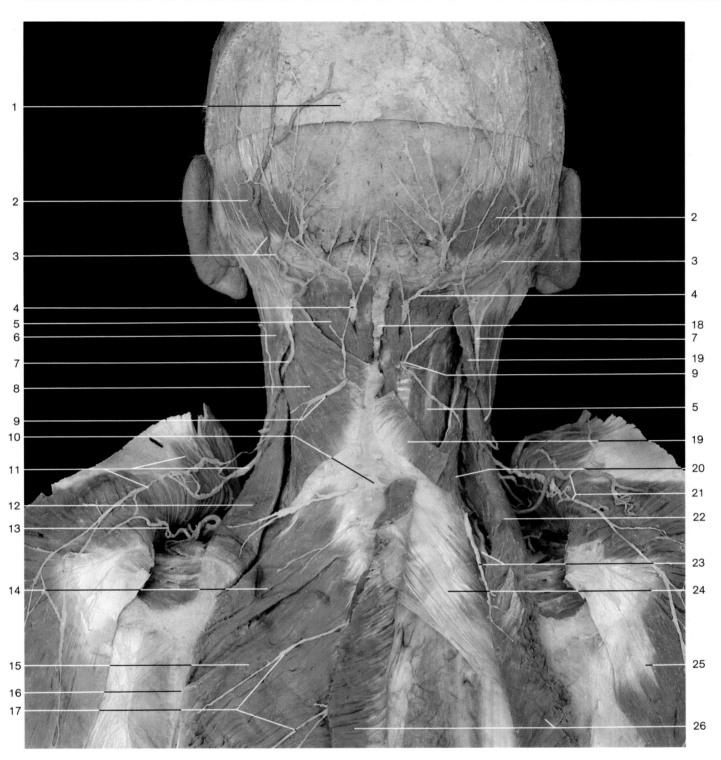

**Dorsal aspect of the neck II. Deeper layer.** The left trapezius muscle has been divided and reflected. On the right, trapezius, rhomboid, and splenius muscles have been divided. Right levator scapulae muscle has been slightly reflected.

1  Galea aponeurotica
2  Occipital belly of occipitofrontalis muscle
3  Occipital artery
4  Greater occipital nerve (C$_2$)
5  Semispinalis capitis muscle
6  Sternocleidomastoid muscle
7  Lesser occipital nerve
8  Left splenius capitis muscle
9  Third occipital nerve (C$_3$)
10 Spinous process of vertebra prominens (C$_7$)

11 Left trapezius muscle and accessory nerve
12 Levator scapulae muscle
13 Superficial branch of transverse cervical artery
14 Rhomboid minor muscle
15 Rhomboid major muscle
16 Medial margin of scapula
17 Medial branches of dorsal rami of spinal nerves
18 Ligamentum nuchae
19 Splenius capitis muscle (divided)

20 Splenius cervicis muscle
21 Right accessory nerve and superficial branch of transverse cervical artery
22 Right levator scapulae muscle
23 Dorsal scapular nerve and deep branch of transverse cervical artery
24 Serratus posterior superior muscle
25 Right trapezius muscle (divided and reflected)
26 Right rhomboid major muscle (divided and reflected)

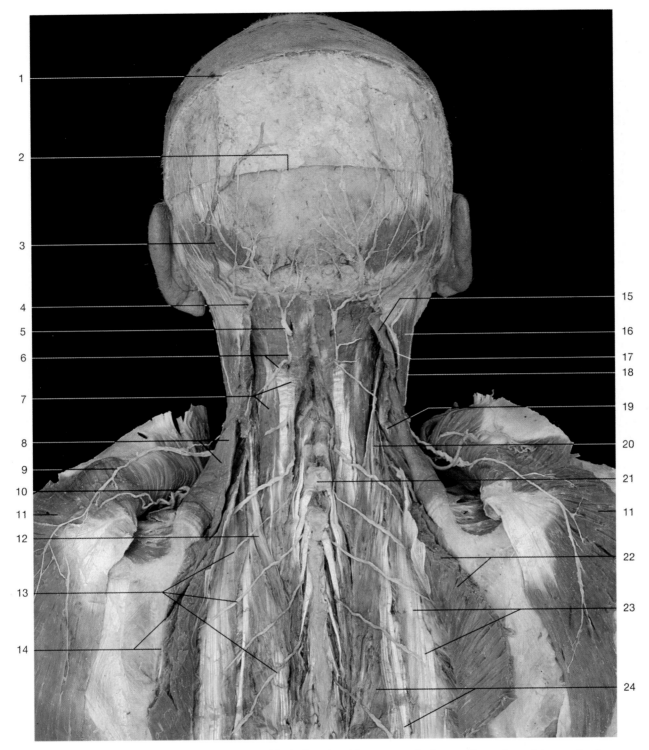

**Dorsal aspect of the neck III. Deepest layer. Nuchal region.** Trapezius, splenius capitis, and cervicis muscles have been divided and partly removed or reflected.

| | | | |
|---|---|---|---|
| 1 | Skin of scalp | 9 | Accessory nerve (n. XI) |
| 2 | Galea aponeurotica | 10 | Superficial cervical artery |
| 3 | Occipital belly of occipitofrontalis | 11 | Trapezius muscle (reflected) |
| | muscle | 12 | Longissimus cervicis muscle |
| 4 | Occipital artery | 13 | Medial cutaneous branches of |
| 5 | Greater occipital nerve | | dorsal rami of spinal nerves |
| 6 | Third occipital nerve | 14 | Medial margin of scapula |
| 7 | Semispinalis capitis muscle | 15 | Splenius capitis muscle (divided) |
| 8 | Levator scapulae muscle | 16 | Sternocleidomastoid muscle |

17  Lesser occipital nerve
18  Great auricular nerve
19  Splenius cervicis muscle
20  Longissimus cervicis muscle
21  Spinous process of seventh cervical
    vertebra (vertebra prominens)
22  Rhomboid muscles (divided)
23  Iliocostalis thoracis muscle
24  Longissimus thoracis muscle

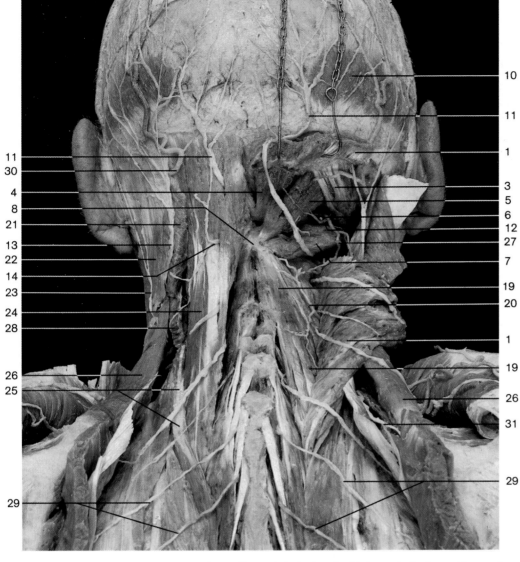

1  Semispinalis capitis muscle (divided)
2  External occipital protuberance
3  Obliquus capitis superior muscle
4  Rectus capitis posterior minor muscle
5  Rectus capitis posterior major muscle
6  Vertebral artery
7  Obliquus capitis inferior muscle
8  Spinous process of axis
9  Third cervical vertebra
10  Occipital belly of occipitofrontalis muscle
11  Greater occipital nerve
12  Suboccipital nerve ($C_1$)
13  Lesser occipital nerve
14  Third occipital nerve ($C_3$)
15  Mastoid process and splenius capitis muscle
16  Atlas
17  Axis
18  Spinous process of third cervical vertebra
19  Right semispinalis cervicis muscle
20  Deep cervical artery
21  Left splenius capitis muscle (divided)
22  Left sternocleidomastoid muscle
23  Great auricular nerve
24  Left semispinalis capitis muscle
25  Left longissimus cervicis muscle
26  Levator scapulae muscle
27  Muscular branch of vertebral artery
28  Left semispinalis cervicis muscle (divided)
29  Medial branches of dorsal rami of spinal nerves
30  Occipital artery
31  Dorsal scapular nerve

**Dorsal aspect of the neck IV. Deepest layer. Suboccipital triangle.** Right semispinalis capitis muscle divided and reflected.

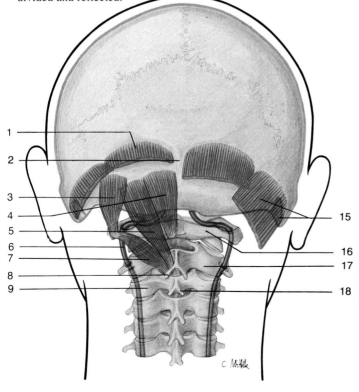

**Suboccipital triangle and position of the vertebral artery** (schematic drawing).

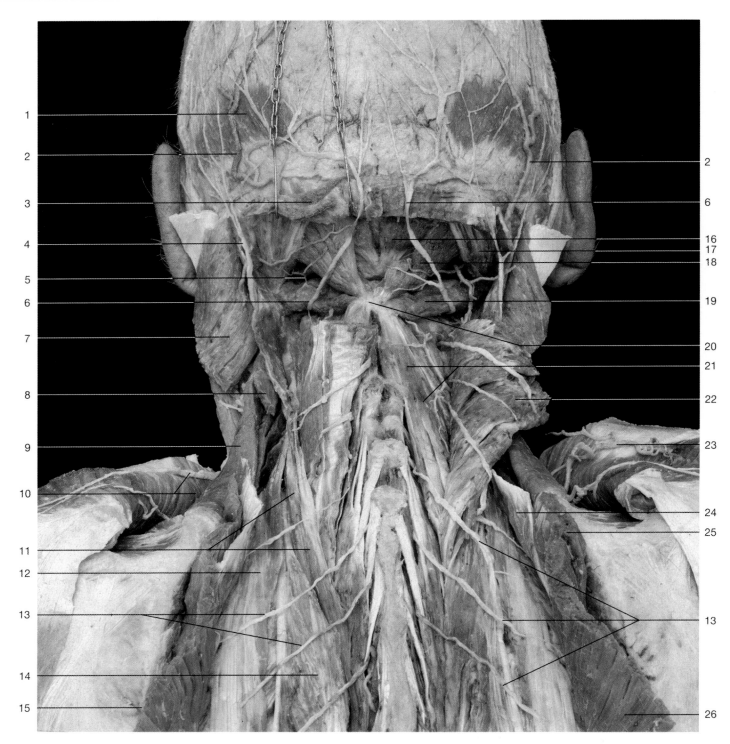

**Dorsal aspect of the neck V. Nuchal region. Deepest layer.** Dissection of suboccipital triangle on both sides.

 1  Occipital belly of occipitofrontalis muscle
 2  Occipital artery
 3  Insertion of semispinalis capitis muscle (divided)
 4  Lesser occipital nerve (from cervical
    plexus)
 5  Suboccipital nerve (C$_1$)
 6  Greater occipital nerve (C$_2$)
 7  Splenius capitis muscle (reflected)
 8  Splenius cervicis muscle
 9  Levator scapulae muscle
10  Accessory nerve (n. XI), trapezius muscle

11  Longissimus cervicis muscle
12  Iliocostalis cervicis muscle
13  Medial cutaneus branches of dorsal rami
    of spinal nerves (C$_7$, C$_8$)
14  Longissimus thoracis muscle
15  Medial margin of scapula
16  Rectus capitis posterior minor muscle
17  Obliquus capitis superior muscle
18  Rectus capitis posterior major muscle
19  Obliquus capitis inferior muscle
20  Spinous process of axis

21  Semispinalis cervicis muscle
22  Semispinalis capitis muscle
    (divided and reflected)
23  Transverse cervical artery
    (superficial branch)
24  Serratus posterior superior muscle
    (divided and reflected)
25  Rhomboid minor muscle
    (divided and reflected)
26  Rhomboid major muscle
    (divided and reflected)

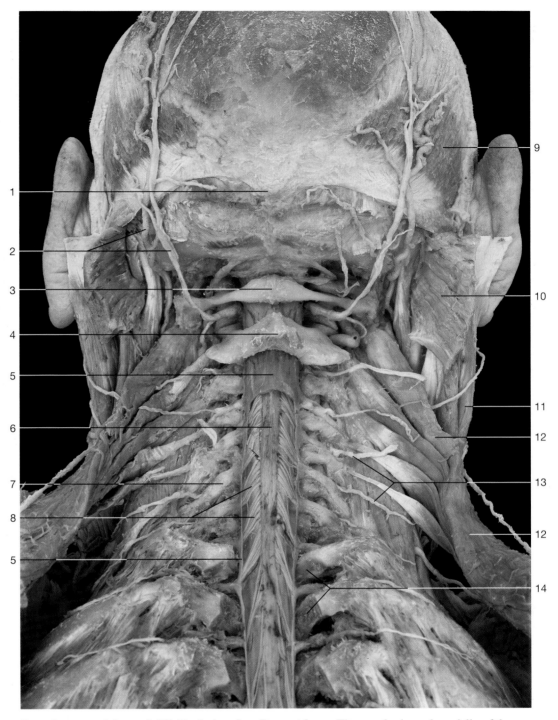

**Dorsal aspect of the neck VI. Nuchal region. Deepest layer.** The vertebral canal caudally of the atlas and axis has been opened to show the spinal cord (dura mater has been partly removed).

1  Protuberantia occipitalis externa
2  Greater occipital nerve (C₂) and occipital artery
3  Atlas (posterior arch)
4  Axis (posterior arch)
5  Dura mater
6  Spinal cord
7  Spinal ganglion
8  Posterior root filaments (fila radicularia posterior)
9  Occipital belly of occipitofrontalis muscle
10  Splenius capitis muscle (cut and reflected)
11  Sternocleidomastoid muscle
12  Levator scapulae muscle
13  Posterior branches of spinal nerves
14  Arches of cervical vertebrae (cut)

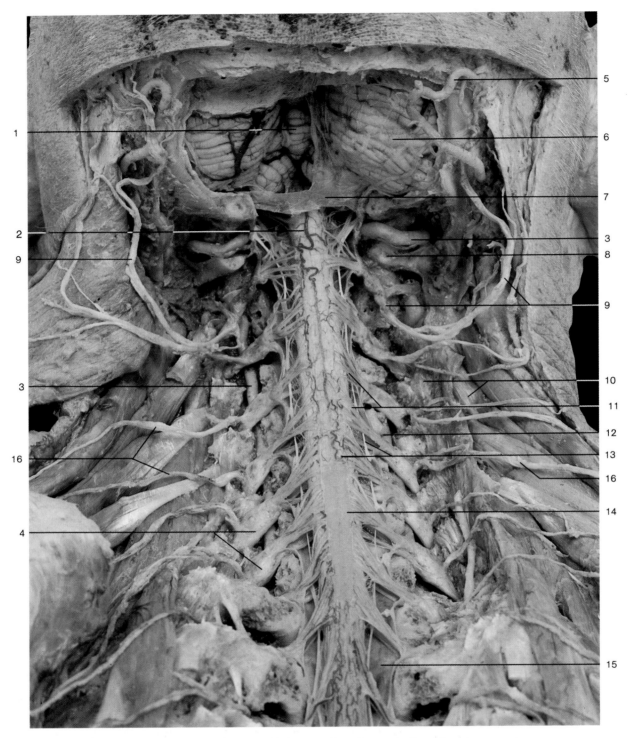

**Neck, deepest layer. Spinal cord and medulla oblongata** (dorsal aspect). Cranial cavity opened.

1  Vermis of the cerebellum
2  Medulla oblongata and posterior spinal artery
3  Vertebral artery
4  Spinal ganglion
5  Occipital artery
6  Cerebellum
7  Cerebellomedullary cistern
8  Atlas

9  Greater occipital nerve (C$_2$)
10  Levator scapulae muscle and intertransverse ligament
11  Dorsal roots of spinal nerves
12  Vertebral arch
13  Denticulate ligament and arachnoid mater
14  Area where pia mater has been removed
15  Dura mater
16  Dorsal rami of spinal nerves

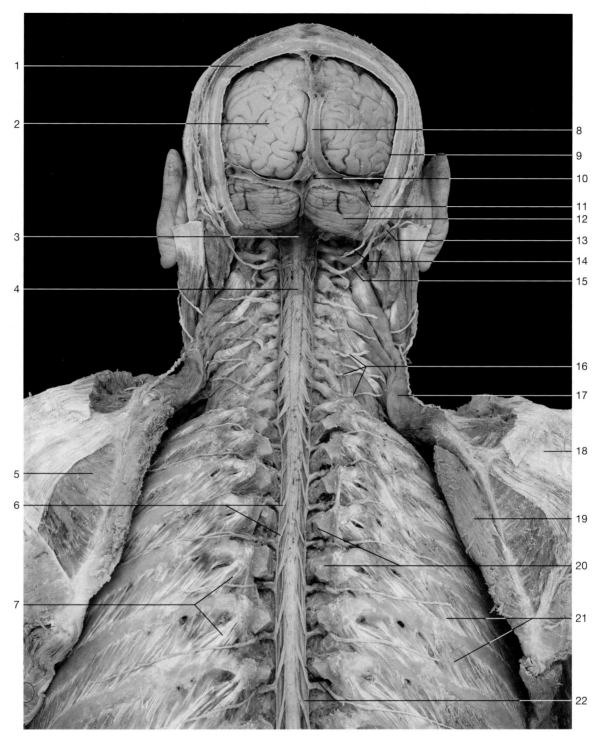

**Neck, deepest layer. Dissection of medulla oblongata and spinal cord** in relation to the brain (dorsal aspect).

1  Calvaria
2  Left hemisphere of the brain
3  Cerebellomedullary cistern
4  Spinal cord
5  Scapula with infraspinous muscle
6  Root filaments (fila radicularia posterior)
7  Levatores costarum muscles
8  Falx cerebri with sinus sagittalis superior
9  Subarachnoidal space
10  Confluens sinuum
11  Transverse sinus

12  Cerebellum
13  Occipital artery
14  Suboccipital nerve (C$_1$)
15  Greater occipital nerve (C$_2$)
16  Posterior branches of spinal nerves
17  Levator scapulae muscle
18  Deltoid muscle
19  Rhomboid muscles
20  Vertebral arches (cut)
21  External intercostal muscle
22  Dura mater

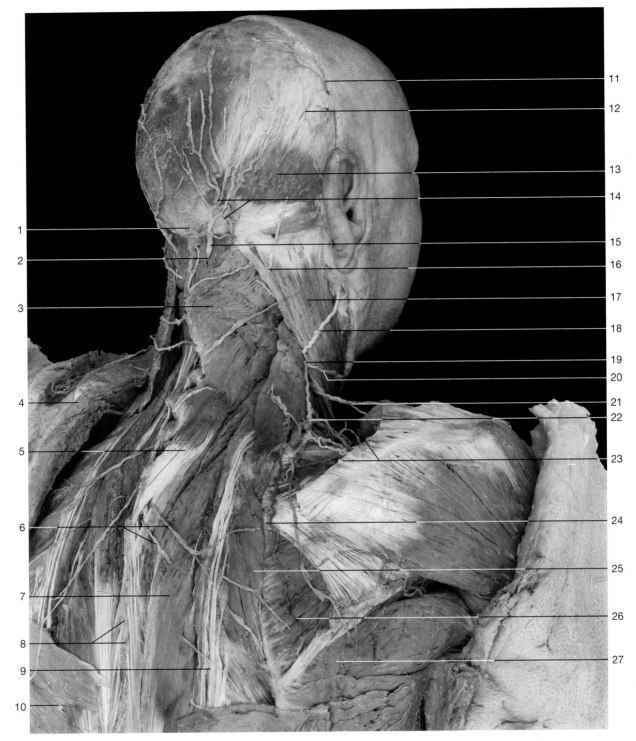

**Dissection of neck and back, deeper layer** (oblique-lateral aspect after removal of trapezius muscle).

 1  Protuberantia occipitalis externa
 2  Semispinalis capitis muscle
 3  Splenius capitis muscle
 4  Scapula
 5  Splenius cervicis muscle
 6  Posterior branches of spinal nerves
 7  Longissimus muscle
 8  Spinous processes of thoracic vertebrae
 9  Iliocostalis muscle
10  Latissimus dorsi muscle
11  Epidermis of the head (scalp)
12  Galea aponeurotica
13  Occipital belly of occipitofrontalis muscle
14  Occipital artery

15  Greater occipital nerve (C$_2$)
16  Lesser occipital nerve
17  Sternocleidomastoid muscle
18  Great auricular nerve
19  Punctum nervosum
20  Transverse cervical nerve
21  Supraclavicular nerves
22  Accessory nerve (n. XI)
23  Trapezius muscle (cut edge)
24  Medial margin of scapula
25  Rhomboid muscle
26  Infraspinous muscle
27  Teres major muscle

# 4  Thoracic Organs

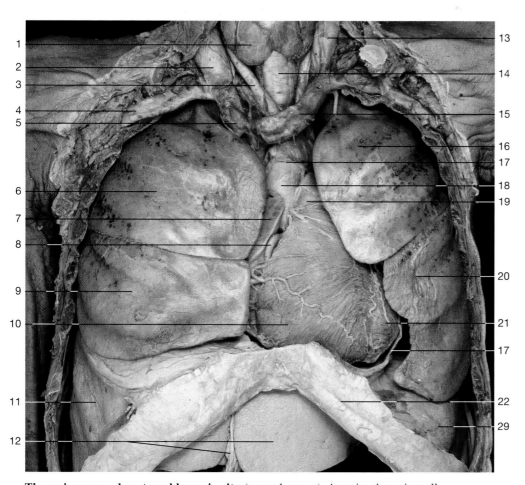

| | |
|---|---|
| 1 | Thyroid gland |
| 2 | Internal jugular vein |
| 3 | Right common carotid artery |
| 4 | Right axillary vein |
| 5 | Right brachiocephalic vein |
| 6 | Superior lobe of right lung |
| 7 | Right atrium |
| 8 | Right coronary artery |
| 9 | Middle lobe of right lung |
| 10 | Right ventricle |
| 11 | Diaphragm |
| 12 | Liver (left lobe) and falciform ligament |
| 13 | Left internal jugular vein |
| 14 | Trachea |
| 15 | Left brachiocephalic vein |
| 16 | Superior lobe of left lung |
| 17 | Cut edge of pericardium |
| 18 | Ascending aorta |
| 19 | Pulmonary trunk |
| 20 | Inferior lobe of left lung |
| 21 | Left ventricle |
| 22 | Costal margin |
| 23 | Right pulmonary artery |
| 24 | Esophagus |
| 25 | Descending aorta |
| 26 | Pericardium |
| 27 | Aortic valve |
| 28 | Thymus |
| 29 | Diaphragm |

**Thoracic organs, heart, and lungs in situ** (ventral aspect). Anterior thoracic wall, parietal pleura, and pericardium have been removed.

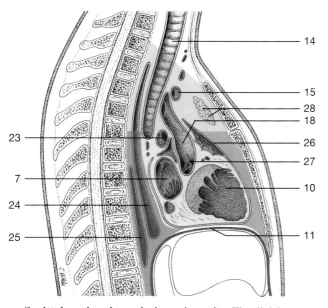

**Sagittal section through thoracic cavity.** The divisions of the mediastinum are indicated by colors.

| Divisions of mediastinum | Main content |
|---|---|
| Superior mediastinum (yellow) | Trachea, brachiocephalic veins, thymus, aortic arch, esophagus, thoracic duct |
| Middle mediastinum (light blue) | Heart, ascending aorta, pulmonary trunk, pulmonary veins, phrenic nerves |
| Posterior mediastinum (red) | Esophagus with vagus nerves, descending aorta, thoracic duct, sympathetic trunks |
| Anterior mediastinum (pink) | Small vessels, connective and fatty tissue, and thymus in the child |

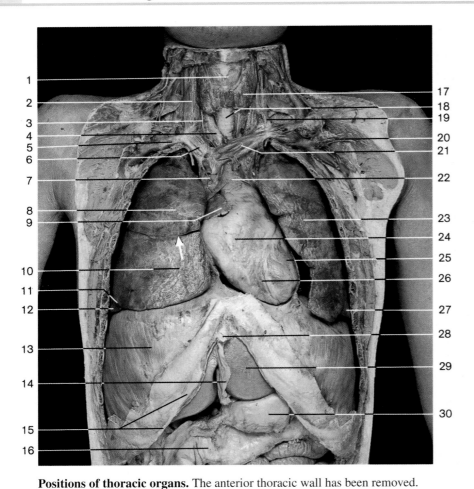

1  Cricothyroid muscle
2  Right internal jugular vein
3  Vagus nerve
4  Right common carotid artery
5  Right subclavian vein
6  Right brachiocephalic vein
7  Superior vena cava
8  Upper lobe of right lung
9  Right auricle
10  Middle lobe of right lung
11  Oblique fissure of right lung
12  Lower lobe of right lung
13  Diaphragm
14  Falciform ligament
15  Costal margin
16  Transverse colon
17  Thyroid gland
18  Trachea
19  Left internal jugular vein
20  Left cephalic vein
21  Left brachiocephalic vein
22  Pericardium (cut edge)
23  Upper lobe of left lung
24  Right ventricle
25  Left ventricle
26  Anterior interventricular sulcus
27  Lower lobe of left lung
28  Xiphoid process
29  Liver
30  Stomach
31  Pectoralis major muscle

**Positions of thoracic organs.** The anterior thoracic wall has been removed.
Arrow: horizontal fissure of right lung.

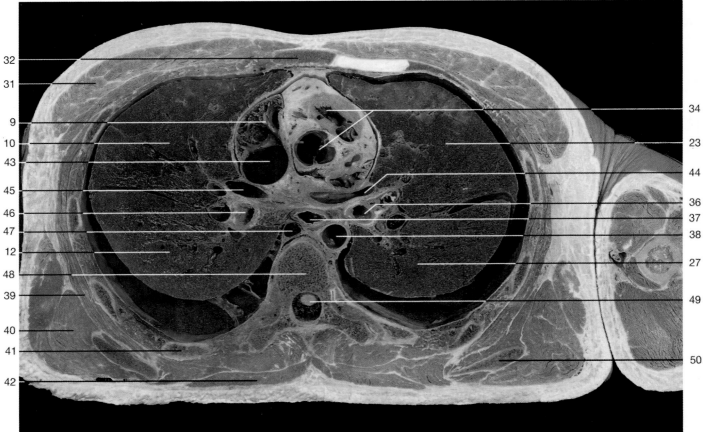

**Horizontal section through the thorax** at the level of the seventh thoracic vertebra (from below).

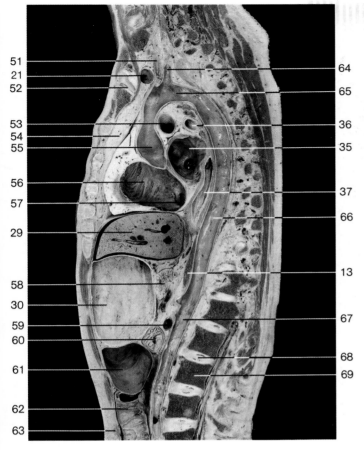

**Sagittal section through the left thorax,** 2 cm lateral to the median plane.

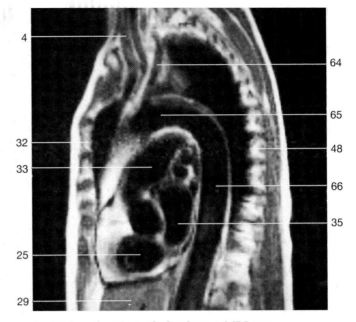

**Sagittal section through the thorax.** MRI scan.

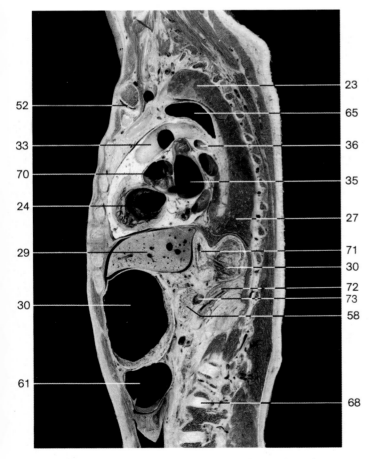

**Sagittal section through the left thorax,** 3.5 cm lateral to the median plane.

32 Sternum
33 Pulmonary trunk
34 Left ventricle and bulb of aorta
35 Left atrium
36 Left main bronchus
37 Esophagus
38 Descending aorta
39 Serratus anterior muscle
40 Teres major muscle
41 Rib
42 Trapezius muscle
43 Right atrium
44 Left pulmonary vein
45 Right pulmonary vein
46 Right main bronchus
47 Azygos vein
48 Body of vertebra
49 Spinal cord
50 Scapula
51 Left common carotid artery
52 Sternoclavicular articulation with disc
53 Right pulmonary artery
54 Remnants of thymus
55 Aortic bulb
56 Right atrium
57 Entrance of inferior vena cava in right atrium
58 Pancreas
59 Left renal vein
60 Duodenum
61 Transverse colon (dilated)
62 Small intestine
63 Umbilicus
64 Left subclavian artery
65 Aortic arch
66 Thoracic aorta
67 Abdominal aorta
68 Intervertebral disc
69 Body of lumbar vertebra
70 Aortic valve
71 Cardia of stomach
72 Suprarenal gland
73 Splenic vein

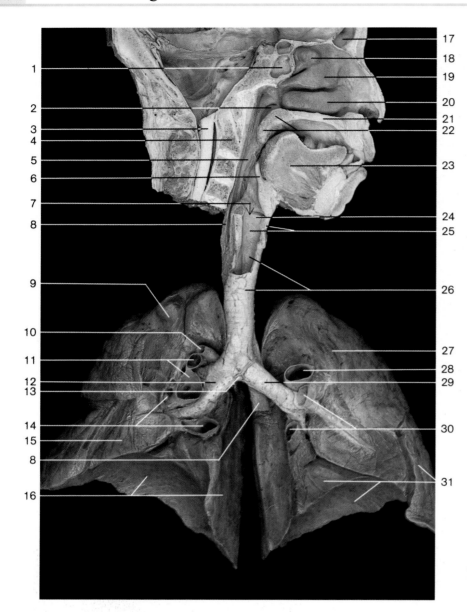

1　Sphenoid sinus
2　Pharyngeal opening of auditory tube
3　Spinal cord
4　Dens of axis
5　Oropharynx (oropharyngeal isthmus)
6　Epiglottis
7　Entrance of larynx
8　Esophagus
9　Upper lobe of right lung
10　Azygos vein
11　Branches of pulmonary artery
12　Right main bronchus
13　Bifurcation of trachea
14　Tributaries of right pulmonary veins
15　Middle lobe of right lung
16　Lower lobe of right lung
17　Frontal sinus
18　Superior nasal concha
19　Middle nasal concha
20　Inferior nasal concha
21　Hard palate
22　Soft palate with uvula
23　Tongue
24　Vocal fold
25　Larynx
26　Trachea
27　Upper lobe of left lung
28　Left pulmonary artery
29　Left main bronchus
30　Left pulmonary veins
31　Lower lobe of left lung

**Respiratory system.** The lungs have been fixed in expiration and turned laterally. Head bisected and turned laterally.

▷ **To page 247**

1　Nasal cavity
2　Pharynx
3　Larynx (thyroid cartilage)
4　Trachea
5　Upper lobe of right lung
6　Bifurcation of trachea
7　Right main bronchus
8　Horizontal fissure of right lung
9　Middle lobe of right lung
10　Oblique fissures of lungs
11　Lower lobe of right lung
12　Clavicle
13　Upper lobe of left lung
14　Left main bronchus
15　Bronchi supplying bronchopulmonary
　　segments
16　Lower lobe of left lung
17　Costal margin
18　Hyoid bone
19　Right superior lobe bronchus
20　Right middle lobe bronchus
21　Right inferior lobe bronchus
22　Left superior lobe bronchus
23　Left inferior lobe bronchus
24　Segmental bronchi
25　Branches of pulmonary arteries
26　Branches of pulmonary veins

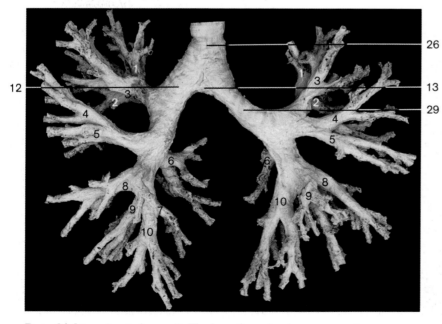

**Bronchial tree** (ventral aspect). The lung tissue has been removed. The bronchopulmonary segments are numbered 1–10.

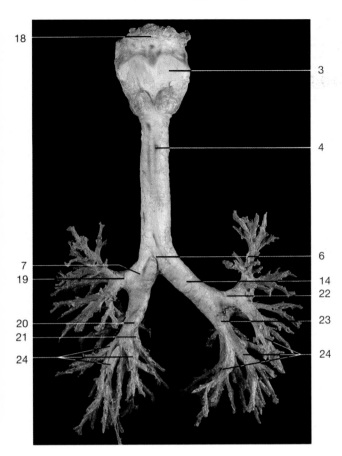

**Larynx, trachea, and bronchial tree** (anterior aspect).

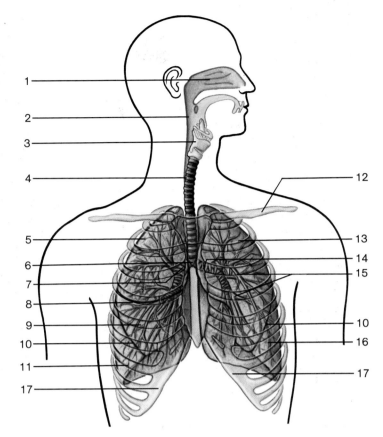

**Organization and positions of respiratory organs** (schematic drawing).

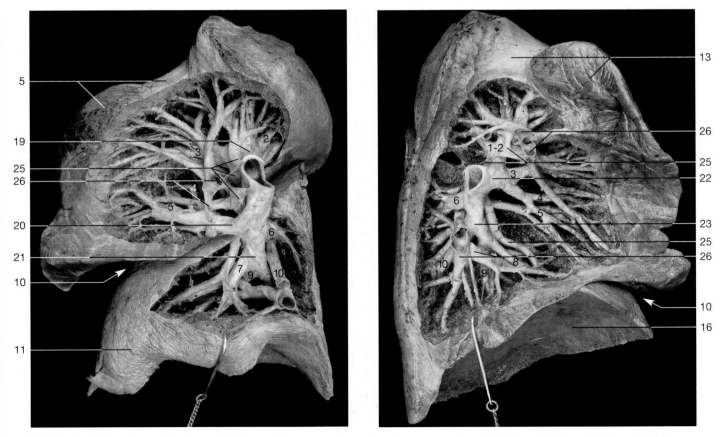

**Mediastinal dissection of the bronchial tree,** pulmonary veins, and pulmonary arteries of right lung (left) and left lung (right) (medial aspect). Segmental bronchi are numbered 1–10.

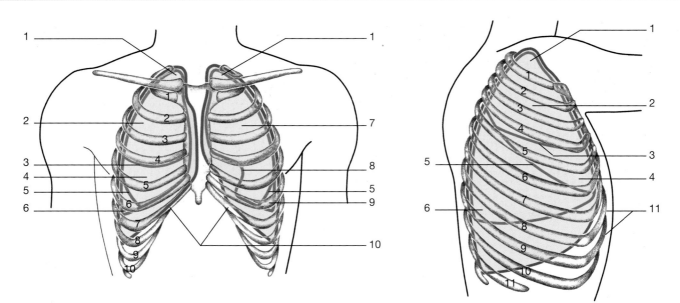

**Surface projections of lungs and pleura on the thoracic wall.** Left: anterior aspect; right: right-lateral aspect.
Red = margins of the lung; blue = margins of pleura. The numbers indicate ribs.

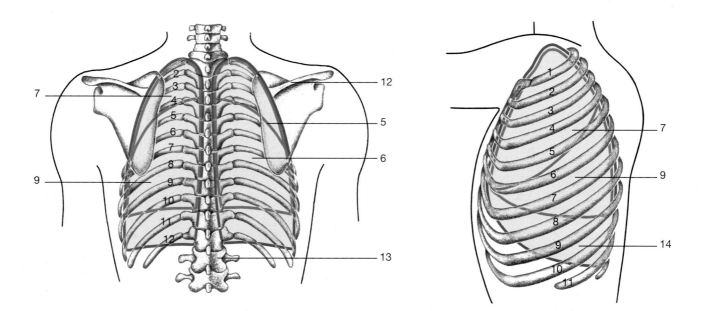

**Surface projections of lungs and pleura on thoracic wall.** Left: posterior aspect; right: left-lateral aspect.
Red = margins of lung; blue = margins of pleura. The numbers indicate ribs.

| | | |
|---|---|---|
| 1 Apex of lung | 6 Lower lobe of right lung | 11 Costal margin |
| 2 Upper lobe of right lung | 7 Upper lobe of left lung | 12 Spine of scapula |
| 3 Horizontal fissure of right lung | 8 Cardiac notch of left lung | 13 First lumbar vertebra |
| 4 Middle lobe of right lung | 9 Lower lobe of left lung | 14 Space between border of lung and pleura |
| 5 Oblique fissures of lungs | 10 Infrasternal angle | (costodiaphragmatic recess) |

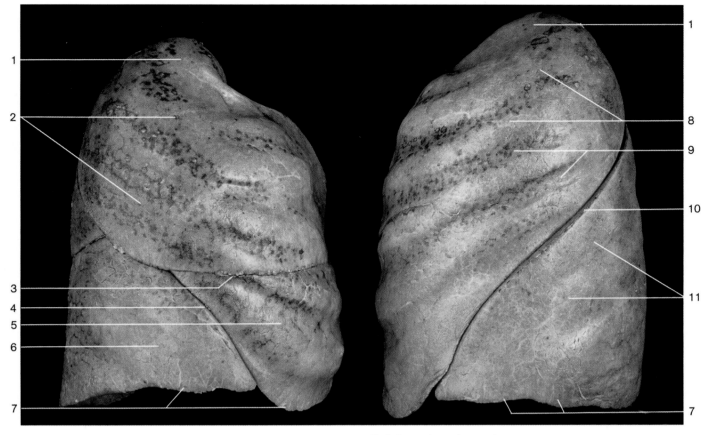

**Right lung** (lateral aspect).

**Left lung** (lateral aspect).

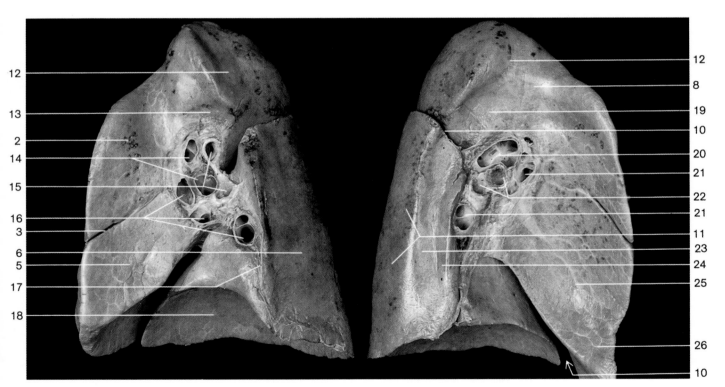

**Right lung** (medial aspect).

**Left lung** (medial aspect).

| | | | |
|---|---|---|---|
| 1 Apex of lung | 8 Upper lobe of left lung | 15 Bronchi | 22 Left secondary bronchi |
| 2 Upper lobe of right lung | 9 Impressions of ribs | 16 Right pulmonary veins | 23 Groove of thoracic aorta |
| 3 Horizontal fissure of right lung | 10 Oblique fissure of left lung | 17 Pulmonary ligament | 24 Groove of esophagus |
| 4 Oblique fissure of right lung | 11 Lower lobe of left lung | 18 Diaphragmatic surface | 25 Cardiac impression |
| 5 Middle lobe of right lung | 12 Groove of subclavian artery | 19 Groove of aortic arch | 26 Lingula |
| 6 Lower lobe of right lung | 13 Groove of azygos arch | 20 Left pulmonary artery | |
| 7 Inferior border | 14 Branches of right pulmonary artery | 21 Branches of left pulmonary veins | |

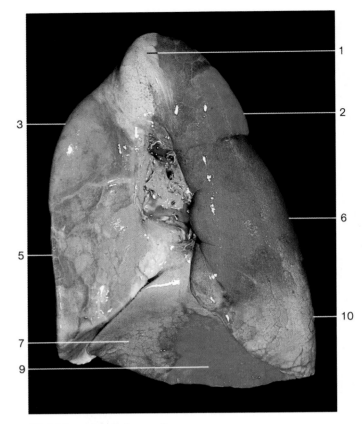

**Right lung** (medial aspect).

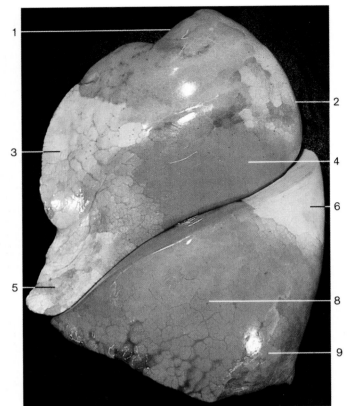

**Left lung** (medial aspect).

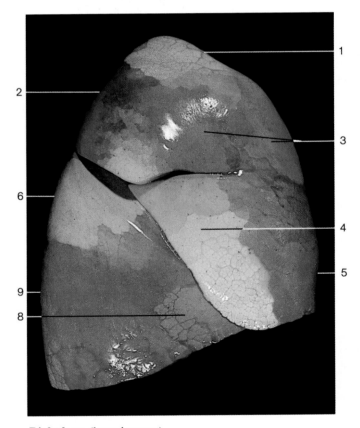

**Right lung** (lateral aspect).

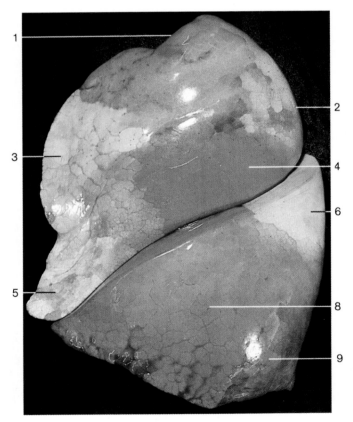

**Left lung** (lateral aspect).

The bronchopulmonary segments of the lungs are differentiated by the various colors. Notice that there is no segment in the left lung that corresponds to the seventh segment of the right lung. Compare with the schematic drawing on the facing page.

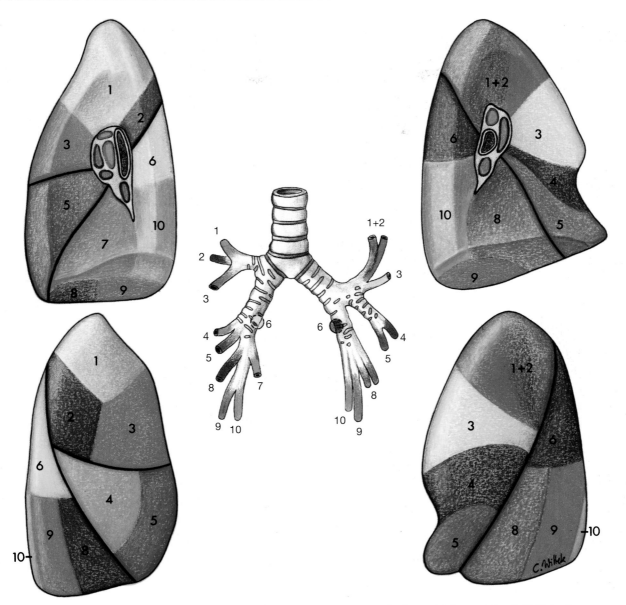

**Distribution of bronchopulmonary segments of the lungs and their relation to the bronchial tree** (after J. F. Huber).

The bronchopulmonary segments are morphologically and functionally separate independent respiratory units of the lung tissue. Each segment is surrounded by connective tissue that is continuous with the visceral pleura. The segmental bronchi in a segment are central, closely accompanied by branches of the pulmonary arteries, whereas the tributaries of the pulmonary veins run **between** the segments. Thus, the veins serve two adjacent segments that drain for the most part into more than one vein. A bronchopulmonary segment is therefore not a complete vascular unit, but segmentation is the result of a specific architecture of the lung vasculature.

| Right lung | | Left lung | | |
|---|---|---|---|---|
| 1 Apical segment | Upper lobe bronchus | 1+2 Apico-posterior segment | Superior division | Upper lobe bronchus |
| 2 Posterior segment | | | | |
| 3 Anterior segment | | 3 Anterior segment | | |
| 4 Lateral segment | Middle lobe bronchus | 4 Superior lingular segment | Inferior division | |
| 5 Medial segment | | 5 Inferior lingular segment | | |
| 6 Superior (apical) segment | Lower lobe bronchus | 6 Superior (apical) segment | Lower lobe bronchus | |
| 7 Medial basal segment | | 7 Absent | | |
| 8 Anterior basal segment | | 8 Anteromedial basal segment | | |
| 9 Lateral basal segment | | 9 Lateral basal segment | | |
| 10 Posterior basal segment | | 10 Posterior basal segment | | |

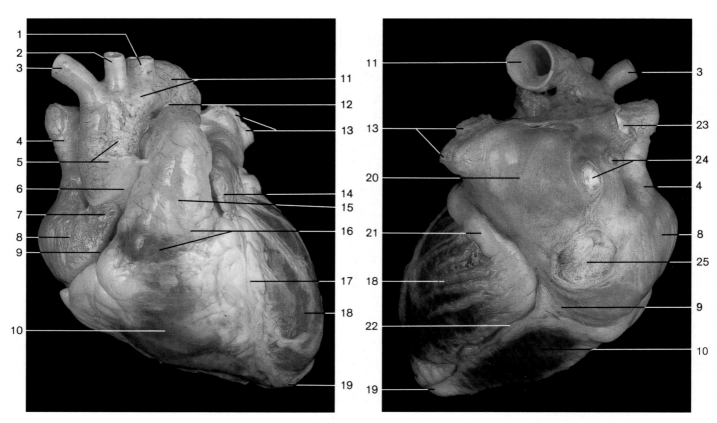

**Heart** of 30-year-old woman (anterior aspect).

**Heart** of 30-year-old woman (oblique-posterior view).

| | | |
|---|---|---|
| 1  Left subclavian artery | 9  Coronary sulcus | 18  Left ventricle |
| 2  Left common carotid artery | 10  Right ventricle | 19  Apex of the heart |
| 3  Brachiocephalic trunk | 11  Aortic arch | 20  Left atrium |
| 4  Superior vena cava | 12  Ligamentum arteriosum | 21  Epicardial fat overlying coronary sinus |
| 5  Ascending aorta | 13  Left pulmonary veins | 22  Posterior interventricular sulcus |
| 6  Bulb of the aorta | 14  Left auricle | 23  Right pulmonary artery |
| 7  Right auricle | 15  Pulmonary trunk | 24  Right pulmonary veins |
| 8  Right atrium | 16  Sinus of pulmonary trunk | 25  Inferior vena cava |
| | 17  Anterior interventricular sulcus | |

**Position of heart** and its vessels within the thorax (schematic drawing).

1  Right brachiocephalic vein
2  Superior vena cava
3  Ascending aorta
4  Right atrium
5  Right ventricle
6  Inferior vena cava
7  Left internal jugular vein
8  Left common carotid artery
9  Left axillary artery and vein
10  Left brachiocephalic vein
11  Pulmonary trunk
12  Left auricle
13  Left ventricle
14  Descending aorta

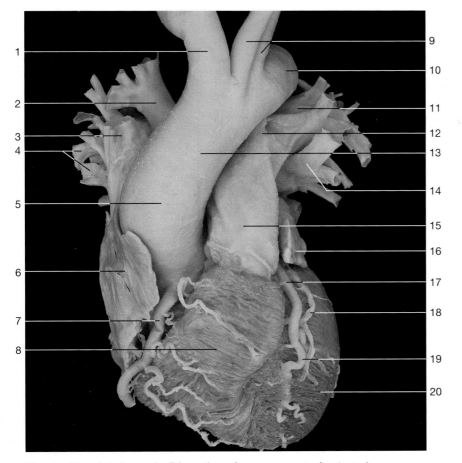

1 Brachiocephalic trunk
2 Right pulmonary artery
3 Superior vena cava
4 Right pulmonary veins
5 Ascending aorta
6 Right atrium
7 Right coronary artery
8 Right ventricle
9 Left common carotid artery and left subclavian artery
10 Descending aorta (thoracic part)
11 Ligamentum arteriosum (remnant of ductus arteriosus Botalli)
12 Left pulmonary artery
13 Aortic arch
14 Left pulmonary veins
15 Pulmonary trunk
16 Left atrium
17 Left coronary artery
18 Diagonal branch of left coronary artery
19 Interventricular branch of left coronary artery
20 Left ventricle
21 Right brachiocephalic vein
22 Thoracic wall
23 Liver
24 Aortic valve
25 Chordae tendineae
26 Papillary muscles
27 Stomach

**Heart with related vessels. Dissection of coronary arteries** (anterior aspect, systolic phase of heart action).

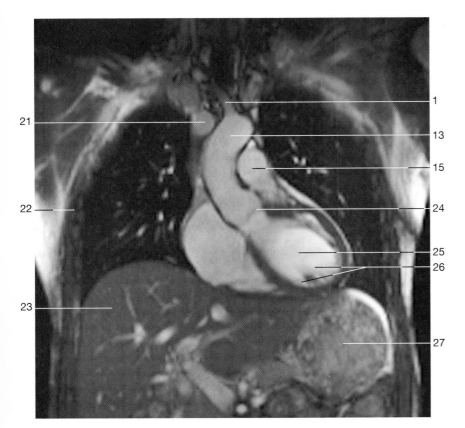

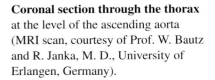

**Coronal section through the thorax** at the level of the ascending aorta (MRI scan, courtesy of Prof. W. Bautz and R. Janka, M. D., University of Erlangen, Germany).

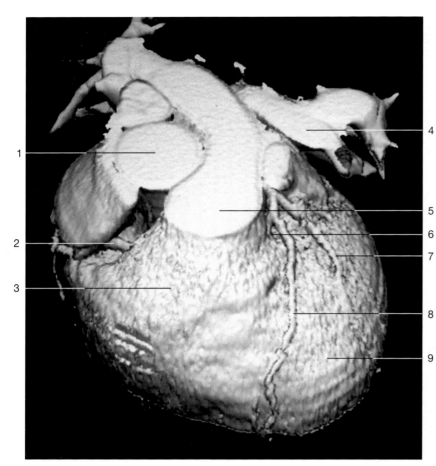

| | |
|---|---|
| 1 | Ascending aorta |
| 2 | Right coronary artery |
| 3 | Right ventricle |
| 4 | Left atrium |
| 5 | Pulmonary trunk |
| 6 | Septal branch of left coronary artery |
| 7 | Diagonal branch |
| 8 | Anterior interventricular branch of left coronary artery |
| 9 | Left ventricle |
| 10 | Aortic root |
| 11 | Superior vena cava |
| 12 | Circumflex branch of left coronary artery |
| 13 | Sternum |

**Human heart** (3-D reconstruction of electron beam CT scans as "Shaded Surface Display"[1]).

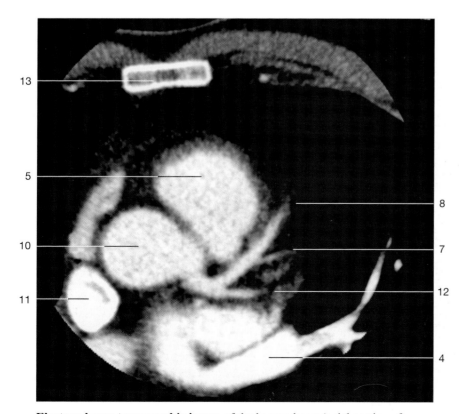

**Electron beam tomographic image** of the human heart (axial section after injection of contrast medium[1]).

[1]  Courtesy of Drs. W. Moshage, S. Achenbach, and D. Ropers, Dept. of Internal Medicine II (Chairman: Prof. W. G. Daniel), University of Erlangen-Nürnberg, Germany.

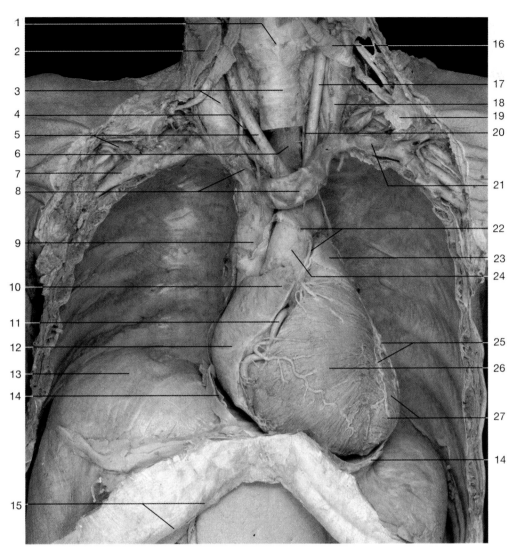

1  Larynx (thyroid cartilage)
2  Sternocleidomastoid muscle
   (divided)
3  Trachea (divided) and right
   internal jugular vein
4  Vagus nerve
5  Right common carotid
   artery and cephalic vein
6  Esophagus
7  Right axillary vein
8  Right and left
   brachiocephalic veins
9  Superior vena cava
10 Right auricle
11 Right coronary artery
12 Right atrium
13 Diaphragm
14 Pericardium (cut edges)
15 Costal margin
16 Omohyoid muscle
17 Left common carotid artery
18 Left internal jugular vein
19 Clavicle (divided)
20 Left recurrent laryngeal
   nerve
21 Subclavian vein
22 Pericardial reflection
23 Pulmonary trunk
24 Ascending aorta
25 Anterior interventricular
   sulcus and anterior
   interventricular branch of
   left coronary artery
26 Right ventricle
27 Left ventricle
28 Aortic valve
29 Tricuspid or right
   atrioventricular valve
30 Inferior vena cava
31 Pulmonary veins
32 Pulmonary valve
33 Left atrioventricular
   (bicuspid or mitral) valve

**Heart and related vessels in situ** (anterior aspect). Anterior thoracic wall, pericardium, and epicardium have been removed; trachea divided.

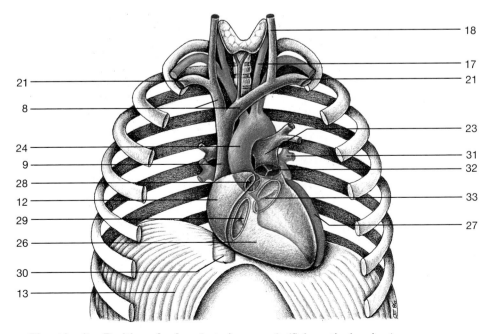

**Heart in situ. Position of valves** (anterior aspect). (Schematic drawing.)

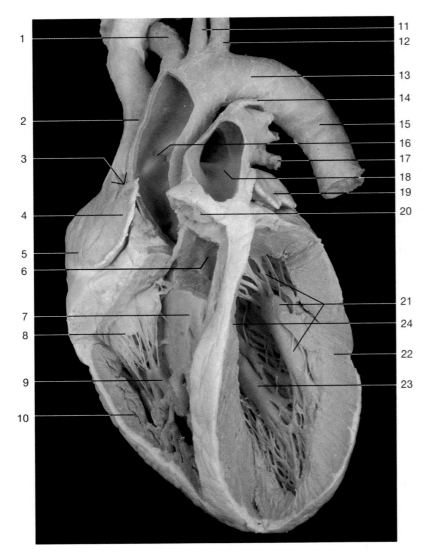

1    Brachiocephalic trunk
2    Superior vena cava
3    Sulcus terminalis
4    Right auricle
5    Right atrium
6    Aortic valve
7    Conus arteriosus (interventricular septum)
8    Right atrioventricular (tricuspid) valve
9    Anterior papillary muscle
10   Myocardium of right ventricle
11   Left common carotid artery
12   Left subclavian artery
13   Aortic arch
14   Ligamentum arteriosum (remnant of ductus
     arteriosus)
15   Thoracic aorta (descending aorta)
16   Ascending aorta
17   Left pulmonary vein
18   Pulmonary trunk
19   Left auricle
20   Pulmonic valve
21   Anterior papillary muscle with chordae
     tendineae
22   Myocardium of left ventricle
23   Posterior papillary muscle
24   Interventricular septum
25   Right and left brachiocephalic veins
26   Chordae tendineae
27   Papillary muscles of right ventricle
28   Left atrium
29   Infundibulum
30   Anterior papillary muscle of left ventricle
31   Left atrioventricular (bicuspid or mitral) valve
     and chordae tendineae
32   Apex of heart
33   Inferior vena cava
34   Liver
35   Aorta (pars abdominalis)

**Anterior aspect of the heart.** Dissection of the four valves.

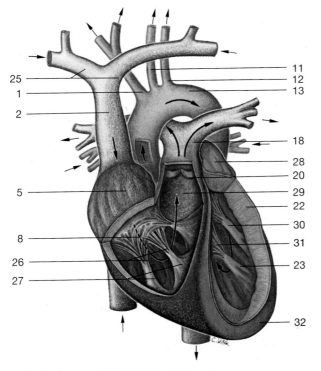

**Circulation within the heart** (anterior aspect;
arrows = direction of blood flow).

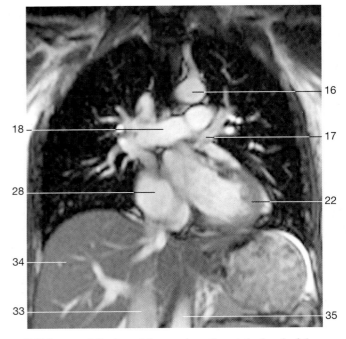

**MRI scan of the heart** (coronal section at the level of the
left atrium; courtesy of Prof W. Bautz and R. Janka, M. D.,
University of Erlangen, Germany).

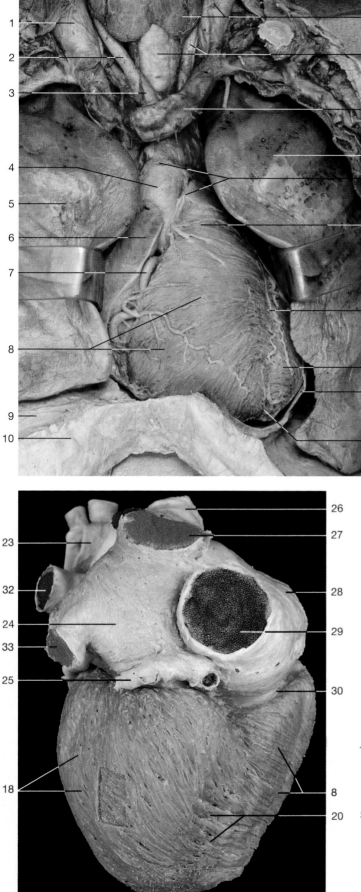

**Heart in situ. Myocardium and coronary arteries** (anterior aspect).

1 Internal jugular vein
2 Common carotid artery
3 Brachiocephalic trunk
4 Ascending aorta
5 Right lung
6 Right auricle
7 Right coronary artery
8 Myocardium of right ventricle
9 Diaphragm
10 Costal margin
11 Thyroid gland and internal jugular vein
12 Trachea and left common carotid artery
13 Left brachiocephalic vein
14 Left lung
15 Pericardium (cut edge)
16 Pulmonary trunk
17 Anterior interventricular artery
18 Myocardium of left ventricle
19 Muscular vortex (right ventricle)
20 Posterior interventricular sulcus
21 Anterior interventricular sulcus
22 Muscular vortex (left ventricle)
23 Aortic arch
24 Left atrium
25 Coronary sinus
26 Superior vena cava
27 Right pulmonary vein
28 Right atrium
29 Inferior vena cava
30 Coronary sulcus
31 Myocardium of left ventricle
32 Left pulmonary artery
33 Left pulmonary vein
34 Apex of heart

**Heart** (posterior aspect). The myocardium of the left ventricle has been fenestrated to show the muscle fiber bundles of the deeper layer with their more circular course.

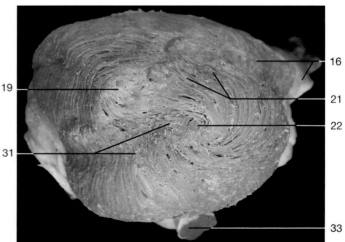

**Vortex of cardiac muscle fibers** (from below).

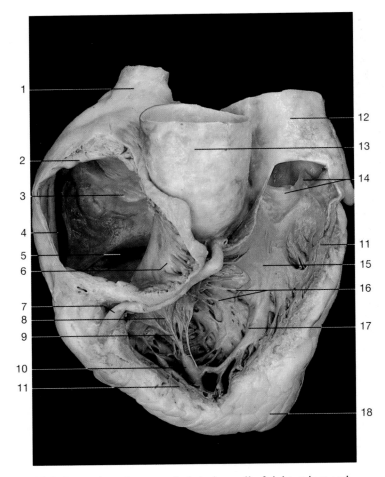

1   Superior vena cava
2   Crista terminalis
3   Fossa ovalis
4   Opening of inferior vena cava
5   Opening of coronary sinus
6   Right auricle
7   Right coronary artery and coronary sulcus
8   Anterior cusp of tricuspid valve
9   Chordae tendineae
10  Anterior papillary muscle
11  Myocardium
12  Pulmonary trunk
13  Ascending aorta
14  Pulmonic valve
15  Conus arteriosus (interventricular septum)
16  Septal papillary muscles
17  Septomarginal or moderator band
18  Apex of heart
19  Left auricle
20  Aortic valve
21  Left ventricle
22  Pulmonary veins
23  Position of fossa ovalis
24  Left atrium
25  Left atrioventricular (bicuspid or mitral) valve
26  Right atrium
27  Pericardium
28  Posterior papillary muscle
29  Right ventricle
30  Interventricular septum

**Right heart** (anterior aspect). Anterior wall of right atrium and ventricle removed.

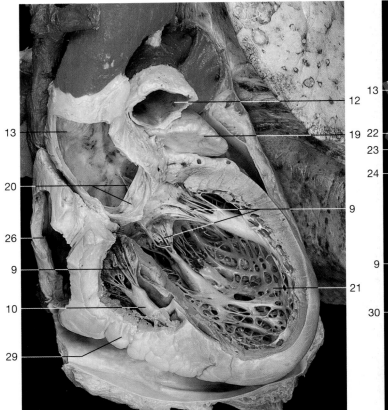

**Heart, left ventricle with mitral valve, papillary muscles, and aortic valve** (anterior portion of the heart removed).

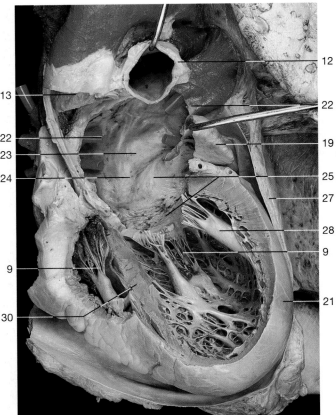

**Heart, left ventricle, and atrium** (opened) showing the posterior part of the mitral valve with papillary muscles.

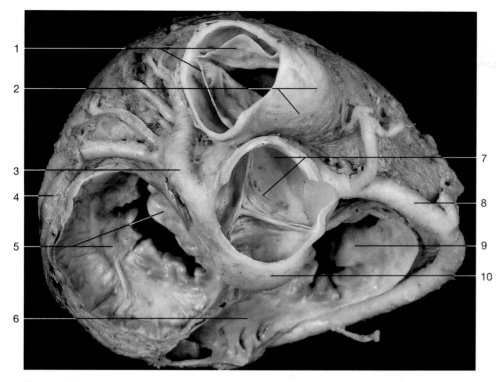

1  Pulmonic valve
2  Sinus of pulmonary trunk
3  Left coronary artery
4  Great cardiac vein
5  Left atrioventricular (mitral) valve
6  Coronary sinus
7  Aortic valve
8  Right coronary artery
9  Right atrioventricular (tricuspid) valve
10  Bulb of aorta
11  Anterior semilunar cusp of pulmonic valve
12  Left semilunar cusp of pulmonic valve
13  Right semilunar cusp of pulmonic valve
14  Left semilunar cusp of aortic valve
15  Right semilunar cusp of aortic valve
16  Posterior semilunar cusp of aortic valve
17  Right atrium
18  Anterior cusp of tricuspid valve
19  Chordae tendineae
20  Trabeculae carneae
21  Interventricular septum
22  Septal cusp of tricuspid valve
23  Anterior papillary muscle
24  Myocardium of right ventricle

**Valves of heart** (superior aspect). Left and right atria removed. Dissection of coronary arteries. Above: anterior wall of the heart.

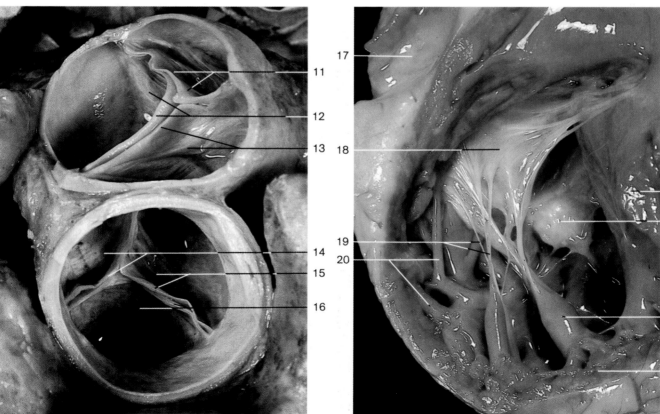

**Pulmonic and aortic valves** (from above). Anterior wall of the heart at the top. Both valves are closed.

**Right atrioventricular (tricuspid) valve** (anterior aspect after removal of the anterior wall of the right ventricle).

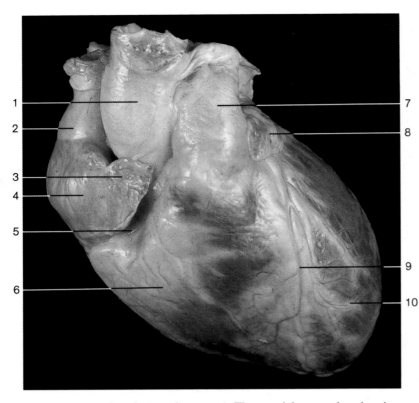

1   Ascending aorta
2   Superior vena cava
3   Right auricle
4   Right atrium
5   Coronary sulcus
6   Right ventricle
7   Pulmonary trunk
8   Left auricle
9   Anterior interventricular sulcus
10  Left ventricle
11  Right pulmonary artery
12  Sulcus terminalis with sino-atrial node
13  Line indicating plane of position of valves
14  Myocardium of right atrium
15  Inferior vena cava
16  Valve of pulmonary trunk
17  Tricuspid valve
18  Myocardium of right ventricle

**Heart,** fixed in **diastole** (anterior aspect). The ventricles are relaxed, atria contracted.

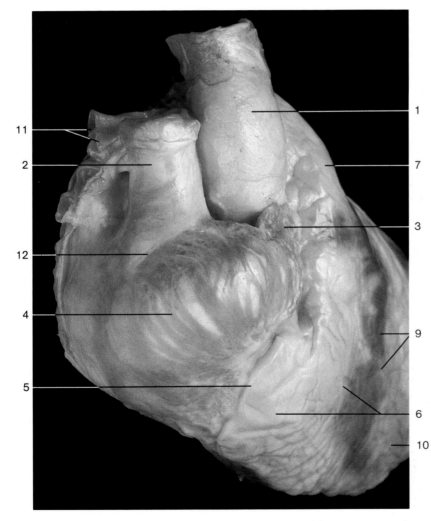

**Heart,** fixed in **systole** (anterolateral aspect). The ventricles are contracted, atria dilated.

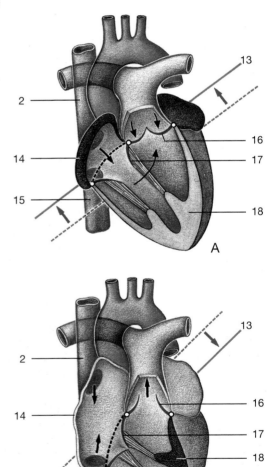

**Morphological changes during heart movements.** Note the changes in position of the valves (red arrows). Contracted portions of heart are indicated in black.

A. **Diastole:** muscles of the ventricles relaxed, atrioventricular valves open, semilunar valves closed.

B. **Systole:** muscles of ventricles contracted, atrioventricular valves closed, semilunar valves open.

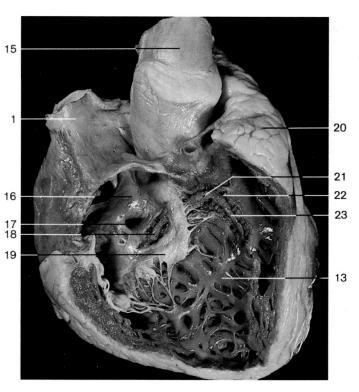

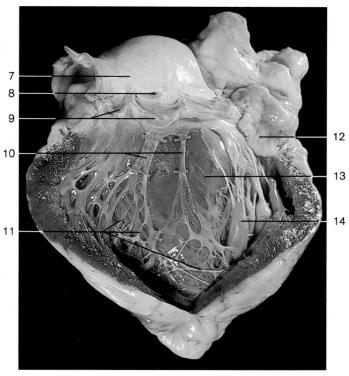

**Right ventricle,** dissection of **atrioventricular node, atrioventricular bundle (bundle of His),** and right limb or bundle branch (probes).

**Left ventricle,** dissection of the left limb or bundle branch of conducting system (probes).

| | | | |
|---|---|---|---|
| 1 | Superior vena cava | 5 | Muscle fiber bundles of right atrium |
| 2 | Sulcus terminalis | 6 | Coronary sulcus (with right coronary artery) |
| 3 | Bulb of aorta | 7 | Aortic sinus |
| 4 | Sinu-atrial node (arrows) | 8 | Entrance to left coronary artery |

9   Aortic valve
10   Branches of left bundle branch
11   Purkinje fibers
12   Left auricle
13   Interventricular septum
14   Papillary muscles
15   Ascending aorta
16   Right atrium
17   Opening of coronary sinus
18   Atrioventricular node
19   Septal cusp of tricuspid valve
20   Pulmonary trunk
21   Atrioventricular bundle (bundle of His)
22   Bifurcation of atrioventricular bundle
23   Right bundle branch
24   Inferior vena cava
25   Left atrium
26   Left bundle branch
27   Papillary muscles with Purkinje fibers

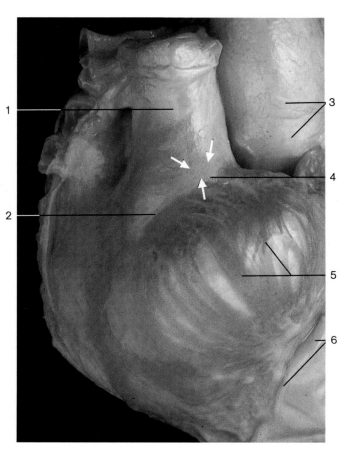

**Right atrium,** anterior wall, showing the location of the **sinu-atrial node** (arrows).

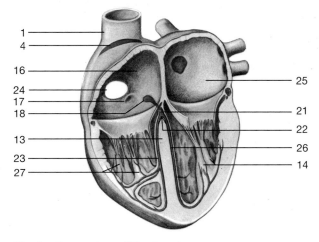

**Conducting system of the heart** (schematic drawing).

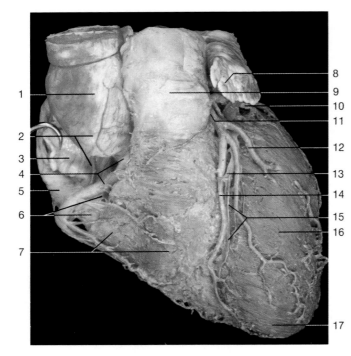

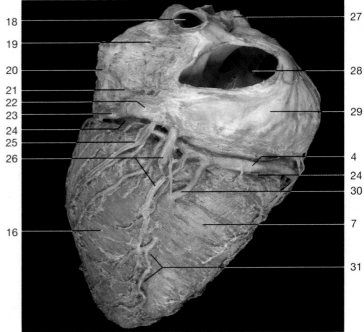

**Coronary arteries** (anterior aspect). The epicardium and subepicardial fatty tissue have been removed. The arteries have been injected with red resin from the aorta.

**Right coronary artery and veins of the heart** (dorsal aspect). The epicardium and subepicardial fatty tissue have been removed.

1   Ascending aorta
2   Aortic bulb and (in the above specimen) sinu-atrial branch of right coronary artery
3   Right auricle
4   Right coronary artery
5   Right atrium
6   Coronary sulcus
7   Right ventricle
8   Left auricle
9   Pulmonary trunk
10  Circumflex branch of left coronary artery
11  Left coronary artery
12  Diagonal branch of left artery
13  Great cardiac vein
14  Anterior interventricular artery
15  Anterior interventricular sulcus
16  Left ventricle
17  Apex of heart
18  Right pulmonary vein
19  Left atrium
20  Left pulmonary veins
21  Oblique vein of left atrium (Marshall's vein)
22  Coronary sinus
23  Great cardiac vein
24  Coronary sulcus (posterior portion)
25  Posterior vein of left ventricle
26  Middle cardiac vein
27  Left pulmonary artery
28  Inferior vena cava
29  Right atrium
30  Posterior interventricular branch of right coronary artery
31  Posterior interventricular sulcus
32  Superior vena cava
33  Right marginal branch
34  Branch of sinu-atrial node
35  Minimal cardiac veins
36  Small cardiac vein

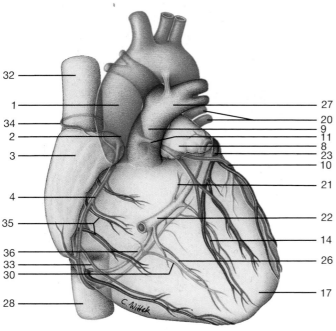

**Vessels of the heart.** Coronary arteries (red) and veins (blue) of the heart (anterior aspect).

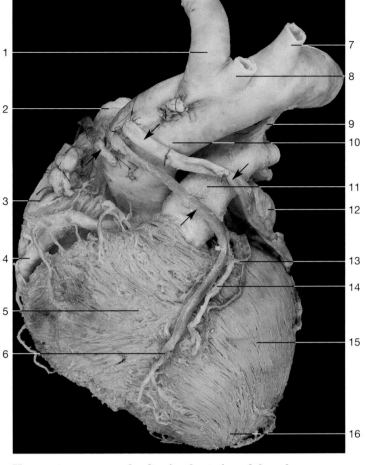

1   Brachiocephalic trunk
2   Superior vena cava
3   Right atrium
4   Right coronary artery
5   Right ventricle
6   Connection of one of the bypass vessels with the
    anterior interventricular artery
7   Left subclavian artery
8   Left common carotid artery
9   Ductus arteriosus (Botalli) (still open)
10  Ascending aorta with three bypass vessels implanted
11  Pulmonary trunk
12  Left atrium
13  Circumflex branch of left coronary artery
14  Anterior interventricular branch of left coronary artery
15  Left ventricle
16  Apex of heart
17  Sternum
18  Right ventricle
19  Liver
20  Spinal cord
21  Trachea
22  Aorta
23  Body of thoracic vertebrae
24  Pulmonary artery
25  Inferior vena cava
26  Hepatic vein

**Heart, coronary vessels after implantation of three bypass vessels** (anterior aspect). The ductus arteriosus (9) is still open.

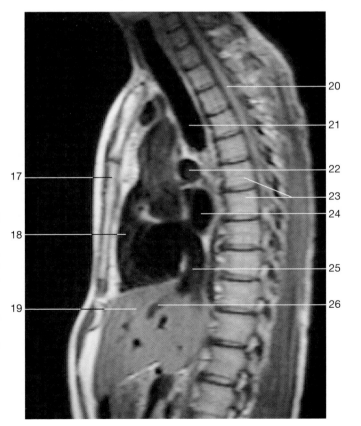

**Sagittal section through the thoracic cavity** (MRI scan, courtesy of Prof. W. Bautz and R. Janka, M. D., University of Erlangen, Germany).

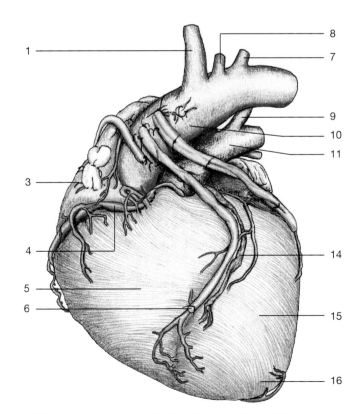

**Heart, coronary vessels after implantation of three bypass vessels** (yellow) (schematic drawing of the specimen above).

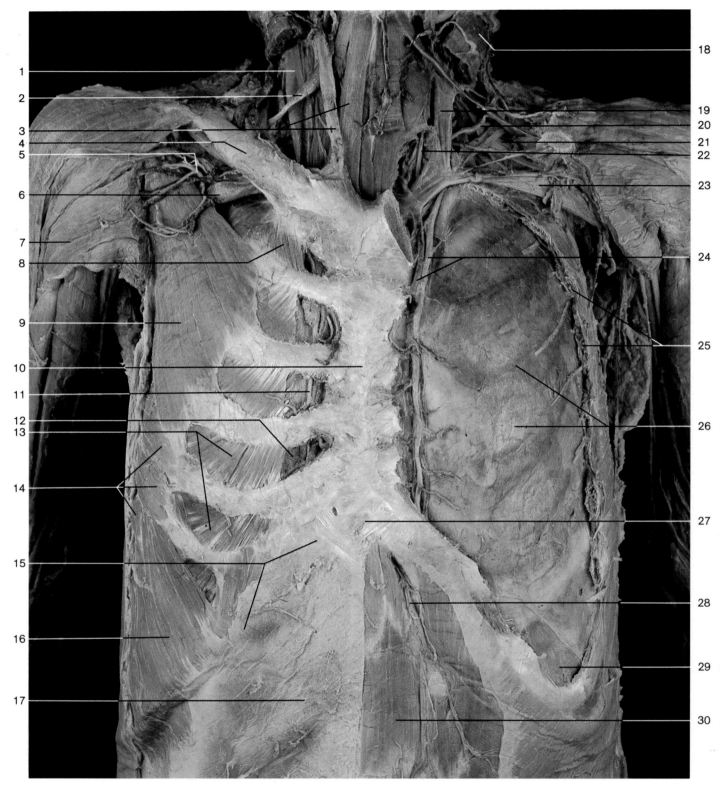

**Thoracic wall and organs** (ventral aspect). The left clavicle and ribs have been partially removed, and the right intercostal spaces have been opened to show the internal thoracic vein and artery.

| | | | | | |
|---|---|---|---|---|---|
| 1 | Right internal jugular vein | 11 | Right internal thoracic artery and vein | 21 | Brachial plexus |
| 2 | Omohyoid muscle | 12 | Fascicles of transversus thoracis muscle | 22 | Vagus nerve |
| 3 | Sternohyoid muscle and external jugular vein | 13 | Internal intercostal muscles | 23 | Left axillary vein |
| 4 | Clavicle | 14 | Serratus anterior muscle | 24 | Left internal thoracic artery and vein |
| 5 | Thoraco-acromial artery | 15 | Costal margin | 25 | Ribs and thoracic wall (cut) |
| 6 | Right subclavian vein | 16 | External abdominal oblique muscle | 26 | Costal pleura |
| 7 | Pectoralis major muscle | 17 | Anterior sheath of rectus abdominis muscle | 27 | Xiphoid process |
| 8 | External intercostal muscle | 18 | Sternocleidomastoid muscle | 28 | Superior epigastric artery |
| 9 | Pectoralis minor muscle | 19 | Left internal jugular vein | 29 | Diaphragm |
| 10 | Body of sternum | 20 | Transverse cervical artery | 30 | Rectus abdominis muscle |

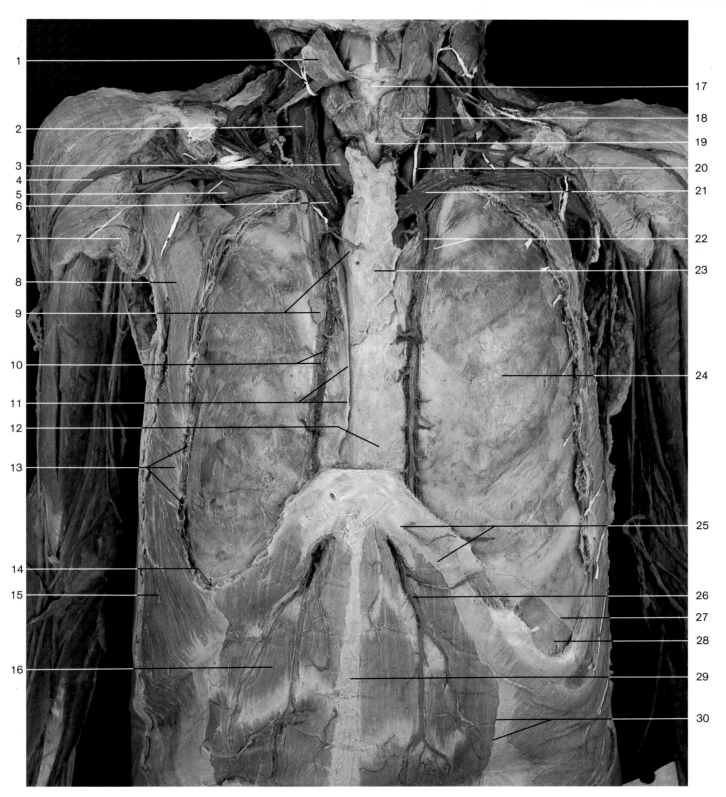

**Thoracic organs, anterior mediastinum, and pleura.** Ribs, clavicle, and sternum have been partly removed.
Red = arteries; blue = veins; green = lymph vessels and nodes.

1  Sternothyroid muscle and its nerve
   (a branch of the ansa cervicalis)
2  Right internal jugular vein
3  Right common carotid artery
4  Cephalic vein
5  Right subclavian vein
6  Right brachiocephalic vein
7  Pectoralis major muscle (divided)
8  Pectoralis minor muscle (divided)
9  Parasternal lymph nodes
10  Internal thoracic artery and vein

11  Anterior margin of costal pleura
12  Pericardium
13  Fifth and sixth ribs (divided)
    and serratus anterior muscle
14  Costodiaphragmatic recess
15  External abdominal oblique muscle
16  Rectus abdominis muscle
17  Larynx (thyroid cartilage)
18  Thyroid gland
19  Trachea
20  Left vagus nerve

21  Left brachiocephalic vein
22  Left internal thoracic artery and vein
23  Thymus
24  Costal pleura
25  Costal margin
26  Superior epigastric artery
27  Margin of costal pleura
28  Diaphragm
29  Linea alba
30  Cut edge of anterior sheath of rectus
    abdominis muscle

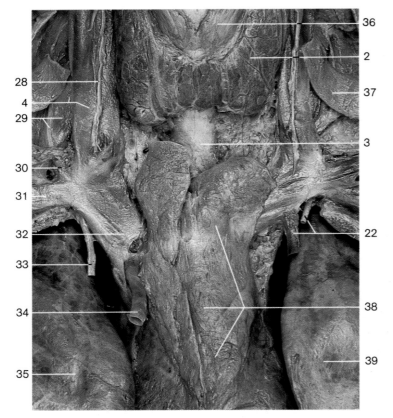

The **thymus** above the heart, showing its position and size.

1  Larynx (thyroid cartilage)
2  Thyroid gland
3  Trachea
4  Internal jugular vein
5  Brachial plexus
6  Right brachiocephalic vein and common carotid
   artery
7  Right phrenic nerve
8  Ascending aorta
9  Pectoralis minor muscle (divided)
10 Pulmonary trunk (covered by pericardium)
11 Costal pleura
12 Pericardium and heart
13 Serratus anterior muscle
14 Xiphoid process
15 Costal margin
16 External abdominal oblique muscle
17 Sternothyroid muscle (divided and reflected)
18 Vagus nerve
19 Left common carotid artery
20 Left sympathetic trunk
21 Left recurrent laryngeal nerve
22 Left internal thoracic artery and vein (divided)
23 Margin of costal pleura
24 Intercostal nerves and vessels
25 Superior epigastric artery
26 Rectus abdominis muscle
27 Diaphragm
28 Ansa cervicalis
29 Phrenic nerve and scalenus anterior muscle
30 External jugular vein (divided)
31 Right subclavian vein
32 Right brachiocephalic vein
33 Internal thoracic artery (divided)
34 Internal thoracic vein (divided)
35 Right lung
36 Cricothyroid muscle
37 Omohyoid muscle
38 Thymus
39 Left lung

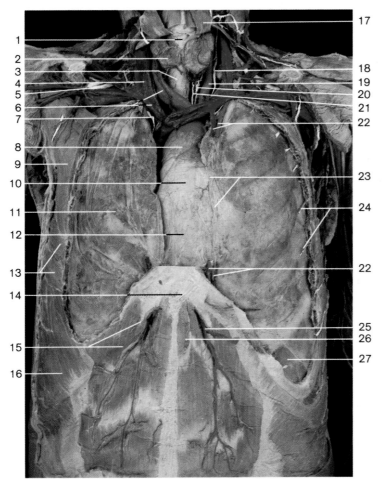

**Thoracic organs** (ventral aspect). The internal thoracic vessels have been removed, and the anterior margins of the pleura and lungs
have been slightly reflected to display the **anterior** and **middle mediastinum,** including the **heart** and **great vessels.**

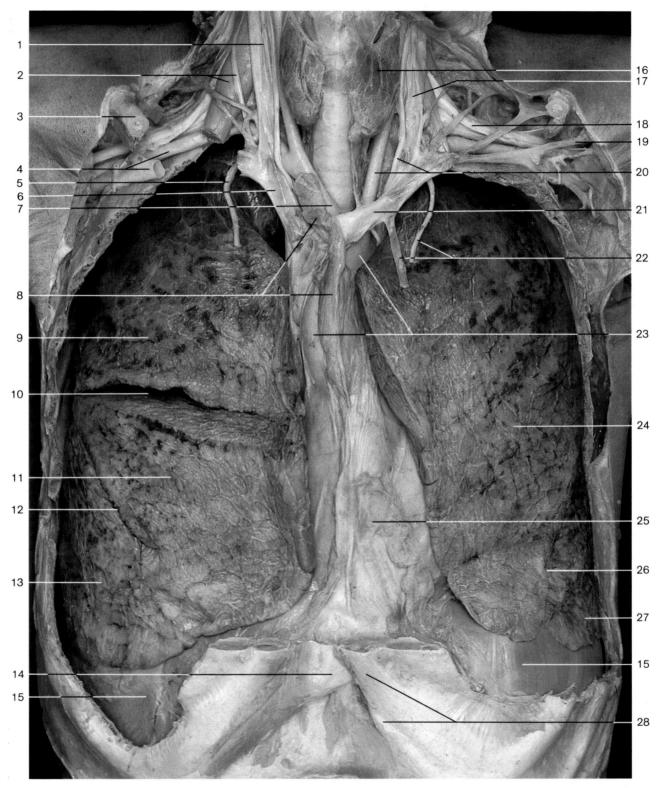

**Thoracic organs** (ventral aspect). The pleura has been opened and the lungs exposed. Remnants of the thymus and pericardium are seen.

1  Right internal jugular vein
2  Phrenic nerve and scalenus anterior muscle
3  Clavicle (divided)
4  Right subclavian artery and vein
5  Internal thoracic artery
6  Right brachiocephalic vein
7  Brachiocephalic trunk
8  Thymus (atrophic)
9  Upper lobe of right lung
10  Horizontal fissure of right lung (incomplete)

11  Middle lobe of right lung
12  Oblique fissure of right lung
13  Lower lobe of right lung
14  Xiphoid process
15  Diaphragm
16  Thyroid gland
17  Left internal jugular vein
18  Brachial plexus
19  Left cephalic vein

20  Left common carotid artery and vagus nerve
21  Left brachiocephalic vein
22  Internal thoracic artery and vein (divided)
23  Ascending aorta and aortic arch
24  Upper lobe of left lung
25  Pericardium
26  Oblique fissure of left lung
27  Lower lobe of left lung
28  Costal margin

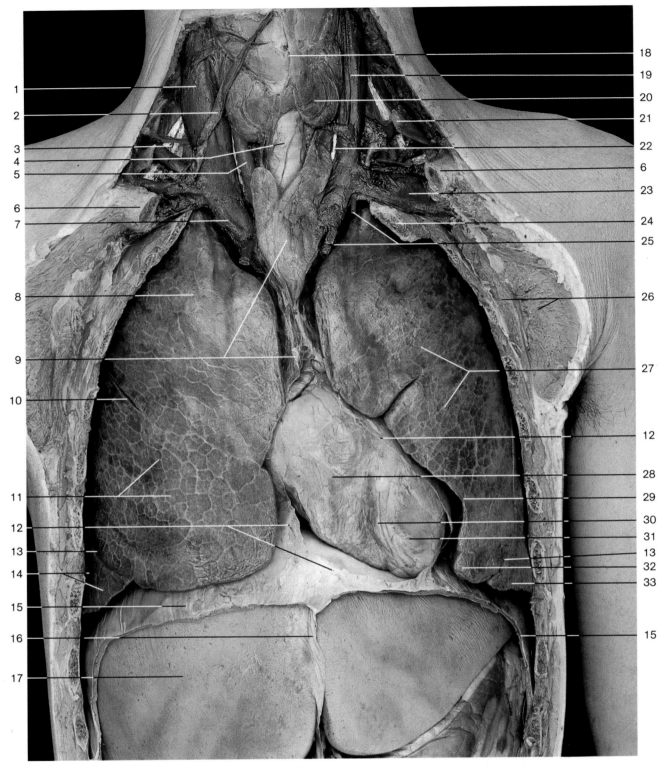

**Thoracic organs** (ventral aspect). The thoracic wall, costal pleura, pericardium, and diaphragm have been partly removed.

| | | |
|---|---|---|
| 1 Internal jugular vein | 13 Oblique fissure of lung | 25 Internal thoracic artery and vein |
| 2 External jugular vein (displaced medially) | 14 Lower lobe of right lung | 26 Pectoralis major and pectoralis minor muscles |
| 3 Brachial plexus | 15 Diaphragm | (cut edges) |
| 4 Trachea | 16 Falciform ligament | 27 Upper lobe of left lung |
| 5 Right common carotid artery | 17 Liver | 28 Right ventricle |
| 6 Clavicle (divided) | 18 Location of larynx | 29 Cardiac notch of left lung |
| 7 Right brachiocephalic vein | 19 Left internal jugular vein | 30 Interventricular sulcus of heart |
| 8 Upper lobe of right lung | 20 Thyroid gland | 31 Left ventricle |
| 9 Thymus (atrophic) | 21 Omohyoid muscle (divided) | 32 Lingula |
| 10 Horizontal fissure of right lung | 22 Vagus nerve | 33 Lower lobe of left lung |
| 11 Middle lobe of right lung | 23 Left subclavian vein | |
| 12 Pericardium (cut edges) | 24 First rib (divided) | |

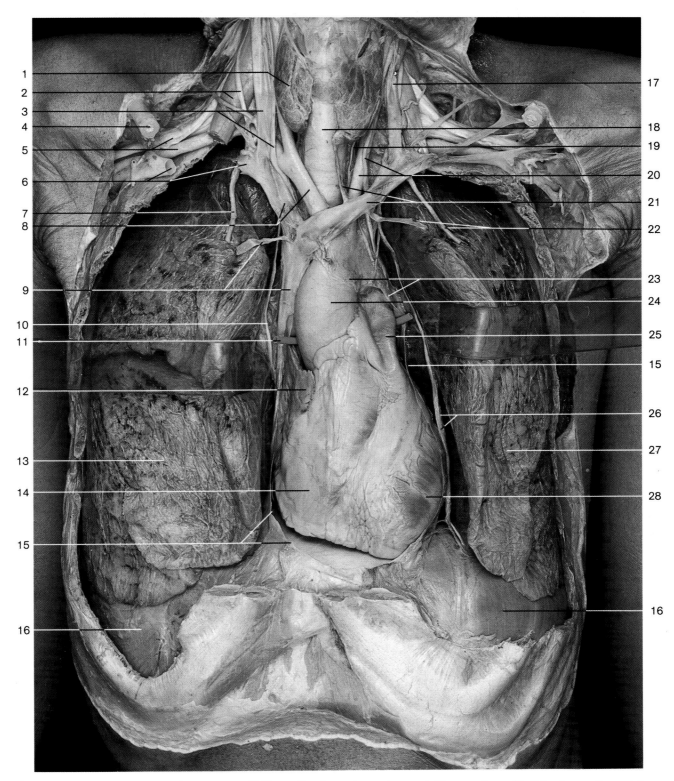

**Thoracic organs, position of the heart, middle mediastinum** (ventral aspect). The anterior wall of the thorax, the costal pleura, and the pericardium have been removed and the lungs slightly reflected.

| | | |
|---|---|---|
| 1 Thyroid gland | 11 Transverse pericardial sinus (probe) | 21 Left brachiocephalic vein and inferior thyroid vein |
| 2 Phrenic nerve and scalenus anterior muscle | 12 Right auricle | |
| 3 Vagus nerve and internal jugular vein | 13 Middle lobe of right lung | 22 Left internal thoracic artery and vein (divided) |
| 4 Clavicle (divided) | 14 Right ventricle | |
| 5 Brachial plexus and subclavian artery | 15 Cut edge of pericardium | 23 Upper margin of pericardial sac |
| 6 Subclavian vein | 16 Diaphragm | 24 Ascending aorta |
| 7 Internal thoracic artery | 17 Internal jugular vein | 25 Pulmonary trunk |
| 8 Brachiocephalic trunk and right brachiocephalic vein | 18 Trachea | 26 Left phrenic nerve and left pericardiacophrenic artery and vein |
| | 19 Left recurrent laryngeal nerve | |
| 9 Superior vena cava and thymic vein | 20 Left common carotid artery and vagus nerve | 27 Upper lobe of left lung |
| 10 Right phrenic nerve | | 28 Left ventricle |

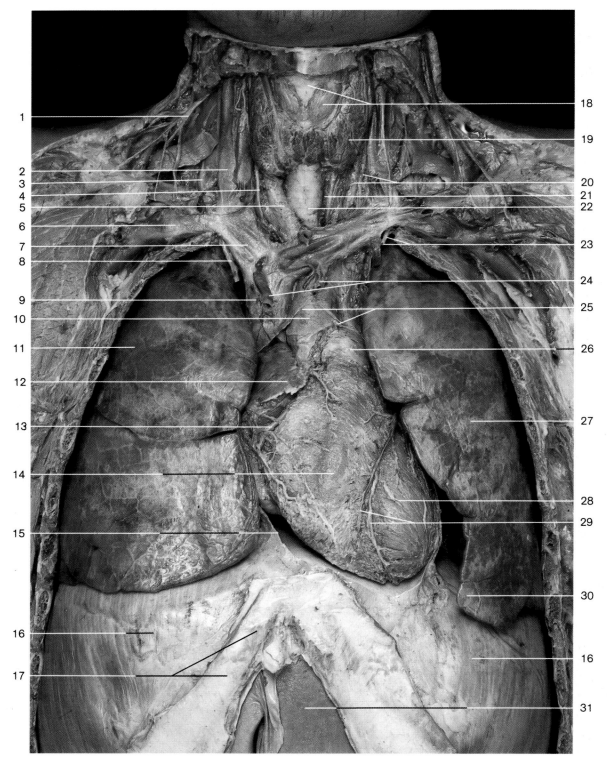

**Thoracic organs, position of heart, dissection of coronary vessels in situ** (ventral aspect). The anterior wall of thorax, costal pleura, and pericardium have been removed.

| | | |
|---|---|---|
| 1 Intermediate supraclavicular nerve | 13 Right coronary artery and | 21 Left recurrent laryngeal nerve |
| 2 Internal jugular vein | small cardiac vein | 22 Trachea |
| 3 Right phrenic nerve | 14 Right ventricle | 23 Left internal thoracic artery and vein (divided) |
| 4 Right vagus nerve | 15 Cut edge of pericardium | 24 Thymic veins |
| 5 Right common carotid artery | 16 Diaphragm | 25 Margin of pericardial sac |
| 6 Right subclavian vein | 17 Costal margin | 26 Pulmonary trunk |
| 7 Right brachiocephalic vein | 18 Larynx (cricothyroid muscle and thyroid | 27 Left lung |
| 8 Right internal thoracic artery | cartilage) | 28 Left ventricle |
| 9 Superior vena cava | 19 Thyroid gland | 29 Anterior interventricular artery and vein |
| 10 Ascending aorta | 20 Left common carotid artery and | 30 Lingula |
| 11 Right lung | left vagus nerve | 31 Liver |
| 12 Right atrium | | |

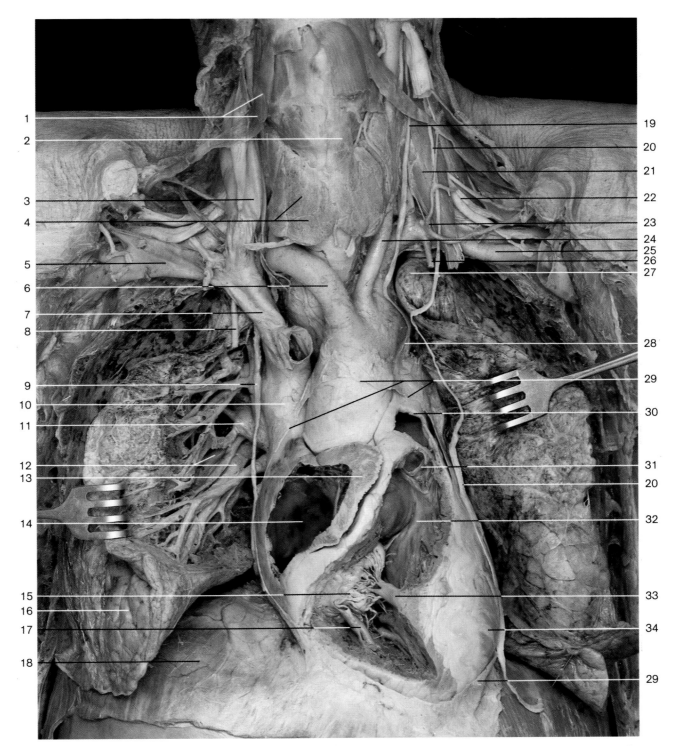

**Thoracic organs, heart with valves in situ** (ventral aspect). Anterior wall of thorax, pleura, and anterior portion of pericardium have been removed. The right atrium and ventricle have been opened to show the right atrioventricular and pulmonary valves.

| | | | | | |
|---|---|---|---|---|---|
| 1 | Omohyoid muscle | 13 | Right auricle | 24 | Left common carotid artery |
| 2 | Pyramidal lobe of thyroid gland | 14 | Right atrium | 25 | Left subclavian artery |
| 3 | Internal jugular vein | 15 | Right atrioventricular (tricuspid) valve | 26 | Left internal thoracic artery |
| 4 | Thyroid gland | 16 | Right lung | 27 | Apex of left lung |
| 5 | Right subclavian vein | 17 | Posterior papillary muscle | 28 | Left recurrent laryngeal nerve |
| 6 | Brachiocephalic trunk | 18 | Diaphragm | 29 | Cut edge of pericardium |
| 7 | Right brachiocephalic vein | 19 | Left vagus nerve | 30 | Pulmonary trunk (fenestrated) |
| 8 | Right internal thoracic artery | 20 | Left phrenic nerve | 31 | Pulmonic valve |
| 9 | Right phrenic nerve | 21 | Scalenus anterior muscle | 32 | Supraventricular crest |
| 10 | Superior vena cava | 22 | Brachial plexus | 33 | Anterior papillary muscle |
| 11 | Pulmonary vein | 23 | Thyrocervical trunk | 34 | Left ventricle |
| 12 | Branches of pulmonary artery | | | | |

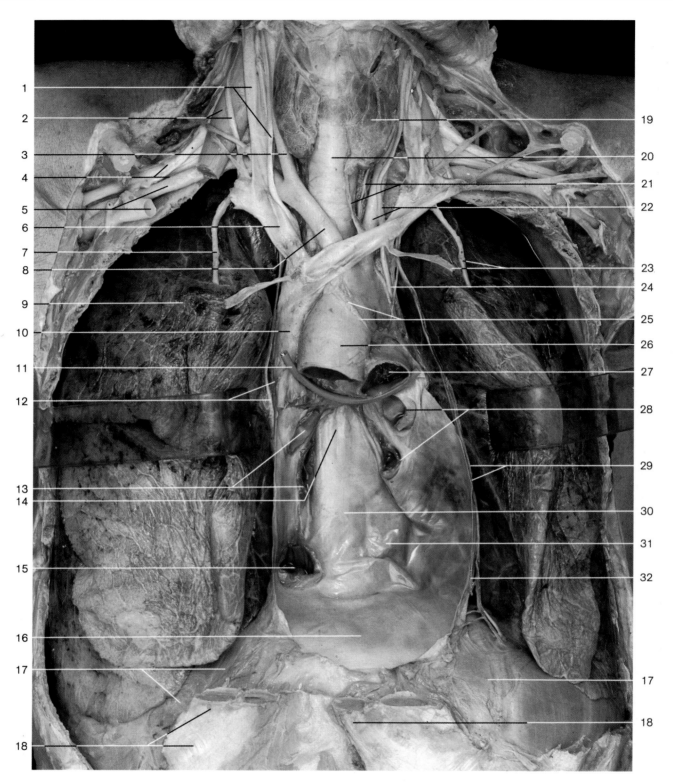

**Thoracic organs, pericardium, and mediastinum** (ventral aspect). Anterior wall of thorax and heart have been removed and the lungs slightly reflected. Note probe within transverse pericardial sinus.

| | | | |
|---|---|---|---|
| 1 | Right internal jugular vein and right vagus nerve | 12 | Right phrenic nerve and right pericardiacophrenic artery and vein |
| 2 | Right phrenic nerve and scalenus anterior muscle | 13 | Right pulmonary veins |
| 3 | Right common carotid artery | 14 | Oblique sinus of pericardium |
| 4 | Brachial plexus | 15 | Inferior vena cava |
| 5 | Right subclavian artery and vein | 16 | Diaphragmatic part of pericardium |
| 6 | Right brachiocephalic vein | 17 | Diaphragm |
| 7 | Right internal thoracic artery (divided) | 18 | Costal margin |
| 8 | Brachiocephalic trunk | 19 | Thyroid gland |
| 9 | Upper lobe of right lung | 20 | Trachea |
| 10 | Superior vena cava | 21 | Left recurrent laryngeal nerve and inferior thyroid vein |
| 11 | Transverse pericardial sinus (probe) | | |

| | |
|---|---|
| 22 | Left common carotid artery and left vagus nerve |
| 23 | Left internal thoracic artery and vein (divided) |
| 24 | Vagus nerve at aortic arch |
| 25 | Cut edge of pericardium |
| 26 | Ascending aorta |
| 27 | Pulmonary trunk (divided) |
| 28 | Left pulmonary veins |
| 29 | Left phrenic nerve and left pericardiacophrenic artery and vein |
| 30 | Contour of esophagus beneath pericardium |
| 31 | Contour of aorta beneath pericardium |
| 32 | Pericardium (cut edge) |

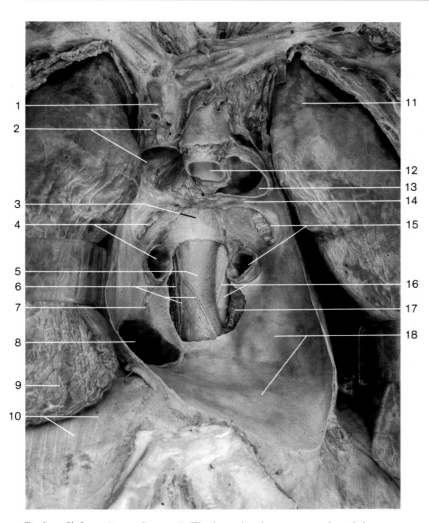

1   Internal thoracic vein
2   Superior vena cava
3   Oblique sinus of pericardium
4   Right pulmonary veins
5   Esophagus
6   Branches of right vagus nerve
7   Mesocardium
8   Inferior vena cava
9   Middle lobe of right lung
10  Diaphragm
11  Upper lobe of left lung
12  Ascending aorta
13  Pulmonary trunk
14  Transverse pericardial sinus
15  Left pulmonary veins
16  Descending aorta and left vagus nerve
17  Left lung (adjacent to pericardium)
18  Pericardium
19  Left subclavian artery
20  Vagus nerve
21  Left recurrent laryngeal nerve
22  Descending aorta
23  Pulmonary artery
24  Left atrium
25  Left ventricle
26  Coronary sinus
27  Left common carotid artery
28  Brachiocephalic trunk
29  Azygos arch
30  Right atrium
31  Right ventricle
32  Aortic arch

**Pericardial sac** (ventral aspect). The heart has been removed, and the posterior wall of the pericardium has been opened to show the adjacent esophagus and aorta.

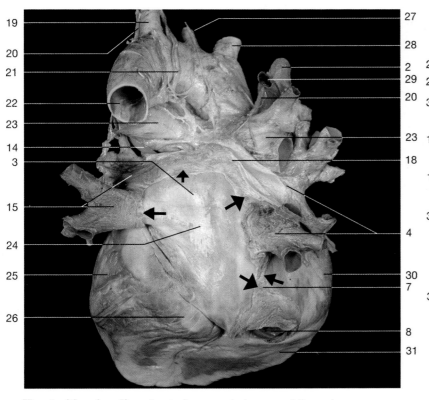

**Heart with epicardium** (posterior aspect). Arrows: oblique sinus.

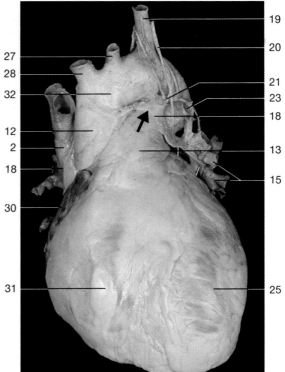

**Heart with epicardium** (anterior aspect). Arrow: pericardial reflection.

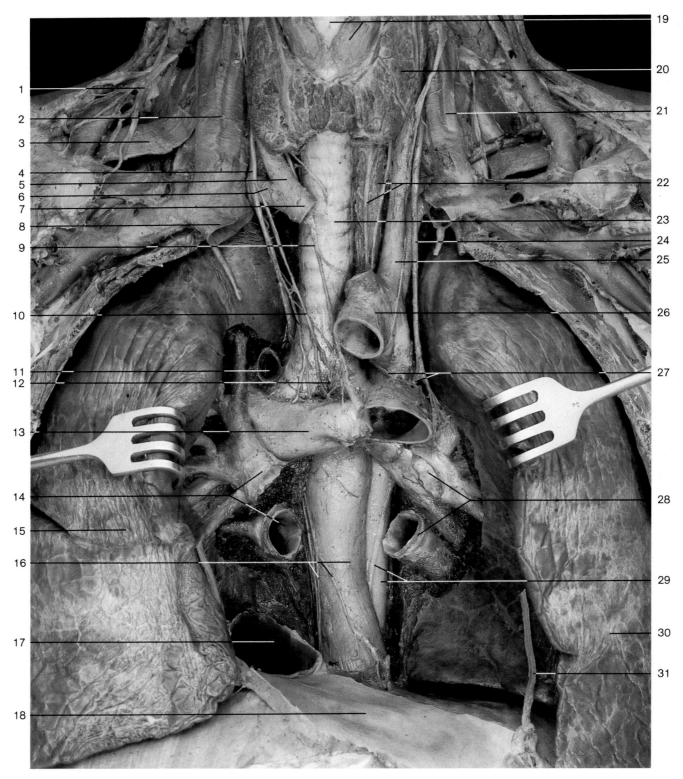

**Mediastinal organs** after removal of heart and pericardium (ventral aspect). Both lungs have been slightly reflected.

| | | |
|---|---|---|
| 1 Supraclavicular nerves | 11 Azygos arch (divided) | 22 Esophagus and left recurrent |
| 2 Internal jugular vein | 12 Bifurcation of trachea | laryngeal nerve |
| 3 Omohyoid muscle | 13 Right pulmonary artery | 23 Trachea |
| 4 Right vagus nerve | 14 Right pulmonary veins | 24 Left vagus nerve |
| 5 Right common carotid artery | 15 Right lung | 25 Left common carotid artery |
| 6 Right subclavian artery | 16 Esophagus and branches | 26 Aortic arch |
| 7 Brachiocephalic trunk | of right vagus nerve | 27 Left recurrent laryngeal nerve |
| 8 Right brachiocephalic vein | 17 Inferior vena cava | branching off from vagus nerve |
| 9 Superior cervical cardiac branch | 18 Pericardium | 28 Left pulmonary veins |
| of vagus nerve | 19 Larynx (thyroid cartilage, cricothyroid muscle) | 29 Thoracic aorta and left vagus nerve |
| 10 Inferior cervical cardiac branches | 20 Thyroid gland | 30 Left lung |
| of vagus nerve | 21 Internal jugular vein | 31 Left phrenic nerve (divided) |

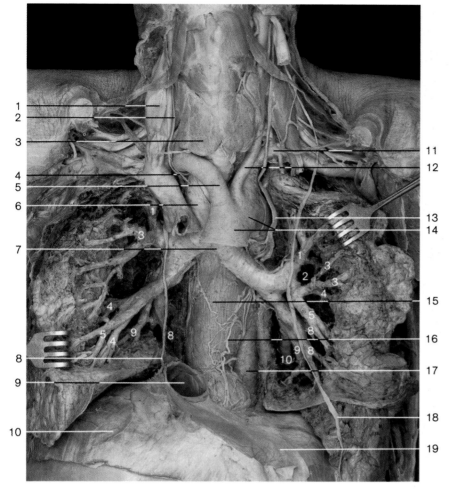

1   Internal jugular vein
2   Right vagus nerve
3   Thyroid gland
4   Right recurrent laryngeal nerve
5   Brachiocephalic trunk
6   Trachea
7   Bifurcation of trachea
8   Right phrenic nerve
9   Inferior vena cava
10  Diaphragm
11  Left subclavian artery
12  Left common carotid artery
13  Left vagus nerve
14  Aortic arch
15  Esophagus
16  Esophageal plexus
17  Thoracic aorta
18  Left phrenic nerve
19  Pericardium at the central tendon of
    diaphragm
20  Right pulmonary artery
21  Left pulmonary artery
22  Tracheal lymph nodes
23  Superior tracheobronchial lymph nodes
24  Bronchopulmonary lymph nodes

**Bronchial tree in situ** (ventral aspect). Heart and pericardium have been
removed; the bronchi of the bronchopulmonary segments are dissected.
1–10 = numbers of segments (cf. p. 246 and 251).

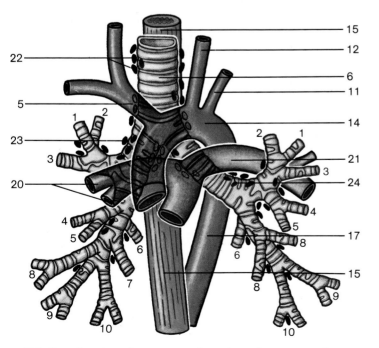

**Relation of aorta, pulmonary trunk, and esophagus to trachea
and bronchial tree** (schematic drawing).
1–10 = number of segments (cf. p. 246 and 251).

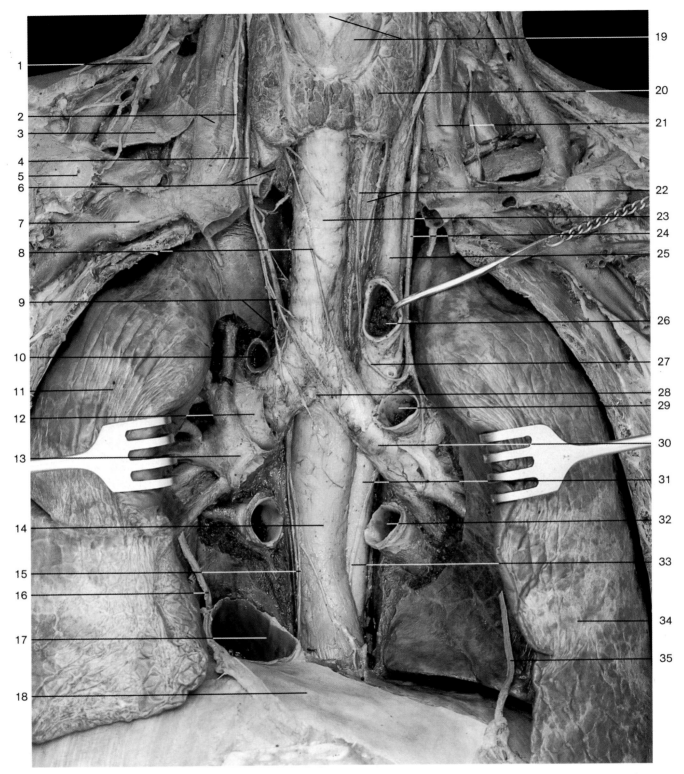

**Organs of posterior mediastinum** (ventral aspect). The heart with the pericardium has been removed, and the lungs and aortic arch have been slightly reflected to show the vagus nerves and their branches.

| | | |
|---|---|---|
| 1 Supraclavicular nerves | 12 Right pulmonary artery | 24 Left vagus nerve |
| 2 Right internal jugular vein with ansa cervicalis | 13 Right pulmonary veins | 25 Left common carotid artery |
| 3 Omohyoid muscle | 14 Esophagus | 26 Aortic arch |
| 4 Right vagus nerve | 15 Esophageal plexus | 27 Left recurrent laryngeal nerve |
| 5 Clavicle | 16 Right phrenic nerve (divided) | 28 Bifurcation of trachea |
| 6 Right subclavian artery and recurrent laryngeal nerve | 17 Inferior vena cava | 29 Left pulmonary artery |
| 7 Right subclavian vein | 18 Pericardium covering the diaphragm | 30 Left primary bronchus |
| 8 Superior cervical cardiac branch of vagus nerve | 19 Larynx (thyroid cartilage and cricothyroid muscle) | 31 Descending aorta |
| 9 Inferior cervical cardiac branch of vagus nerve | 20 Thyroid gland | 32 Left pulmonary veins |
| 10 Azygos arch (divided) | 21 Left internal jugular vein | 33 Branch of left vagus nerve |
| 11 Right lung | 22 Esophagus and left recurrent laryngeal nerve | 34 Left lung |
| | 23 Trachea | 35 Left phrenic nerve (divided) |

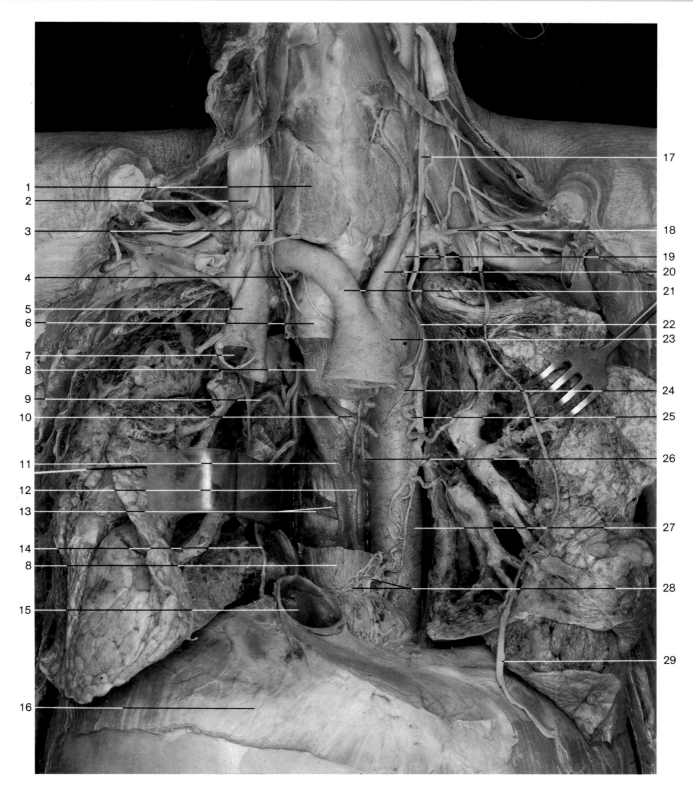

**Mediastinal organs** (ventral aspect). Heart and distal part of esophagus have been removed to display the vessels and nerves of the posterior mediastinum.

| | | |
|---|---|---|
| 1 Thyroid gland | 11 Azygos vein | 21 Brachiocephalic trunk |
| 2 Right internal jugular vein | 12 Thoracic duct | 22 Left vagus nerve |
| 3 Right vagus nerve | 13 Posterior intercostal artery and vein | 23 Aortic arch |
| 4 Point where right recurrent laryngeal nerve | (in front of the vertebral column) | 24 Left recurrent laryngeal nerve |
| is branching off the vagus nerve | 14 Right phrenic nerve | 25 Left bronchial artery |
| 5 Right brachiocephalic vein | 15 Inferior vena cava | 26 Lymph node |
| 6 Trachea | 16 Diaphragm | 27 Thoracic aorta |
| 7 Left brachiocephalic vein (reflected) | 17 Left vagus nerve | 28 Esophageal plexus |
| 8 Esophagus | 18 Thyrocervical trunk | 29 Left phrenic nerve |
| 9 Right bronchial artery | 19 Left subclavian artery | |
| 10 Posterior intercostal artery | 20 Left common carotid artery | |

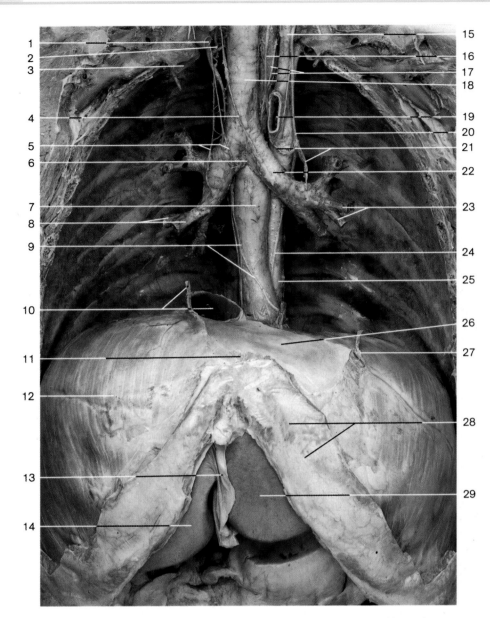

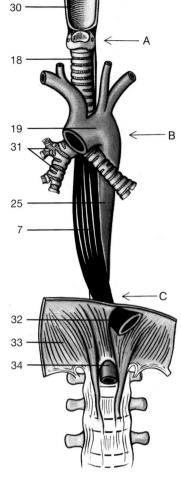

**Diaphragm and organs of mediastinum** (anterior aspect). Heart and lungs have been removed; the costal margin remains in place. Note the different courses of left and right vagus.

**Organs of posterior mediastinum** (ventral aspect). (Schematic drawing.) Three regions in which the esophagus is narrowed are shown:
A: at the level of the cricoid cartilage;
B: at the level of the aortic arch;
C: at the level of the diaphragm.

| | |
|---|---|
| 1 | Right subclavian artery |
| 2 | Right recurrent laryngeal nerve |
| 3 | Right brachiocephalic vein |
| 4 | Superior cervical cardiac nerve |
| 5 | Inferior cervical cardiac nerves and pulmonary branches |
| 6 | Bifurcation of trachea |
| 7 | Esophagus (thoracic part) |
| 8 | Bronchi of lateral and medial segments of middle lobe |
| 9 | Esophageal plexus and branches of right vagus nerve |
| 10 | Inferior vena cava and right phrenic nerve (cut) |
| 11 | Sternal part of diaphragm |
| 12 | Costal part of diaphragm |
| 13 | Falciform ligament of liver |

| | |
|---|---|
| 14 | Liver (quadrate lobe) |
| 15 | Left common carotid artery |
| 16 | Left recurrent laryngeal nerve |
| 17 | Esophageal branches of left vagus nerve and esophagus |
| 18 | Trachea |
| 19 | Aortic arch |
| 20 | Left vagus nerve |
| 21 | Left recurrent laryngeal nerve with inferior cardiac nerve |
| 22 | Left primary bronchus |
| 23 | Superior and inferior lingular bronchi |
| 24 | Esophageal plexus of left vagus nerve |
| 25 | Descending aorta |
| 26 | Central tendon of diaphragm covered with pericardium |
| 27 | Left phrenic nerve (divided) |

| | |
|---|---|
| 28 | Costal margin |
| 29 | Liver, left lobe |
| 30 | Pharynx |
| 31 | Secondary bronchi |
| 32 | Esophagus (abdominal part) |
| 33 | Diaphragm |
| 34 | Abdominal aorta |

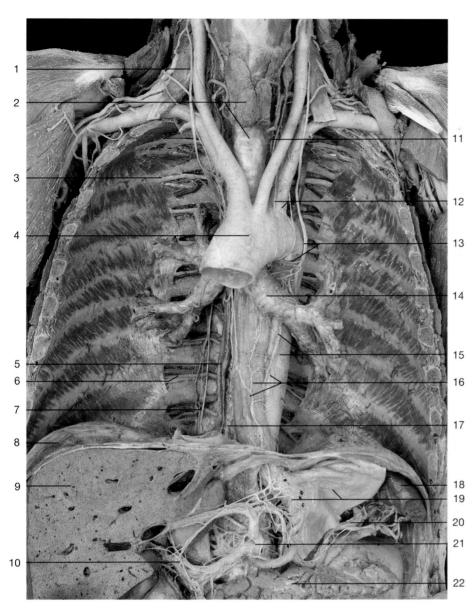

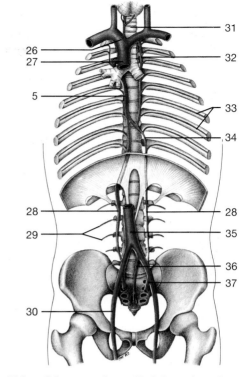

**Organs of posterior mediastinum** (anterior aspect).

**Veins of the posterior wall of thoracic and abdominal cavity** (schematic drawing).

1  Right vagus nerve
2  Thyroid gland and trachea
3  Intercostal nerve
4  Aortic arch
5  Azygos vein
6  Posterior intercostal artery
7  Greater splanchnic nerve
8  Diaphragm
9  Liver
10  Proper hepatic artery and hepatic plexus
11  Left recurrent laryngeal nerve
12  Inferior cervical cardiac nerves
13  Left vagus nerve and left recurrent laryngeal nerve
14  Left primary bronchus
15  Thoracic aorta and left vagus nerve
16  Esophagus and esophageal plexus
17  Thoracic duct
18  Spleen
19  Anterior gastric plexus and stomach (divided)
20  Splenic artery and splenic plexus
21  Celiac trunk and celiac plexus
22  Pancreas
23  Ramus communicans
24  Sympathetic trunk and sympathetic ganglion
25  Posterior intercostal vein and artery and intercostal nerve
26  Right brachiocephalic vein
27  Superior vena cava
28  Ascending lumbar vein
29  Lumbar veins
30  Right external iliac vein
31  Trachea
32  Accessory hemiazygos vein
33  Posterior intercostal veins
34  Hemiazygos vein
35  Inferior vena cava
36  Median sacral vein
37  Internal iliac vein

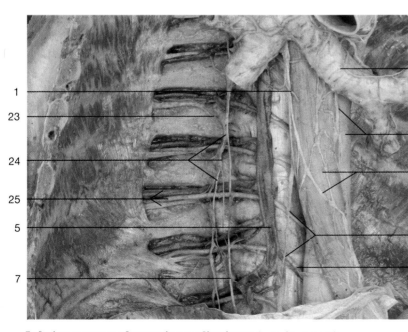

**Inferior segment of posterior mediastinum** (anterior aspect).

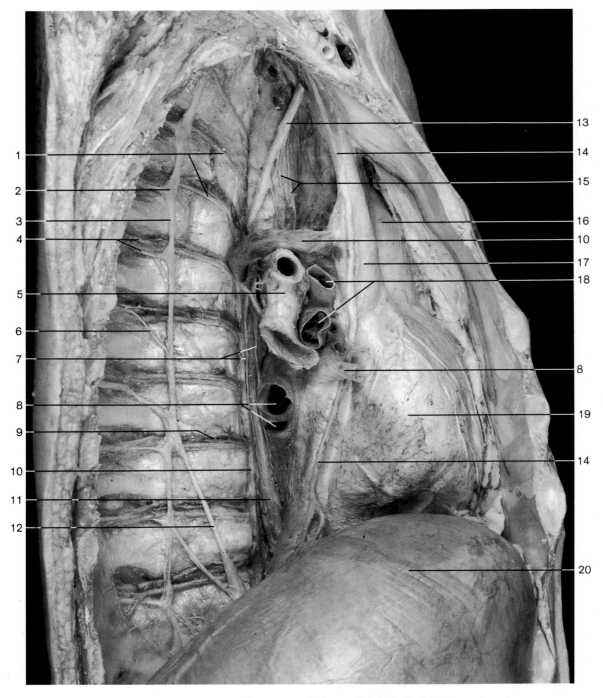

**Mediastinal organs** (right lateral aspect). Right lung and pleura of right half of the thorax have been removed.

| | |
|---|---|
| 1 | Posterior intercostal arteries |
| 2 | Ganglion of sympathetic trunk |
| 3 | Sympathetic trunk |
| 4 | Vessels and nerves of the intercostal space (from above: posterior intercostal vein and artery and intercostal nerve) |
| 5 | Right primary bronchus |
| 6 | Ramus communicans of sympathetic trunk |
| 7 | Esophageal plexus (branches of right vagus nerve) |
| 8 | Pulmonary veins |
| 9 | Posterior intercostal vein |
| 10 | Azygos vein |
| 11 | Esophagus |
| 12 | Greater splanchnic nerve |
| 13 | Right vagus nerve |
| 14 | Right phrenic nerve |
| 15 | Inferior cervical cardiac branches of vagus nerve |
| 16 | Aortic arch |
| 17 | Superior vena cava |
| 18 | Right pulmonary artery |
| 19 | Heart with pericardium |
| 20 | Diaphragm |

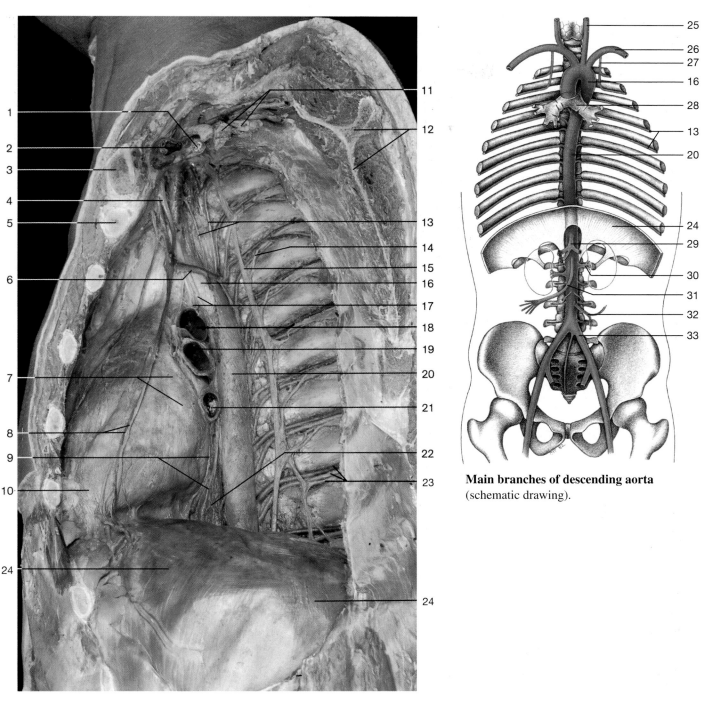

**Organs of posterior and superior mediastinum** (left lateral aspect).

**Main branches of descending aorta** (schematic drawing).

| | | |
|---|---|---|
| 1 | Subclavian artery | 12 | Scapula (divided) | 23 | Posterior intercostal artery and vein and intercostal nerve |
| 2 | Subclavian vein | 13 | Posterior intercostal arteries | 24 | Diaphragm |
| 3 | Clavicle (divided) | 14 | White ramus communicans of sympathetic trunk | 25 | Common carotid artery |
| 4 | Left vagus nerve | 15 | Sympathetic trunk | 26 | Subclavian artery |
| 5 | First rib (divided) | 16 | Aortic arch | 27 | Highest intercostal artery |
| 6 | Left superior intercostal vein | 17 | Left vagus nerve and left recurrent laryngeal nerve | 28 | Bifurcation of trachea |
| 7 | Left atrium with pericardium | 18 | Left pulmonary artery | 29 | Celiac trunk |
| 8 | Left phrenic nerve and pericardiacophrenic artery and vein | 19 | Left primary bronchus | 30 | Renal artery |
| 9 | Esophageal plexus (branches derived from left vagus nerve) | 20 | Thoracic aorta | 31 | Superior mesenteric artery |
| 10 | Apex of heart with pericardium | 21 | Pulmonary vein | 32 | Inferior mesenteric artery |
| 11 | Brachial plexus | 22 | Esophagus (thoracic part) | 33 | Common iliac artery |

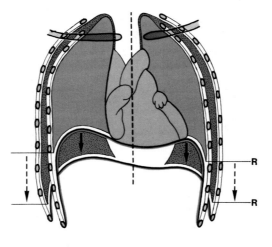

1   Superior vena cava
2   Right atrium
3   Right ventricle
4   Costal part of diaphragm
5   Costal margin
6   Position of costodiaphragmatic recess
7   Lateral arcuate ligament
8   Medial arcuate ligament
9   Right crus of lumbar part of diaphragm
10  Quadratus lumborum muscle
11  Ascending aorta
12  Pulmonary trunk
13  Left ventricle
14  Pericardium, diaphragm
15  Esophageal hiatus and abdominal
     part of esophagus (cut)
16  Lumbar part of diaphragm
17  Aortic hiatus
18  Psoas major muscle
19  Lumbar vertebra

**Diaphragm in situ** (anterior aspect). Anterior walls of thoracic and abdominal cavities have been removed. Natural position of the heart above the central tendon on the diaphragm is shown.

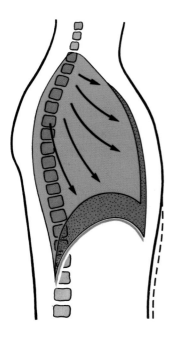

**Changes in the position of the diaphragm and thoracic cage during respiration.** Left: lateral aspect; right: anterior aspect. During inspiration the diaphragm moves downwards and the lower part of the thoracic cage expands forward and laterally, causing the costodiaphragmatic recess (R) to enlarge (cf. dotted arrows).

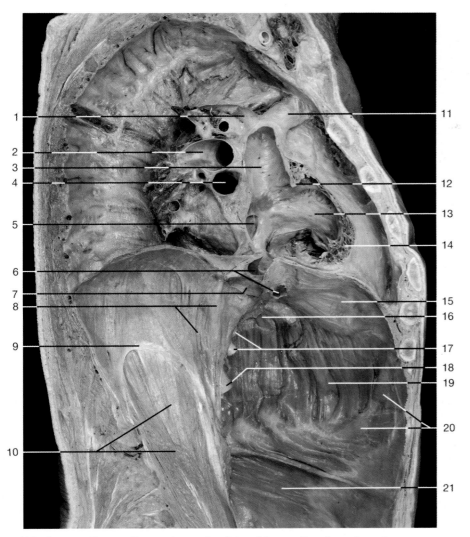

1 Azygos venous arch
2 Right pulmonary artery
3 Superior vena cava
4 Right pulmonary vein
5 Fossa ovalis
6 Hepatic veins
7 Inferior vena cava
8 Right crus of lumbar part of diaphragm
9 Medial arcuate ligament
10 Psoas major muscle
11 Left brachiocephalic vein
12 Terminal crista
13 Right atrium
14 Right auricle
15 Central tendon of diaphragm
16 Esophagus
17 Celiac trunk and superior mesenteric artery
18 Aorta
19 Costal part of diaphragm
20 Costal margin
21 Transversus abdominis muscle

**Diaphragm.** Paramedian section to the right of the median plane through thoracic and upper abdominal cavity. The plane passes through the superior and inferior vena cava just to the right of the vertebral bodies. Most of the heart remains in situ to the left of this plane (specimen is viewed from the right side).

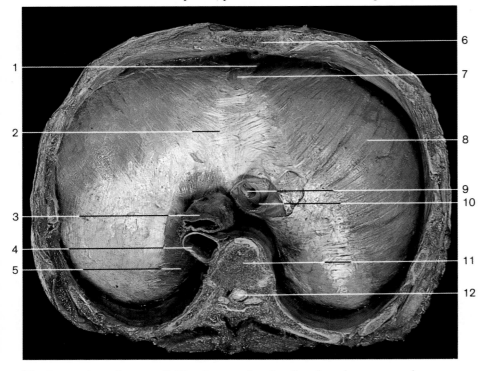

1 Sternocostal triangle
2 Central tendon (from above)
3 Esophagus
4 Aorta
5 Lumbar part of diaphragm
6 Sternum
7 Sternal part of diaphragm
8 Costal part of diaphragm
9 Entrance of hepatic veins
10 Inferior vena cava
11 Body of 9th thoracic vertebra
12 Spinal cord

**Diaphragm** (superior aspect). The pleura and pericardium have been removed.

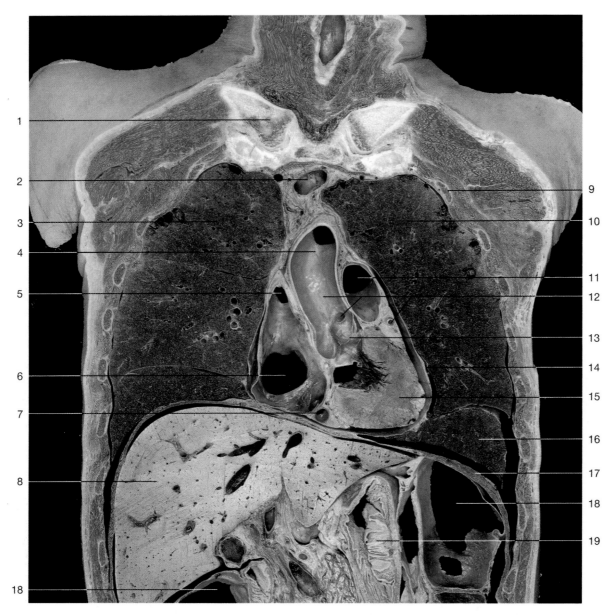

**Coronal section through the thorax** at the level of ascending aorta (anterior aspect).

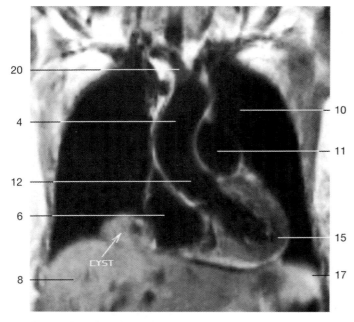

**Coronal section through the thorax** at the level of ascending aorta. (MRI scan.)

1   Clavicle
2   Left brachiocephalic vein
3   Superior lobe of right lung
4   Aortic arch
5   Superior vena cava
6   Right atrium (entrance of inferior vena cava)
7   Coronary sinus
8   Liver
9   Second rib
10  Superior lobe of left lung
11  Pulmonary trunk
12  Ascending aorta and left coronary artery
13  Aortic valve
14  Pericardium
15  Myocardium of left ventricle
16  Lower lobe of left lung
17  Diaphragm
18  Colic flexures
19  Stomach
20  Brachiocephalic trunk

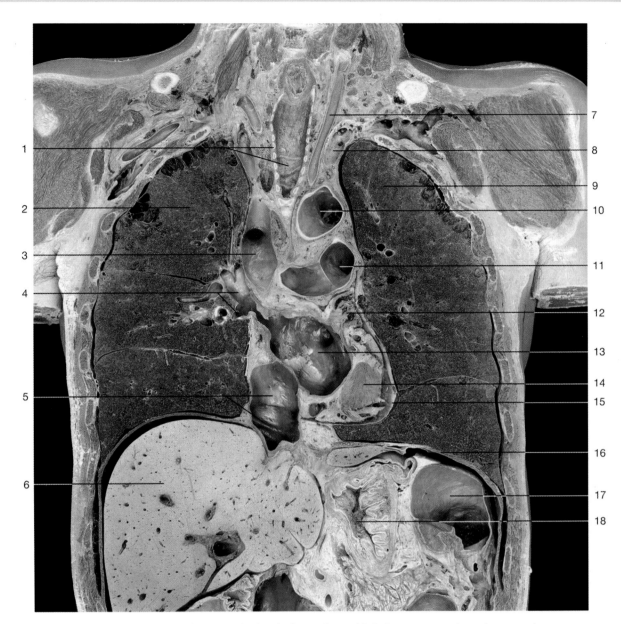

**Coronal section through the thorax** at the level of superior and inferior vena cava (anterior aspect).

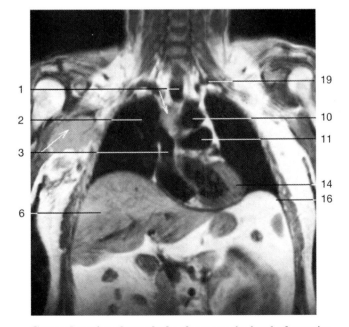

**Coronal section through the thorax** at the level of superior vena cava. Arrows = Metastases of tumor. (MRI scan.)

1   Trachea
2   Upper lobe of right lung
3   Superior vena cava
4   Right pulmonary veins
5   Inferior vena cava and right atrium
6   Liver
7   Left common carotid artery
8   Left subclavian vein
9   Upper lobe of left lung
10  Aortic arch
11  Left pulmonary artery
12  Left auricle
13  Left atrium with orifices
    of pulmonary veins
14  Left ventricle (myocardium)
15  Pericardium
16  Diaphragm
17  Left colic flexure
18  Stomach
19  Left subclavian artery

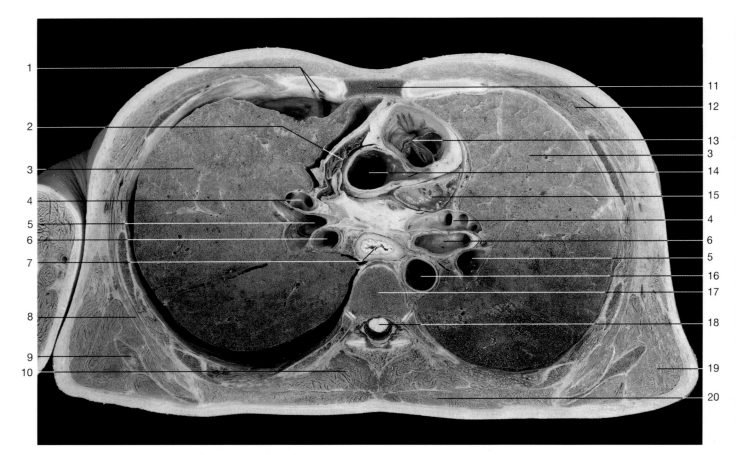

**Horizontal section through the thorax** at level 1 (from below).

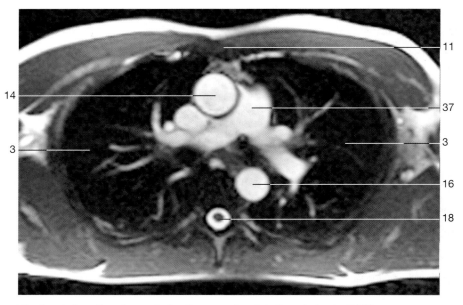

**Horizontal section through the thorax** at level 1 (from below). (MRI scan, courtesy of Prof. W. Bautz and R. Janka, M. D., University of Erlangen, Germany.)

|  |  |  |  |
|---|---|---|---|
| 1 | Internal thoracic artery and vein | 12 | Pectoralis major and minor muscles |
| 2 | Right atrium | 13 | Conus arteriosus (right ventricle), |
| 3 | Lung |  | pulmonic valve |
| 4 | Pulmonary artery | 14 | Ascending aorta and left coronary artery |
| 5 | Pulmonary vein |  | (only in upper figure) |
| 6 | Primary bronchus | 15 | Left atrium |
| 7 | Esophagus | 16 | Descending aorta |
| 8 | Serratus anterior muscle | 17 | Thoracic vertebra |
| 9 | Scapula | 18 | Spinal cord |
| 10 | Longissimus thoracis muscle | 19 | Latissimus dorsi muscle |
| 11 | Sternum | 20 | Trapezius muscle |

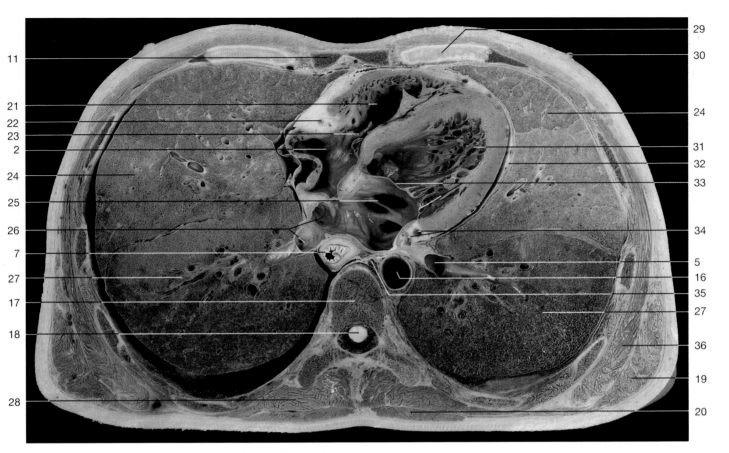

**Horizontal section through the thorax** at level 2 (from below).

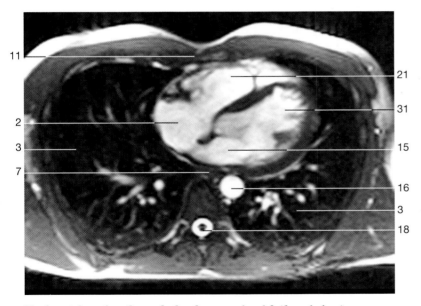

**Horizontal section through the thorax** at level 2 (from below).
(MRI scan, courtesy of Prof. W. Bautz and R. Janka, M. D., University of
Erlangen, Germany.)

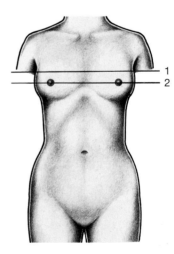

**Levels of sections.**

| | | | |
|---|---|---|---|
| 21 | Right ventricle | 31 | Left ventricle |
| 22 | Right coronary artery | 32 | Pericardium |
| 23 | Right atrioventricular valve | 33 | Left atrioventricular valve |
| 24 | Lung (upper lobe) | 34 | Left coronary artery and coronary sinus |
| 25 | Left atrium | 35 | Accessory hemiazygos vein |
| 26 | Pulmonary veins | 36 | Serratus anterior muscle |
| 27 | Lung (lower lobe) | 37 | Pulmonary trunk |
| 28 | Erector muscle of spine | | |
| 29 | Third costal cartilage | | |
| 30 | Nipple | | |

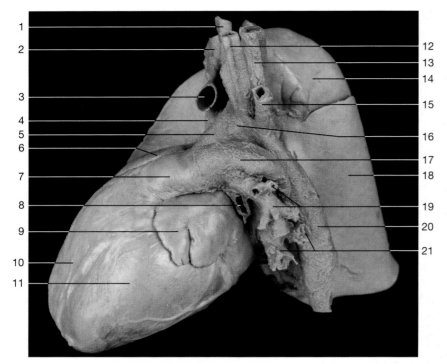

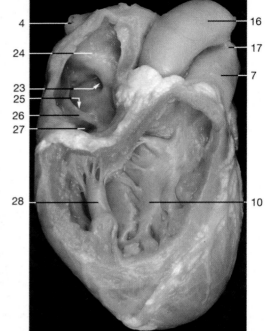

**Heart and right lung of the fetus** (viewed from left side). The left lung has been removed. Note the ductus arteriosus (Botalli).

**Heart of the fetus** (anterior aspect). Right atrium and ventricle opened.

| Shunts in the fetal circulation system | | |
|---|---|---|
| 1. Ductus venosus (of Arantius) | between umbilical vein and inferior vena cava | bypass of liver circulation |
| 2. Foramen ovale | between right and left atrium | bypass of pulmonary circulation |
| 3. Ductus arteriosus (Botalli) | between pulmonary trunk and aorta | |

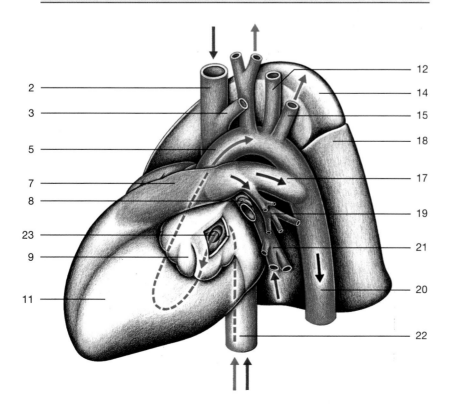

 1  Right common carotid artery
 2  Right brachiocephalic vein
 3  Left brachiocephalic vein
 4  Superior vena cava
 5  Ascending aorta
 6  Right auricle
 7  Pulmonary trunk
 8  Left primary bronchus
 9  Left auricle
10  Right ventricle
11  Left ventricle
12  Left common carotid artery
13  Trachea
14  Superior lobe of right lung
15  Left subclavian artery
16  Aortic arch
17  Ductus arteriosus (Botalli)
18  Inferior lobe of right lung
19  Left pulmonary artery with branches to the left lung
20  Descending aorta
21  Left pulmonary veins
22  Inferior vena cava
23  Foramen ovale
24  Right atrium
25  Opening of inferior vena cava
26  Valve of inferior vena cava (Eustachian valve)
27  Opening of coronary sinus
28  Anterior papillary muscle of right ventricle

◁ **Heart of the fetus** (schematic drawing). Direction of blood flow indicated by arrows. Note the change in oxygenation of blood after ductus arteriosus entry into aorta.

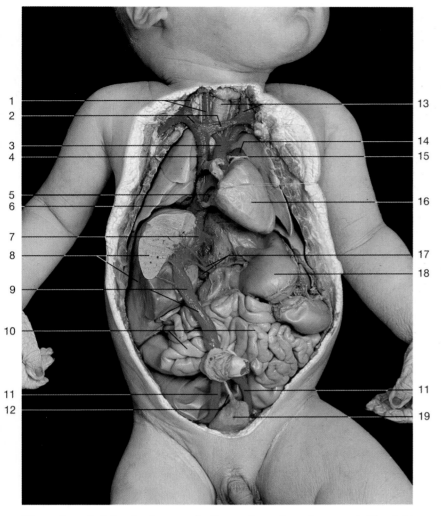

1  Internal jugular vein and right common carotid artery
2  Right and left brachiocephalic vein
3  Aortic arch
4  Superior vena cava
5  Foramen ovale
6  Inferior vena cava
7  Ductus venosus
8  Liver
9  Umbilical vein
10  Small intestine
11  Umbilical artery
12  Urachus
13  Trachea and left internal jugular vein
14  Left pulmonary artery
15  Ductus arteriosus (Botalli)
16  Right ventricle
17  Hepatic arteries (red) and portal vein (blue)
18  Stomach
19  Urinary bladder
20  Portal vein
21  Pulmonary veins
22  Descending aorta
23  Placenta

**Thoracic and abdominal organs in the newborn** (anterior aspect). The right atrium has been opened to show the foramen ovale. The left lobe of the liver has been removed.

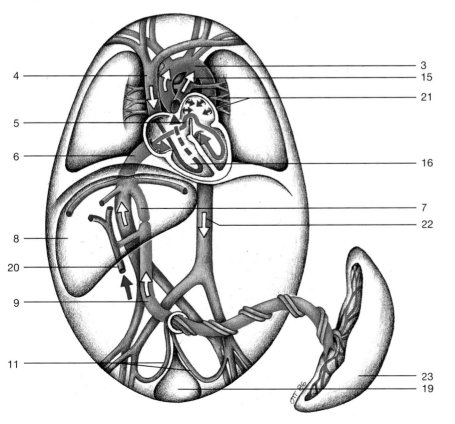

◁ **Fetal circulatory system** (schematic drawing). The oxygen gradient is indicated by color.

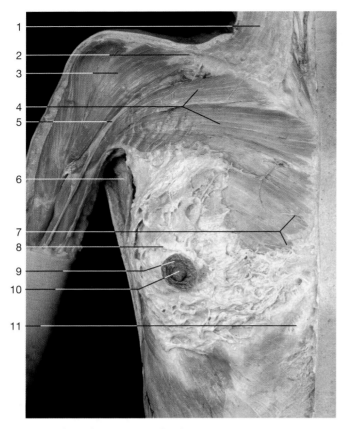

**Dissection of mammary gland** (anterior aspect).

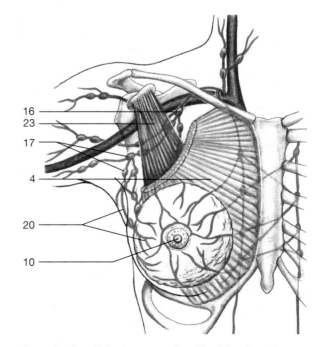

**Dissection of mammary gland and axillary lymph nodes.**

| | | |
|---|---|---|
| 1 | Platysma muscle | |
| 2 | Clavicle | |
| 3 | Deltoid muscle | |
| 4 | Pectoralis major muscle | |
| 5 | Deltopectoral groove and cephalic vein | |
| 6 | Latissimus dorsi muscle | |
| 7 | Medial mammarian branches of intercostal nerves | |

| | |
|---|---|
| 8 | Breast tissue |
| 9 | Areola |
| 10 | Nipple (papilla) |
| 11 | Costal margin |
| 12 | Pectoral fascia |
| 13 | Mammary gland |
| 14 | Serratus anterior muscle (insertion) |
| 15 | Lactiferous sinus |

| | |
|---|---|
| 16 | Apical lymph nodes |
| 17 | Axillary lymph nodes |
| 18 | Intercostobrachial nerve |
| 19 | Lateral thoracic vein |
| 20 | Lymph vessels |
| 21 | Serratus anterior muscle |
| 22 | Medial branches of intercostal arteries |
| 23 | Pectoralis minor muscle |

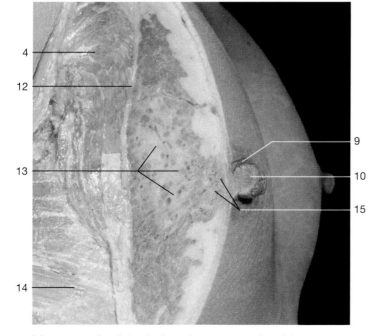

**Mammary gland** (sagittal section; pregnant female).

**Lymphatics of the breast and axilla.** Most lymph vessels drain into the axillary lymph nodes.

# 5 Abdominal Organs

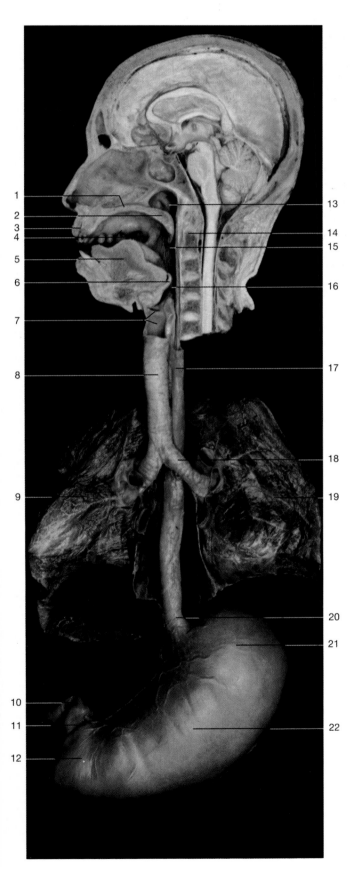

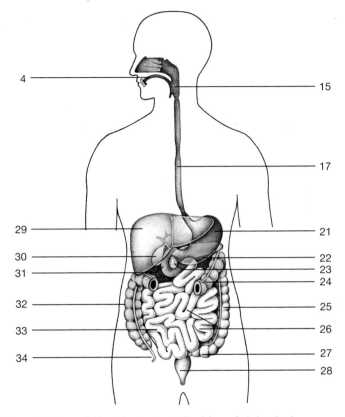

**Organization of digestive system.** Position of abdominal organs.

| | | | |
|---|---|---|---|
| 1 | Hard palate | 19 | Left lung |
| 2 | Soft palate with uvula | 20 | Abdominal part of esophagus |
| 3 | Vestibule of the mouth | | and cardia |
| 4 | Oral cavity proper | 21 | Fundus of stomach |
| 5 | Tongue | 22 | Body of stomach |
| 6 | Epiglottis | 23 | Pancreas |
| 7 | Vocal ligament and larynx | 24 | Transverse colon (divided) |
| 8 | Trachea | 25 | Descending colon |
| 9 | Right lung | 26 | Jejunum |
| 10 | Superior part of duodenum | 27 | Sigmoid colon |
| 11 | Pylorus | 28 | Rectum |
| 12 | Pyloric antrum | 29 | Liver |
| 13 | Nasopharynx | 30 | Gallbladder |
| 14 | Dens of axis | 31 | Duodenum |
| 15 | Oropharynx | 32 | Ascending colon |
| 16 | Laryngopharynx | 33 | Ileum |
| 17 | Esophagus (thoracic part) | 34 | Vermiform appendix |
| 18 | Left primary bronchus | | |

◁ **Survey of upper portion of digestive system.**
Oral cavity, pharynx, esophagus, and stomach.

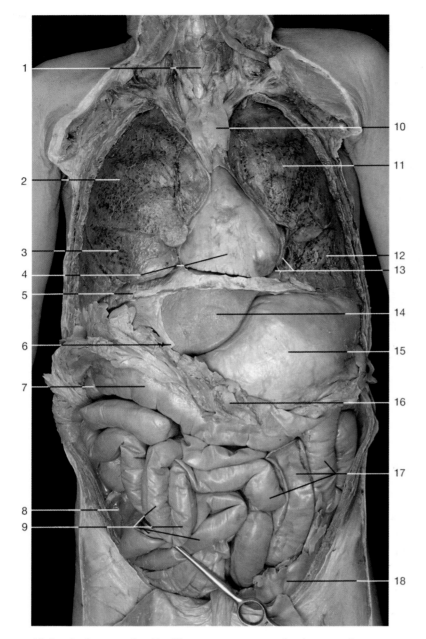

1   Thyroid gland
2   Upper lobe of right lung
3   Middle lobe of right lung
4   Heart
5   Diaphragm
6   Round ligament of liver (ligamentum teres)
7   Transverse colon
8   Cecum
9   Small intestine (ileum)
10  Thymus
11  Upper lobe of left lung
12  Lower lobe of left lung
13  Pericardium (cut edge)
14  Liver (left lobe)
15  Stomach
16  Greater omentum
17  Small intestine (jejunum)
18  Sigmoid colon
19  Rectus abdominis muscle
20  Small intestine (section)
21  Rib
22  Common bile duct, duodenum, and pancreas
23  Inferior vena cava
24  Liver
25  Body of second lumbar vertebra
26  Right kidney
27  Cauda equina and dura mater
28  Linea alba
29  Stomach and pylorus
30  Superior mesenteric artery and vein
31  Abdominal aorta
32  Left renal artery and vein
33  Left kidney
34  Psoas major muscle
35  Deep muscles of the back
36  Pancreas adjacent to lesser sac
    (bursa omentalis)
37  Falciform ligament with ligamentum teres

**Abdominal organs in situ.** The greater omentum has been partly removed or reflected.

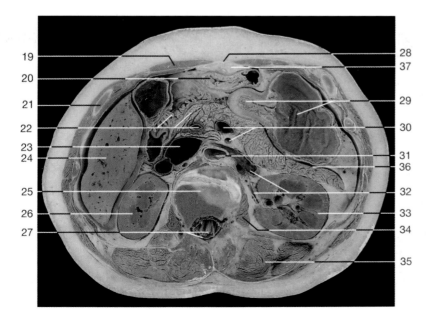

**Transverse section through the abdominal cavity** at the level of the second lumbar vertebra (from below).

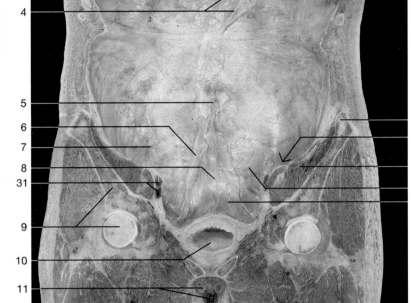

**Anterior abdominal wall** with pelvic cavity and thigh (frontal section, male) (internal aspect).

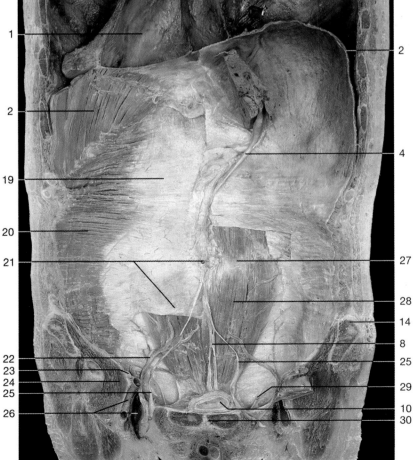

1 Left ventricle with pericardium
2 Diaphragm
3 Remnant of liver
4 Ligamentum teres
   (free margin of falciform ligament)
5 Site of umbilicus
6 Medial umbilical fold
   (containing the obliterated umbilical artery)
7 Lateral umbilical fold (containing inferior
   epigastric artery and vein)
8 Median umbilical fold
   (containing remnant of urachus)
9 Head of femur and pelvic bone
10 Urinary bladder
11 Root of penis
12 Falciform ligament of liver
13 Rib (divided)
14 Iliac crest (divided)
15 Site of deep inguinal ring and
   lateral inguinal fossa
16 Iliopsoas muscle (divided)
17 Medial inguinal fossa
18 Supravesical fossa
19 Posterior layer of rectus sheath
20 Transversus abdominis muscle
21 Umbilicus and arcuate line
22 Inferior epigastric artery
23 Femoral nerve
24 Iliopsoas muscle
25 Remnant of umbilical artery
26 Femoral artery and vein
27 Tendinous intersection of rectus abdominis
   muscle
28 Rectus abdominis muscle
29 Interfoveolar ligament
30 Pubic symphysis (divided)
31 External iliac artery and vein

**Anterior abdominal wall** (male) (internal aspect). The peritoneum and parts of the posterior layer of rectus sheath have been removed. Dissection of inferior epigastric arteries and veins.

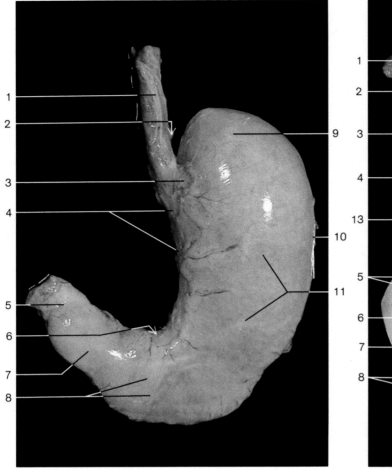

**Stomach** (ventral aspect).

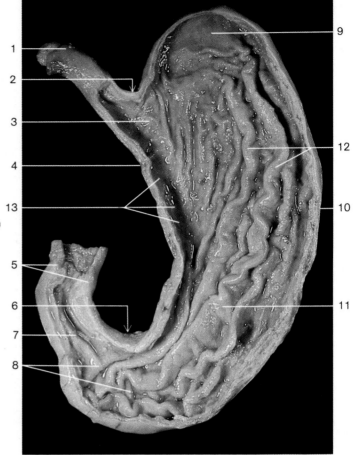

**Mucosa of posterior wall of stomach** (ventral aspect).

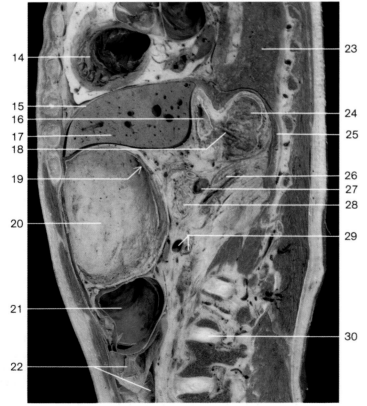

**Parasagittal section through upper part of left abdominal cavity** 3.5 cm lateral to median plane.

1　Esophagus
2　Cardial notch
3　Cardial part of stomach
4　Lesser curvature of stomach
5　Pyloric sphincter
6　Angular notch (incisura angularis)
7　Pyloric canal
8　Pyloric antrum
9　Fundus of stomach
10　Greater curvature of stomach
11　Body of stomach
12　Folds of mucous membrane (gastric rugae)
13　Gastric canal
14　Right ventricle of heart
15　Diaphragm (cut edge)
16　Abdominal portion of esophagus
17　Liver
18　Cardial part of stomach (cut edge)
19　Position of pyloric canal
20　Body of stomach
21　Transverse colon
22　Small intestine
23　Lung (cut edge)
24　Fundus of stomach (section)
25　Lumbar portion of diaphragm (cut edge)
26　Suprarenal gland
27　Splenic vein
28　Pancreas
29　Superior mesenteric artery and vein
30　Intervertebral disc

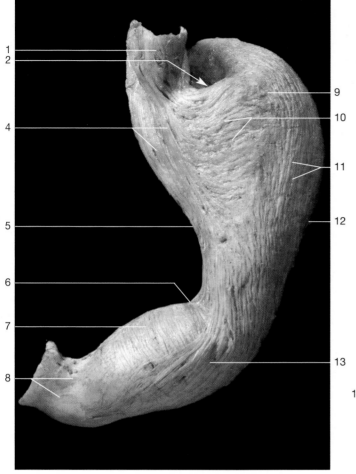

**Muscular coat of stomach,** outer layer (ventral aspect).

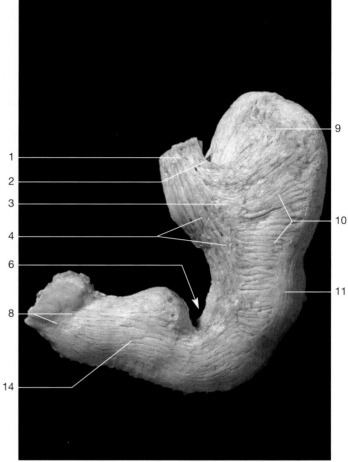

**Muscular coat of stomach,** middle layer (ventral aspect).

1   Esophagus (abdominal part)
2   Cardial notch
3   Cardial part of stomach
4   Longitudinal muscle layer at lesser curvature of stomach
5   Lesser curvature
6   Incisura angularis
7   Circular muscle layer of pyloric part of stomach
8   Pyloric sphincter muscle
9   Fundus of stomach
10  Circular muscle layer of fundus of stomach
11  Longitudinal muscle layer of greater curvature of stomach
12  Greater curvature of stomach
13  Longitudinal muscle layer (transition from body to pyloric part of stomach)
14  Pyloric part of stomach
15  Oblique muscle fibers

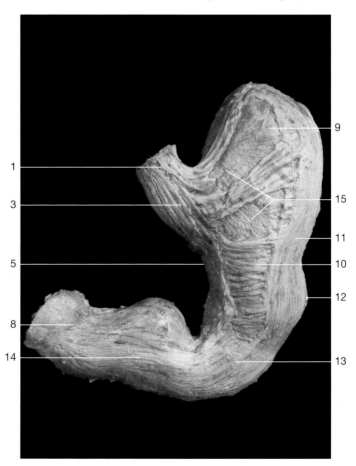

**Muscular coat of stomach,** inner layer (ventral aspect).

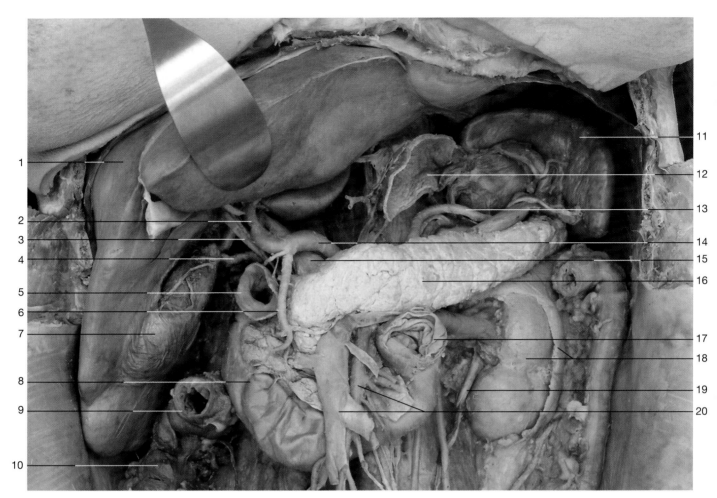

**Upper abdominal organs.** Pancreas, duodenum, and left kidney are shown. Stomach and transverse colon have been removed, liver elevated; superior mesenteric vein is slightly enlarged.

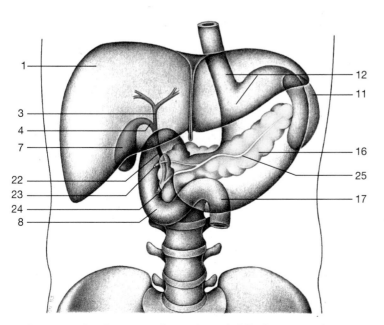

**Pancreas, duodenum, and extrahepatic bile ducts** (anterior aspect, schematic drawing).

1  Liver
2  Hepatic artery proper
3  Hepatic duct
4  Cystic duct
5  Pylorus
6  Gastroduodenal artery
7  Gallbladder
8  Duodenum
9  Transverse colon (cut)
10 Ascending colon
11 Spleen
12 Cardia
13 Splenic artery
14 Common hepatic artery
15 Portal vein
16 Pancreas (body)
17 Duodenojejunal flexure
18 Kidney (with capsula adiposa)
19 Ureter
20 Superior mesenteric artery and vein
21 Aorta (abdominal part)
22 Common bile duct
23 Lesser duodenal papilla
24 Greater duodenal papilla
25 Pancreatic duct

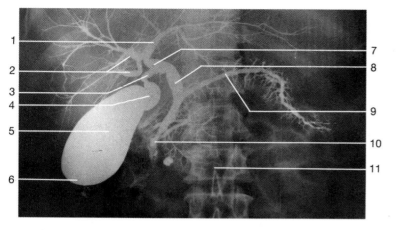

1  Left hepatic duct
2  Right hepatic duct
3  Cystic duct
4  Neck of gallbladder
5  Body of gallbladder
6  Fundus of gallbladder
7  Common hepatic duct
8  Common bile duct
9  Pancreatic duct
10  Greater duodenal papilla
11  Second lumbar vertebra
12  Folds of mucous membrane of gallbladder
13  Muscular coat of gallbladder
14  Neck of gallbladder (opened)
15  Cystic duct with spiral fold
16  Lesser duodenal papilla
17  Accessory pancreatic duct
18  Uncinate process
19  Plica circularis of duodenum (Kerckring's fold)
20  Head of pancreas
21  Body of pancreas
22  Tail of pancreas
23  Descending part of duodenum
24  Incisure of pancreas

**Radiograph of biliary ducts, gallbladder, and pancreatic duct** (anterior-posterior view).

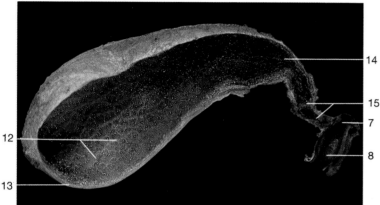

**Isolated gallbladder and cystic duct** (anterior aspect).
The gallbladder has been opened to display the mucous membrane.

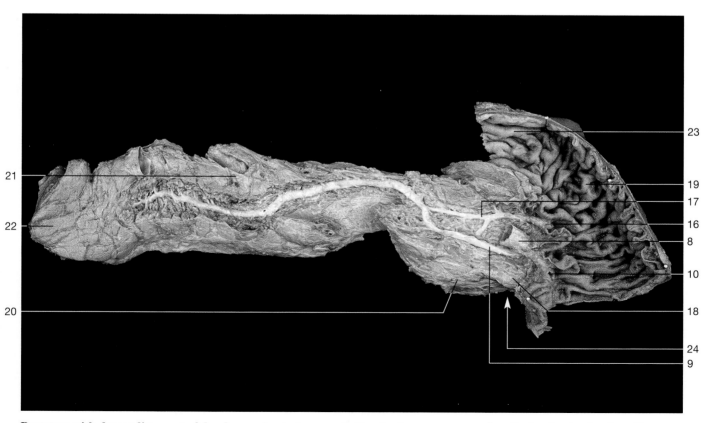

**Pancreas with descending part of duodenum** (posterior aspect). The duodenum was opened to display the duodenal papillae. Pancreatic duct has been dissected, the common bile duct has been divided. The sphincter of Oddi is shown.

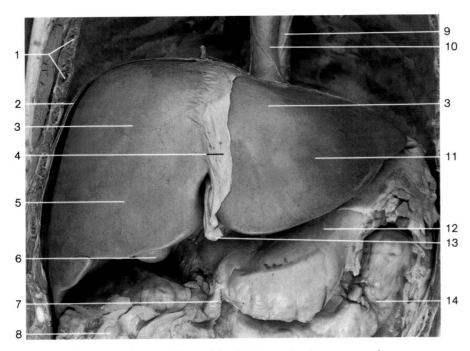

**Liver in situ** (ventral aspect). Part of the diaphragm has been removed.

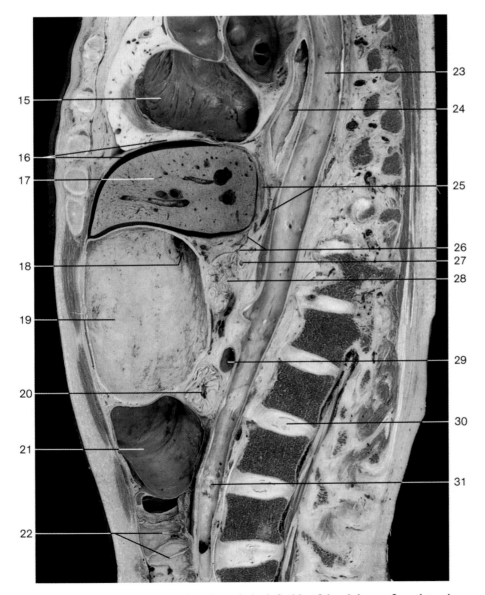

**Liver in situ.** Parasagittal section through the left side of the abdomen 2 cm lateral to median plane.

1   Ribs (cut edges)
2   Diaphragm
3   Diaphragmatic surface of liver
4   Falciform ligament of liver
5   Right lobe of liver
6   Fundus of gallbladder
7   Gastrocolic ligament
8   Greater omentum
9   Aorta
10  Esophagus
11  Left lobe of liver
12  Stomach
13  Ligamentum teres
14  Transverse colon
15  Right atrium of heart
16  Central tendon and sternal
    portion of diaphragm
17  Liver (cut edge)
18  Entrance to duodenum (pylorus)
19  Stomach
20  Duodenum
21  Transverse colon
    (divided, dilated)
22  Small intestine
23  Thoracic aorta
    (longitudinally divided)
24  Esophagus
    (longitudinally divided)
25  Esophageal hiatus of diaphragm
26  Omental bursa (lesser sac)
27  Splenic artery
28  Pancreas
29  Left renal vein
30  Intervertebral disc
31  Abdominal aorta
    (longitudinally divided)

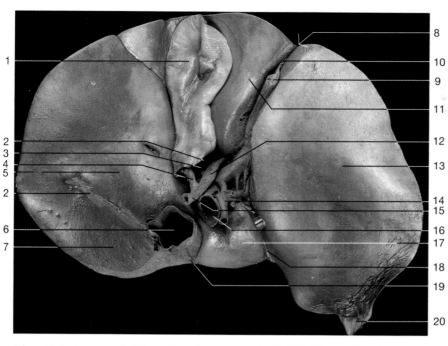

1   Fundus of gallbladder
2   Peritoneum (cut edges)
3   Cystic artery
4   Cystic duct
5   Right lobe of liver
6   Inferior vena cava
7   Bare area of liver
8   Notch for ligamentum teres and
    falciform ligament
9   Ligamentum teres
10  Falciform ligament of liver
11  Quadrate lobe of liver
12  Common hepatic duct
13  Left lobe of liver
14  Hepatic artery proper ⎫
15  Common bile duct      ⎬  Portal triad
16  Portal vein           ⎭
17  Caudate lobe of liver
18  Ligamentum venosum
19  Ligament of inferior vena cava
20  Appendix fibrosa (left triangular
    ligament)
21  Coronary ligament of liver
22  Hepatic veins
23  Porta hepatis

**Liver** (inferior aspect). Dissection of porta hepatis. Gallbladder partly collapsed. Ventral margin of liver above.

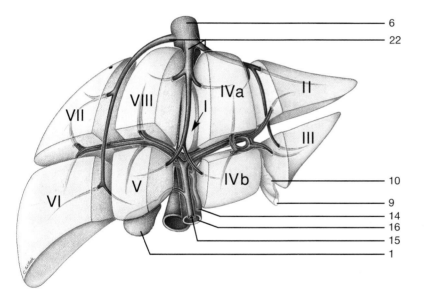

**Segmentation of the liver** (anterior aspect). Liver segments indicated by Roman numerals.

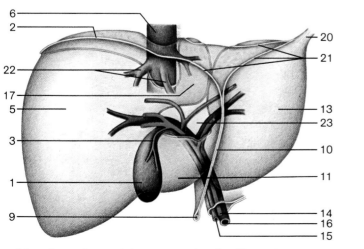

**Liver** (ventral aspect) (transparent drawing illustrating margins of peritoneal folds).

It should be noted that the anatomical left and right lobes of the liver do not reflect the internal distribution of the hepatic artery, portal vein, and biliary ducts. With these structures, used as criteria, the left lobe includes both the caudate and quadrate lobes, and thus the line dividing the liver into left and right functional lobes passes through the gallbladder and inferior vena cava. The three main hepatic veins drain segments of the liver that have no visible external markings.

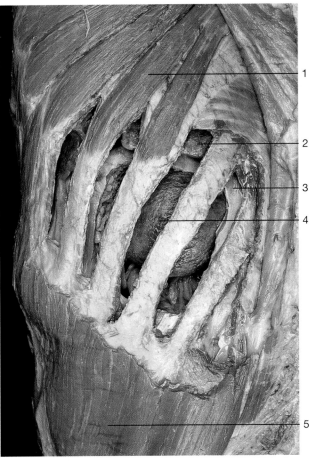

1   Serratus anterior muscle
2   Left lung
3   Diaphragm
4   Spleen
5   External abdominal oblique muscle
6   Gastrosplenic ligament
7   Splenic artery
8   Pancreas tail
9   Superior margin of spleen
10  Anterior border of spleen
11  Liver
12  Hepatic artery proper
13  Cystic duct
14  Gallbladder
15  Lesser duodenal papilla (probe)
16  Greater duodenal papilla (probe)
17  Duodenum (fenestrated)
18  Cardia
19  Pancreas and pancreatic duct
20  Kidney (with capsula adiposa, capsular fat, adipose tissue)
21  Common bile duct
22  Superior mesenteric artery and vein
23  Ureter
24  Aorta with celiac trunk
25  Suprarenal gland
26  Inferior mesenteric vein

**Location of the spleen in situ** (left-lateral aspect).
Intercostal spaces and diaphragm have been fenestrated.

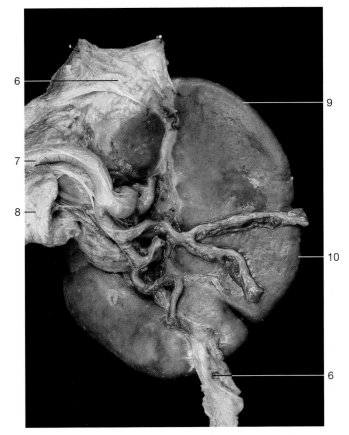

**Spleen** (visceral surface), hilum of spleen with vessels,
nerves, and ligaments.

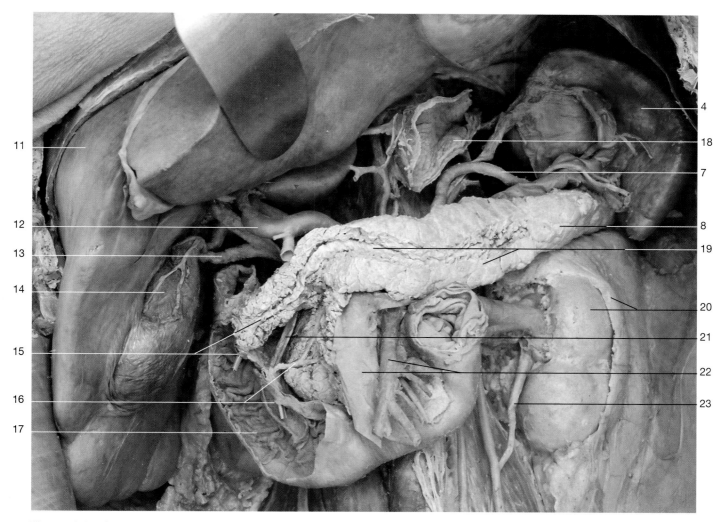

**Upper abdominal organs** (anterior aspect). Stomach and transverse colon have been removed, the duodenum fenestrated. The liver has been elevated to show the extrahepatic bile ducts. In this case the accessory pancreatic duct represents the main excretory duct of the pancreas.

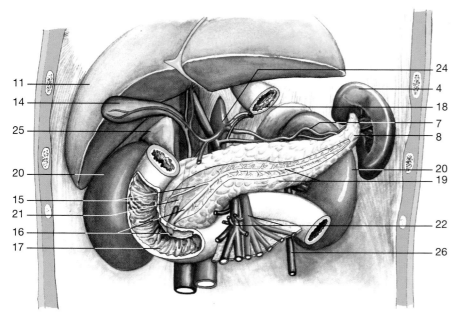

**Upper abdominal organs** (anterior aspect). The schematic drawing shows the most common situation of the pancreatic ducts.

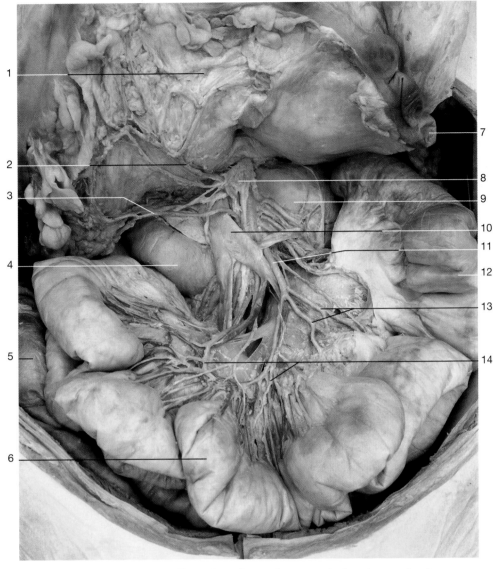

1  Greater omentum
2  Middle colic artery
3  Right colic artery
4  Duodenum
5  Ascending colon
6  Ileum
7  Transverse colon
8  Celiac ganglion
9  Duodenojejunal flexure
10  Superior mesenteric vein
11  Superior mesenteric
    artery
12  Jejunum
13  Jejunal arteries
14  Ileal arteries
15  Liver
16  Celiac trunk and
    abdominal aorta
17  Gallbladder
18  Pancreas
19  Ileocolic artery
20  Stomach
21  Spleen
22  Left colic flexure
23  Appendicular artery
24  Vermiform appendix

**Vessels of abdominal organs, dissection of superior mesenteric artery and vein.**
Greater omentum and transverse colon are reflected.

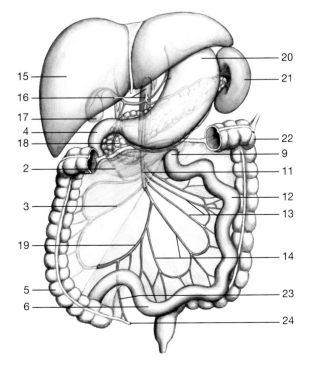

**Main branches of superior mesenteric artery**
(schematic drawing).

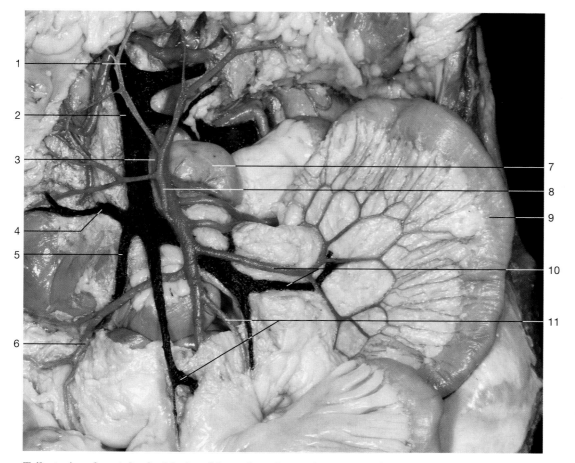

**Tributaries of portal vein** (blue) **and branches of superior mesenteric artery** (red) (anterior aspect).

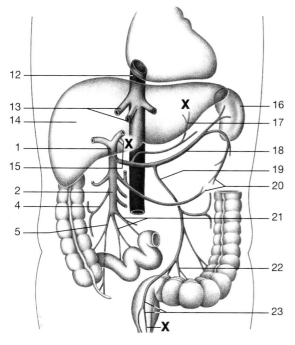

**Main tributaries of portal vein** (blue).
Inferior vena cava = violet; X = sites of portocaval anastomoses.

1   Portal vein
2   Superior mesenteric vein
3   Superior mesenteric artery
4   Right colic vein
5   Ileocolic vein
6   Ileocolic artery
7   Duodenojejunal flexure
8   Middle colic artery
9   Jejunum
10  Jejunal arteries and veins
11  Ileal arteries and veins
12  Inferior vena cava
13  Hepatic veins
14  Liver
15  Para-umbilical veins
    (located within the
    ligamentum teres)
16  Spleen
17  Left gastric vein with
    esophageal branches
18  Splenic vein
19  Inferior mesenteric vein
20  Gastro-omental veins
21  Ileal veins
22  Sigmoid veins
23  Superior rectal vein

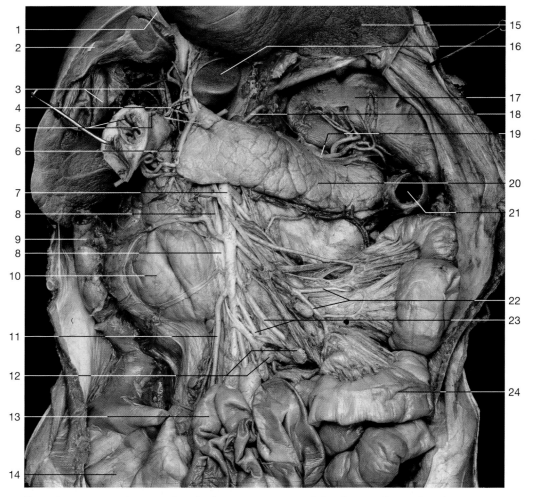
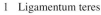

1   Ligamentum teres
2   Liver
3   Gallbladder and common bile duct
4   Hepatic artery proper and portal vein
5   Right gastric artery and pylorus
6   Gastroduodenal artery
7   Superior mesenteric artery
8   Superior mesenteric vein
9   Ascending colon
10   Duodenum
11   Ileocolic artery
12   Lymph nodes
13   Ileum
14   Cecum
15   Left lobe of liver
16   Caudate lobe of liver
17   Spleen
18   Left gastric artery
19   Splenic artery
20   Pancreas
21   Left colic flexure (cut)
22   Jejunal arteries
23   Ileal arteries
24   Jejunum
25   Middle colic artery
26   Right colic artery
27   Appendicular artery
28   Transverse mesocolon
29   Duodenojejunal flexure
30   Inferior mesenteric artery
31   Left colic artery
32   Sigmoid arteries
33   Superior rectal artery
34   Inferior vena cava
35   Abdominal aorta
36   Descending colon
37   Ileum
38   Sigmoid colon
39   Vermiform appendix
40   Cecum

**Superior mesenteric artery in relation to pancreas and duodenum.** Stomach and transverse colon have been removed and the liver elevated. Note the location of the spleen. A yellow probe is inserted through the omental foramen.

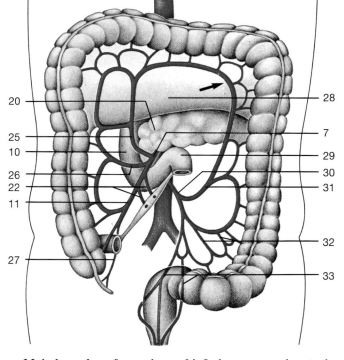

**Main branches of superior and inferior mesenteric arteries** (schematic drawing). Arrow = Riolan's anastomosis.

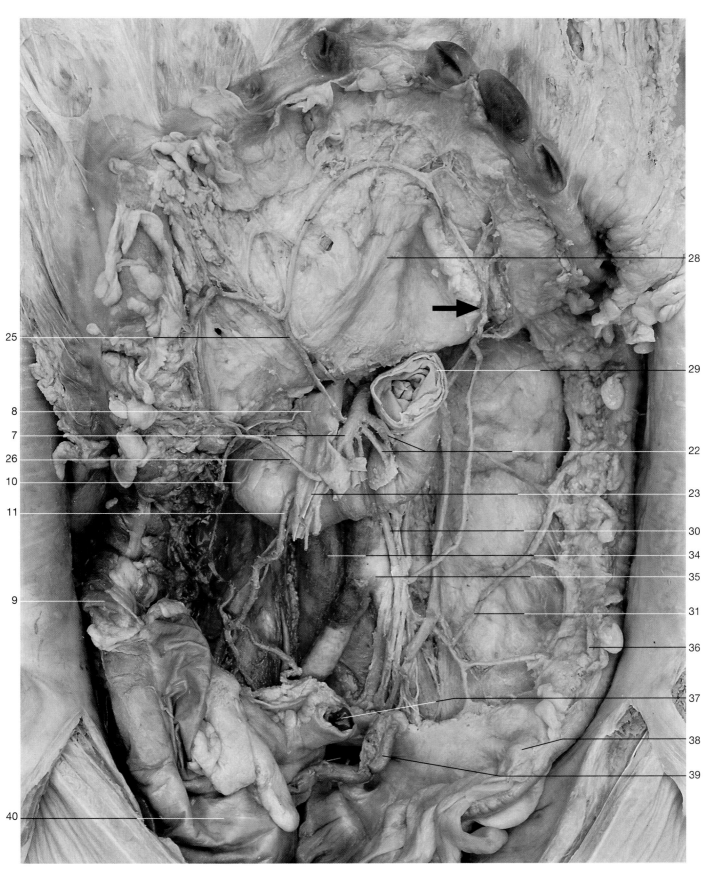

**Vessels of the retroperitoneal organs. Direction of the inferior mesenteric artery** and its anastomosis with the middle colic artery (arrow = Riolan's anastomosis). Greater omentum and transverse colon have been reflected, the intestine partly removed. The normally retrocecally located vermiform appendix has been replaced anteriorly. The right common iliac artery is partly obstructed by a blood thrombus.

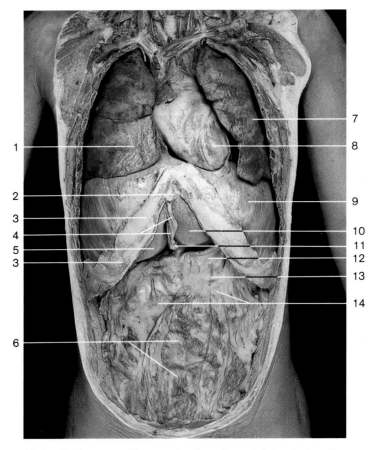

1   Middle lobe of right lung
2   Xiphoid process
3   Costal margin
4   Falciform ligament of liver
5   Quadrate lobe of liver
6   Greater omentum
7   Upper lobe of left lung
8   Heart
9   Diaphragm
10  Left lobe of liver
11  Ligamentum teres
12  Stomach
13  Gastrocolic ligament
14  Transverse colon
15  Taenia coli
16  Appendices epiploicae
17  Cecum
18  Taenia coli
19  Ileum
20  Transverse mesocolon
21  Jejunum
22  Sigmoid colon
23  Position of root of mesentery
24  Vermiform appendix
25  Duodenojejunal flexure
26  Mesentery

**Abdominal organs.** The anterior thoracic and abdominal walls have been removed.

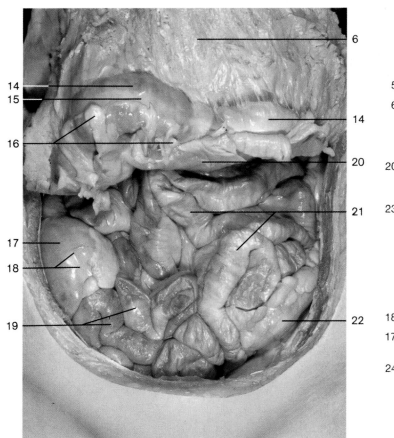

**Abdominal organs.** The greater omentum, which is fixed to the transverse colon, has been raised.

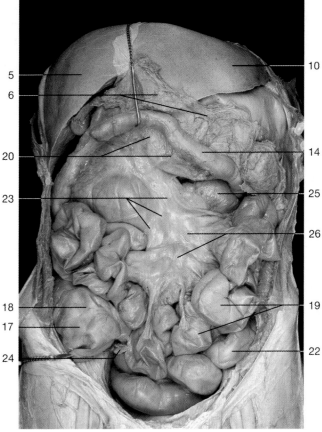

**Abdominal organs** (anterior aspect). The transverse colon has been reflected.

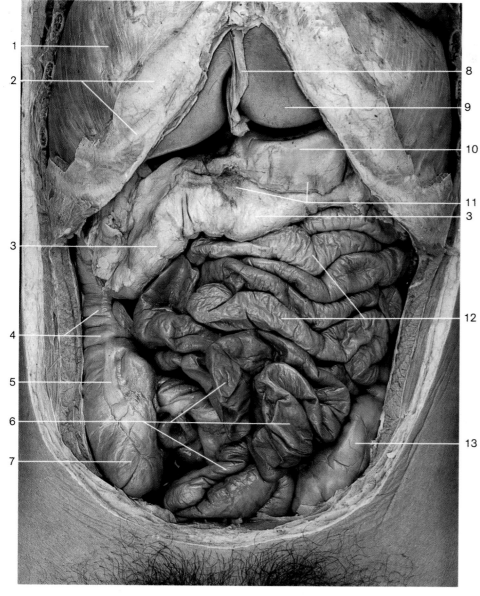

1   Diaphragm
2   Costal margin
3   Transverse colon
4   Ascending colon with haustra
5   Free taenia of cecum
6   Ileum
7   Cecum
8   Falciform ligament of liver
9   Liver
10  Stomach
11  Gastrocolic ligament
12  Jejunum
13  Sigmoid colon
14  Vermiform appendix
15  Terminal ileum
16  Meso-appendix
17  Mesentery

**Abdominal organs in situ.** The greater omentum has been removed.

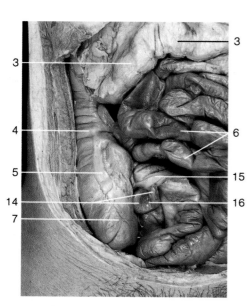

**Ascending colon, cecum, and vermiform appendix** (detail of the preceding figure).

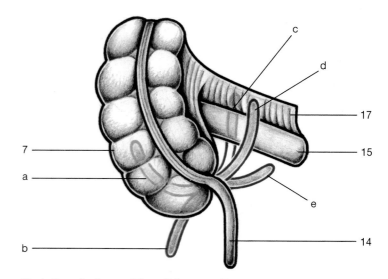

**Variations in the position of the vermiform appendix.**
a = retrocecal; b = paracolic; c = retro-ileal; d = pre-ileal;
e = subcecal.

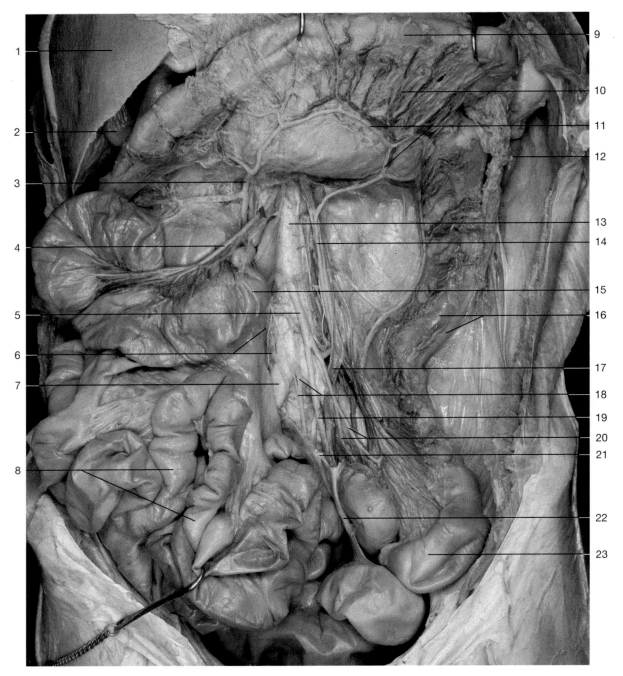

**Abdominal organs. Dissection of inferior mesenteric artery and autonomic plexus.** The transverse colon with mesocolon has been raised and the small intestine reflected.

| | |
|---|---|
| 1 Liver | 12 Spleen |
| 2 Gallbladder | 13 Abdominal aorta |
| 3 Middle colic artery | 14 Left colic artery |
| 4 Jejunal artery | 15 Duodenojejunal flexure |
| 5 Inferior mesenteric artery | 16 Descending colon (free taenia of colon) |
| 6 Sympathetic nerves and ganglia | 17 Inferior mesenteric vein |
| 7 Right common iliac artery | 18 Superior hypogastric plexus |
| 8 Small intestine (ileum) | 19 Superior rectal artery |
| 9 Transverse colon (reflected) | 20 Sigmoid arteries |
| 10 Transverse mesocolon | 21 Peritoneum (cut edge) |
| 11 Anastomosis between middle and left colic artery | 22 Sigmoid mesocolon |
| | 23 Sigmoid colon |

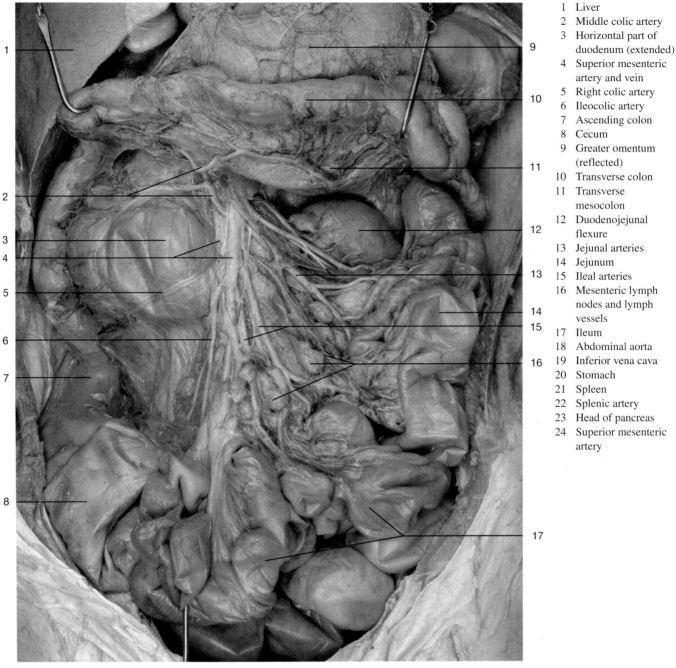

1 Liver
2 Middle colic artery
3 Horizontal part of duodenum (extended)
4 Superior mesenteric artery and vein
5 Right colic artery
6 Ileocolic artery
7 Ascending colon
8 Cecum
9 Greater omentum (reflected)
10 Transverse colon
11 Transverse mesocolon
12 Duodenojejunal flexure
13 Jejunal arteries
14 Jejunum
15 Ileal arteries
16 Mesenteric lymph nodes and lymph vessels
17 Ileum
18 Abdominal aorta
19 Inferior vena cava
20 Stomach
21 Spleen
22 Splenic artery
23 Head of pancreas
24 Superior mesenteric artery

**Abdominal organs. Superior mesenteric artery. Mesenteric lymph nodes.** Transverse colon reflected.

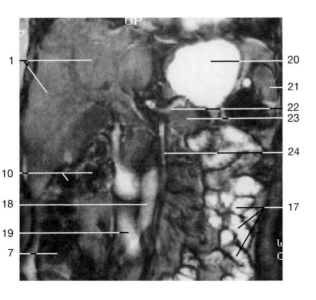

**Frontal section through the abdominal cavity.** (MRI scan: the intestinal tract and vessels are filled with a paramagnetic substance [Gadolinium]; courtesy of Dr. W. Rödl, Erlangen, Germany.)

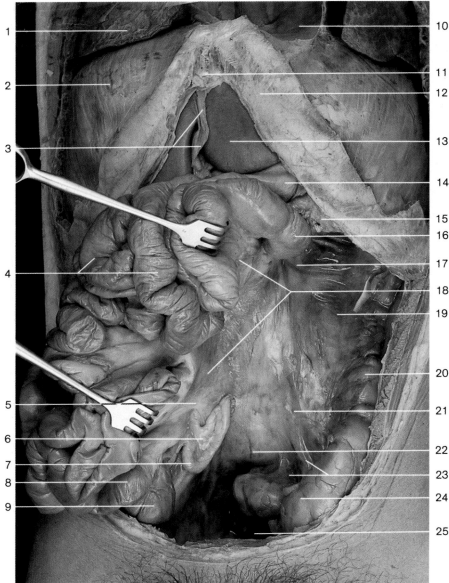

1   Lung
2   Diaphragm
3   Falciform ligament of liver
4   Jejunum
5   Ileocecal fold
6   Meso-appendix
7   Vermiform appendix
8   Ileocecal junction
9   Cecum
10  Pericardial sac
11  Xiphoid process
12  Costal margin
13  Liver
14  Stomach
15  Transverse colon
16  Duodenojejunal flexure
17  Inferior duodenal fold
18  Mesentery
19  Position of left kidney
20  Descending colon
21  Position of left common iliac artery
22  Sacral promontory
23  Sigmoid mesocolon
24  Sigmoid colon
25  Rectum
26  Beginning of jejunum
27  Peritoneum of posterior
    abdominal wall
28  Transverse mesocolon
29  Superior duodenal fold
30  Superior duodenal recess
31  Retroduodenal recess
32  Free taenia of ascending colon
33  Ileocecal valve
34  Frenulum of ileocecal valve
35  Orifice of vermiform
    appendix (probe)
36  Ileocolic artery
37  Vermiform appendix with
    appendicular artery
38  Ascending colon

**Abdominal cavity.** Mesenteries. The small intestine has been reflected laterally to demonstrate the mesentery.

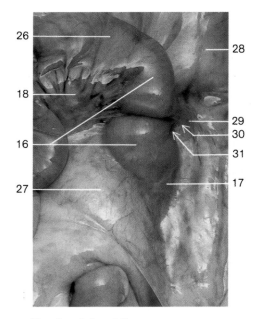

**Duodenojejunal flexure**
(enlargement of preceding figure).

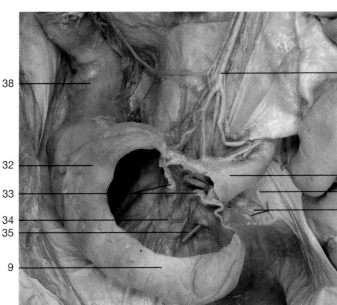

**Ileocecal valve** (ventral aspect). The cecum and terminal part of the ileum have been opened.

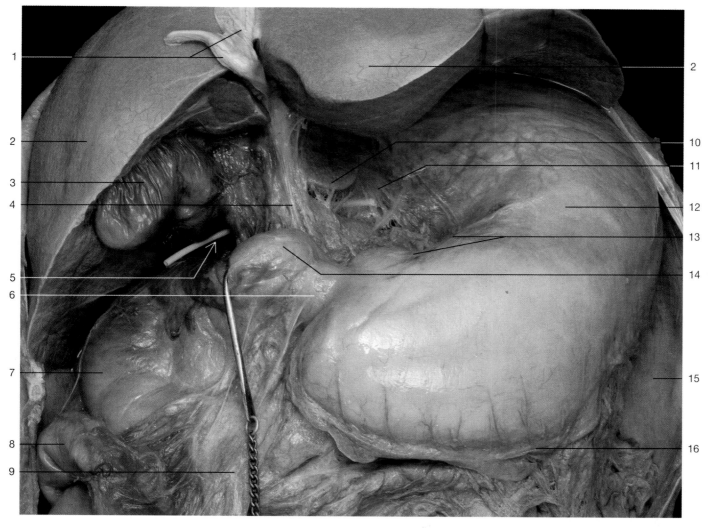

**Upper abdominal organs.** Thorax and anterior part of diaphragm have been removed and the liver raised to display the lesser omentum. A probe has been inserted into the epiploic foramen and lesser sac.

1   Falciform ligament and ligamentum teres
2   Liver
3   Gallbladder (fundus)
4   Hepatoduodenal ligament
5   Epiploic foramen (probe)
6   Pylorus
7   Descending part of duodenum
8   Right colic flexure
9   Gastrocolic ligament
10  Caudate lobe of liver (behind lesser omentum)
11  Lesser omentum
12  Stomach
13  Lesser curvature of stomach
14  Superior part of duodenum
15  Diaphragm
16  Greater curvature of stomach with gastro-omental
    vessels
17  Twelfth thoracic vertebra
18  Right kidney
19  Right suprarenal gland
20  Inferior vena cava
21  Falciform ligament of liver
22  Abdominal aorta
23  Spleen
24  Lienorenal ligament
25  Gastrosplenic ligament
26  Pancreas
27  Lesser sac

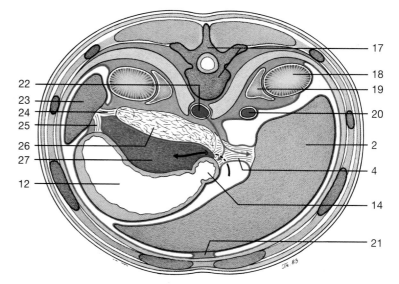

**Horizontal section through omental bursa** above the level of epiploic foramen (black arrow). Viewed from above. Red arrows: routes of the arterial branches of celiac trunk to liver, stomach, duodenum, and pancreas (posterior aspect).

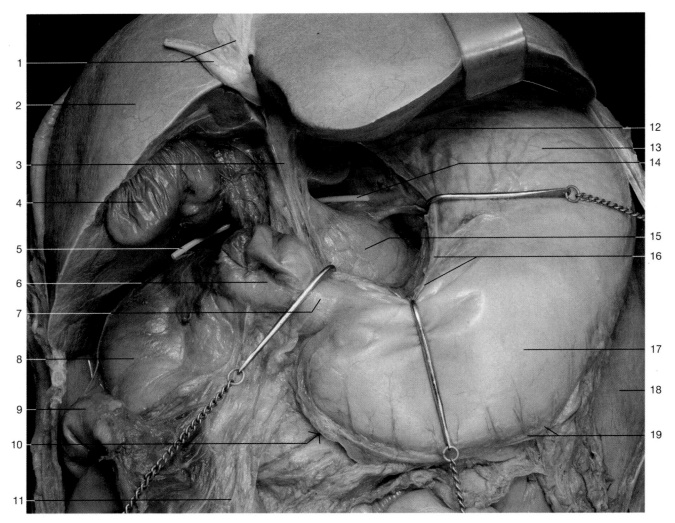

**Upper abdominal organs, lesser sac,** omental bursa (anterior aspect). Lesser omentum partly removed, liver and stomach slightly reflected.

| | | | |
|---|---|---|---|
| 1 | Falciform ligament and ligamentum teres | 18 | Diaphragm |
| 2 | Liver | 19 | Greater curvature with gastro-omental |
| 3 | Hepatoduodenal ligament | | vessels |
| 4 | Gallbladder | 20 | Head of pancreas and gastropancreatic fold |
| 5 | Probe within the epiploic foramen | 21 | Spleen |
| 6 | Superior part of duodenum | 22 | Tail of pancreas |
| 7 | Pylorus | 23 | Left colic flexure |
| 8 | Descending part of duodenum | 24 | Root of transverse mesocolon |
| 9 | Right colic flexure | 25 | Transverse mesocolon |
| 10 | Gastrocolic ligament | 26 | Gastrocolic ligament (cut edge) |
| 11 | Greater omentum | 27 | Transverse colon |
| 12 | Caudate lobe of liver | 28 | Umbilicus |
| 13 | Fundus of stomach | 29 | Small intestine |
| 14 | Probe at the level of the vestibule of lesser sac | 30 | Lesser omentum |
| | (through epiploic foramen) | 31 | Lesser sac (omental bursa) |
| 15 | Head of pancreas | 32 | Duodenum |
| 16 | Lesser curvature of stomach | 33 | Mesentery |
| 17 | Body of stomach | 34 | Sigmoid colon |

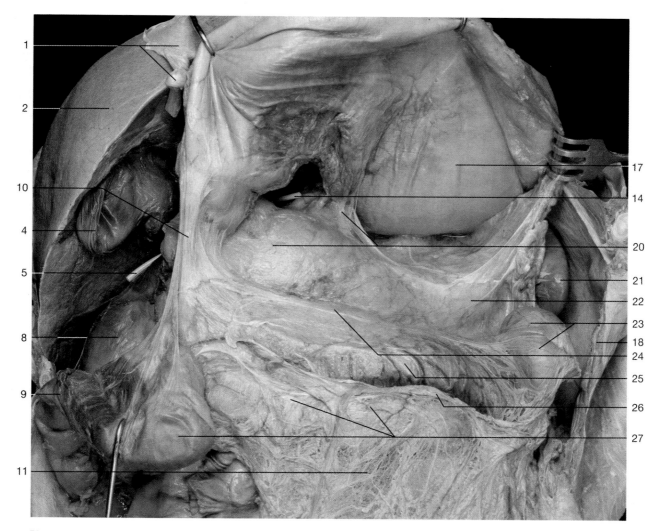

**Upper abdominal organs, lesser sac,** omental bursa (anterior aspect). The gastrocolic ligament has been divided and the whole stomach raised to display the posterior wall of the lesser sac.

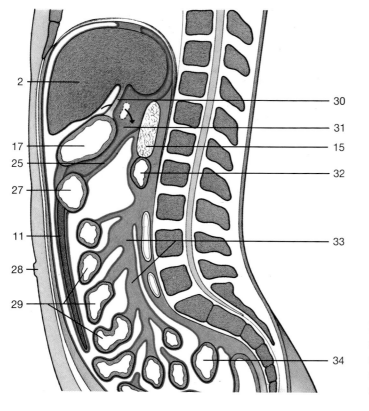

**Midsagittal section through abdominal cavity,** demonstrating the site of lesser sac (blue). (Schematic drawing.) The epiploic foramen, entrance to the lesser sac, is indicated by an arrow. Red = peritoneum.

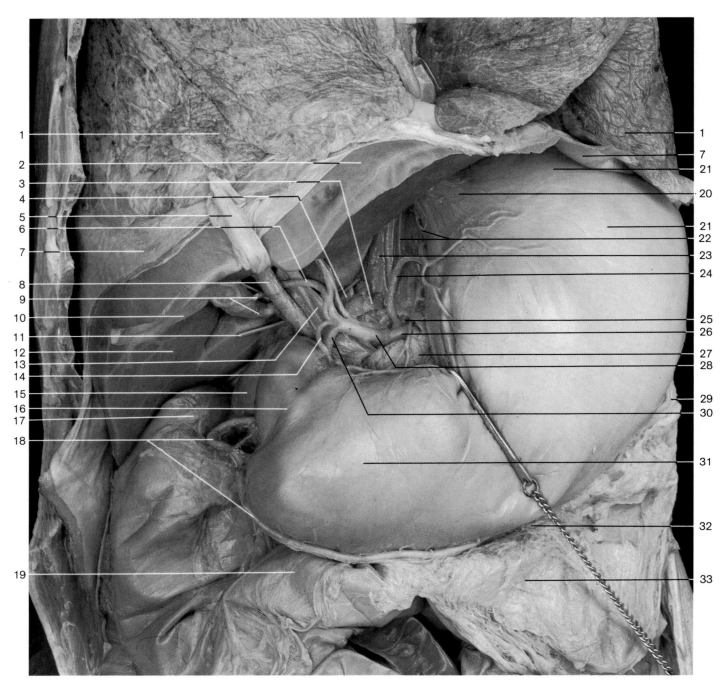

**Arteries of upper abdominal organs; dissection of celiac trunk.** The lesser omentum has been removed and the lesser curvature of the stomach reflected to display the branches of the celiac trunk. The probe is situated within the epiploic foramen.

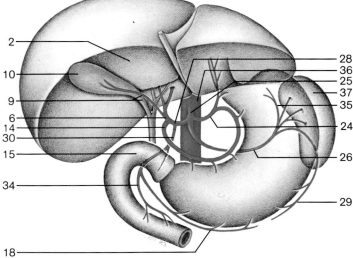

**Branches of celiac trunk** (schematic drawing).

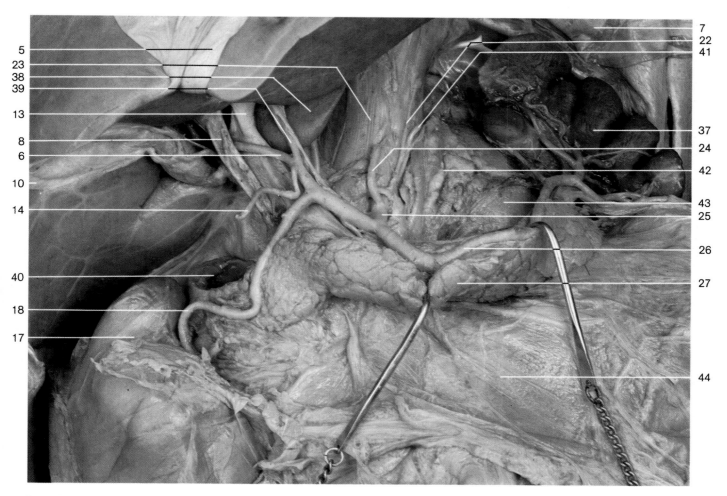

**Branches of celiac trunk; blood supply of liver, pancreas, and spleen.** The stomach, superior part of duodenum, and celiac ganglion have been removed to reveal the anterior aspect of the posterior wall of the lesser sac (omental bursa) and the vessels and ducts of the hepatoduodenal ligament. The pancreas has been slightly reflected anteriorly.

| | | | |
|---|---|---|---|
| 1 | Lung | 23 | Lumbar part of diaphragm |
| 2 | Liver (visceral surface) | 24 | Left gastric artery |
| 3 | Lymph node | 25 | Celiac trunk |
| 4 | Inferior vena cava | 26 | Splenic artery |
| 5 | Ligamentum teres (reflected) | 27 | Pancreas |
| 6 | Right branch of hepatic artery proper | 28 | Common hepatic artery |
| 7 | Diaphragm | 29 | Left gastro-omental (gastro-epiploic) artery |
| 8 | Common hepatic duct (dilated) | 30 | Gastroduodenal artery |
| 9 | Cystic duct and artery | 31 | Pyloric part of stomach |
| 10 | Gallbladder | 32 | Greater curvature of stomach |
| 11 | Probe in epiploic foramen | 33 | Gastrocolic ligament |
| 12 | Right lobe of liver | 34 | Superior pancreaticoduodenal artery |
| 13 | Portal vein | 35 | Short gastric arteries |
| 14 | Right gastric artery | 36 | Aorta |
| 15 | Duodenum | 37 | Spleen |
| 16 | Pylorus | 38 | Caudate lobe of liver |
| 17 | Right colic flexure | 39 | Left branch of hepatic artery proper |
| 18 | Right gastro-omental (gastro-epiploic) artery | 40 | Descending part of duodenum (cut) |
| 19 | Transverse colon | 41 | Left inferior phrenic artery |
| 20 | Abdominal part of esophagus (cardiac part of stomach) | 42 | Suprarenal gland |
| 21 | Fundus of stomach | 43 | Kidney |
| 22 | Esophageal branches of left gastric artery | 44 | Transverse mesocolon |

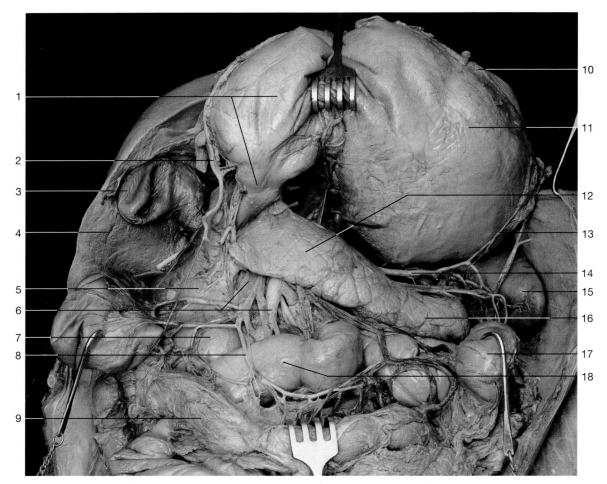

**Pancreas and extrahepatic bile ducts in situ** (anterior aspect). The gastrocolic ligament has been divided, the transverse colon and the stomach replaced to display the pancreas and superior mesenteric vessels.

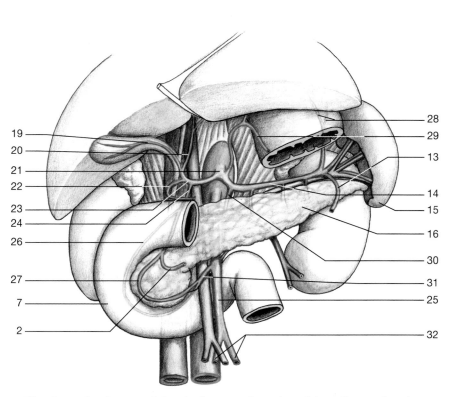

**Blood supply of upper abdominal organs** (branches of the celiac trunk and superior mesenteric artery). (Schematic drawing.)

1   Stomach (pyloric part) and pylorus
2   Right gastro-omental (gastro-epiploic) artery
3   Fundus of gallbladder
4   Liver (right lobe)
5   Head of pancreas
6   Superior mesenteric artery and vein
7   Duodenum
8   Middle colic artery
9   Transverse colon
10  Greater curvature of stomach
    (remnants of gastrocolic ligament)
11  Body of stomach
12  Body of pancreas
13  Left gastro-omental (gastro-epiploic) artery
14  Splenic artery
15  Spleen
16  Tail of pancreas
17  Left colic flexure
18  Jejunum
19  Cystic artery
20  Hepatic artery proper
21  Celiac trunk
22  Right gastric artery
23  Common hepatic artery
24  Gastroduodenal artery
25  Superior mesenteric artery
26  Superior posterior pancreaticoduodenal artery
27  Superior anterior pancreaticoduodenal artery
28  Short gastric arteries
29  Left gastric artery
30  Posterior pancreatic branch of splenic artery
31  Inferior pancreaticoduodenal artery
32  Jejunal arteries

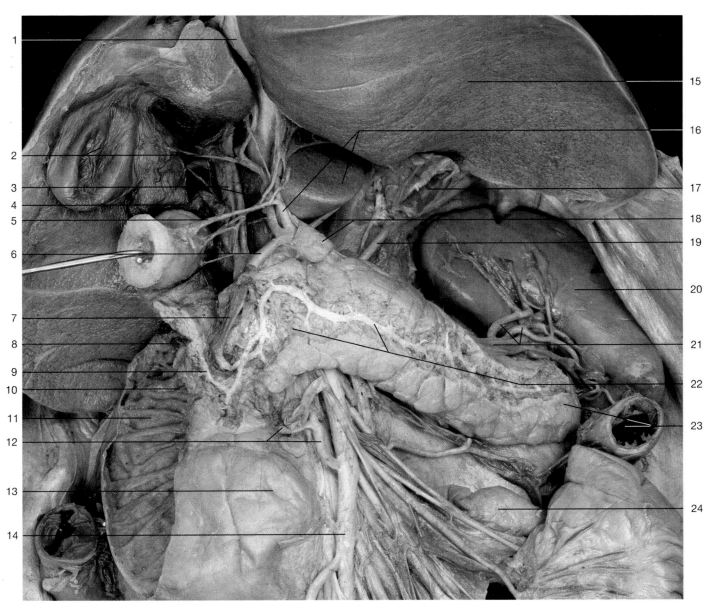

**Posterior abdominal wall with duodenum, pancreas, and spleen** (anterior aspect). Dissection of pancreatic and common bile duct. The stomach has been removed, the liver raised, and the duodenum anteriorly opened.

1  Ligamentum teres
2  Gallbladder and cystic artery
3  Common hepatic duct and portal vein
4  Cystic duct
5  Right gastric artery (pylorus with superior part of duodenum, cut and reflected)
6  Gastroduodenal artery
7  Common bile duct
8  Probe within the minor duodenal papilla
9  Accessory pancreatic duct
10 Probe within the major duodenal papilla
11 Descending part of duodenum (opened)
12 Middle colic artery and inferior pancreaticoduodenal artery

13 Horizontal part of duodenum (distended)
14 Superior mesenteric artery
15 Liver (left lobe)
16 Caudate lobe of liver and hepatic artery proper
17 Abdominal part of esophagus (cut)
18 Probe in epiploic foramen and lymph node
19 Left gastric artery
20 Spleen
21 Splenic vein and branches of splenic artery
22 Pancreatic duct and head of pancreas
23 Left colic flexure and tail of pancreas
24 Duodenojejunal flexure

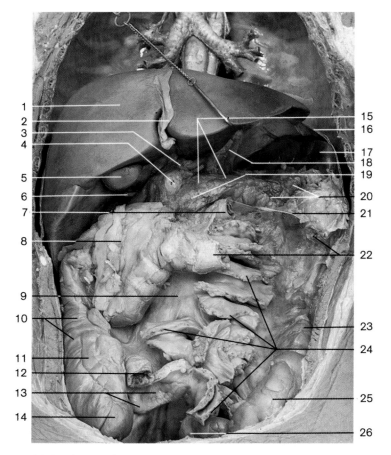

**Abdominal cavity** after removal of stomach, jejunum, ileum, and part of the transverse colon. Liver has been slightly raised.

1   Liver
2   Falciform ligament
3   Hepatoduodenal ligament
4   Pylorus (divided)
5   Gallbladder
6   Probe within the epiploic foramen
7   Duodenojejunal flexure (divided)
8   Greater omentum
9   Root of mesentery
10  Ascending colon
11  Free colic taenia
12  End of ileum (divided)
13  Vermiform appendix with meso-appendix
14  Cecum
15  Pancreas and site of lesser sac
16  Diaphragm
17  Spleen
18  Cardia (part of stomach, divided)
19  Head of pancreas
20  Body and tail of pancreas
21  Transverse mesocolon
22  Transverse colon (divided)
23  Descending colon
24  Cut edge of mesentery
25  Sigmoid colon
26  Rectum
27  Attachment of bare area of liver
28  Inferior vena cava
29  Kidney
30  Attachment of right colic flexure
31  Root of transverse mesocolon
32  Junction between descending and horizontal
     parts of duodenum
33  Bare surface for ascending colon
34  Ileocecal recess
35  Retrocecal recess
36  Root of meso-appendix
37  Superior recess        ⎫
38  Isthmus (opening)      ⎬  of lesser sac
39  Splenic recess         ⎭  (omental bursa)
40  Superior duodenal recess
41  Inferior duodenal recess
42  Bare surface for descending colon
43  Paracolic recesses
44  Root of mesentery
45  Root of mesosigmoid
46  Intersigmoid recess
47  Hepatic veins
48  Duodenojejunal flexure
49  Attachment of left colic flexure
50  Esophagus
51  Entrance to lesser sac through the epiploic
     foramen

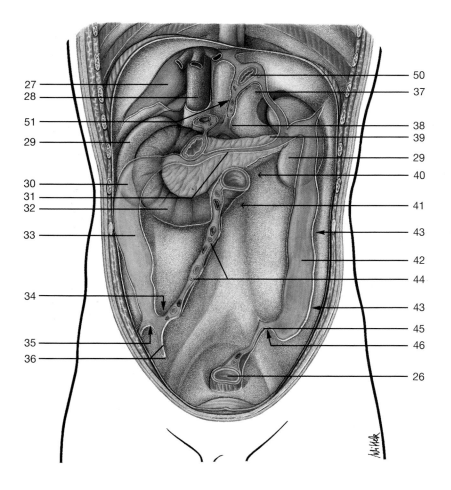

**Peritoneal reflections from organs and the position of root of mesentery and peritoneal recesses on the posterior abdominal wall** (schematic drawing).

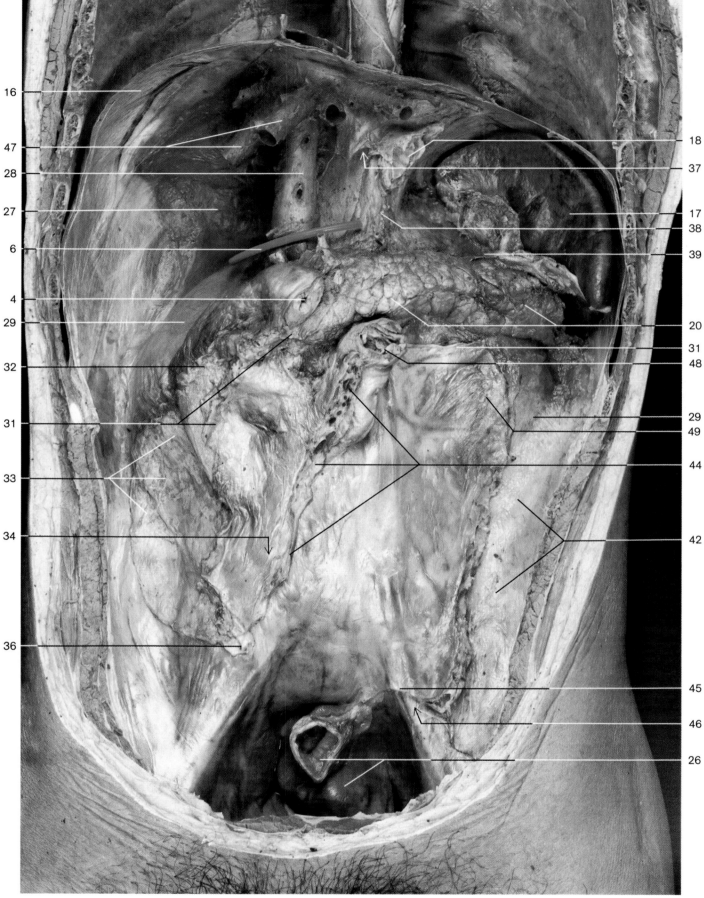

**Peritoneal recesses on the posterior abdominal wall.** The liver, stomach, jejunum, ileum, and colon have been removed. The duodenum, pancreas, and spleen have been left in place.

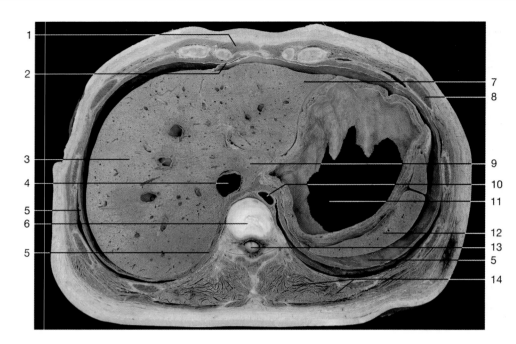

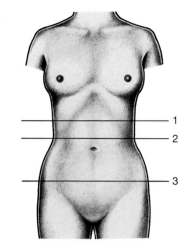

**Horizontal section through the abdominal cavity** at level 1 (from below).

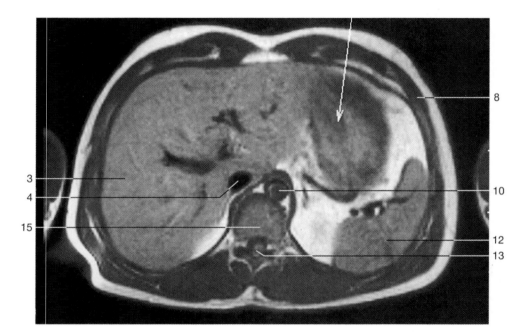

**Horizontal section through the abdominal cavity.** MRI scan, corresponding to level 1. Arrow: stomach.

| 1 | Rectus abdominis muscle | 20 | Greater duodenal papilla |
|---|---|---|---|
| 2 | Falciform ligament | 21 | Duodenum |
| 3 | Liver (right lobe) | 22 | Suprarenal gland and ureter |
| 4 | Inferior vena cava | 23 | Kidney |
| 5 | Diaphragm | 24 | Round ligament of liver |
| 6 | Intervertebral disc | 25 | Superior mesenteric artery and vein |
| 7 | Liver (left lobe) | 26 | Psoas major muscle |
| 8 | Rib | 27 | Descending colon |
| 9 | Liver (caudate lobe) | 28 | Quadratus lumborum muscle |
| 10 | Abdominal (descending) aorta | 29 | Cauda equina |
| 11 | Stomach | 30 | Right renal vein |
| 12 | Spleen | 31 | Small intestine |
| 13 | Spinal cord | 32 | Iliacus muscle |
| 14 | Longissimus and iliocostalis muscles | 33 | Ilium |
| 15 | Body of vertebra | 34 | Ileocecal valve |
| 16 | Rectus abdominis muscle | 35 | Cecum |
| 17 | External abdominal oblique muscle | 36 | Common iliac artery and vein |
| 18 | Transverse colon | 37 | Gluteus medius muscle |
| 19 | Head of pancreas | 38 | Vertebral canal and dura mater |

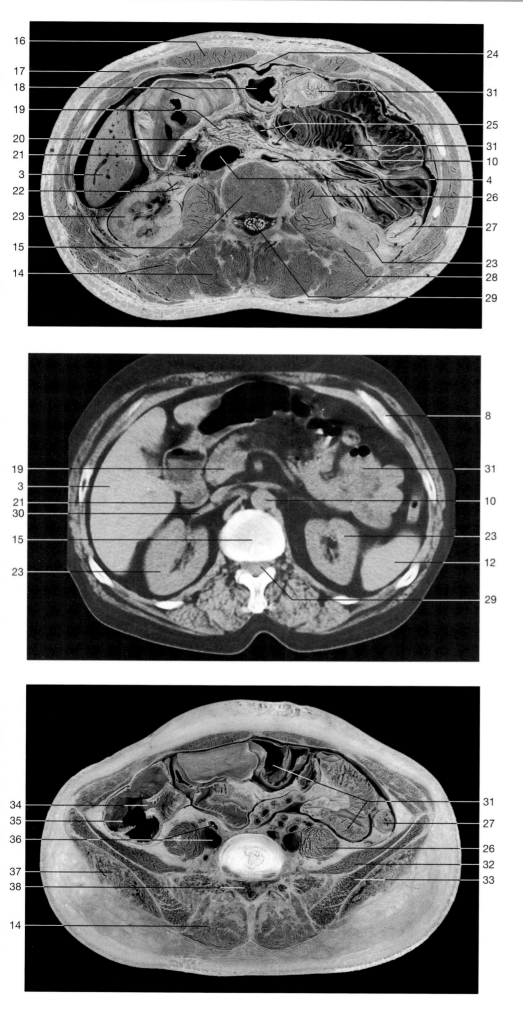

**Horizontal section through the abdominal cavity** at the level of greater duodenal papilla (from below).

**Horizontal section through the abdominal cavity.** CT scan, corresponding to level 2.

**Horizontal section through the abdominal cavity** at level 3 (from below).

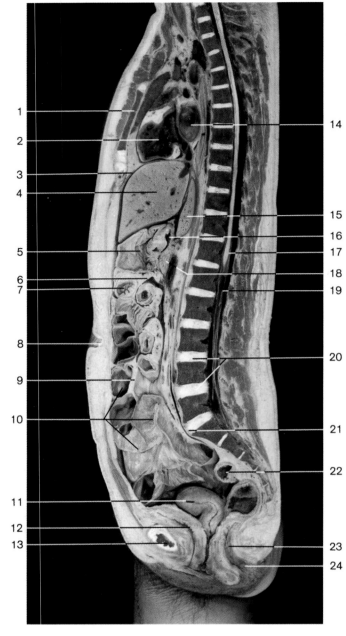

**Midsagittal section through the trunk** (female).

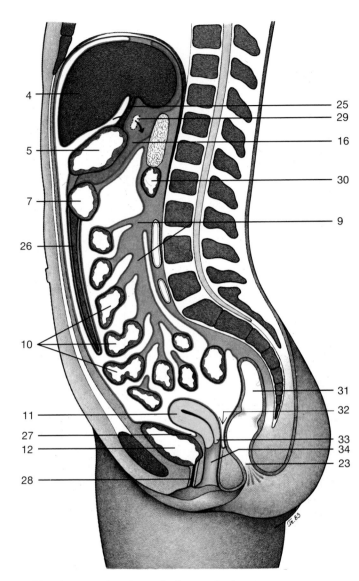

**Midsagittal section through the trunk** (female).
(Schematic drawing.)
Blue = omental bursa; red = peritoneum.

| | | | | |
|---|---|---|---|---|
| 1 | Sternum | 13 | Pubic symphysis | 24 Anus |
| 2 | Right ventricle of heart | 14 | Left atrium of heart | 25 Lesser omentum |
| 3 | Diaphragm | 15 | Caudate lobe of liver | 26 Greater omentum |
| 4 | Liver | 16 | Omental bursa or lesser sac | 27 Vesico-uterine pouch |
| 5 | Stomach | 17 | Conus medullaris | 28 Urethra |
| 6 | Transverse mesocolon | 18 | Pancreas | 29 Epiploic (omental) foramen |
| 7 | Transverse colon | 19 | Cauda equina | 30 Duodenum |
| 8 | Umbilicus | 20 | Intervertebral discs | 31 Rectum |
| 9 | Mesentery | | (lumbar vertebral column) | 32 Recto-uterine pouch |
| 10 | Small intestine | 21 | Sacral promontory | 33 Vaginal part of |
| 11 | Uterus | 22 | Sigmoid colon | cervix of uterus |
| 12 | Urinary bladder | 23 | Anal canal | 34 Vagina |

# 6 Retroperitoneal Organs

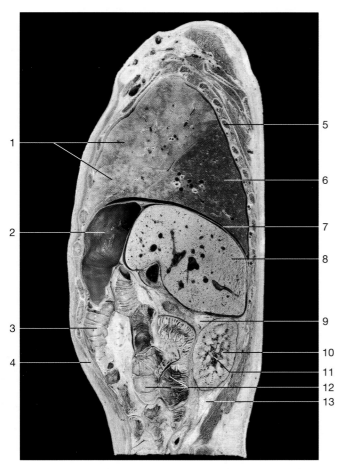

**Parasagittal section through the thoracic and abdominal cavities** (medial aspect, 6 cm right of median plane).

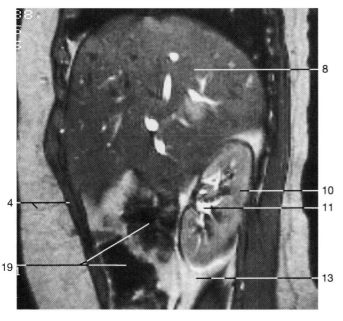

**Parasagittal section through the abdominal cavity.**
(MRI scan, courtesy of Prof. W. Rödl, Erlangen, Germany.)

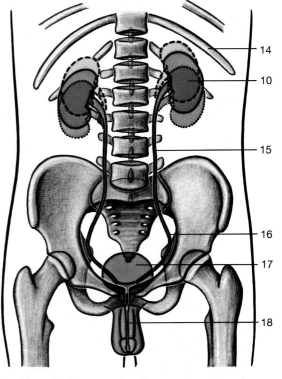

**Position of kidneys and urinary system** (anterior view). The excursions of the kidneys with the respiratory movements of the diaphragm are indicated (schematic drawing).

1   Right lung (superior and middle lobes)
2   Transverse colon
3   Jejunum
4   Abdominal wall
5   Fourth rib
6   Right lung (inferior lobe)
7   Diaphragm
8   Liver
9   Suprarenal gland
10  Kidney
11  Renal pelvis
12  Small intestine
13  Perirenal fatty tissue
14  Eleventh rib
15  Ureter (abdominal part)
16  Ureter (pelvic part)
17  Urinary bladder
18  Urethra
19  Colon

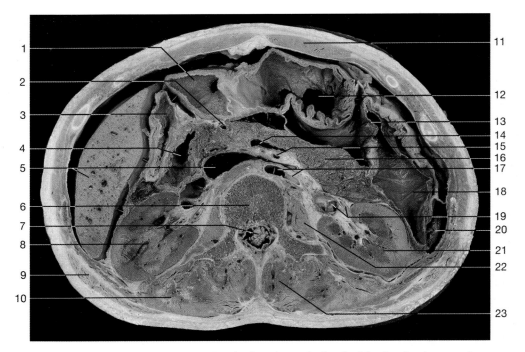

1 Pyloric antrum
2 Gastroduodenal artery
3 Descending part of duodenum
4 Vestibule of lesser sac
5 Inferior vena cava and liver
6 Body of first lumbar vertebra
7 Cauda equina
8 Right kidney
9 Latissimus dorsi muscle
10 Iliocostalis muscle
11 Rectus abdominis muscle
12 Stomach
13 Lesser sac
14 Splenic vein
15 Superior mesenteric artery
16 Pancreas
17 Aorta and left renal artery
18 Transverse colon
19 Renal artery and vein
20 Spleen
21 Left kidney
22 Psoas major muscle
23 Multifidus muscle
24 Margin of lung
25 Margin of pleura
26 Renal pelvis
27 Left ureter
28 Descending colon
29 Rectum
30 Right suprarenal gland
31 Twelfth rib
32 Ascending colon
33 Right ureter
34 Cecum
35 Vermiform appendix
36 Urinary bladder
37 Liver
38 Anterior layer of renal fascia
39 Duodenum
40 Perirenal fatty tissue
41 Posterior layer of renal fascia
42 Abdominal cavity

**Horizontal section through the abdominal cavity** at the level of the first lumbar vertebra (from below).

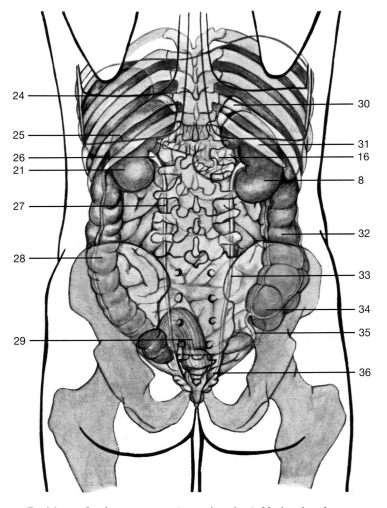

**Positions of urinary organs** (posterior view). Notice that the upper part of the kidney reaches the level of the margin of pleura and lung.

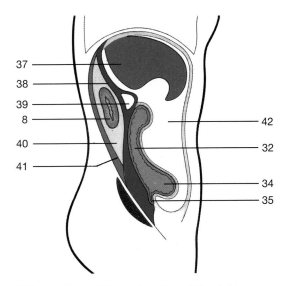

**Retroperitoneal tissue,** location of the right kidney (schematic drawing).
Yellow = adipose capsule of kidney.

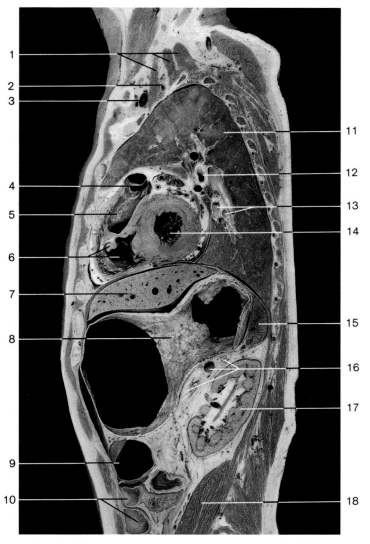

1  Scalenus anterior, medius, and posterior muscles
2  Left subclavian artery
3  Left subclavian vein
4  Pulmonic valve
5  Arterial cone
6  Right ventricle of heart
7  Liver
8  Stomach
9  Transverse colon
10  Small intestine
11  Left lung
12  Left main bronchus
13  Branches of pulmonary vein
14  Left ventricle of heart
15  Spleen
16  Splenic artery and vein and pancreas
17  Left kidney
18  Psoas major muscle
19  Inferior vena cava
20  Renal vein
21  Body of twelfth thoracic vertebra and vertebral canal
22  Right kidney
23  Superior mesenteric artery
24  Superior mesenteric vein
25  Pancreas
26  Abdominal aorta
27  Left psoas major and quadratus lumborum muscles
28  Anterior layer of renal fascia  ⎫
29  Posterior layer of renal fascia  ⎬ of Gerota
30  Perirenal fatty tissue
31  Abdominal cavity
32  Descending and sigmoid colon

**Parasagittal section through the thoracic and abdominal cavities** at the level of the left kidney (5.5 cm left of median plane).

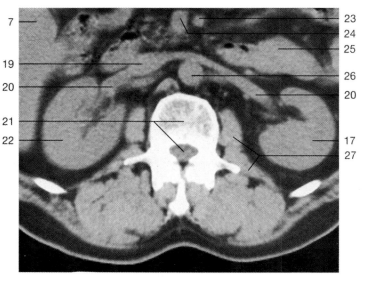

**Horizontal section through the retroperitoneal region** at level of 12th thoracic vertebra. (CT scan, from below.)

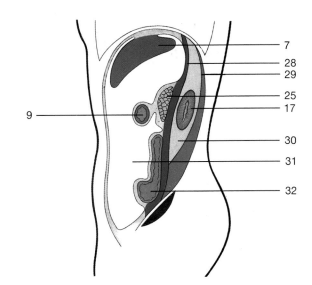

**Retroperitoneal tissue,** position of left kidney (schematic drawing).

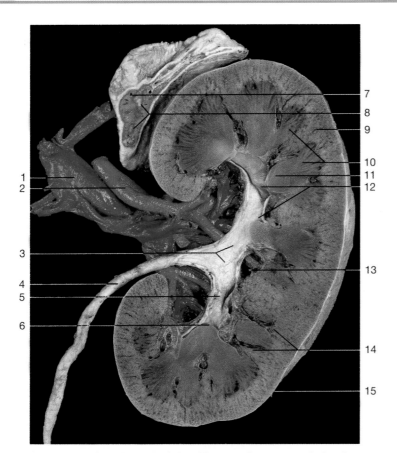

1   Renal vein
2   Renal artery
3   Renal pelvis
4   Abdominal part of ureter
5   Major renal calyx
6   Cribriform area of renal papilla
7   Cortex of suprarenal gland
8   Medulla of suprarenal gland
9   Cortex of kidney
10  Medulla of kidney
11  Renal papilla
12  Minor renal calyx
13  Renal sinus
14  Renal columns
15  Fibrous capsule of kidney

**Coronal section through right kidney and suprarenal gland**
(posterior view). The renal pelvis has been opened and the fatty
tissue removed to display the renal vessels.

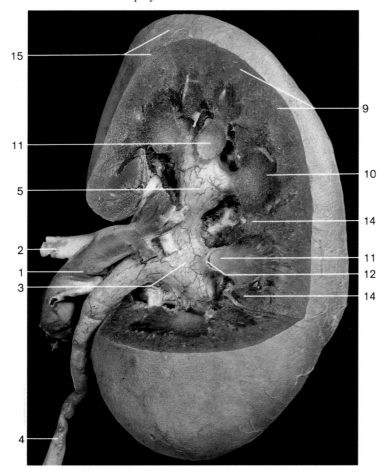

**Right kidney** (posterior view). Partial coronal section to expose
internal aspect of the kidney.

Each kidney can be divided into five segments
supplied by individual interlobar arteries
considered as end arteries. Thus, obstruc-
tion leads to infarcts marking the trace of
segment borders. The anterior kidney surface reveals four segments, the posterior
only three (Nos. 1, 4, and 5).

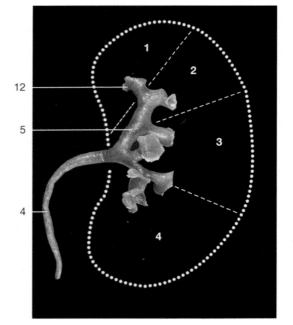

**Cast of renal pelvis and calices.**
1–4 = Renal segments on anterior surface.

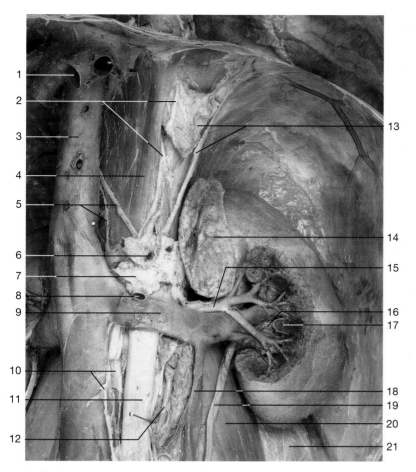

1 Hepatic vein
2 Anterior and posterior vagal trunk
3 Inferior vena cava
4 Lumbar part of diaphragm
5 Right greater and lesser splanchnic nerves
6 Celiac trunk
7 Celiac ganglion and plexus
8 Superior mesenteric artery
9 Left renal vein
10 Right sympathetic trunk and ganglion
11 Abdominal aorta
12 Left sympathetic trunk
13 Esophagus (cut),
   left greater splanchnic nerve
14 Left suprarenal gland
15 Left renal artery
16 Renal pelvis
17 Renal papilla with minor calyx
18 Left testicular vein
19 Left ureter
20 Psoas major muscle
21 Quadratus lumborum muscle
22 Glomerulus
23 Afferent arteriole of glomerulus
24 Glomeruli
25 Radiating cortical artery
26 Subcortical or arcuate artery
27 Subcortical or arcuate vein
28 Interlobular vein
29 Interlobular artery
30 Interlobar artery and vein
31 Vessels of renal capsule
32 Efferent arteriole of glomerulus
33 Vasa recta of renal medulla
34 Spiral arteries of renal pelvis

**Left kidney and suprarenal gland in situ.** The anterior cortical layer of the kidney has been removed to display the renal pelvis and papillae.

**Glomeruli** (210×). Scanning electron micrograph showing glomeruli and associated arteries.

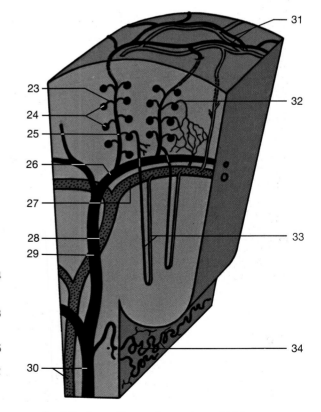

**Architecture of vascular system of kidney** (schematic drawing).

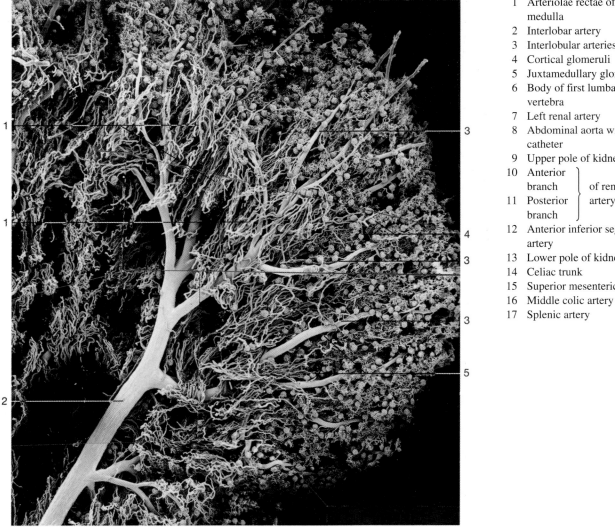

1   Arteriolae rectae of renal medulla
2   Interlobar artery
3   Interlobular arteries
4   Cortical glomeruli
5   Juxtamedullary glomeruli
6   Body of first lumbar vertebra
7   Left renal artery
8   Abdominal aorta with catheter
9   Upper pole of kidney
10  Anterior branch ⎫ of renal
11  Posterior branch ⎬ artery
12  Anterior inferior segmental artery
13  Lower pole of kidney
14  Celiac trunk
15  Superior mesenteric artery
16  Middle colic artery
17  Splenic artery

**Resin cast of kidney arteries.** (Scanning electron micrograph.)

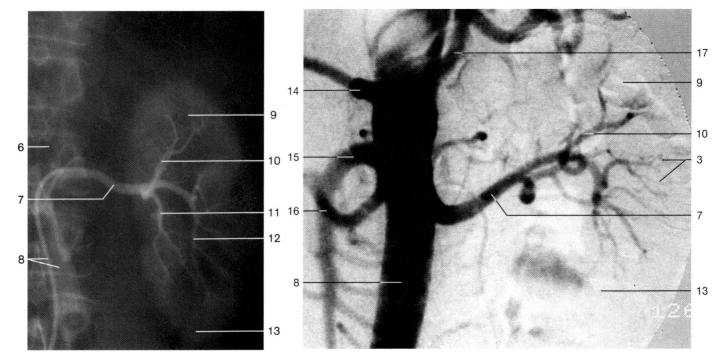

**Left kidney.** (Arteriogram.)                    **Abdominal aorta.** (Subtraction angiograph.)

1  Diaphragm
2  Hepatic veins
3  Inferior vena cava
4  Common hepatic artery
5  Suprarenal gland
6  Celiac trunk
7  Right renal vein
8  Kidney
9  Abdominal aorta
10  Subcostal nerve
11  Iliohypogastric nerve
12  Central tendon of
    diaphragm
13  Inferior phrenic artery
14  Cardic part of stomach
15  Spleen
16  Splenic artery
17  Superior renal artery
18  Superior mesenteric artery
19  Psoas major muscle
20  Inferior mesenteric artery
21  Ureter
22  Superior suprarenal
    artery
23  Upper capsular artery
24  Anterior branch of renal
    artery
25  Perforating artery
26  Lower capsular artery
27  Ureter
28  Right inferior phrenic artery
29  Left inferior phrenic artery
30  Middle suprarenal artery
31  Inferior suprarenal artery
32  Posterior branch of renal
    artery
33  Left testicular (or ovarian)
    artery
34  Renal artery

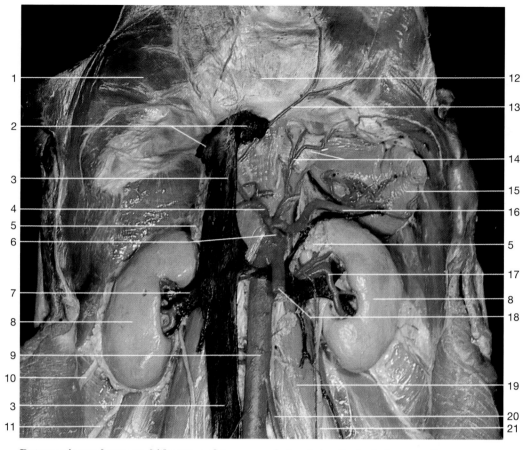

**Retroperitoneal organs, kidneys, and suprarenal glands in situ** (anterior aspect).
Red = arteries; blue = veins.

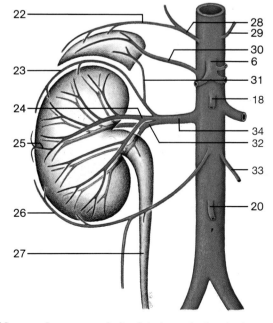

**Arteries of kidney and suprarenal gland** (schematic drawing).

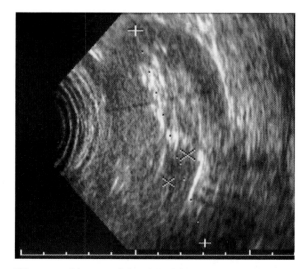

**Ultrasound image of the right kidney** (upper and lower border of the kidney marked by crosses; × = small cortical cyst).

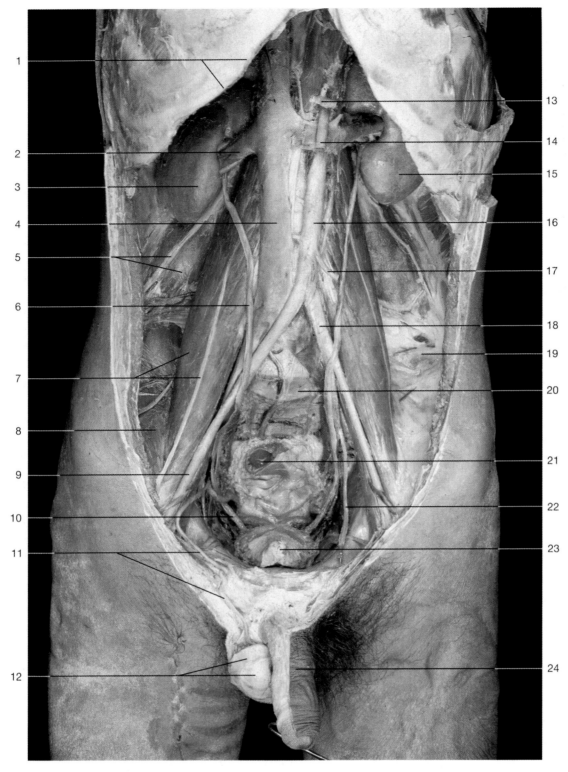

**Retroperitoneal organs, urinary system in the male** (anterior view). The peritoneum has been removed.

| | | |
|---|---|---|
| 1 Costal arch | 8 Iliacus muscle | 17 Inferior mesenteric artery |
| 2 Right renal vein | 9 External iliac artery | 18 Common iliac artery |
| 3 Right kidney | 10 Ureter (pelvic part) | 19 Iliac crest |
| 4 Inferior vena cava | 11 Ductus deferens | 20 Sacral promontory |
| 5 Iliohypogastric nerve and | 12 Testis and epididymis | 21 Rectum (cut) |
| quadratus lumborum muscle | 13 Celiac trunk | 22 Medial umbilical ligament |
| 6 Ureter (abdominal part) | 14 Superior mesenteric artery | 23 Urinary bladder |
| 7 Psoas major muscle and | 15 Left kidney | 24 Penis |
| genitofemoral nerve | 16 Abdominal aorta | |

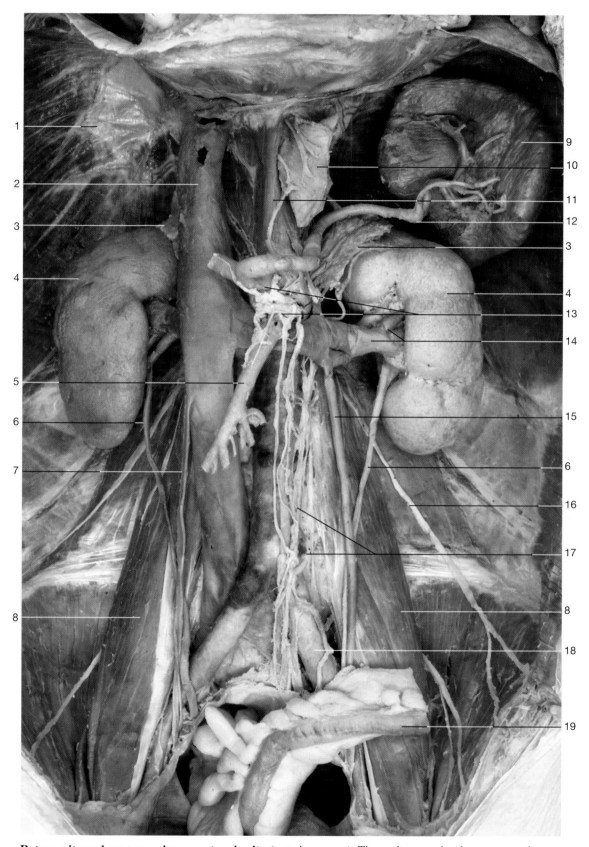

**Retroperitoneal organs, urinary system in situ** (anterior aspect). The peritoneum has been removed. Note the autonomic plexus and ganglia at the abdominal aorta.

| | | | |
|---|---|---|---|
| 1 Diaphragm | 7 Right spermatic vein | 11 Abdominal aorta | 16 Ilio-inguinal nerve |
| 2 Inferior vena cava | 8 Psoas major | 12 Splenic artery | 17 Superior hypogastric |
| 3 Suprarenal gland | muscle | 13 Celiac trunk and | plexus and ganglion |
| 4 Kidney | 9 Spleen | celiac ganglion | 18 Left common iliac |
| 5 Superior mesenteric artery | 10 Cardiac part of | 14 Renal artery and vein | artery |
| 6 Ureter | stomach | 15 Left spermatic vein | 19 Sigmoid colon |

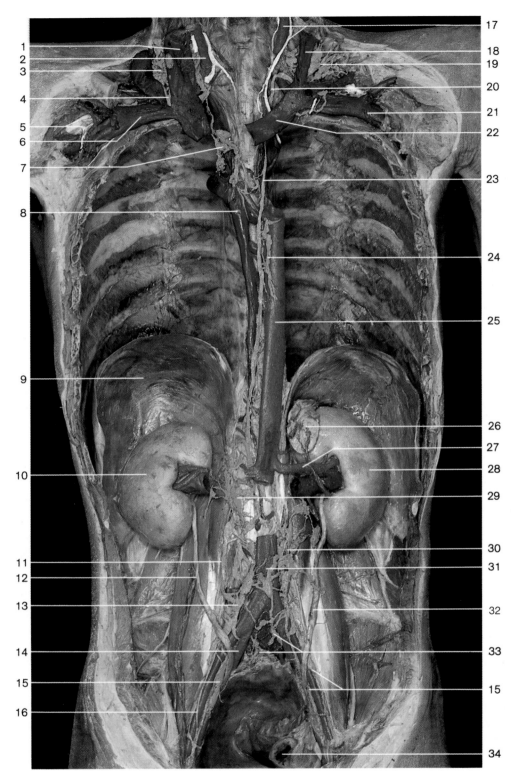

**Lymph vessels and lymph nodes of the posterior wall of thoracic and abdominal cavities**
(anterior aspect). Green = lymph vessels and nodes; blue = veins; red = arteries; white = nerves.

| | | | |
|---|---|---|---|
| 1 | Internal jugular vein | 9 | Diaphragm | 18 | Internal jugular vein | 27 | Left renal artery |
| 2 | Right common carotid | 10 | Right kidney | 19 | Deep cervical lymph nodes | 28 | Left kidney |
| | artery and right vagus nerve | 11 | Right lumbar trunk | 20 | Thoracic duct entering | 29 | Cisterna chyli |
| 3 | Jugulo-omohyoid lymph | 12 | Right ureter | | left jugular angle | 30 | Lumbar lymph nodes |
| | node | 13 | Common iliac lymph nodes | 21 | Left subclavian vein | 31 | Abdominal aorta |
| 4 | Right lymphatic duct | 14 | Right internal iliac artery | 22 | Left brachiocephalic vein | 32 | Left ureter |
| 5 | Subclavian trunk | 15 | External iliac lymph nodes | 23 | Thoracic duct | 33 | Sacral lymph nodes |
| 6 | Right subclavian vein | 16 | Right external iliac artery | 24 | Mediastinal lymph nodes | 34 | Rectum (cut edge) |
| 7 | Bronchomediastinal trunk | 17 | Left common carotid artery | 25 | Thoracic aorta | | |
| 8 | Azygos vein | | and left vagus nerve | 26 | Left suprarenal gland | | |

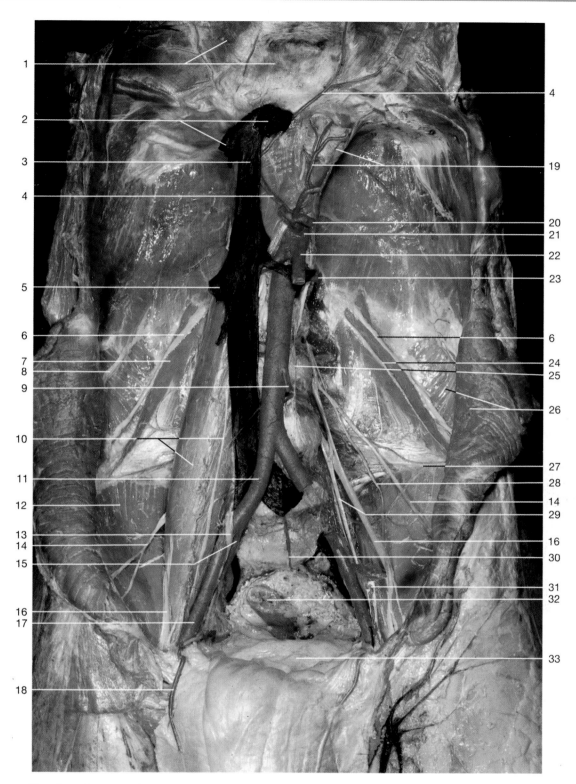

**Vessels and nerves of posterior abdominal wall** (anterior aspect). Part of the left psoas major muscle has been removed to display the lumbar plexus. Red = arteries; blue = veins.

1  Diaphragm
2  Hepatic veins
3  Inferior vena cava
4  Inferior phrenic artery
5  Right renal vein
6  Iliohypogastric nerve
7  Quadratus lumborum muscle
8  Subcostal nerve
9  Inferior mesenteric artery
10  Right genitofemoral nerve and psoas major muscle

11  Common iliac artery
12  Iliacus muscle
13  Right ureter (divided)
14  Lateral femoral cutaneous nerve
15  Internal iliac artery
16  Femoral nerve
17  External iliac artery
18  Inferior epigastric artery
19  Cardiac part of stomach and esophageal branches of left gastric artery

20  Splenic artery
21  Celiac trunk
22  Superior mesenteric artery
23  Left renal artery
24  Ilio-inguinal nerve
25  Sympathetic trunk
26  Transversus abdominis muscle
27  Iliac crest
28  Left genitofemoral nerve
29  Left obturator nerve
30  Median sacral artery

31  Psoas major muscle (divided) with supplying artery
32  Rectum (cut)
33  Urinary bladder

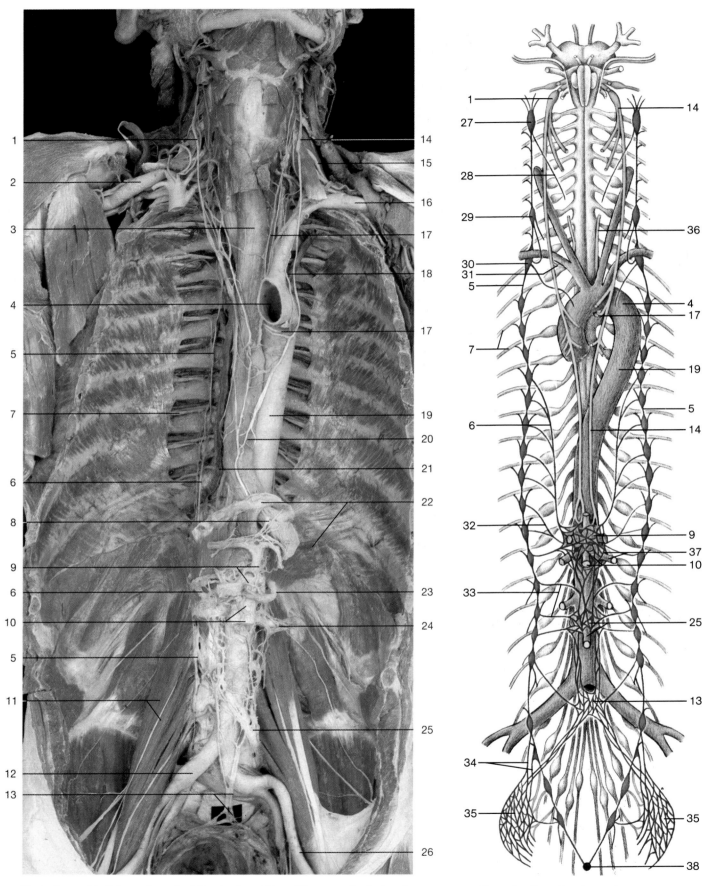

**Posterior wall of thoracic and abdominal cavities with sympathetic trunk, vagus nerve, and autonomic ganglia** (anterior view). Thoracic and abdominal organs removed, except for the esophagus and aorta.

**Organization of autonomic nervous system** (after Mattuschka). (Schematic drawing.) Yellow = parasympathetic nerves; green = sympathetic nerves.

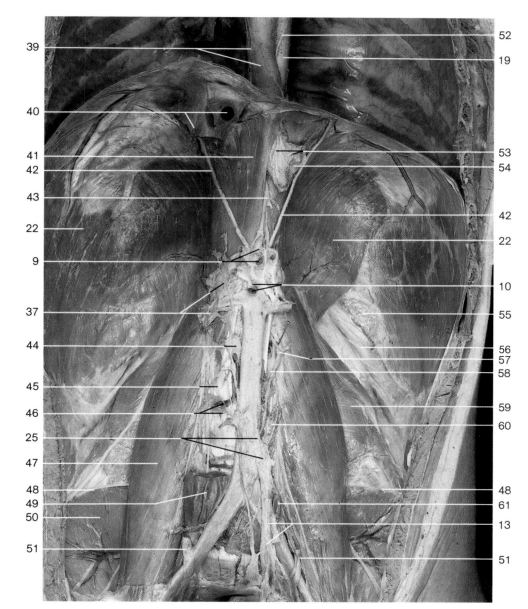

**Ganglia and plexus of the autonomic nervous system within the retroperitoneal space** (anterior view). The kidneys and the inferior vena cava with its tributaries have been removed (compare pp. 282 and 283).

1  Right vagus nerve
2  Right subclavian artery
3  Esophagus
4  Aortic arch
5  Sympathetic trunk
6  Greater splanchnic nerve
7  Intercostal nerve
8  Abdominal part of esophagus and vagal trunk
9  Celiac trunk with celiac ganglion
10  Superior mesenteric artery and ganglion
11  Psoas major muscle and genitofemoral nerve
12  Common iliac artery
13  Superior hypogastric plexus and ganglion
14  Left vagus nerve
15  Brachial plexus

16  Left subclavian artery
17  Left recurrent laryngeal nerve
18  Inferior cervical cardiac nerve
19  Thoracic aorta
20  Esophageal plexus
21  Azygos vein
22  Diaphragm
23  Splenic artery
24  Left renal artery and plexus
25  Inferior mesenteric ganglion and artery
26  Left external iliac artery
27  Superior cervical ganglion of sympathetic trunk
28  Superior cardiac branch of sympathetic trunk
29  Middle cervical ganglion of sympathetic trunk
30  Inferior cervical ganglion of sympathetic trunk

31  Right recurrent laryngeal nerve
32  Lesser splanchnic nerve
33  Lumbar splanchnic nerves
34  Sacral splanchnic nerves
35  Inferior hypogastric ganglion and plexus
36  Left recurrent laryngeal nerve
37  Aorticorenal plexus and renal artery
38  Ganglion impar
39  Esophagus with branches of vagus nerve
40  Hepatic veins
41  Right crus of diaphragm
42  Inferior phrenic artery
43  Right vagus nerve entering the celiac ganglion
44  Right lumbar lymph trunk
45  Lumbar part of right sympathetic trunk

46  Lumbar artery and vein
47  Psoas major muscle
48  Iliac crest
49  Inferior vena cava
50  Iliacus muscle
51  Ureter
52  Left vagus nerve forming the esophageal plexus
53  Left vagus nerve forming the gastric plexus
54  Esophagus continuing into the cardiac part of stomach
55  Lumbocostal triangle
56  Position of twelfth rib
57  Left lumbar lymph trunk
58  Ganglion of sympathetic trunk
59  Quadratus lumborum muscle
60  Lumbar part of left sympathetic trunk
61  Iliac lymph vessels

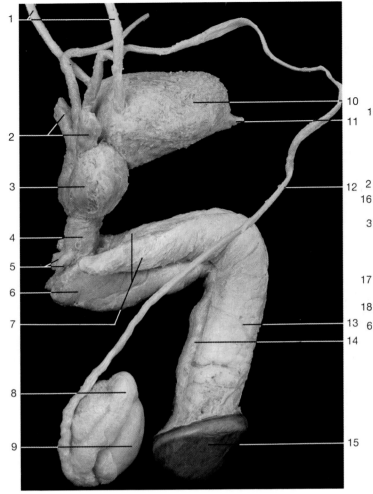

**Male genital organs** isolated (right lateral aspect).

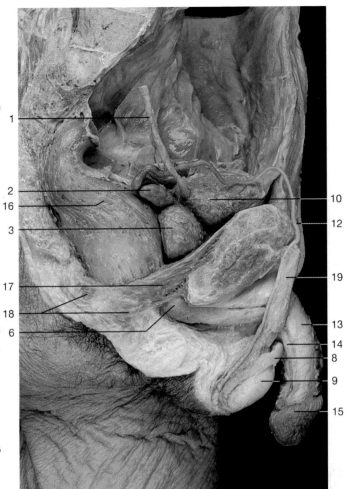

**Male genital organs** in situ (right lateral aspect).

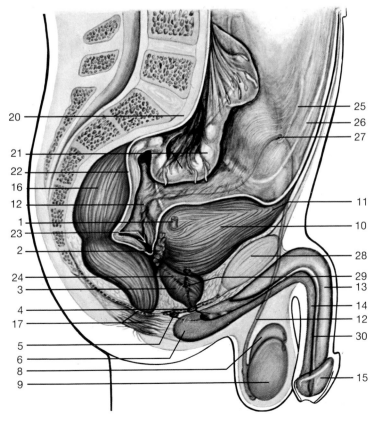

**Positions of male genital organs** (right lateral aspect).
(Schematic drawing.)

1  Ureter
2  Seminal vesicle
3  Prostate gland
4  Urogenital diaphragm and membranous part of urethra
5  Bulbo-urethral or Cowper's gland
6  Bulb of penis
7  Left and right crus penis
8  Epididymis
9  Testis
10 Urinary bladder
11 Apex of urinary bladder
12 Ductus deferens
13 Corpus cavernosum of penis
14 Corpus spongiosum of penis
15 Glans penis
16 Ampulla of rectum
17 Levator ani muscle
18 Anal canal and external anal sphincter muscle
19 Spermatic cord (cut)
20 Sacral promontory
21 Sigmoid colon
22 Peritoneum (cut edge)
23 Rectovesical pouch
24 Ejaculatory duct
25 Lateral umbilical fold
26 Medial umbilical fold
27 Deep inguinal ring and ductus deferens
28 Pubic symphysis
29 Prostatic part of urethra
30 Spongy urethra

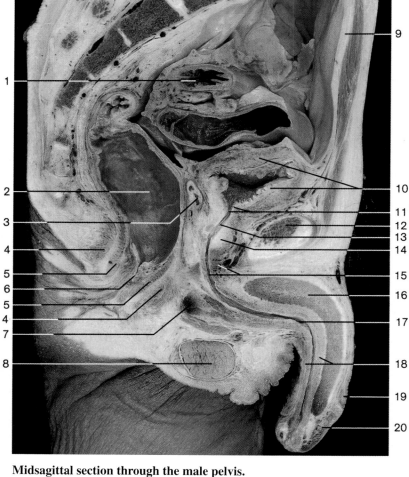

1  Sigmoid colon
2  Ampulla of rectum
3  Ampulla of ductus deferens
4  External anal sphincter muscle
5  Internal anal sphincter muscle
6  Anal canal
7  Bulb of penis
8  Testis (cut surface)
9  Median umbilical ligament
10  Urinary bladder
11  Internal urethral orifice and sphincter
12  Pubic symphysis
13  Prostatic part of urethra
14  Prostate gland
15  Membranous part of urethra and external
    urethral sphincter
16  Corpus cavernosum of penis
17  Spongy urethra
18  Corpus spongiosum of penis
19  Foreskin or prepuce
20  Glans penis
21  Kidney
22  Renal pelvis
23  Abdominal part of ureter
24  Pelvic part of ureter
25  Seminal vesicle
26  Ejaculatory duct
27  Bulbo-urethral or Cowper's gland
28  Ductus deferens
29  Epididymis
30  Umbilicus
31  Trigone of bladder and ureteric orifice
32  Navicular fossa of urethra
33  External urethral orifice
34  Testis

**Midsagittal section through the male pelvis.**

**Male urogenital system** (schematic drawing).

The **prostate** is located between the bladder and urogenital diaphragm. The penis includes the **urethra** and thus serves for both ejaculation and micturition. The internal (involuntary) and external (voluntary) urethral sphincters are widely separated. The **ureter** having crossed the ductus deferens enters the urinary bladder at its base. The peritoneum is reflected off the posterior surface of the bladder onto the rectum, thus forming the rectovesical pouch.

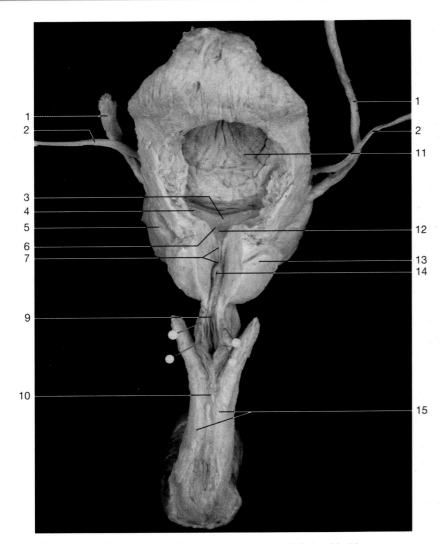

1 Ureter
2 Ductus deferens
3 Interureteric fold
4 Ureteric orifice
5 Seminal vesicle
6 Trigone of bladder
7 Prostatic urethra with seminal colliculus
  and urethral crest
8 Deep transverse perineal muscle
9 Membranous urethra
10 Spongy urethra
11 Mucous membrane of urinary bladder
12 Internal urethral orifice and uvula of bladder
13 Prostate
14 Prostatic utricle
15 Right and left corpus cavernosum of penis
16 Ejaculatory duct
17 Sphincter urethrae muscle
18 Median umbilical fold with remnant of urachus
19 Medial umbilical fold with remnant of
   umbilical artery
20 Urinary bladder
21 Rectovesical pouch
22 Rectum
23 Sacrum
24 Deep iliac circumflex artery
25 Deep inguinal ring and ductus deferens
26 External iliac artery and vein
27 Femoral nerve
28 Obturator nerve and internal iliac artery
29 Ilium and sacrum
30 Inferior epigastric artery
31 Iliopsoas muscle

**Male urogenital organs,** isolated (anterior view). Urinary bladder, prostate, and urethra have been opened. The urinary bladder is contracted.

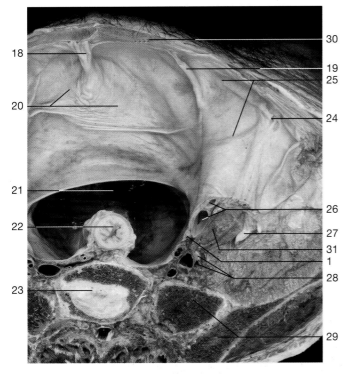

**Pelvic cavity in the male** (viewed from above).

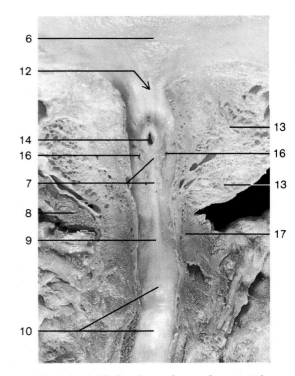

**Posterior half of male urethra and prostate** in continuity with neck of bladder (anterior view).

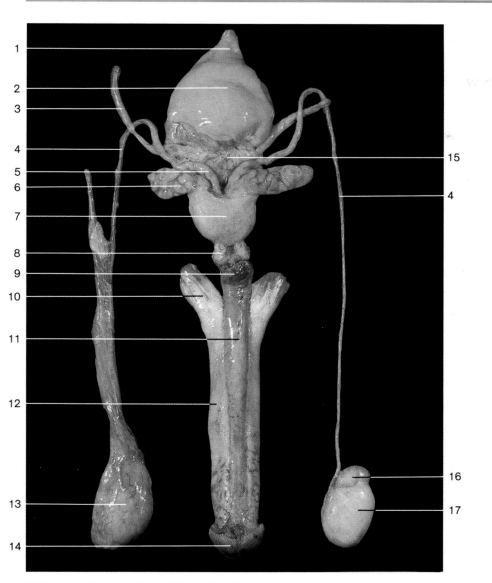

1   Apex of urinary bladder with urachus
2   Urinary bladder
3   Ureter
4   Ductus deferens
5   Ampulla of ductus deferens
6   Seminal vesicle
7   Prostate
8   Bulbo-urethral or Cowper's gland
9   Bulb of penis
10  Crus penis
11  Corpus spongiosum of penis
12  Corpus cavernosum of penis
13  Testis and epididymis with coverings
14  Glans penis
15  Fundus of bladder
16  Head of epididymis
17  Testis
18  Mucous membrane of bladder
19  Trigone of bladder
20  Ureteric orifice
21  Internal urethral orifice
22  Seminal colliculus
23  Prostate
24  Prostatic urethra
25  Membranous urethra
26  Spongy (penile) urethra
27  Skin of penis
28  Deep dorsal vein of penis (unpaired)
29  Dorsal artery of penis (paired)
30  Tunica albuginea of corpora cavernosa
31  Septum of penis
32  Deep artery of penis
33  Tunica albuginea of corpus spongiosum
34  Deep fascia of penis

**Male genital organs,** isolated (posterior view).

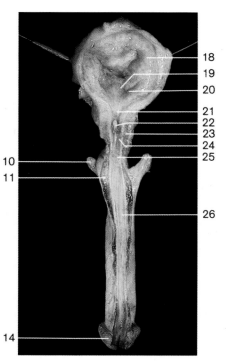

**Urinary bladder, urethra, and penis** (anterior view, opened longitudinally).

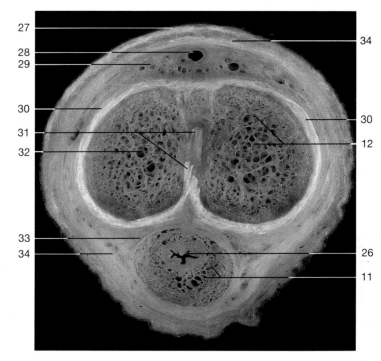

**Cross section of penis** (inferior aspect).

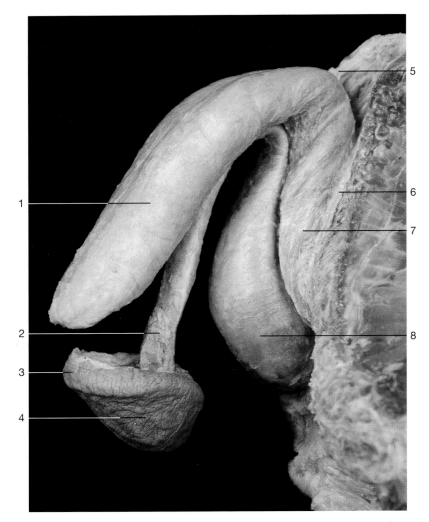

1   Corpus cavernosum of penis
2   Corpus spongiosum of penis
3   Corona of glans penis
4   Glans penis
5   Suspensory ligament of penis
6   Inferior pubic ramus
7   Crus penis
8   Bulb of penis
9   Deep dorsal vein of penis
10  Septum pectiniforme
11  Dorsal artery of penis
12  Bulbo-urethral or Cowper's gland
13  Urinary bladder
14  Seminal vesicle
15  Ampulla of ductus deferens
16  Ductus deferens
17  Membranous urethra
18  Prostate
19  Ureter

**Male external genital organs** (lateral view). The corpus spongiosum of the penis with the glans penis has been isolated and reflected.

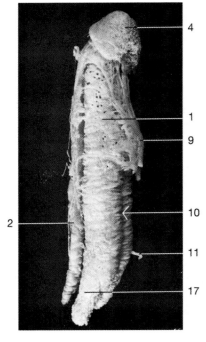

**Resin cast of erected penis.**

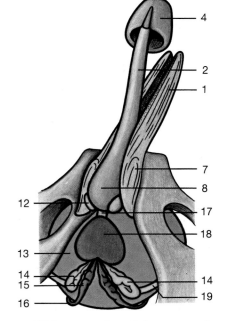

**Male external genital organs and accessory glands** (schematic drawing).

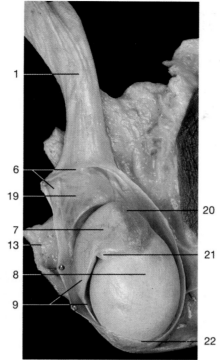

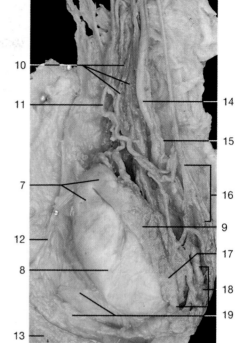

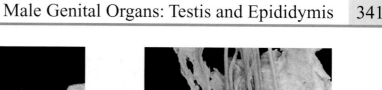

**Testis and epididymis with investing layers** (lateral view).

1 Spermatic cord covered with cremasteric fascia
2 Cremaster muscle
3 Position of epididymis
4 Internal spermatic fascia
5 Position of testis
6 Internal spermatic fascia with adjacent investing layers of testis (cut surface)
7 Head of epididymis

**Testis and epididymis** (lateral view). The tunica vaginalis has been opened.

8 Testis with tunica vaginalis (visceral layer)
9 Body of epididymis
10 Pampiniform venous plexus (anterior veins)
11 Testicular artery
12 Tunica vaginalis (parietal layer, cut edge)
13 Skin and dartos muscle (reflected)

**Testis, epididymis, and spermatic cord.** Dissection of spermatic cord and ductus deferens (left side, posterolateral aspect).

14 Ductus deferens
15 Artery of ductus deferens
16 Posterior veins of pampiniform plexus
17 Tail of epididymis
18 Transition of epididymal duct to ductus deferens and venous plexus
19 Parietal layer of tunica vaginalis
20 Appendix of epididymis
21 Appendix of testis
22 Gubernaculum testis

**Longitudinal section through testis and epididymis.** The left figure shows the testicular septa after removal of the seminiferous tubules.

1 Spermatic cord (cut surface)
2 Head of epididymis (cut surface)
3 Septa of testis
4 Mediastinum testis
5 Tunica albuginea
6 Superior pole of testis
7 Convoluted seminiferous tubules
8 Inferior pole of testis

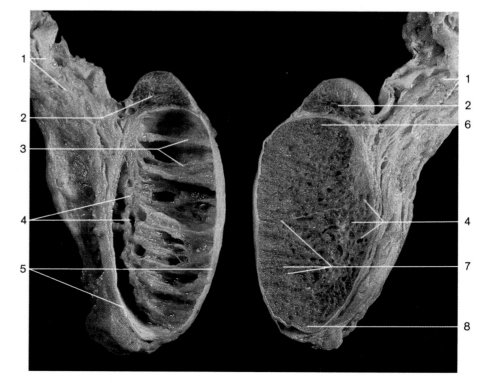

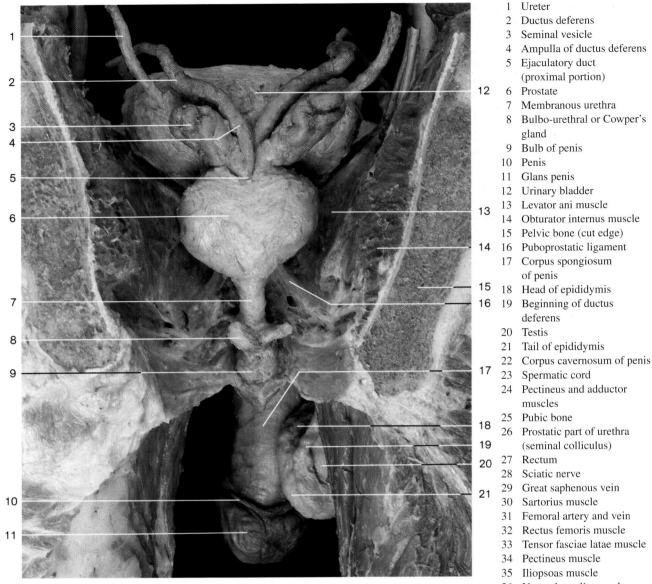

1  Ureter
2  Ductus deferens
3  Seminal vesicle
4  Ampulla of ductus deferens
5  Ejaculatory duct
   (proximal portion)
6  Prostate
7  Membranous urethra
8  Bulbo-urethral or Cowper's
   gland
9  Bulb of penis
10 Penis
11 Glans penis
12 Urinary bladder
13 Levator ani muscle
14 Obturator internus muscle
15 Pelvic bone (cut edge)
16 Puboprostatic ligament
17 Corpus spongiosum
   of penis
18 Head of epididymis
19 Beginning of ductus
   deferens
20 Testis
21 Tail of epididymis
22 Corpus cavernosum of penis
23 Spermatic cord
24 Pectineus and adductor
   muscles
25 Pubic bone
26 Prostatic part of urethra
   (seminal colliculus)
27 Rectum
28 Sciatic nerve
29 Great saphenous vein
30 Sartorius muscle
31 Femoral artery and vein
32 Rectus femoris muscle
33 Tensor fasciae latae muscle
34 Pectineus muscle
35 Iliopsoas muscle
36 Vastus lateralis muscle
37 Obturator externus muscle
38 Femur
39 Ischial tuberosity
40 Gluteus maximus muscle

**Accessory glands of male genital organs in situ.** Coronal section through the pelvic cavity. Posterior aspect of urinary bladder, prostate, and seminal vesicles.

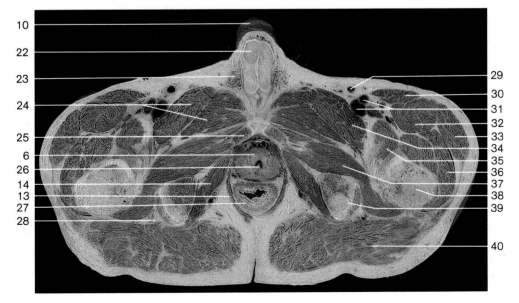

**Horizontal section through pelvic cavity at level of prostate.**

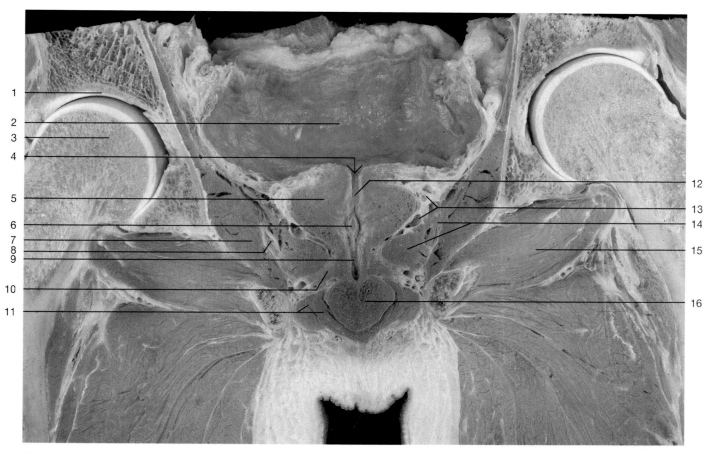

**Coronal section through pelvic cavity** at the level of prostate and hip joint (anterior aspect).

| | | |
|---|---|---|
| 1 Acetabulum of hip joint | 10 Deep transverse perineus muscle | 19 Seminal vesicle |
| 2 Urinary bladder | 11 Crus penis and ischiocavernosus muscle | 20 Internal anal sphincter muscle |
| 3 Head of femur | 12 Prostatic part of urethra | 21 External anal sphincter muscle |
| 4 Internal urethral orifice | 13 Prostatic plexus | 22 Anus |
| 5 Prostate | 14 Levator ani muscle | 23 Psoas major muscle |
| 6 Seminal colliculus | 15 Obturator externus muscle | 24 Intervertebral disc |
| 7 Obturator internus muscle | 16 Bulb of penis | 25 Ilium |
| 8 Ischiorectal fossa | 17 Ampulla of rectum | 26 Ligament of the head of the femur |
| 9 Membranous urethra | 18 Anal canal | 27 Sacral promontory |

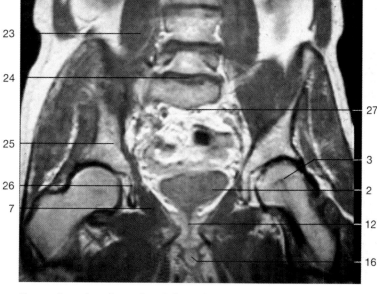

**Coronal section through pelvic cavity.** (MRI scan.)

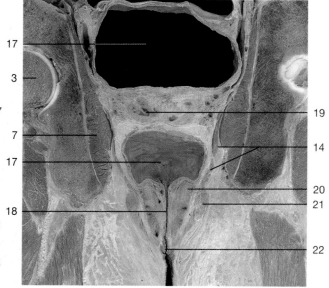

**Coronal section through anal canal.**

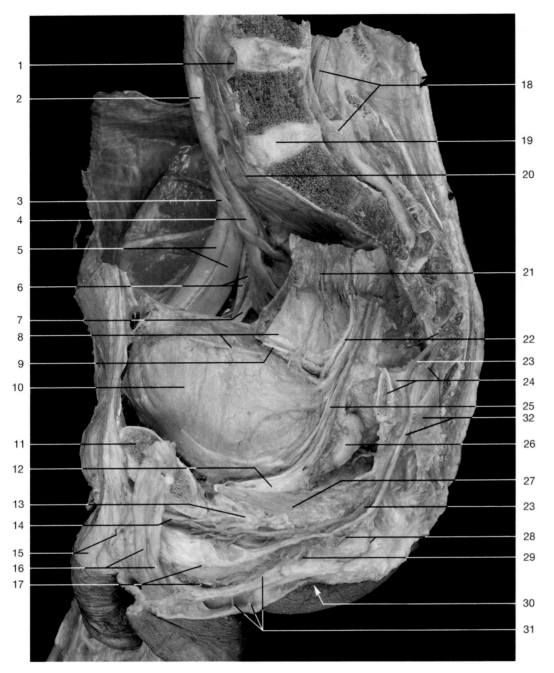

**Pelvic cavity in the male** (right half of parasagittal section). The arteries have been injected with red resin. The parietal layer of peritoneum has been removed. The urinary bladder is filled to a great extent.

1  Left common iliac artery
2  Right common iliac artery
3  Right ureter
4  Right internal iliac artery
5  Right external iliac artery and vein
6  Right obturator artery and nerve
7  Umbilical artery
8  Sigmoid and superior vesical artery
9  Left ductus deferens
10  Urinary bladder
11  Pubic bone (cut)
12  Prostate
13  Vesicoprostatic venous plexus
14  Deep dorsal vein of penis and
     dorsal artery of penis
15  Penis and superficial dorsal vein
16  Spermatic cord and testicular artery
17  Bulb of penis and deep artery of penis

18  Cauda equina and dura mater (divided)
19  Intervertebral disc between fifth
     lumbar vertebra and sacrum
20  Sacral promontory
21  Mesosigmoid
22  Left ureter
23  Left internal pudendal artery
24  Ischial spine (cut), sacrospinal ligament,
     inferior gluteal artery
25  Left inferior vesical artery
26  Seminal vesicle
27  Levator ani muscle
28  Branches of inferior rectal artery
29  Perineal artery
30  Anus
31  Posterior scrotal branches
32  Pudendal nerve and sacrotuberal ligament

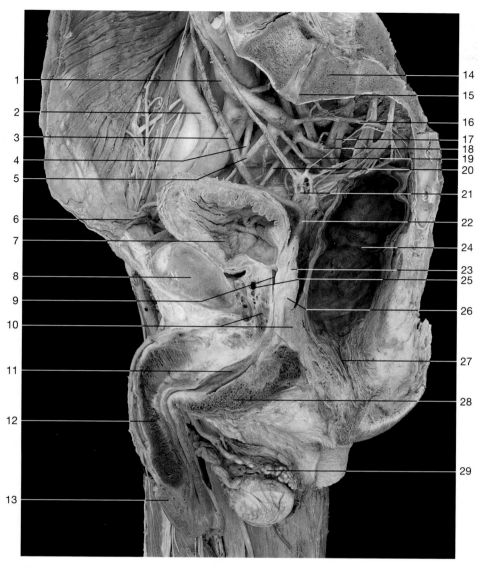

1  Internal iliac artery
2  External iliac artery
3  Ureter
4  Obturator nerve
5  Umbilical artery
6  Anulus inguinalis profundus
   (deep inguinal ring)
7  Urinary bladder (vesica urinaria)
8  Symphysis
9  Prostatic part of urethra
10 Sphincter muscle of urethra
11 Urethra (spongy part)
12 Cavernous body of penis
13 Glans penis
14 Sacrum
15 Promontory
16 Lateral sacral artery
17 Plexus sacralis
18 Inferior gluteal artery
19 Internal pudendal artery
20 Obturator artery
21 Inferior hypogastric plexus
22 Ductus deferens
23 Seminal vesicle (vesicula seminalis)
24 Rectum
25 Prostatic venous plexus
26 Prostate
27 Anal canal
28 Spongy part of penis
29 Pampiniform plexus
30 Testis and epididymis
31 Common iliac artery
32 Umbilical artery
33 Medial umbilical ligament
34 Branches of superior vesical artery
35 Urogenital diaphragm
36 Deep artery of penis
37 Dorsal artery of penis
38 Penis
39 Iliolumbar artery
40 Superior gluteal artery
41 Middle rectal artery
42 Levator ani muscle
43 Inferior rectal artery
44 Inferior vesical artery

**Vessels of the pelvic cavity in the male** (sagittal section, right side, medial aspect).
The gluteus maximus muscle has been removed.

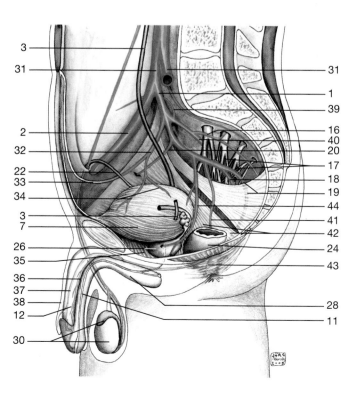

**Main branches of internal iliac artery in the male**
(schematic drawing).

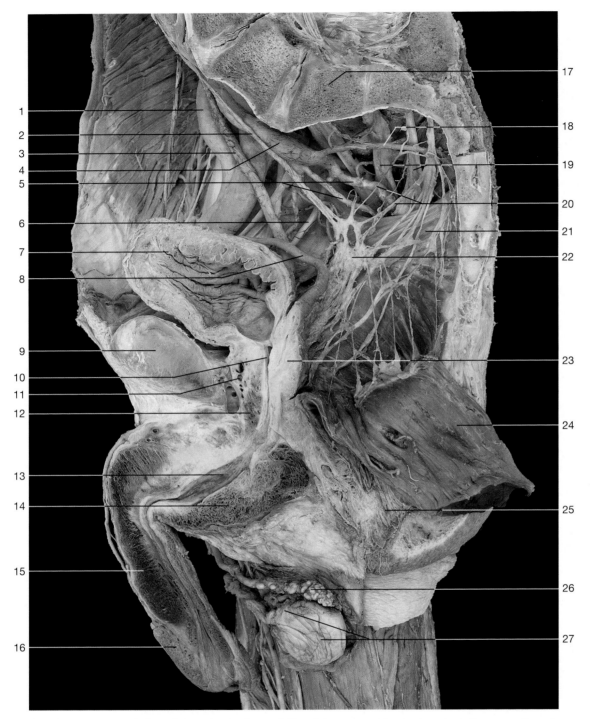

**Vessels and nerves of the pelvic cavity in the male** (medial aspect, midsagittal section). Rectum reflected to display the inferior hypogastric plexus.

1  External iliac artery
2  Right hypogastric nerve
3  Ureter
4  Internal iliac artery
5  Inferior gluteal artery and internal pudendal artery
6  Obturator artery
7  Urinary bladder
8  Ductus deferens
9  Symphysis pubica
10  Prostatic part of urethra
11  Prostatic venous plexus
12  Sphincter urethrae muscle
13  Spongy part of urethra
14  Corpus spongiosum penis
15  Corpus cavernosum penis
16  Glans penis
17  Sacrum
18  Lateral sacral artery
19  Sacral plexus
20  Pelvic splanchnic nerves (nervi erigentes)
21  Levator ani muscle
22  Inferior hypogastric plexus (pelvic plexus)
23  Prostate
24  Rectum (reflected)
25  Anal canal and external anal sphincter
26  Pampiniform plexus continuous with testicular vein
27  Testis and epididymis

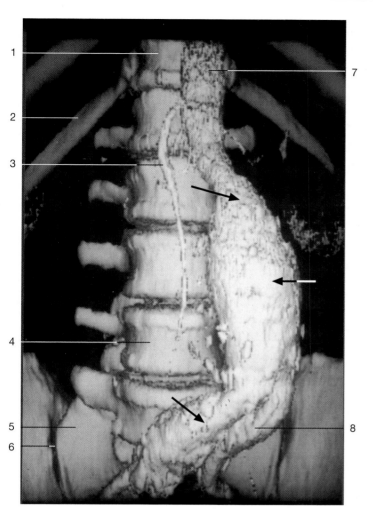

1   Twelfth thoracic vertebra (T$_{12}$)
2   Twelfth rib (rib XII)
3   Inferior mesenteric artery
4   Fourth lumbar vertebra (L$_4$)
5   Sacrum
6   Sacro-iliac articulation
7   Aorta (abdominal part)
8   Left common iliac artery (included into the aneurysm)
9   Aorta with aneurysm
10  Body of lumbar vertebra
11  Intrinsic muscles of the back
12  Thrombotic part of the aneurysm (green)
13  Inferior vena cava (compressed, blue)
14  Iliopsoas muscle
15  Vertebral canal
16  Aneurysm of the aorta (red)

**Abdominal part of the aorta showing an infrarenal aneurysm** with involvement of both iliac arteries (arrows) (3-D reconstruction, courtesy of Prof. H. Rupprecht and Dr. M. Rexer, Klinikum Fürth, Germany).

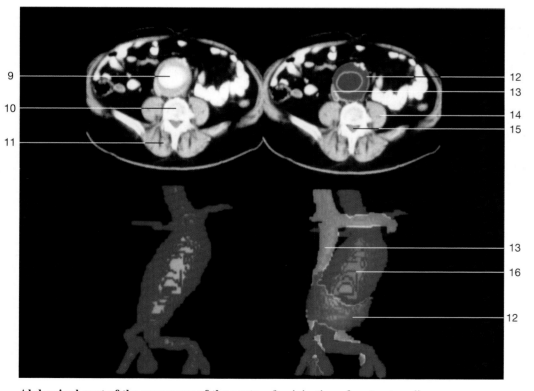

**Abdominal part of the aneurysm of the aorta,** after injection of contrast medium.
Above = horizontal sections through the abdominal cavity, showing different contrast medium concentrations within the aorta and the aneurysm; below = 3-D reconstruction of the aneurysm; red = aorta; green = thrombotic areas; blue = vein (vena cava inferior, partly compressed).

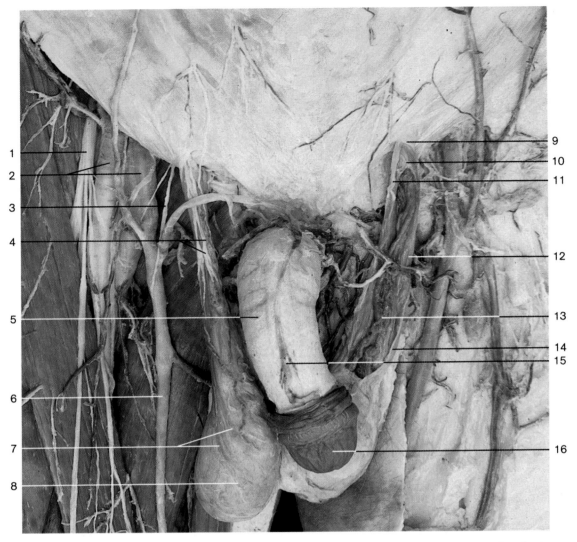

**Male external genital organs with penis, testis, and spermatic cord,** superficial layers (anterior view).

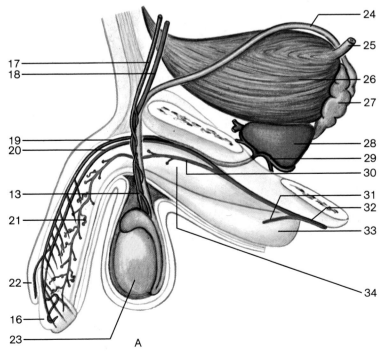

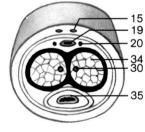

**Vessels of male genital organs** (schematic drawing).
A = lateral aspect; B = cross section of penis.

1  Femoral nerve
2  Femoral artery and vein
3  Femoral branch of genitofemoral nerve
4  Spermatic cord with genital branch
   of genitofemoral nerve
5  Penis with deep fascia
6  Great saphenous vein
7  Cremaster muscle
8  Testis with cremaster muscle
9  Superficial inguinal ring
10 Internal spermatic fascia (cut edge)
11 Ilio-inguinal nerve
12 Left spermatic cord
13 Pampiniform venous plexus
14 External spermatic fascia
15 Superficial dorsal vein of penis
16 Glans penis

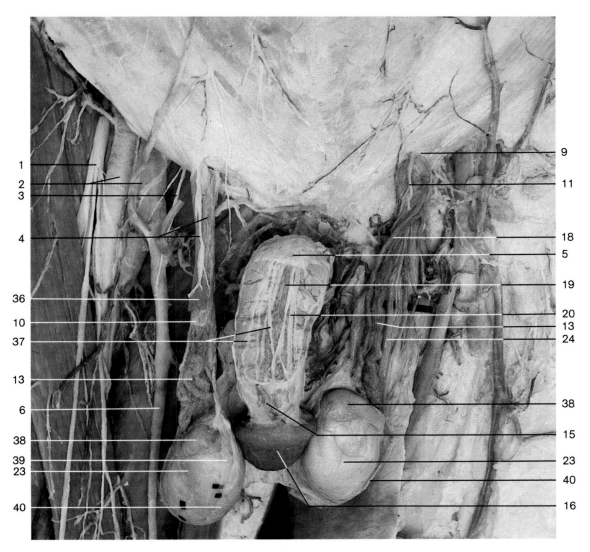

**Male external genital organs with penis, testis, and spermatic cord,** deeper layers (ventral aspect). The deep fascia of the penis has been opened to display the dorsal nerves and vessels.

17 Testicular vein
18 Testicular artery
19 Deep dorsal vein of penis
20 Dorsal artery of penis
21 Helicine arteries
22 Prepuce
23 Testis with tunica albuginea
24 Ductus deferens
25 Ureter
26 Urinary bladder
27 Seminal vesicle
28 Prostate
29 Vesicoprostatic venous plexus
30 Deep artery of penis
31 Artery of bulb of penis
32 Internal pudendal artery
33 Corpus spongiosum of penis
34 Corpus cavernosum of penis
35 Urethra
36 Cremasteric fascia with cremaster muscle
37 Dorsal nerve of penis
38 Epididymis
39 Tunica vaginalis (visceral layer)
40 Tunica vaginalis (parietal layer)
41 Testis with vascular loops

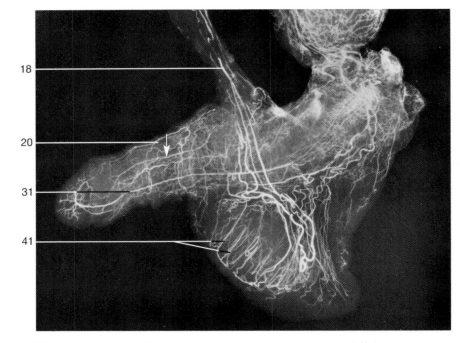

**Male genital organs** (lateral aspect). (Arteriogram.) Arrow = Helicine artery.

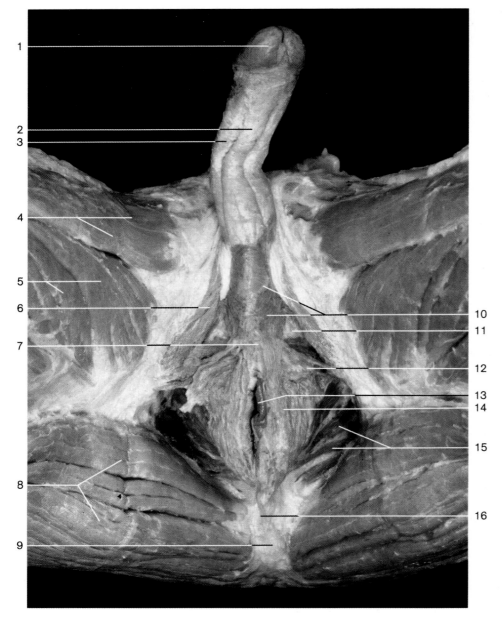

1 Glans penis
2 Corpus spongiosum of penis
3 Corpus cavernosum of penis
4 Gracilis muscle
5 Adductor muscles
6 Ischiocavernosus muscle overlying crus of penis
7 Perineal body
8 Gluteus maximus muscle
9 Coccyx
10 Bulbospongiosus muscle
11 Deep transverse perineus muscle covered by inferior fascia of urogenital diaphragm
12 Superficial transverse perineus muscle
13 Anus
14 External anal sphincter muscle
15 Levator ani muscle
16 Anococcygeal ligament
17 Obturator internus muscle
18 Urethra
19 Deep transverse perineus muscle

**Muscles of urogenital and pelvic diaphragms in the male** (from below).

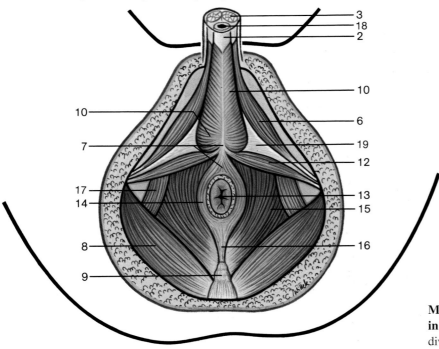

**Muscles of urogenital and pelvic diaphragms in the male** (from below). The penis has been divided (schematic drawing).

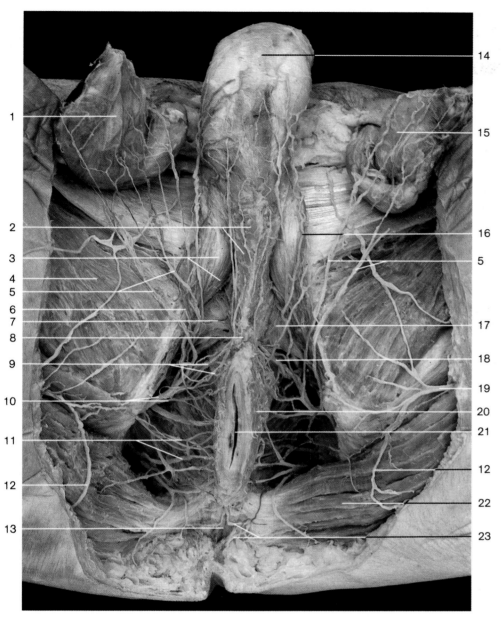

1   Right testis (reflected laterally and upward)
2   Bulbospongiosus muscle
3   Ischiocavernosus muscle
4   Adductor magnus muscle
5   Posterior scrotal nerves and superficial perineal arteries
6   Posterior scrotal artery and vein
7   Right artery of bulb of penis
8   Perineal body
9   Perineal branches of pudendal nerve
10  Pudendal nerve and internal pudendal artery
11  Inferior rectal arteries and nerves
12  Inferior cluneal nerve
13  Coccyx (location)
14  Penis
15  Left testis (reflected laterally)
16  Left posterior scrotal artery
17  Deep transverse perineal muscle
18  Left artery of bulb of penis
19  Posterior femoral cutaneous nerve
20  External anal sphincter muscle
21  Anus
22  Gluteus maximus muscle
23  Anococcygeal nerves
24  Acetabulum (femur removed)
25  Ligament of femoral head
26  Body of ischium (cut)
27  Sciatic nerve
28  Coccygeus muscle
29  Levator ani muscle
    a  iliococcygeus muscle
    b  pubococcygeus muscle
    c  puborectalis muscle
30  Prostatic venous plexus
31  Body of pubis
32  Testis

**Urogenital diaphragm and external genital organs in the male** with vessels and nerves (from below). The testes have been reflected laterally.

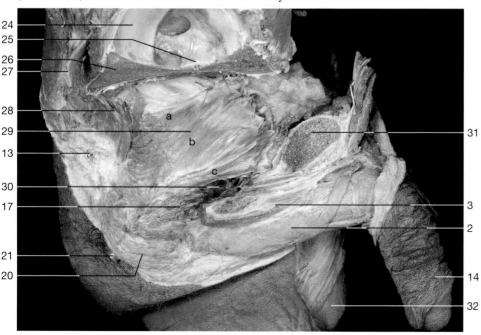

**Pelvic diaphragm and external genital organs** in the male. The right half of the pelvis including the obturator internus muscle and femur have been removed to display the right half of the levator ani muscle.

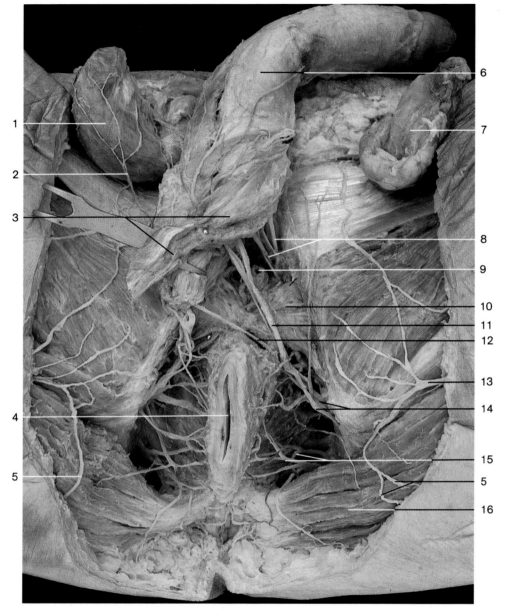

1  Right testis (reflected)
2  Posterior scrotal nerves
3  Left crus penis with ischiocavernosus muscle
4  Anus
5  Inferior cluneal nerves
6  Penis
7  Left testis (reflected)
8  Dorsal artery and nerve of penis
9  Urethra
10  Deep transverse perineus muscle
11  Perineal branch of pudendal nerve
12  Artery of bulb of penis (reflected)
13  Branch of posterior femoral cutaneous nerve
14  Internal pudendal artery and pudendal nerve
15  Inferior rectal arteries and nerves
16  Gluteus maximus muscle
17  Dorsal nerve of penis
18  Posterior femoral cutaneous nerve
19  Perineal branches of pudendal nerve
20  Inferior rectal nerves
21  Bulbospongiosus muscle (inside: dorsal artery of penis)
22  Perineal artery
23  External anal sphincter muscle
24  Inferior rectal artery and veins

**Urogenital diaphragm and external genital organs in the male** (from below). The left crus penis has been isolated and reflected laterally together with the bulb of the penis. The urethra has been cut.

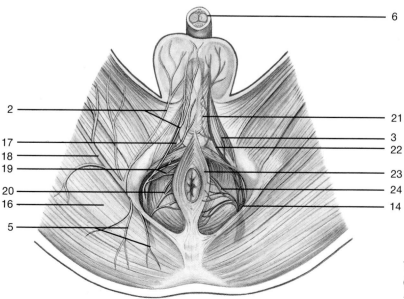

**Urogenital and anal region in the male** (from below). Right side: nerves; left side: arteries and veins.

1  Right testis (reflected)
2  Corpus spongiosum of penis
3  Corpus cavernosum of penis
4  Perineal branch of posterior
   femoral cutaneous nerve
5  Posterior scrotal arteries and
   nerves
6  Deep artery of penis
7  Deep transverse perineal muscle
8  Right perineal nerves
9  Inferior rectal nerves
10 Inferior cluneal nerve
11 Anococcygeal nerves
12 Left spermatic cord
13 Left testis (cut surface)
14 Dorsal artery and nerve of penis
15 Deep dorsal vein of penis
16 Urethra (cut)
17 Artery of bulb of penis
18 Superficial transverse perineus
   muscle
19 Left artery of bulb of penis
20 Perineal branch of pudendal nerve
21 Anus
22 External anal sphincter muscle
23 Gluteus maximus muscle
24 Internal pudendal artery and
   pudendal nerve
25 Sacrotuberous ligament
26 Coccyx
27 Urogenital diaphragm (deep
   transverse perineus muscle)
28 Tendinous center of perineum
   (perineal body)
29 Levator ani muscle
30 Anococcygeal ligament
31 Obturator internus muscle
32 Dorsal artery of penis

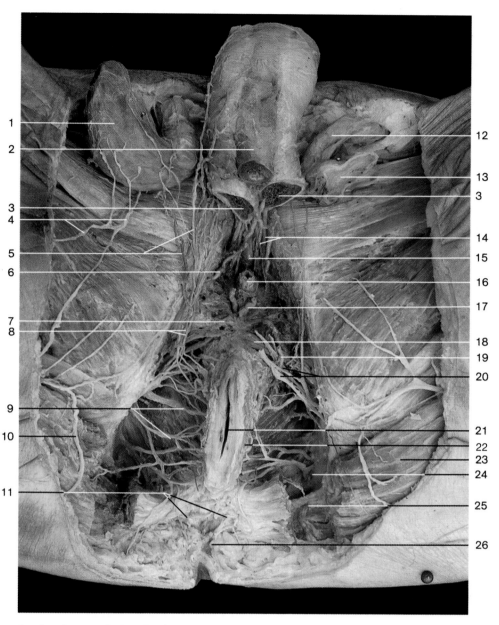

**Anal and urogenital region in the male** (from below). The root of the penis has been cut. Dissection of the urogenital diaphragm.

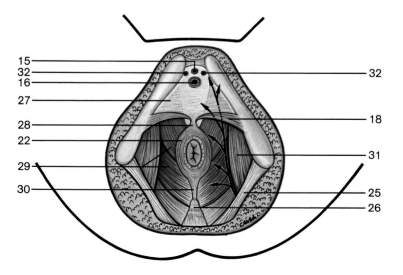

**Urogenital and pelvic diaphragms in the male** (from below). The penis has been removed. The arrows indicate the course of vessels and nerves (schematic drawing).

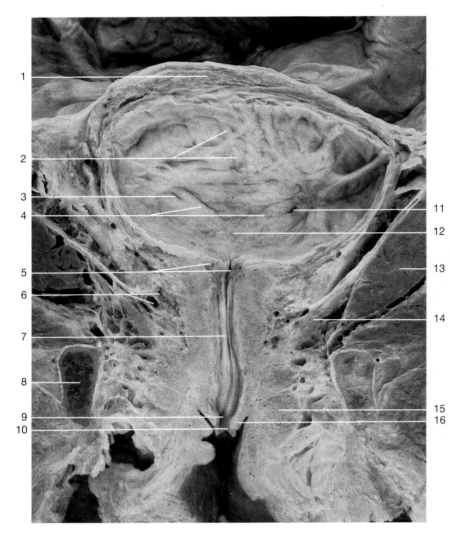

**Coronal section through the female urinary bladder and urethra** (anterior view).

1  Muscular coat of urinary bladder
2  Folds of mucous membrane of urinary bladder
3  Right ureteric orifice
4  Interureteric fold
5  Internal urethral orifice
6  Vesico-uterine venous plexus
7  Urethra
8  Pubic bone (cut edge)
9  External urethral orifice
10  Vestibule of vagina
11  Left ureteric orifice
12  Trigone of bladder
13  Obturator internus muscle
14  Levator ani muscle
15  Bulb of the vestibule
16  Left labium minus
17  Uterine tube
18  Mesosalpinx
19  Ovary
20  Sigmoid colon
21  Saphenous opening
22  Urinary bladder
23  Vesico-uterine pouch
24  Fundus of uterus
25  Recto-uterine pouch (of Douglas)
26  Ampulla of rectum
27  Kidney
28  Abdominal part of ureter
29  Pelvic part of ureter
30  Anal canal
31  Perineum (perineal body)
32  Umbilicus
33  Infundibulum of uterine tube
34  Vaginal portion of cervix of uterus
35  Vagina
36  Pubic symphysis
37  Clitoris
38  Deep transverse perineus muscle

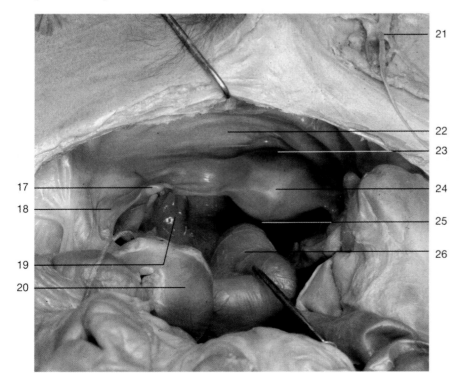

**Female internal genital organs.** Pelvic cavity (from above).

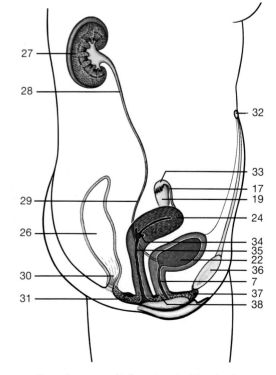

**Female urogenital system** (midsagittal section). (Schematic drawing.)

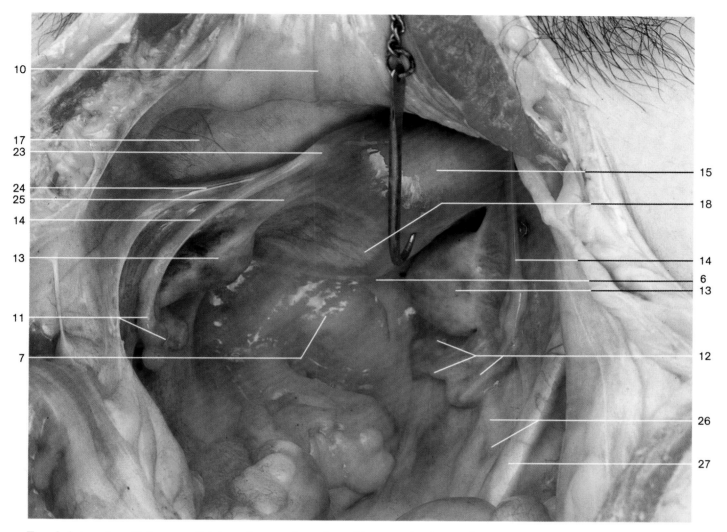

**Female internal genital organs.** Pelvic cavity, seen from above. The uterus has been reflected to the right.

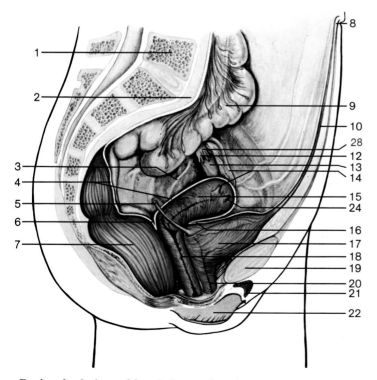

**Regional relations of female internal genital organs**
(medial aspect). (Schematic drawing.)

1 Body of fifth lumbar vertebra
2 Sacral promontory
3 Left ureter
4 Peritoneum (cut edge)
5 Right ureter (divided)
6 Recto-uterine pouch (of Douglas)
7 Rectum
8 Umbilicus
9 Sigmoid colon
10 Median umbilical fold with urachus
11 Ampulla of uterine tube
12 Fimbriae of uterine tube
13 Ovary
14 Uterine tube (isthmus)
15 Uterus
16 Vesico-uterine pouch
17 Urinary bladder
18 Vagina
19 Pubic symphysis
20 Urethra
21 Clitoris
22 Labium minus
23 Insertion of uterine tube at fundus of uterus
24 Round ligament of uterus
25 Ligament of the ovary
26 Suspensory ligament of ovary
27 Right common iliac artery (covered by peritoneum)
28 Infundibulum of uterine tube

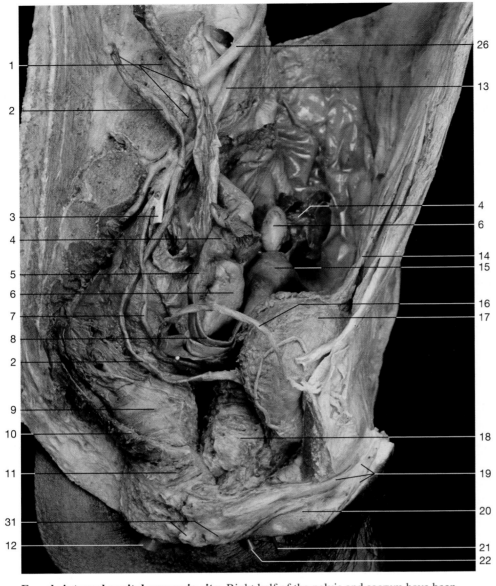

1  Body of fifth lumbar vertebra, suspensory ligament of ovary, and sacral promontory
2  Ureter
3  Medial umbilical ligament (remnant of umbilical artery) (cut)
4  Infundibulum of uterine tube
5  Ampulla of uterine tube
6  Ovary
7  Uterine artery
8  Uterine tube
9  Rectum
10 Levator ani muscle (pelvic diaphragm – cut edge)
11 External anal sphincter muscle
12 Anus (probe)
13 Internal iliac artery
14 Remnant of urachus (median umbilical ligament)
15 Uterus
16 Round ligament of uterus
17 Urinary bladder
18 Vagina
19 Clitoris
20 Labium minus
21 External orifice of urethra (red probe)
22 Vaginal orifice (green probe)
23 Lateral umbilical ligament
24 Inferior epigastric artery
25 Obturator artery, vein, and nerve
26 External iliac artery
27 Recto-uterine pouch (of Douglas)
28 Recto-uterine fold
29 Vesico-uterine pouch
30 Suspensory ligament of ovary
31 Greater vestibular gland and bulb of the vestibule

**Female internal genital organs in situ.** Right half of the pelvis and sacrum have been removed.

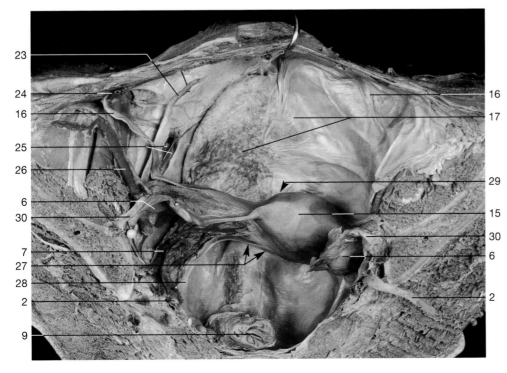

**Female internal genital organs in situ** (seen from above).
The peritoneum at the left half of pelvic cavity has been removed to display uterine tube, vessels, and nerves.

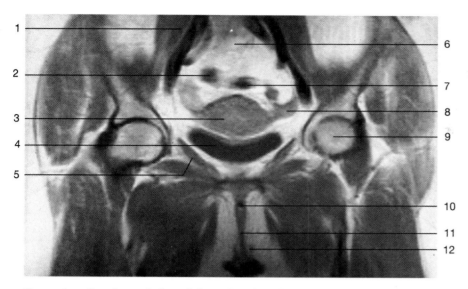

**Coronal section through the pelvic cavity of the female.** (MRI scan.)

1   Psoas major muscle
2   Ampulla of rectum
3   Uterus
4   Urinary bladder
5   Obturator internus muscle
6   Promontory
7   Sigmoid colon
8   Uterine tube
9   Head of femur
10  Urethra
11  Vagina
12  Labium minus
13  Umbilicus
14  Duodenum
15  Ascending part of duodenum
16  Root of mesentery
17  Mesentery
18  Vesico-uterine pouch
19  Urinary bladder (collapsed)
20  Pubic symphysis
21  Anterior fornix of vagina
22  Clitoris
23  Labium minus
24  Labium majus
25  Vertebral canal with cauda equina
26  Intervertebral disc
27  Body of fifth lumbar vertebra
28  Sacral promontory
29  Mesosigmoid
30  Recto-uterine pouch (of Douglas)
31  Posterior fornix of vagina
32  Cervix of uterus
33  External anal sphincter muscle
34  Anal canal
35  Internal anal sphincter muscle
36  Anus
37  Hymen
38  Small intestine
39  Rectus abdominis muscle

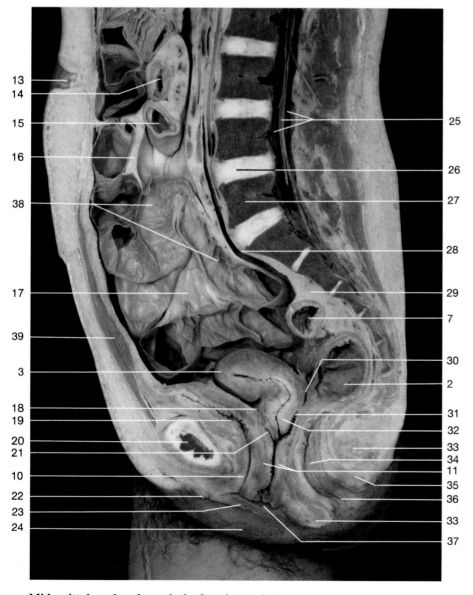

**Midsagittal section through the female trunk.** The urinary bladder is empty;
the position and shape of the uterus are normal.

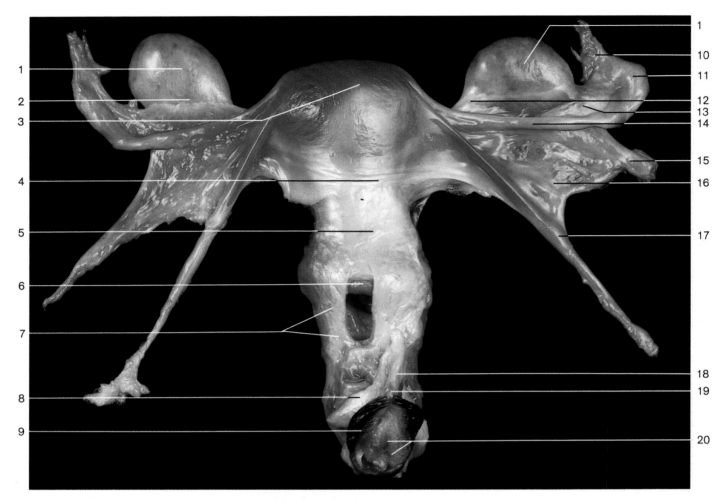

**Female genital organs,** isolated (anterior view). The anterior wall of the vagina has been opened to display the vaginal portion of the cervix.

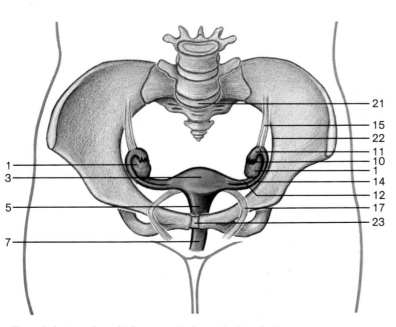

**Female internal genital organs** (schematic drawing).

1  Ovary
2  Mesovarium
3  Fundus of uterus
4  Vesico-uterine pouch
5  Cervix of uterus
6  Vaginal portion of cervix
7  Vagina
8  Crus of clitoris
9  Labium minus
10  Fimbriae of uterine tube
11  Infundibulum of uterine tube
12  Ligament of the ovary
13  Mesosalpinx
14  Uterine tube
15  Suspensory ligament of ovary
    (caudally displaced)
16  Broad ligament of uterus
17  Round ligament of uterus
18  Corpus cavernosum of clitoris
19  Glans of clitoris
20  Hymen, vaginal orifice
21  Promontory
22  Linea terminalis of pelvis
23  Pubic symphysis

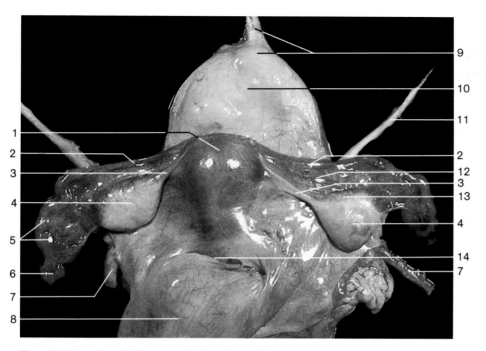

1  Fundus of uterus
2  Uterine tube
3  Ligament of the ovary
4  Ovary
5  Infundibulum of uterine tube
6  Fimbriae of uterine tube
7  Ureter
8  Rectum
9  Apex of urinary bladder and median umbilical ligament
10  Urinary bladder
11  Round ligament of uterus
12  Mesosalpinx
13  Mesovarium
14  Recto-uterine pouch (of Douglas)
15  Suspensory ligament of ovary
16  Scarring of ovary (following ovulation)
17  Abdominal opening of uterine tube
18  Body of uterus
19  Cervical canal
20  Vaginal portion of cervix of uterus (congestion)
21  Vagina
22  Mucous membrane of uterus
23  Anterior fornix of vagina

**Female internal genital organs,** isolated (superior-posterior view).

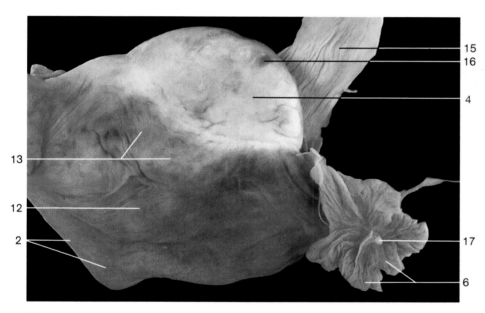

**Right ovary and uterine tube,** isolated (superior-posterior view). The fimbriae of the uterine tube have been reflected to show the abdominal ostium.

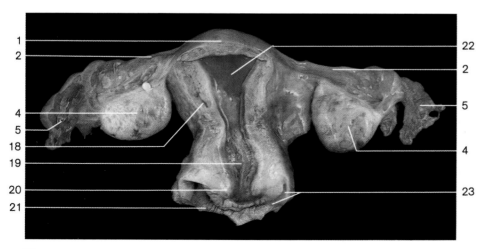

**Uterus and related organs** (posterior view). The posterior wall of the uterus has been opened.

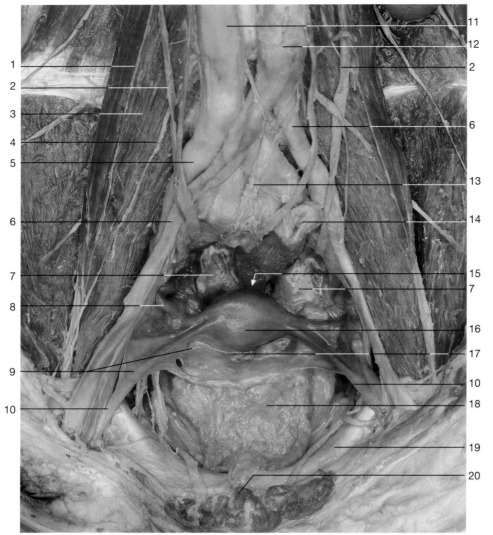

1   Ilio-inguinal nerve
2   Ureter
3   Psoas major muscle
4   Genitofemoral nerve
5   Common iliac vein
6   Common iliac artery
7   Ovary
8   Uterine tube
9   Peritoneum
10  Round ligament of uterus
11  Inferior vena cava
12  Abdominal aorta
13  Superior hypogastric plexus
14  Rectum
15  Recto-uterine pouch
    (of Douglas)
16  Uterus
17  Vesico-uterine pouch
18  Urinary bladder
19  Iliac crest
20  Pubic symphysis
21  Vaginal portion of cervix
    of uterus
22  Vagina
23  Clitoris
24  Corpus cavernosum of clitoris
25  Vaginal orifice
26  Bulb of vestibule
27  Greater vestibular gland
28  Ovarian artery
29  Suspensory ligament of ovary
30  Internal iliac artery
31  Tubal branch of ovarian artery
32  Ovarian branch of ovarian
    artery
33  Uterine artery
34  Ovarian branch of uterine
    artery
35  Artery of round ligament
36  Internal pudendal artery
37  Vaginal artery

**View of the female pelvis** showing uterus, urinary bladder, and uterine ligaments (superior aspect).

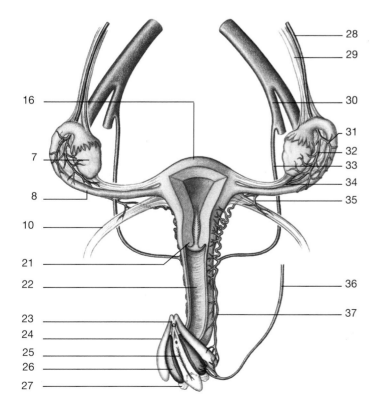

**Arteries of female genital organs** (schematic drawing).

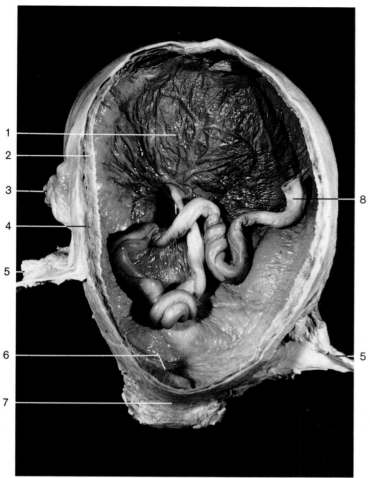

**Fullterm uterus with placenta** (anterior view). The anterior wall of the uterus has been removed to show the location of the placenta.

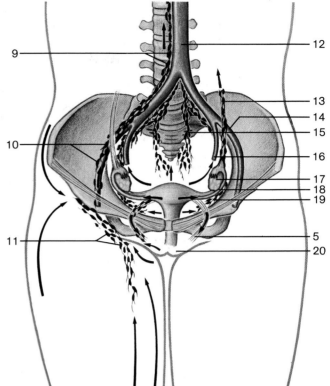

**Main drainage routes of lymph vessels of uterus and its adnexa** (indicated by arrows). (Schematic drawing.) Red = arteries; black = lymph vessels and nodes; yellow = internal genital organs.

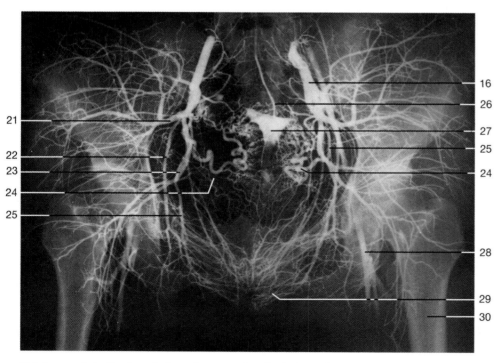

**Pelvic vessels in the female** (anterior-posterior view). (Arteriogram.)

1  Placenta
2  Amnion and chorion
3  Adnexa of uterus
   (uterine tube and ovaries)
4  Myometrium
5  Round ligament of uterus
6  Internal orifice of uterus
7  Cervix of uterus
8  Umbilical cord
9  Lumbar lymph nodes
10  External iliac lymph nodes
11  Inguinal lymph nodes
12  Abdominal aorta
13  Suspensory ligament of ovary
14  External iliac artery
15  Sacral lymph nodes
16  Internal iliac artery
17  Ovary
18  Uterine tube
19  Internal iliac lymph nodes
20  External genital organs
21  Superior gluteal artery
22  Obturator artery
23  Inferior gluteal artery
24  Uterine artery
25  Internal pudendal artery
26  Middle sacral artery
27  Uterine cavity
28  Femoral artery
29  Vessels of labium majus
30  Femur

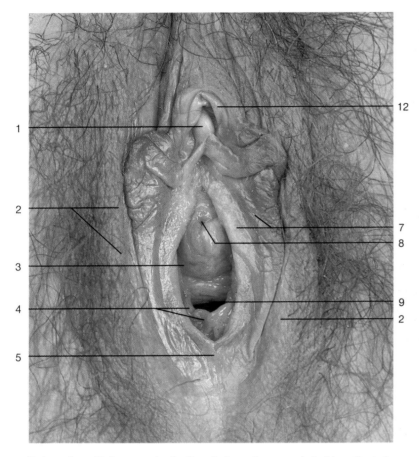

1   Glans of clitoris
2   Labium majus
3   Vestibule of vagina
4   Hymen
5   Posterior labial commissure
6   Body of clitoris
7   Labium minus
8   External orifice of urethra
9   Vaginal orifice
10  Ureter
11  Adnexa of uterus
12  Prepuce of clitoris
13  Crus of clitoris
14  Greater vestibular glands
15  Anus and internal anal sphincter muscle
16  Median umbilical ligament containing urachus
17  Urinary bladder
18  Infundibulum of uterine tube
19  Ovary
20  Ampulla of uterine tube
21  Suspensory ligament of the ovary
22  Bulbospongiosus muscle and bulb of vestibule
23  Central tendon of perineum (perineal body)
24  External anal sphincter muscle

**External genital organs** in the female (anterior aspect). Labia reflected.

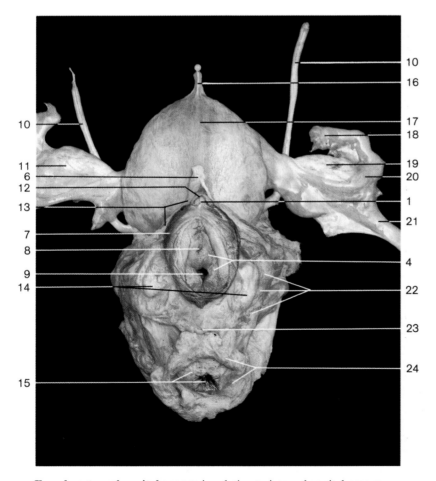

**Female external genital organs** in relation to internal genital organs and urinary system (isolated, anterior aspect).

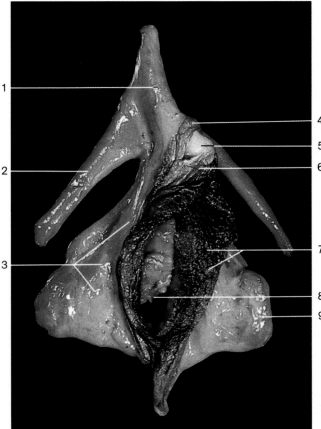

**Cavernous tissue of female external genital organs,** isolated (anterior aspect).

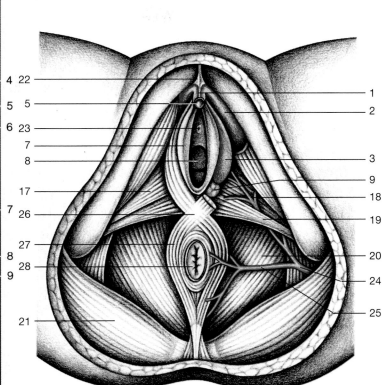

**Urogenital and pelvic diaphragms** (anterior aspect). (Schematic drawing.) Blue = cavernous tissue of clitoris and bulb of vestibule.

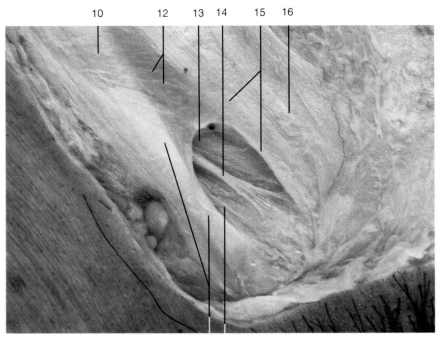

**Inguinal canal and round ligament of uterus in situ** (right side, ventral aspect).

1 Body of clitoris
2 Crus of clitoris
3 Bulb of vestibule
4 Prepuce of clitoris
5 Glans of clitoris
6 Frenulum of clitoris
7 Labium minus
8 Vaginal orifice
9 Greater vestibular gland
10 Lateral crus of superficial inguinal ring
11 Ilio-inguinal nerve
12 Intercrural fibers
13 Superficial inguinal ring
14 Round ligament of uterus
15 Medial crus of superficial inguinal ring
16 Aponeurosis of external abdominal
   oblique muscle
17 Deep transverse perineal muscle with
   fascia
18 Deep artery of clitoris
19 Superficial transverse perineus muscle
20 Levator ani muscle
21 Gluteus maximus muscle
22 Suspensory ligament of clitoris
23 External orifice of urethra
24 Internal pudendal artery
25 Inferior rectal artery
26 Perineal body
27 External anal sphincter muscle
28 Anus

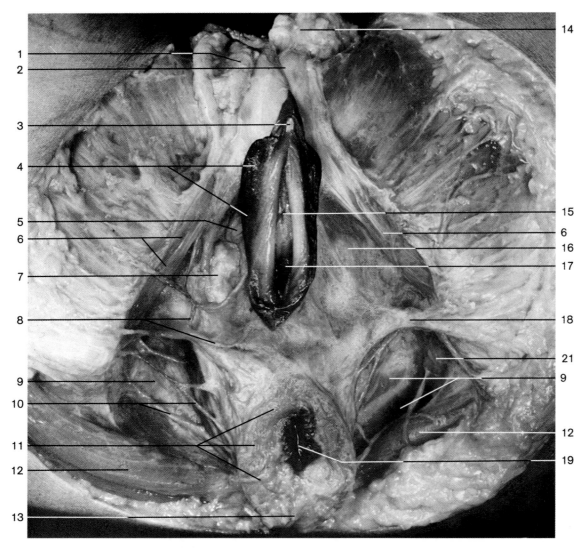

**Female urogenital diaphragm and external genital organs,** superficial layer (from below).

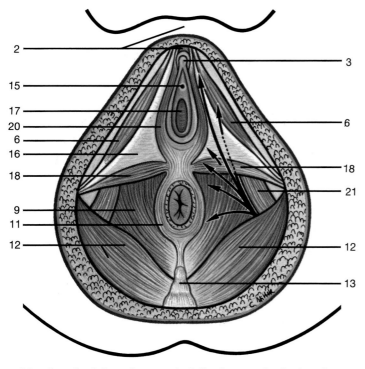

**Muscles of pelvic and urogenital diaphragms in the female**
(from below). (Schematic drawing.)

1   Fatty tissue encasing round ligament
2   Position of pubic symphysis
3   Clitoris
4   Labium minus
5   Bulb of vestibule
6   Ischiocavernosus muscle
7   Greater vestibular gland
8   Perineal branches of pudendal nerve
9   Levator ani muscle
10  Inferior rectal nerves
11  External anal sphincter muscle
12  Gluteus maximus muscle
13  Coccyx
14  Fatty tissue of mons pubis
15  External orifice of urethra
16  Urogenital diaphragm with fascia of deep transverse
    perineus muscle
17  Vaginal orifice
18  Superficial transverse perineal muscle
19  Anus
20  Bulbospongiosus muscle
21  Obturator internus muscle

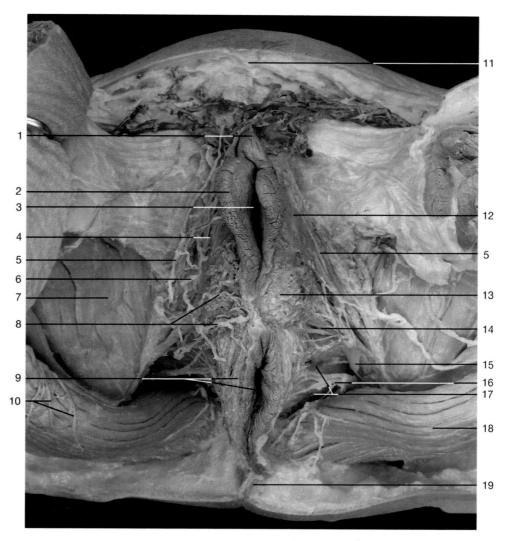

**Urogenital diaphragm and external genital organs in the female,** superficial layer (from below). On the right side the bulb of vestibule has been removed.

1  Prepuce of clitoris
2  Labium minus
3  Vaginal orifice
4  Deep transverse perineus muscle
5  Dorsal nerve of clitoris
6  Posterior labial nerves
7  Great adductor muscle
8  Perineal branches of pudendal nerve
9  Anus and external anal sphincter muscle
10  Inferior cluneal nerves
11  Mons pubis
12  Crus of clitoris with ischiocavernosus muscle
13  Bulb of vestibule
14  Superficial transverse perineus muscle
15  Pudendal nerve and internal pudendal artery
16  Inferior rectal nerves
17  Levator ani muscle
18  Gluteus maximus muscle
19  Anococcygeal ligament
20  External urethral orifice
21  Glans of clitoris

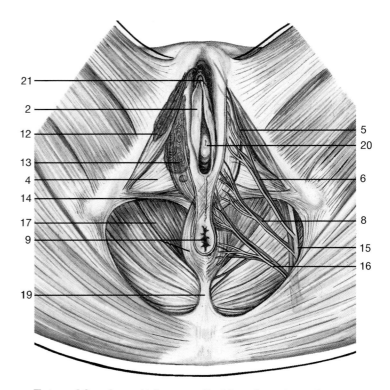

**External female genital organs.** Position of arteries and nerves; bulb of vestibule in blue (schematic drawing).

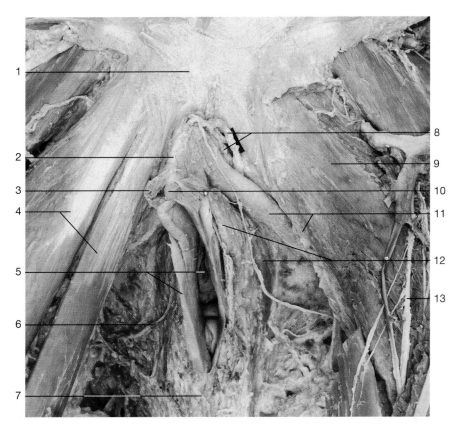

1   Position of pubic symphysis
2   Body of clitoris
3   Prepuce of clitoris
4   Adductor longus and gracilis muscles
5   External orifice of vagina and
    labium minus
6   Posterior labial nerve
7   Perineal body
8   Deep artery of clitoris and
    dorsal nerve of clitoris
9   Adductor brevis muscle
10  Glans of clitoris
11  Crus of clitoris and
    ischiocavernosus muscle
12  Bulb of vestibule and
    bulbospongiosus muscle
13  Anterior branch of obturator nerve
14  Labium minus
15  Vaginal orifice
16  Posterior labial nerves
17  Branches of pudendal nerve
18  External sphincter of anus
19  Anus
20  Bulb of vestibule (divided)
21  Dorsal artery of clitoris
22  Superficial transverse perineus muscle
23  Perineal branch of posterior femoral
    cutaneous nerve
24  Levator ani muscle
25  Pudendal nerve and
    internal pudendal artery
26  Inferior rectal nerves
27  Gluteus maximus muscle
28  Anococcygeal ligament

**External female genital organs** (inferior aspect). The clitoris has been dissected and slightly reflected to the right. The prepuce of clitoris has been divided to display the glans.

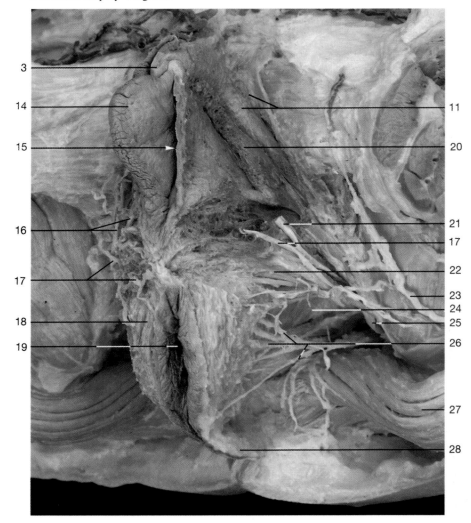

**Urogenital diaphragm and external genital organs in the female** (lateral inferior view). The bulb of vestibule has partly been removed; the left labium minus was cut away.

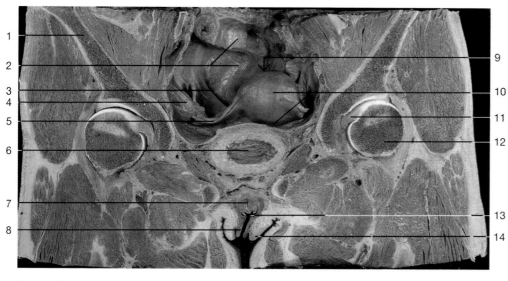

**Coronal section through the pelvic cavity of the female** (cf. MRI scan on page 357).

| | |
|---|---|
| 1 | Ilium |
| 2 | Rectum |
| 3 | Recto-uterine fold |
| 4 | Ovary |
| 5 | Uterine tube |
| 6 | Urinary bladder |
| 7 | Urethra |
| 8 | Labium minus |
| 9 | Recto-uterine pouch of Douglas |
| 10 | Uterus (uterovesical pouch) |
| 11 | Ligament of the head of the femur |
| 12 | Head of femur |
| 13 | Vestibule of vagina |
| 14 | Labium majus |
| 15 | Anal cleft |
| 16 | Coccyx |
| 17 | Rectum |
| 18 | Myometrium of uterus |
| 19 | Uterine cavity |
| 20 | Obturator internus muscle |
| 21 | Iliopsoas muscle |
| 22 | Sartorius muscle |
| 23 | Sciatic nerve and gluteus maximus muscle |
| 24 | Uterine venous plexus |
| 25 | Broad ligament |
| 26 | Small intestine |
| 27 | Femoral artery and vein |
| 28 | Femoral nerve |
| 29 | Pyramidalis muscle |
| 30 | Rectum (anal canal) |
| 31 | Vagina |
| 32 | Urethral sphincter muscle (base of urinary bladder) |
| 33 | Pubic symphysis |
| 34 | Levator ani muscle |
| 35 | Obturator externus muscle |
| 36 | Mons pubis |
| 37 | Pectineus muscle |

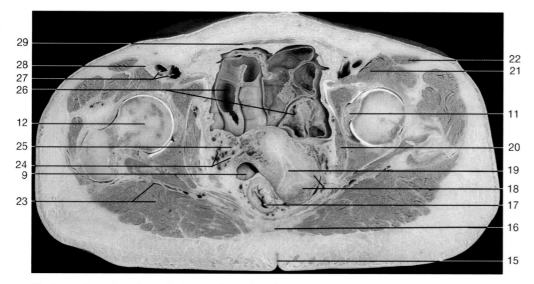

**Horizontal section through the pelvic cavity of the female** at level of uterus (from below). The uterus is retroverted to the left.

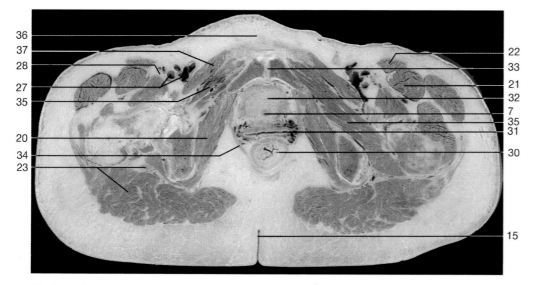

**Horizontal section through the pelvic cavity of the female** at level of the urethral sphincter and vagina (from below).

# 7 Upper Limb

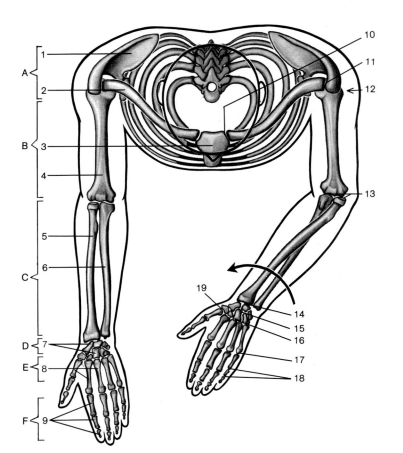

A   Shoulder girdle
B   Arm
C   Forearm
D   Wrist
E   Palm of hand
F   Finger

**Bones**
1   Scapula
2   Clavicle
3   Sternum
4   Humerus
5   Radius
6   Ulna
7   Carpal bones
8   Metacarpal bones
9   Phalanges

**Joints**
10   Sternoclavicular joint
11   Acromioclavicular joint
12   Shoulder joint
13   Elbow joint
14   Wrist joint
15   Midcarpal joint
16   Carpometacarpal joint
17   Metacarpophalangeal joint
18   Interphalangeal joints of the hand
19   Carpometacarpal joint of thumb

**Organization of shoulder girdle and upper limb** (superior aspect). The two positions of the forearm essential to manual skills in the human, supination (right arm) and pronation (left arm), are shown.

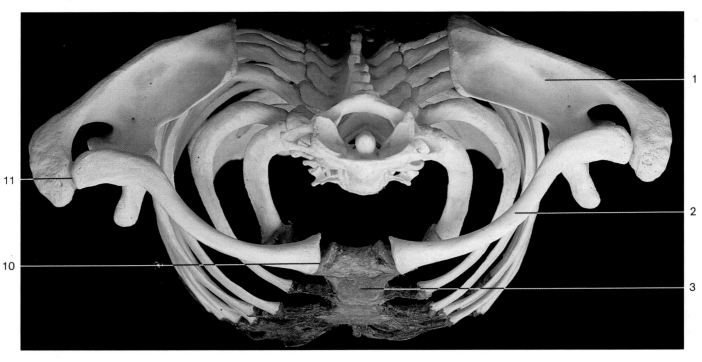

**Bones of shoulder girdle** articulated with the thorax (superior aspect).

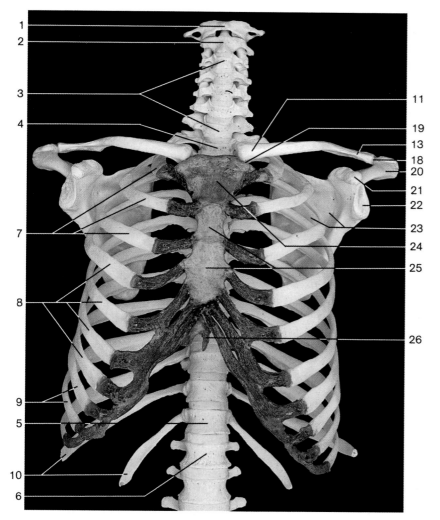

**Skeleton of shoulder girdle and thorax** (anterior aspect).
The cartilaginous parts of the ribs appear dark brown.

**Vertebral column**
1 Atlas
2 Axis
3 Third–seventh cervical vertebrae
4 First thoracic vertebra
5 Twelfth thoracic vertebra
6 First lumbar vertebra

**Ribs**
7 First–third ribs ⎫
8 Fourth–seventh ribs ⎬ True ribs
9 Eighth–tenth ribs ⎫
10 Eleventh and twelfth ribs ⎬ False ribs
   (floating ribs)

**Clavicle**
11 Sternal end
12 Articular facet for sternum
13 Acromial end
14 Articular facet for acromion
15 Impression for costoclavicular ligament
16 Conoid tubercle
17 Trapezoid line
18 Site of acromioclavicular joint
19 Site of sternoclavicular joint

**Scapula**
20 Acromion
21 Coracoid process
22 Glenoid cavity
23 Costal surface

**Sternum**
24 Manubrium
25 Body
26 Xiphoid process

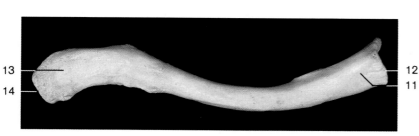

**Right clavicle** (superior aspect).

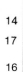
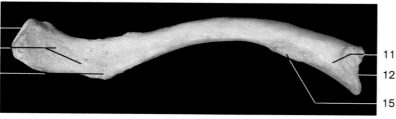

**Right clavicle** (inferior aspect).

Because of his upright posture, man's upper limb has developed a high degree of mobility. The shoulder girdle is to a great extent movable in the thorax and is connected with the trunk only by the sternoclavicular joint. A further characteristic of man's forearm is the capacity for rotation (i.e., pronation and supination).

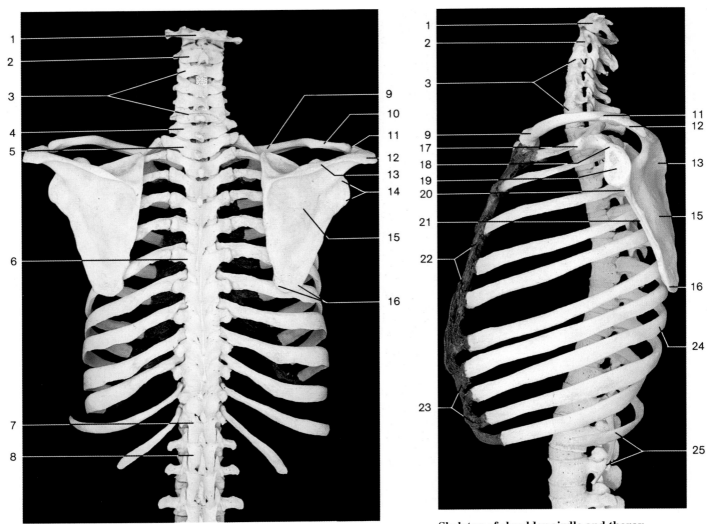

**Skeleton of shoulder girdle and thorax** (posterior view).

**Skeleton of shoulder girdle and thorax**
(lateral view).

**Vertebral column**
1   Atlas
2   Axis
3   Third–sixth cervical vertebrae
4   Seventh vertebra (vertebra prominens)
5   First thoracic vertebra
6   Sixth thoracic vertebra
7   Twelfth thoracic vertebra
8   First lumbar vertebra

**Clavicle**
9   Sternal end
10  Acromial end
11  Site of acromioclavicular joint

**Scapula**
12  Acromion
13  Spine of scapula
14  Lateral angle

15  Posterior surface
16  Inferior angle
17  Coracoid process
18  Supraglenoid tubercle
19  Glenoid cavity
20  Infraglenoid tubercle
21  Lateral margin

**Thorax**
22  Body of sternum
23  Costal arch
24  Angle of ribs
25  Free ribs

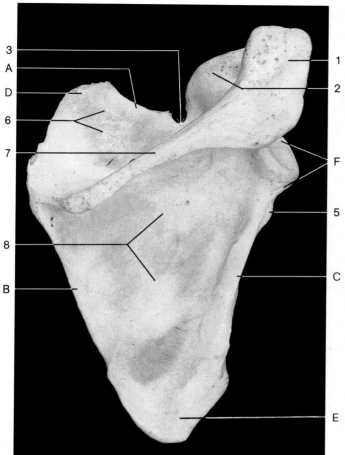

**Right scapula** (posterior aspect).

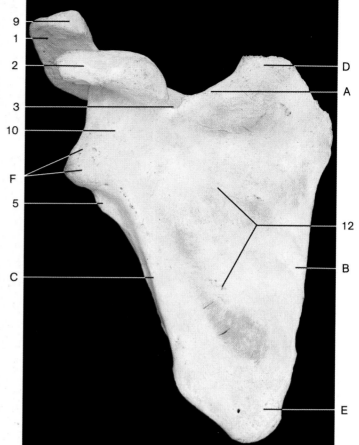

**Right scapula** (anterior aspect, costal surface).

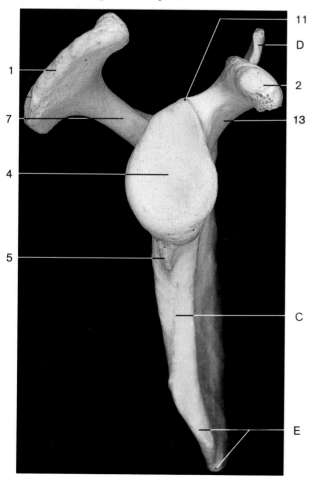

**Right scapula** (lateral aspect).

**Scapula**

A   Superior border
B   Medial border
C   Lateral border
D   Superior angle
E   Inferior angle
F   Lateral angle

1   Acromion
2   Coracoid process
3   Scapular notch
4   Glenoid cavity
5   Infraglenoid tubercle
6   Supraspinous fossa
7   Spine
8   Infraspinous fossa
9   Articular facet for acromion
10  Neck
11  Supraglenoid tubercle
12  Costal (anterior) surface
13  Base of coracoid process

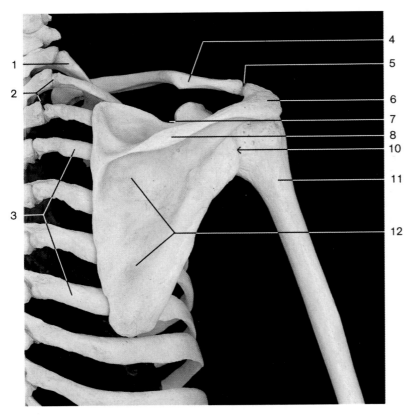

1  1st rib
2  Position of costotransverse joints
3  Fourth–seventh ribs
4  Clavicle
5  Position of acromioclavicular joint
6  Acromion
7  Scapular notch
8  Spine of scapula
9  Head of humerus
10  Glenoid cavity
11  Surgical neck of humerus
12  Posterior surface of scapula
13  Coracoid process
14  Infraglenoid tubercle
15  Greater tubercle of humerus
16  Anatomical neck of humerus

**Bones of shoulder joint** (posterior aspect).

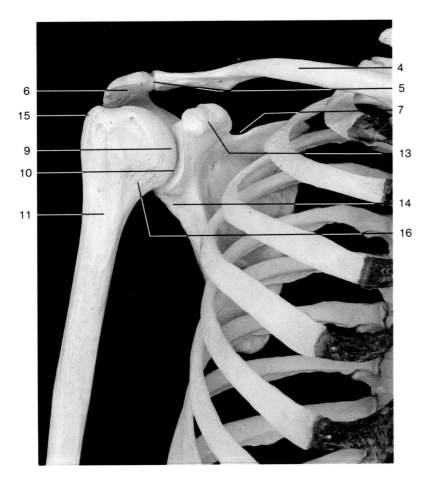

**Bones of shoulder joint** (anterior aspect).

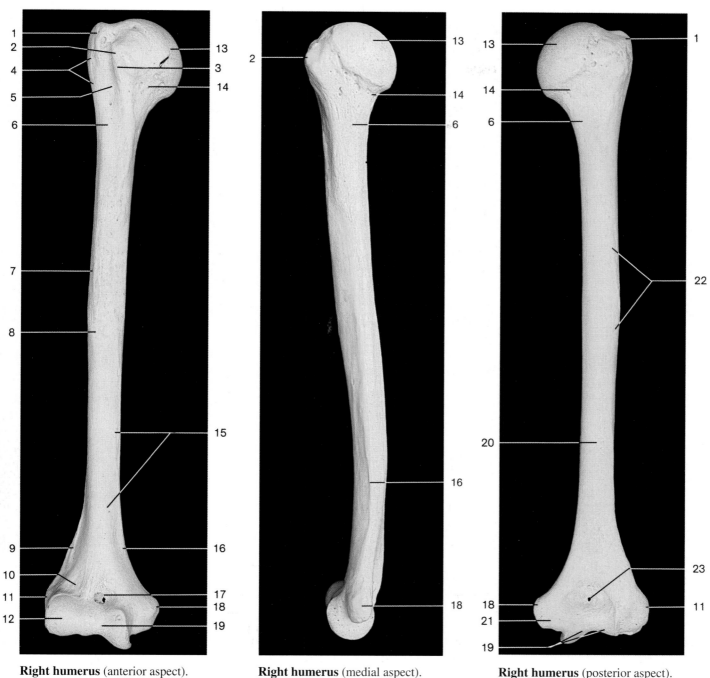

**Right humerus** (anterior aspect).

**Right humerus** (medial aspect).

**Right humerus** (posterior aspect).

**Humerus**

| | | | | | | | |
|---|---|---|---|---|---|---|---|
| 1 | Greater tubercle | 7 | Deltoid tuberosity | 13 | Head | 19 | Trochlea |
| 2 | Lesser tubercle | 8 | Anterolateral surface | 14 | Anatomical neck | 20 | Posterior surface |
| 3 | Crest of lesser tubercle | 9 | Lateral supracondylar ridge | 15 | Anteromedial surface | 21 | Groove for ulnar nerve |
| 4 | Crest of greater tubercle | 10 | Radial fossa | 16 | Medial supracondylar ridge | 22 | Groove for radial nerve |
| 5 | Intertubercular sulcus | 11 | Lateral epicondyle | 17 | Coronoid fossa | 23 | Olecranon fossa |
| 6 | Surgical neck | 12 | Capitulum | 18 | Medial epicondyle | | |

**Radius**
1 Head
2 Articular circumference
3 Neck
4 Radial tuberosity
5 Shaft
6 Anterior surface
7 Styloid process
8 Articular surface
9 Posterior surface
10 Ulnar notch

**Ulna**
11 Trochlear notch
12 Coronoid process
13 Radial notch
14 Ulnar tuberosity
15 Head
16 Articular circumference
17 Styloid process
18 Posterior surface
19 Olecranon

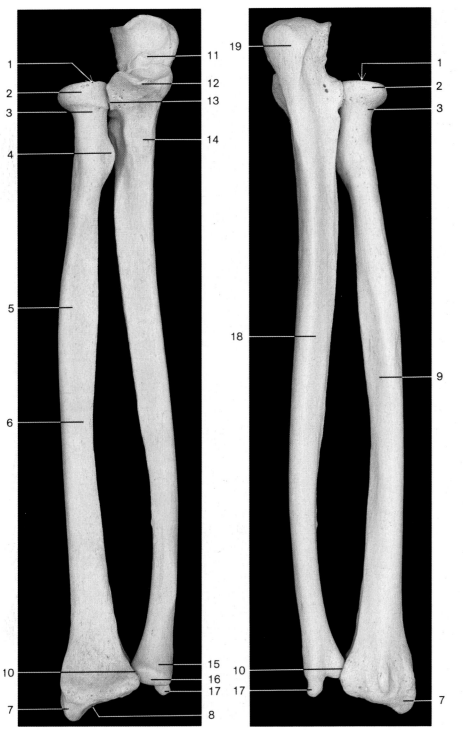

**Bones of right forearm, radius, and ulna** (anterior aspect).

**Bones of right forearm, radius, and ulna** (posterior aspect).

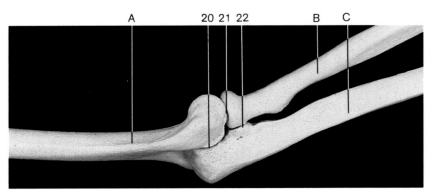

**Bones of right elbow joint** (lateral aspect).

**Articulations at the right elbow**
20 Site of humero-ulnar joint
21 Site of humeroradial joint
22 Site of proximal radio-ulnar joint

A Humerus
B Radius
C Ulna

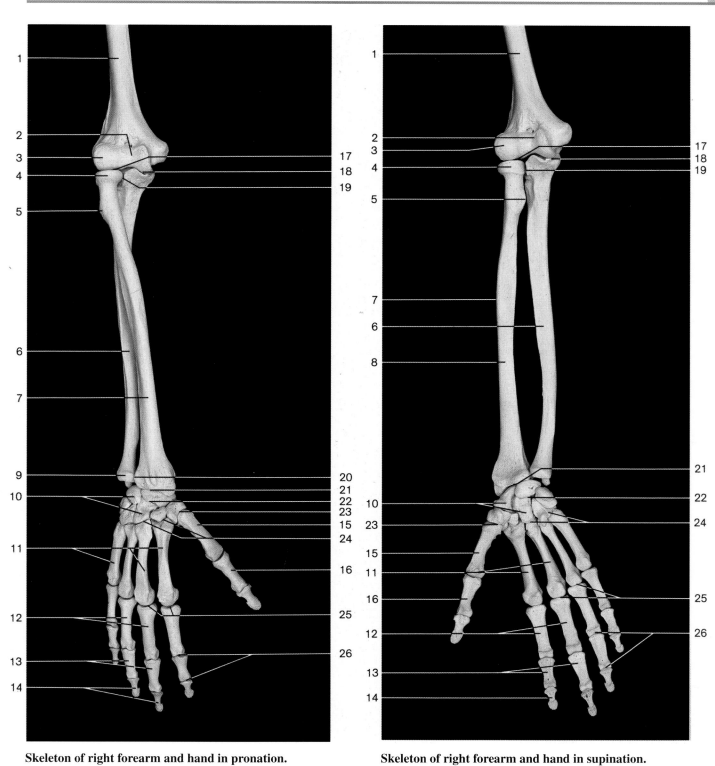

**Skeleton of right forearm and hand in pronation.**

**Skeleton of right forearm and hand in supination.**

| | | | |
|---|---|---|---|
| 1 | Humerus | 12 | Proximal phalanges |
| 2 | Trochlea of humerus | 13 | Middle phalanges |
| 3 | Capitulum of humerus | 14 | Distal phalanges |
| 4 | Articular circumference of radius | 15 | Metacarpal bone of thumb |
| 5 | Radial tuberosity | 16 | Proximal phalanx of thumb |
| 6 | Anterior surface of ulna | | |
| 7 | Posterior surface of radius | | |
| 8 | Anterior surface of radius | | |
| 9 | Articular circumference of ulna | | |
| 10 | Carpal bones | | |
| 11 | Metacarpal bones | | |

**Sites of joints**
17   Humeroradial joint
18   Humero-ulnar joint
19   Proximal radio-ulnar joint
20   Distal radio-ulnar joint
21   Wrist joint
22   Midcarpal joint
23   Carpometacarpal joint of thumb
24   Carpometacarpal joints
25   Metacarpophalangeal joints
26   Interphalangeal joints of the hand

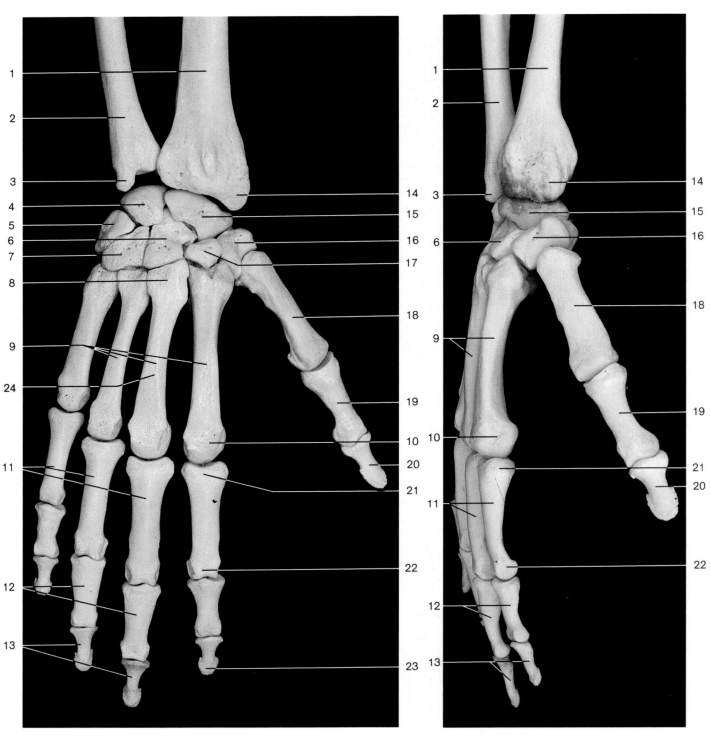

**Skeleton of right wrist and hand** (dorsal aspect).

**Skeleton of right wrist and hand**
(medial aspect).

| | | | | |
|---|---|---|---|---|
| 1 | Radius | 8 | Base of third metacarpal bone | 15 | Scaphoid bone |
| 2 | Ulna | 9 | Metacarpal bones | 16 | Trapezium bone |
| 3 | Styloid process of ulna | 10 | Head of metacarpal bone | 17 | Trapezoid bone |
| 4 | Lunate bone | 11 | Proximal phalanges of hand | 18 | Metacarpal bone of thumb |
| 5 | Triquetral bone | 12 | Middle phalanges of hand | 19 | Proximal phalanx of thumb |
| 6 | Capitate bone | 13 | Distal phalanges of hand | 20 | Distal phalanx of thumb |
| 7 | Hamate bone | 14 | Styloid process of radius | 21 | Base of second proximal phalanx |

1   Radius
2   Ulna
3   Styloid process of ulna
4   Lunate bone ⎫
5   Triquetral bone ⎬ Carpal bones
6   Capitate bone ⎪
7   Hamate bone ⎭

8   Base of third metacarpal bone
9   Metacarpal bones
10  Head of metacarpal bone
11  Proximal phalanges of hand
12  Middle phalanges of hand
13  Distal phalanges of hand
14  Styloid process of radius

15  Scaphoid bone ⎫
16  Trapezium bone ⎬ Carpal bones
17  Trapezoid bone ⎭
18  Metacarpal bone of thumb
19  Proximal phalanx of thumb
20  Distal phalanx of thumb
21  Base of second proximal phalanx

22  Head of second
    proximal phalanx
23  Tuberosity of distal
    phalanx
24  Body of
    third metacarpal
    bone

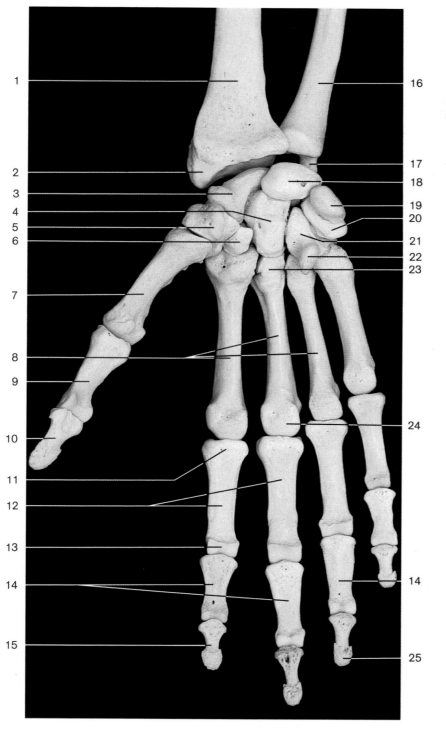

| 1 | Radius |
| 2 | Styloid process of radius |
| 3 | Scaphoid bone |
| 4 | Capitate bone |
| 5 | Trapezium |
| 6 | Trapezoid bone |
| 7 | First metacarpal bone |
| 8 | Second to fourth metacarpal bones |
| 9 | Proximal phalanx of thumb |
| 10 | Distal phalanx of thumb |
| 11 | Base of second proximal phalanx |
| 12 | Proximal phalanges |
| 13 | Head of second proximal phalanx |
| 14 | Middle phalanges |
| 15 | Distal phalanx |
| 16 | Ulna |
| 17 | Styloid process of ulna |
| 18 | Lunate bone |
| 19 | Pisiform bone |
| 20 | Triquetral bone |
| 21 | Hamate bone |
| 22 | Hamulus or hook of hamate bone |
| 23 | Base of third metacarpal bone |
| 24 | Head of metacarpal bone |
| 25 | Tuberosity of distal phalanx |

3–6 Carpal bones

18–22 Carpal bones

**Skeleton of right wrist and hand** (palmar aspect).

The human hand is one of the most admirable structures of the human body. The carpometacarpal joint of the thumb, a saddle joint, enjoys wide mobility, so that the thumb can get in contact with all other fingers, thus enabling the hand to become an instrument for grasping and psychologic expression. During evolution these newly developed functions appeared after the erect posture of the human body was achieved. An inevitable prerequisite for the development of human cultures is not only the differentiation of the brain but also the development of an organ capable of realizing its ideas: the human hand.

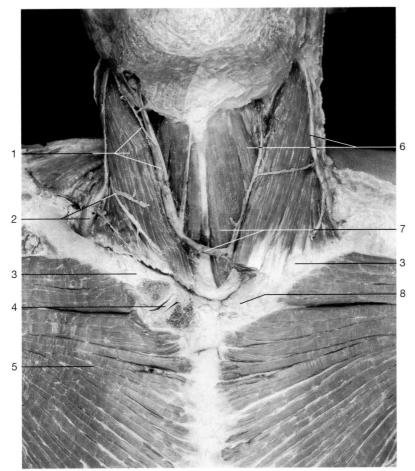

1  Sternocleidomastoid muscle, cervical branch of
   facial nerve, and anterior jugular vein
2  External jugular vein and transverse cervical nerve
   (inferior branch)
3  Clavicle
4  Sternoclavicular joint (opened) with articular disc
5  Pectoralis major muscle
6  Omohyoid muscle and external jugular vein
7  Jugular venous arch and sternohyoid muscle
8  Sternoclavicular joint (not opened)
9  Acromial end of clavicle
10 Acromioclavicular joint
11 Acromion
12 Tendon of supraspinatus muscle
   (attached to the articular capsule)
13 Coraco-acromial ligament
14 Tendon of long head of biceps brachii muscle
15 Tendon of subscapularis muscle
   (attached to the articular capsule)
16 Intertubercular sulcus
17 Articular capsule of shoulder joint
18 Humerus
19 Trapezoid ligament
20 Coracoid process
21 Glenoid labrum
22 Shoulder joint (joint cavity)
23 Scapula
24 Supraspinatus muscle
25 Cartilage of glenoid cavity
26 Tendon of long head of triceps brachii muscle
27 Head of humerus (articular cartilage)
28 Epiphysial line

**Right sternoclavicular joint** (anterior aspect). On the right side the joint
has been opened by a coronal section. Note the articular disc.

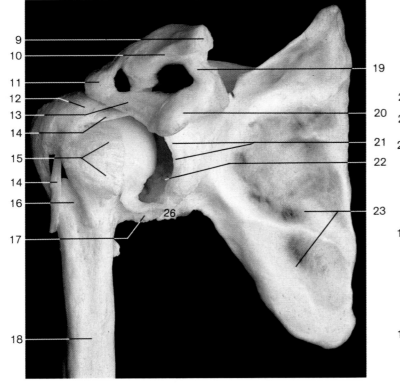

**Right shoulder joint.** The anterior part of the articular capsule has
been removed and the head of the humerus has been slightly
rotated outward to show the cavity of the joint.

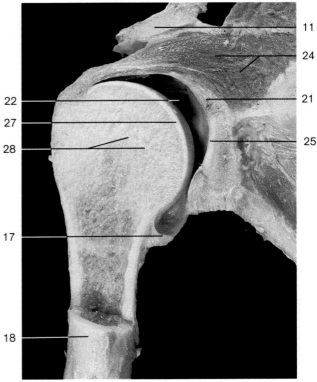

**Coronal section of the right shoulder joint**
(anterior aspect).

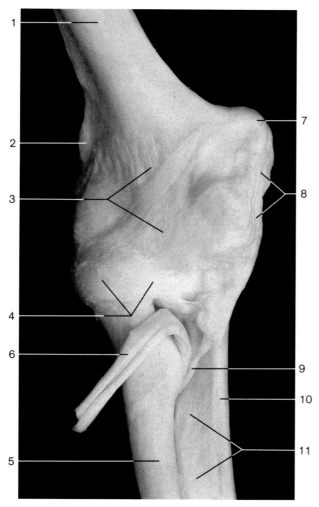

**Ligaments of elbow joint** (anterior aspect).

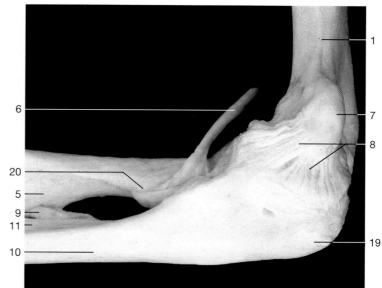

**Elbow joint with collateral ligaments** (medial aspect).

| | | | |
|---|---|---|---|
| 1 | Humerus | 11 | Interosseous membrane |
| 2 | Lateral epicondyle of humerus | 12 | Radial fossa |
| 3 | Articular capsule | 13 | Capitulum of humerus |
| 4 | Anular ligament of proximal radio-ulnar joint | 14 | Head of radius |
| 5 | Radius | 15 | Radial collateral ligament |
| 6 | Tendon of biceps brachii muscle | 16 | Coronoid fossa |
| 7 | Medial epicondyle of humerus | 17 | Trochlea of humerus |
| 8 | Ulnar collateral ligament | 18 | Coronoid process of ulna |
| 9 | Oblique chord | 19 | Olecranon |
| 10 | Ulna | 20 | Radial tuberosity |

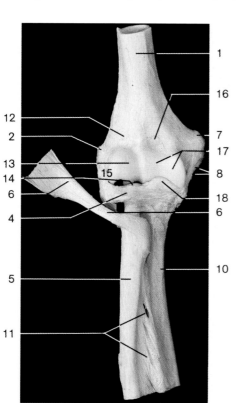

**Elbow joint with ligaments** (anterior aspect). Articular capsule has been removed to show the anular ligament.

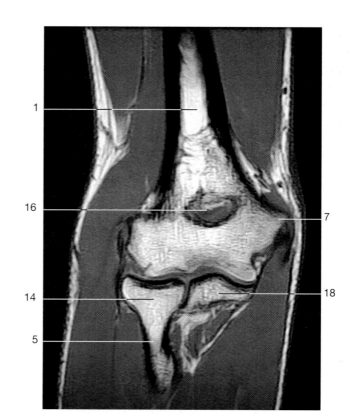

**Coronal section of elbow joint**
(MRI scan, courtesy of Prof. Dr. A. Heuck, Munich).

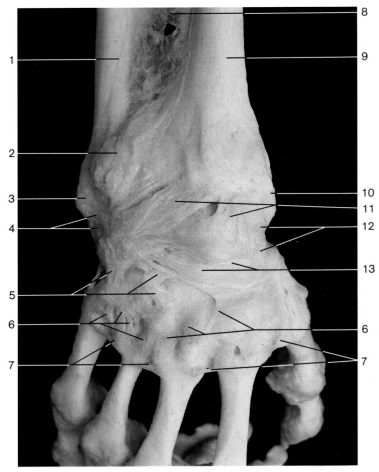

1   Ulna
2   Exostosis (pathological)
3   Head of ulna
4   Ulnar carpal collateral ligament
5   Deep intercarpal ligaments
6   Dorsal carpometacarpal ligaments
7   Dorsal metacarpal ligaments
8   Interosseous membrane
9   Radius
10  Styloid process of radius
11  Dorsal radiocarpal ligament
12  Radial collateral ligament
13  Articular capsule and dorsal intercarpal ligaments
14  Palmar radiocarpal ligament
15  Tendon of flexor carpi radialis muscle (cut)
16  Radiating carpal ligament
17  Palmar carpometacarpal ligaments
18  First metacarpal bone
19  Palmar ulnocarpal ligament
20  Tendon of flexor carpi ulnaris muscle (cut)
21  Pisohamate ligament
22  Pisometacarpal ligament
23  Palmar metacarpal ligaments
24  Fifth metacarpal bone

**Ligaments of hand and wrist** (dorsal aspect).

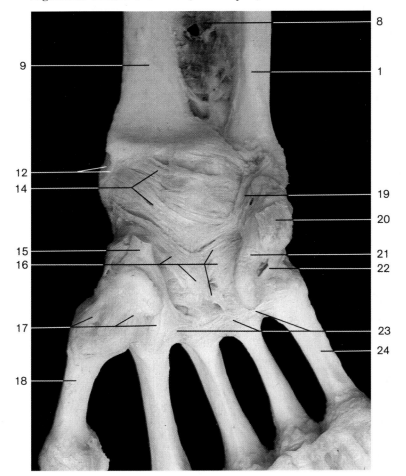

**Ligaments of hand and wrist** (palmar aspect).

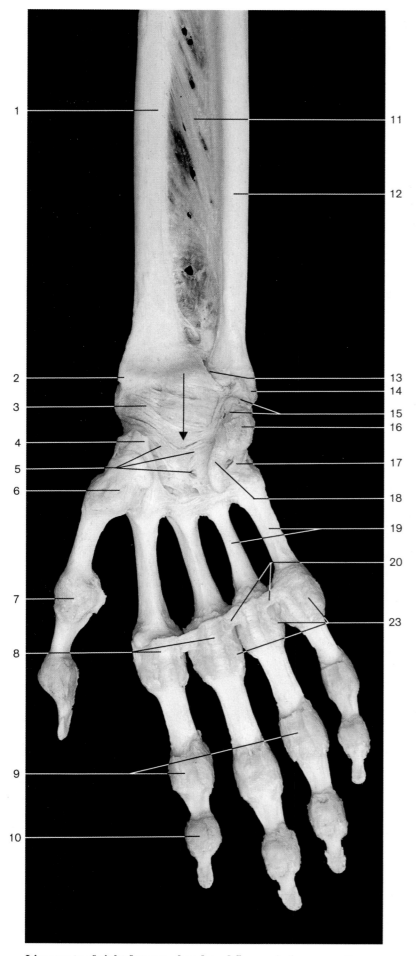

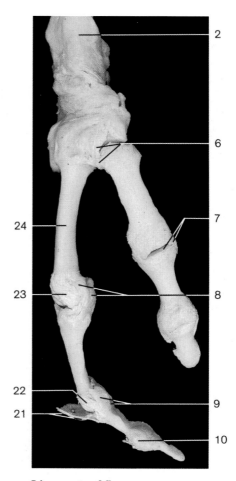

1  Radius
2  Styloid process of radius
3  Palmar radiocarpal ligament
4  Tendon of flexor carpi radialis muscle (cut)
5  Radiating carpal ligament
6  Articular capsule of carpometacarpal
   joint of thumb
7  Articular capsule of metacarpophalangeal
   joint of thumb
8  Palmar ligaments and articular capsule
   of metacarpophalangeal joints
9  Palmar ligaments and articular capsule
   of interphalangeal joints
10  Articular capsule
11  Interosseous membrane
12  Ulna
13  Distal radio-ulnar joint
14  Styloid process of ulna
15  Palmar ulnocarpal ligament
16  Pisiform bone with tendon of flexor
    carpi ulnaris muscle
17  Pisometacarpal ligament
18  Pisohamate ligament
19  Metacarpal bone
20  Deep transverse metacarpal ligament
21  Tendons of extensor muscles and
    articular capsule
22  Collateral ligament of interphalangeal joint
23  Collateral ligaments of
    metacarpophalangeal joints
24  Second metacarpal bone

**Ligaments of right forearm, hand, and fingers** (palmar aspect).
The arrow indicates the location of the carpal tunnel.

**Ligaments of fingers**
(lateral aspect).

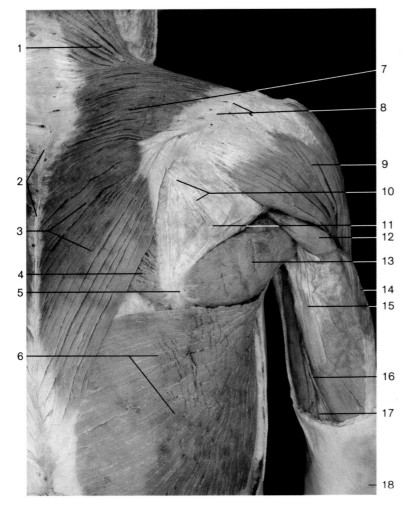

1   Descending fibers of trapezius muscle
2   Spinous processes of thoracic vertebrae
3   Ascending fibers of trapezius muscle
4   Rhomboid major muscle
5   Inferior angle of scapula
6   Latissimus dorsi muscle
7   Transverse fibers of trapezius muscle
8   Spine of scapula
9   Posterior fibers of deltoid muscle
10  Infraspinatus muscle and infraspinous fascia
11  Teres minor muscle and fascia
12  Long head of triceps brachii muscle
13  Teres major muscle
14  Lateral head of triceps brachii muscle
15  Medial head of triceps brachii muscle
16  Medial intermuscular septum
17  Ulnar nerve
18  Olecranon

**Muscles of shoulder and arm,** superficial layer (dorsal aspect).

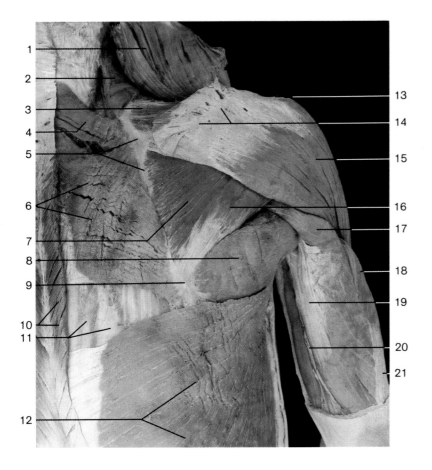

1   Trapezius muscle (reflected)
2   Levator scapulae muscle
3   Supraspinatus muscle
4   Rhomboid minor muscle
5   Medial border of scapula
6   Rhomboid major muscle
7   Infraspinatus muscle
8   Teres major muscle
9   Inferior angle of scapula
10  Cut edge of trapezius muscle
11  Intrinsic muscles of back with fascia
12  Latissimus dorsi muscle
13  Acromion
14  Spine of scapula
15  Deltoid muscle
16  Teres minor muscle
17  Long head of triceps brachii muscle
18  Lateral head of triceps brachii muscle
19  Medial head of triceps brachii muscle
20  Medial intermuscular septum
21  Tendon of triceps brachii muscle

**Muscles of shoulder and arm,** deeper layer (right side, dorsal aspect). The trapezius muscle has been cut near its origin at the vertebral column and reflected upward.

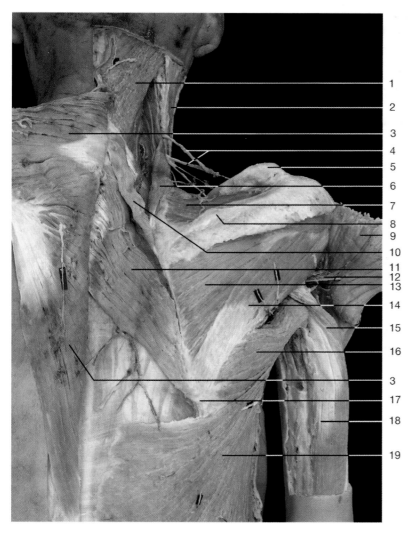

1  Splenius capitis muscle
2  Sternocleidomastoid muscle
3  Trapezius muscle (reflected)
4  Lateral supraclavicular nerves
5  Clavicle
6  Levator scapulae muscle
7  Supraspinatus muscle
8  Spine of scapula
9  Deltoid muscle (reflected)
10  Rhomboid minor muscle
11  Rhomboid major muscle
12  Axillary nerve and posterior
    circumflex humeral artery
13  Infraspinatus muscle
14  Teres minor muscle
15  Long head of triceps brachii muscle
16  Teres major muscle
17  Inferior angle of scapula
18  Triceps brachii muscle
19  Latissimus dorsi muscle

**Muscles of shoulder and arm,** deeper layer, right side (dorsal aspect).
The trapezius and deltoid muscles have been divided and reflected.

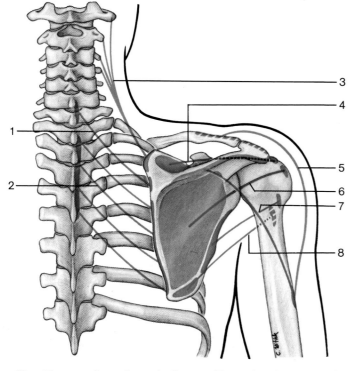

**Shoulder muscles,** schematic diagram illustrating the course of
the main muscles of the dorsal aspect of the shoulder.

1  Rhomboid minor muscle (red)
2  Rhomboid major muscle (red)
3  Levator scapulae muscle (red)
4  Supraspinatus muscle (blue)
5  Deltoid muscle (red)
6  Infraspinatus muscle (blue)
7  Teres minor muscle (red)
8  Teres major muscle (red)

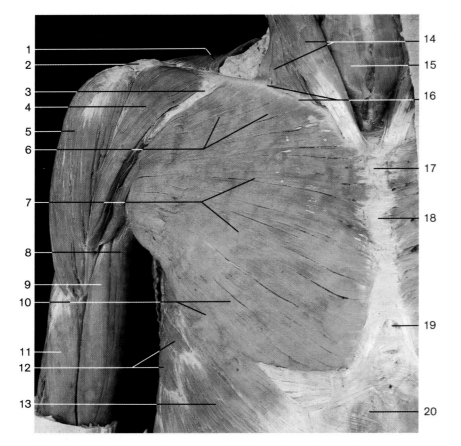

1   Trapezius muscle
2   Acromion
3   Deltopectoral triangle
4   Clavicular part of deltoid muscle
    (anterior fibers)
5   Acromial part of deltoid muscle
    (central fibers)
6   Clavicular part of pectoralis major muscle
7   Sternocostal part of pectoralis major muscle
8   Short head of biceps brachii muscle
9   Long head of biceps brachii muscle
10  Abdominal part of pectoralis major muscle
11  Brachialis muscle
12  Serratus anterior muscle
13  External abdominal oblique muscle
14  Sternocleidomastoid muscle
15  Infrahyoid muscles
16  Clavicle
17  Manubrium sterni
18  Body of sternum
19  Xiphoid process
20  Anterior layer of sheath of rectus
    abdominis muscle

**Muscles of shoulder and arm,** superficial layer (ventral aspect).

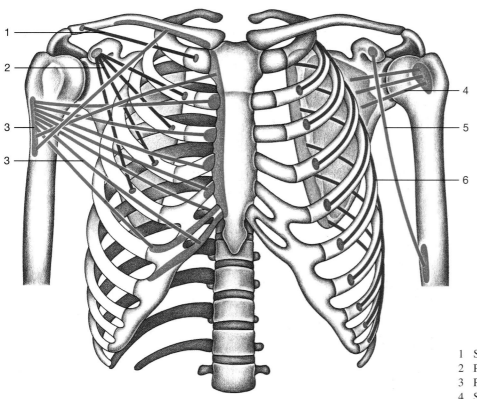

**Arrangement of pectoral and shoulder muscles** (ventral aspect).
(Schematic drawing.)

1   Subclavius muscle (blue)
2   Pectoralis minor muscle (blue)
3   Pectoralis major muscle (red)
4   Subscapularis muscle (red)
5   Coracobrachialis muscle (red)
6   Serratus anterior muscle (green)

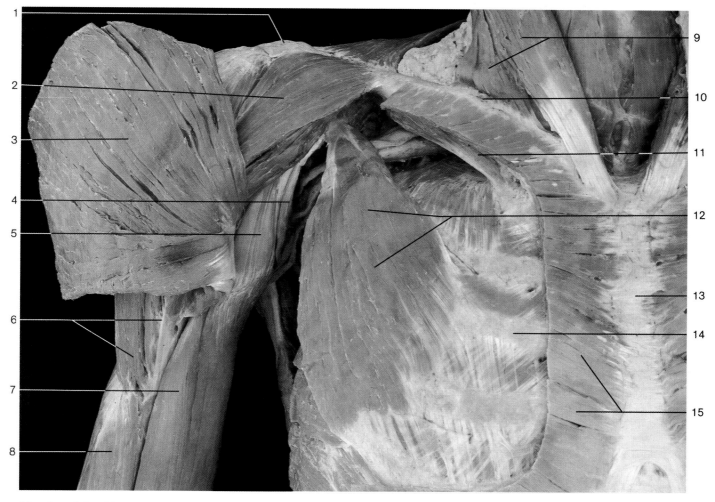

**Muscles of shoulder and arm,** deep layer (ventral aspect).

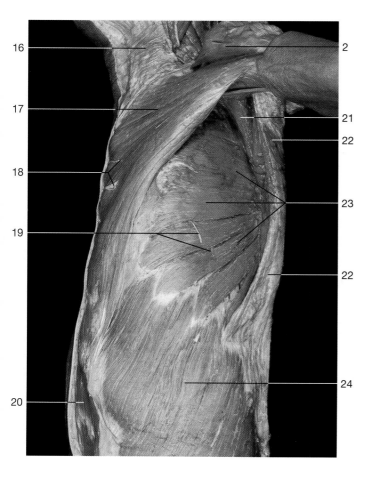

1  Acromion
2  Clavicular part of deltoid muscle
3  Pectoralis major muscle (reflected)
4  Coracobrachialis muscle
5  Short head of biceps brachii muscle
6  Deltoid muscle (insertion on humerus)
7  Long head of biceps brachii muscle
8  Brachialis muscle
9  Sternocleidomastoid muscle
10  Clavicle
11  Subclavius muscle
12  Pectoralis minor muscle
13  Sternum
14  Third rib
15  Pectoralis major muscle
16  Platysma muscle
17  Pectoralis major muscle forming the anterior axillary fold
18  Anterior cutaneous branches of intercostal nerves
19  Lateral cutaneous branches of intercostal nerves
20  Rectus abdominis muscle
21  Subscapularis muscle
22  Latissimus dorsi muscle forming the posterior axillary fold
23  Serratus anterior muscle forming the medial wall of the axilla
24  External abdominal oblique muscle

**Axillary fossa and serratus anterior muscle**
(left side, lateral aspect).

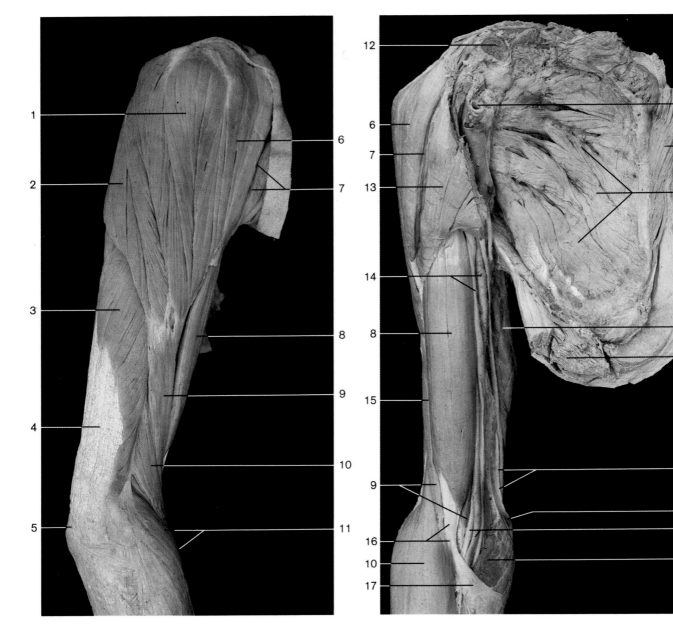

**Muscles of right arm** (lateral aspect).

**Muscles of right arm** (ventral aspect). The arm with the scapula and attached muscles has been removed from the trunk.

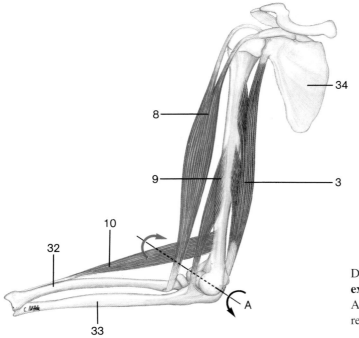

Diagram illustrating the position of the **flexor and extensor muscles of the arm** and their effect on the elbow joint. A = axis; arrows = direction of movements; red = flexion; black = extension.

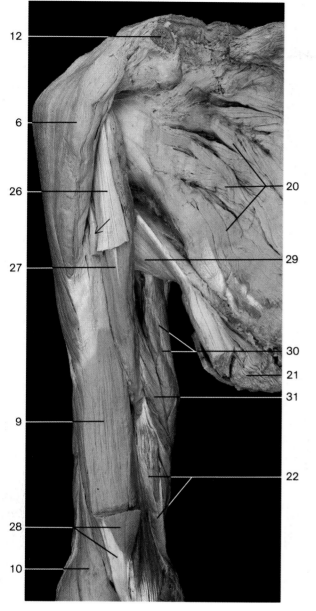

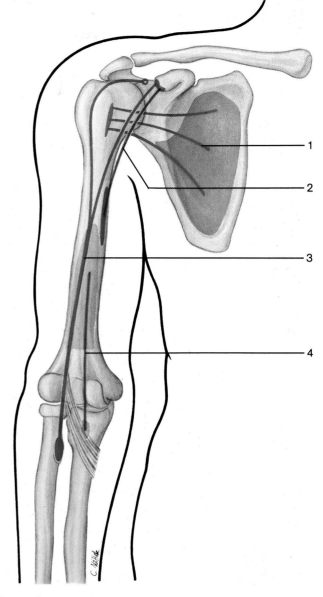

**Flexor muscles of right arm** (ventral aspect).
Part of the biceps brachii muscle has been
removed. Arrow: tendon of long head of biceps
brachii muscle.

**Position and course of flexors of arm** (schematic drawing).

1    Subscapularis muscle (red)
2    Coracobrachialis muscle (blue)
3    Biceps brachii muscle (red)
4    Brachialis muscle (blue)

| | |
|---|---|
| 1    Acromial part of deltoid muscle (central fibers) | 18    Axillary artery |
| 2    Scapular part of deltoid muscle (posterior fibers) | 19    Rhomboid major muscle |
| 3    Triceps brachii muscle | 20    Subscapularis muscle |
| 4    Tendon of triceps brachii muscle | 21    Latissimus dorsi muscle (divided) |
| 5    Olecranon | 22    Medial intermuscular septum |
| 6    Clavicular part of deltoid muscle (anterior fibers) | 23    Medial epicondyle of humerus |
| 7    Deltopectoral groove | 24    Brachial artery and median nerve |
| 8    Biceps brachii muscle | 25    Pronator teres muscle |
| 9    Brachialis muscle | 26    Tendon of short head of biceps brachii muscle |
| 10    Brachioradialis muscle | 27    Coracobrachialis muscle |
| 11    Extensor carpi radialis longus muscle | 28    Distal part of biceps brachii muscle |
| 12    Clavicle (divided) | 29    Teres major muscle |
| 13    Pectoralis major muscle | 30    Long head of triceps brachii muscle |
| 14    Medial intermuscular septum with vessels and nerves | 31    Medial head of triceps brachii muscle |
| 15    Lateral intermuscular septum | 32    Radius |
| 16    Tendon of biceps brachii muscle | 33    Ulna |
| 17    Bicipital aponeurosis | 34    Scapula |

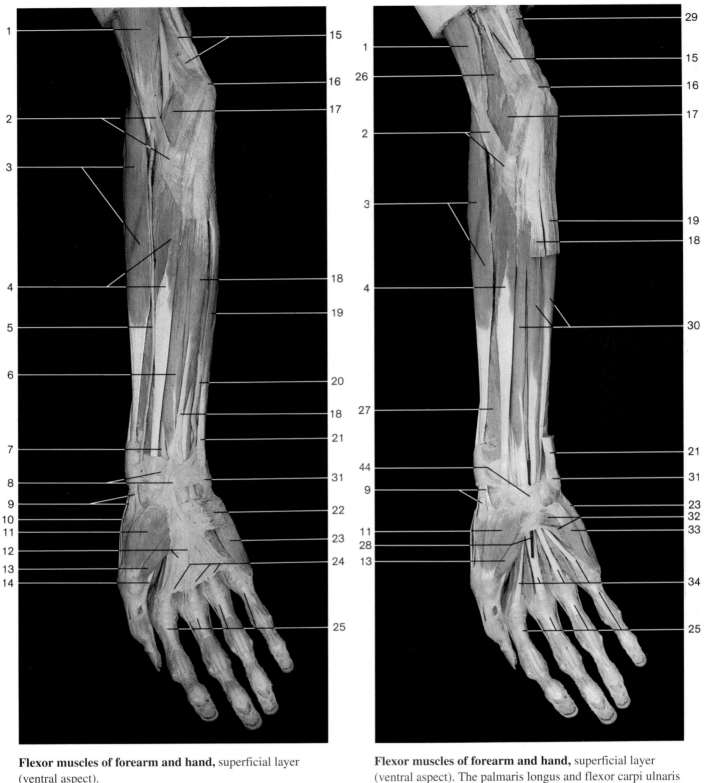

**Flexor muscles of forearm and hand,** superficial layer (ventral aspect).

**Flexor muscles of forearm and hand,** superficial layer (ventral aspect). The palmaris longus and flexor carpi ulnaris muscles have been removed.

1   Biceps brachii muscle
2   Bicipital aponeurosis
3   Brachioradialis muscle
4   Flexor carpi radialis muscle
5   Radial artery
6   Flexor digitorum superficialis muscle
7   Median nerve
8   Antebrachial fascia and tendon of palmaris longus muscle
9   Tendon of abductor pollicis longus muscle
10  Tendon of extensor pollicis brevis muscle
11  Abductor pollicis brevis muscle

12  Palmar aponeurosis
13  Superficial head of flexor pollicis brevis muscle
14  Tendon of flexor pollicis longus muscle
15  Medial intermuscular septum
16  Medial epicondyle of humerus
17  Humeral head of pronator teres muscle
18  Palmaris longus muscle
19  Flexor carpi ulnaris muscle
20  Ulnar artery
21  Tendon of flexor carpi ulnaris muscle
22  Palmaris brevis muscle

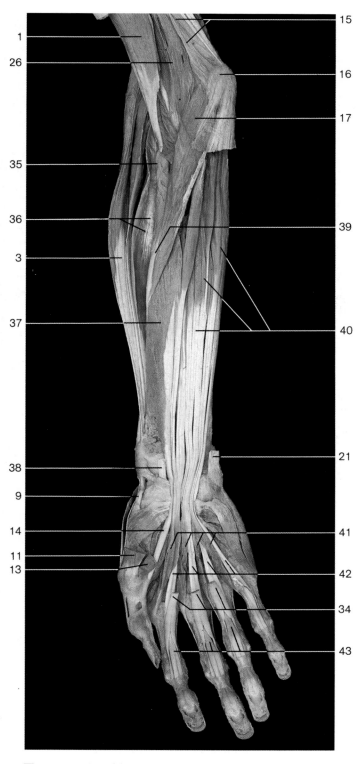

**Flexor muscles of forearm and hand,** middle layer (ventral aspect). The palmaris longus, flexor carpi radialis, and ulnaris muscles have been removed. The flexor retinaculum has been divided.

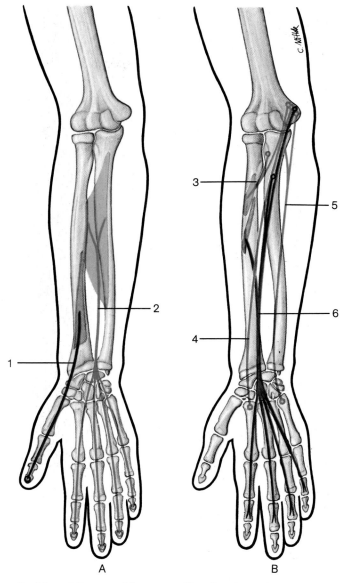

**Position of flexors of fingers and hand** (schematic drawing).

A   Deep layer
B   Superficial layer

1   Flexor pollicis longus muscle (blue)
2   Flexor digitorum profundus muscle (red)
3   Pronator teres muscle (red)
4   Flexor carpi radialis muscle (red)
5   Flexor carpi ulnaris muscle (red)
6   Flexor digitorum superficialis muscle (blue)

23   Abductor digiti minimi muscle
24   Transverse fasciculi of palmar aponeurosis
25   Digital fibrous sheaths of tendons of flexor digitorum muscle
26   Brachialis muscle
27   Flexor pollicis longus muscle
28   Carpal tunnel (canalis carpi, probe)
29   Triceps brachii muscle
30   Flexor digitorum superficialis muscle
31   Pisiform bone
32   Opponens digiti minimi muscle
33   Flexor digiti minimi brevis muscle
34   Tendons of flexor digitorum superficialis muscle

35   Supinator muscle
36   Extensor carpi radialis brevis muscle
37   Flexor pollicis longus muscle
38   Tendon of flexor carpi radialis muscle
39   Pronator teres muscle (insertion of radius)
40   Flexor digitorum profundus muscle
41   Lumbrical muscles
42   Tendons of flexor digitorum profundus muscle
43   Tendons of flexor digitorum profundus muscle having passed through the divided tendons of the flexor digitorum superficialis muscle
44   Flexor retinaculum

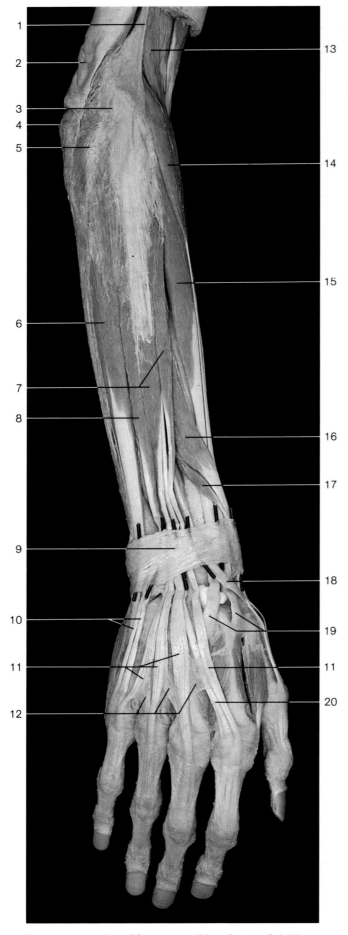

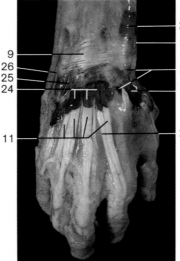

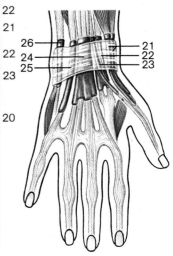

**Synovial sheaths of extensor tendons.** The sheaths have been injected with blue gelatin.

**Synovial sheaths of extensor tendons** on the back of the right wrist (indicated in blue). Notice the six tunnels for the passage of the extensor tendons beneath the extensor retinaculum (semischematic drawing).

1   Lateral intermuscular septum
2   Tendon of triceps brachii muscle
3   Lateral epicondyle of humerus
4   Olecranon
5   Anconeus muscle
6   Extensor carpi ulnaris muscle
7   Extensor digitorum muscle
8   Extensor digiti minimi muscle
9   Extensor retinaculum
10  Tendons of extensor digiti minimi muscle
11  Tendons of extensor digitorum muscle
12  Intertendinous connections
13  Brachioradialis muscle
14  Extensor carpi radialis longus muscle
15  Extensor carpi radialis brevis muscle
16  Abductor pollicis longus muscle
17  Extensor pollicis brevis muscle
18  Tendon of extensor pollicis longus muscle
19  Tendons of both extensor carpi radialis longus
    and extensor carpi radialis brevis muscles
20  Tendon of extensor indicis muscle
21  First tunnel:    Abductor pollicis longus muscle
                     Extensor pollicis brevis muscle
22  Second tunnel: Extensor carpi radialis longus and brevis muscles
23  Third tunnel:    Extensor pollicis longus muscle
24  Fourth tunnel:   Extensor digitorum muscle
                     Extensor indicis muscle
25  Fifth tunnel:    Extensor digiti minimi muscle
26  Sixth tunnel:    Extensor carpi ulnaris muscle

**Extensor muscles of forearm and hand,** superficial layer (dorsal aspect). Tunnels for extensor tendons indicated by probes.

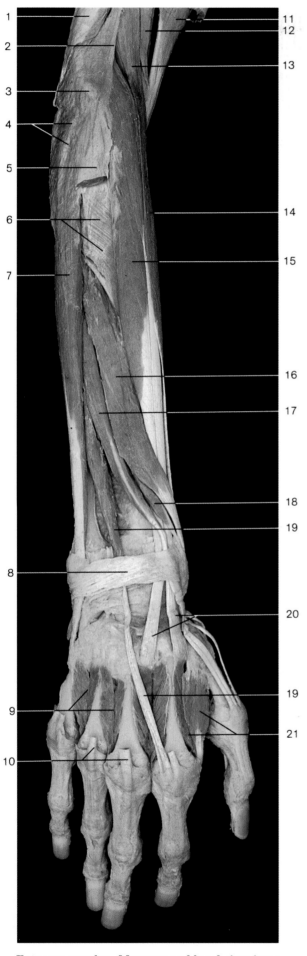

1   Triceps brachii muscle
2   Lateral intermuscular septum
3   Lateral epicondyle of humerus
4   Anconeus muscle
5   Extensor digitorum and extensor digiti minimi muscles (cut)
6   Supinator muscle
7   Extensor carpi ulnaris muscle
8   Extensor retinaculum
9   Third and fourth dorsal interosseous muscles
10  Tendons of extensor digitorum muscle (cut)
11  Biceps brachii muscle
12  Brachialis muscle
13  Brachioradialis muscle
14  Extensor carpi radialis longus muscle
15  Extensor carpi radialis brevis muscle
16  Abductor pollicis longus muscle
17  Extensor pollicis longus muscle
18  Extensor pollicis brevis muscle
19  Extensor indicis muscle
20  Tendons of the extensor carpi radialis longus
    and extensor carpi radialis brevis muscles
21  First dorsal interosseous muscle

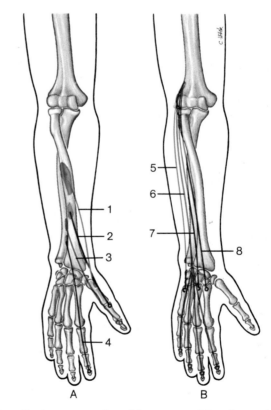

**Position of extensor muscles of forearm and hand**
(semischematic drawing).

**Extensor muscles of forearm and hand,** deep layer
(dorsal aspect).

A  Extensors of thumb

1   Abductor pollicis longus muscle
    (red)
2   Extensor pollicis brevis muscle
    (blue)
3   Extensor pollicis longus muscle
    (red)
4   Extensor indicis muscle
    (blue)

B  Extensors of fingers and hand

5   Extensor carpi ulnaris muscle
    (blue)
6   Extensor digitorum muscle
    (red)
7   Extensor carpi radialis brevis
    muscle (blue)
8   Extensor carpi radialis longus
    muscle (blue)

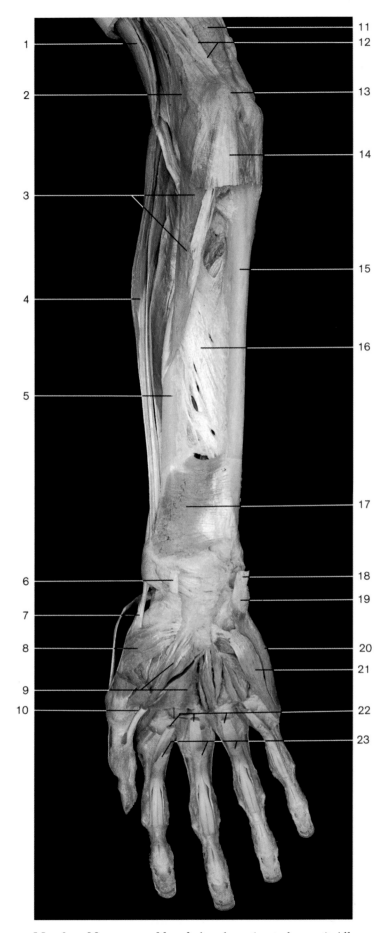

1   Biceps brachii muscle
2   Brachialis muscle
3   Pronator teres muscle
4   Brachioradialis muscle
5   Radius
6   Tendon of flexor carpi radialis muscle
7   Tendon of abductor pollicis longus muscle
8   Opponens pollicis muscle
9   Adductor pollicis muscle
10  Tendon of flexor pollicis longus muscle
11  Triceps brachii muscle
12  Medial intermuscular septum
13  Medial epicondyle of humerus
14  Common flexor mass (divided)
15  Ulna
16  Interosseous membrane
17  Pronator quadratus muscle
18  Tendon of flexor carpi ulnaris muscle
19  Pisiform bone
20  Abductor digiti minimi muscle
21  Flexor digiti minimi brevis muscle
22  Tendons of flexor digitorum profundus muscle
23  Tendons of flexor digitorum superficialis muscle
24  Flexor retinaculum
25  Hypothenar muscles
26  Thenar muscles
27  Common synovial sheath of flexor tendons
28  Synovial sheath of tendon of flexor pollicis longus muscle
29  Digital synovial sheaths of flexor tendons

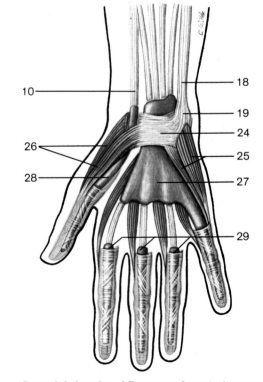

**Muscles of forearm and hand,** deep layer (ventral aspect). All flexors have been removed to display the pronator quadratus and pronator teres muscles together with the interosseous membrane. Forearm in supination.

**Synovial sheaths of flexor tendons** (palmar aspect of right hand). (Semischematic drawing.)

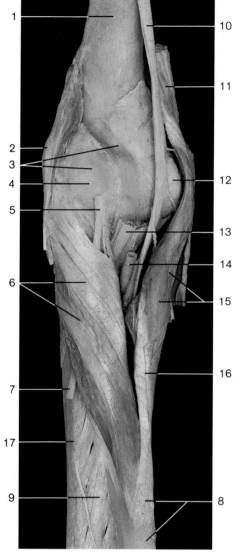

**Right supinator and elbow joint**
(anterior aspect). Forearm in pronation.

1   Humerus
2   Lateral epicondyle of humerus
3   Articular capsule
4   Position of capitulum of humerus
5   Deep branch of radial nerve
6   Supinator muscle
7   Entrance of deep branch of radial nerve to extensor muscles
8   Radius and insertion of pronator teres muscle
9   Interosseous membrane
10  Median nerve
11  Triceps brachii muscle
12  Trochlea of humerus
13  Tendon of biceps brachii muscle
14  Brachial artery
15  Pronator teres muscle
16  Tendon of pronator teres muscle
17  Ulna
18  Pronator quadratus muscle
19  Tendon of flexor carpi radialis muscle
20  Thenar muscles
21  Synovial sheath of tendon of flexor pollicis longus muscle
22  Fibrous sheath of flexor tendons
23  Digital synovial sheath of flexor tendons
24  Flexor digitorum superficialis muscle
25  Tendon of flexor carpi ulnaris muscle
26  Common synovial sheath of flexor tendons
27  Position of pisiform bone
28  Flexor retinaculum
29  Hypothenar muscles

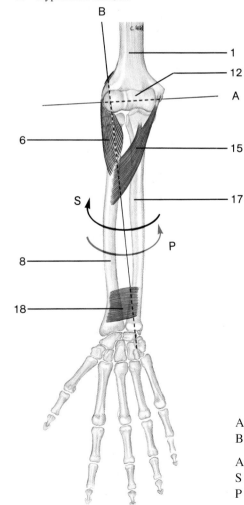

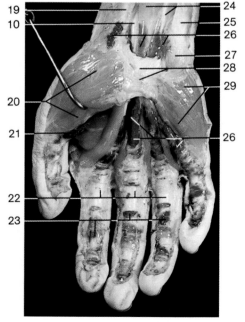

**Synovial sheaths of flexor tendons**
(palmar aspect of right hand). Blue PVA
solution has been injected into the sheaths.

A   Axis of flexion and extension
B   Axis of rotation

Arrows:
S   Supination
P   Pronation

Diagram illustrating the **two axes of the elbow joint.**

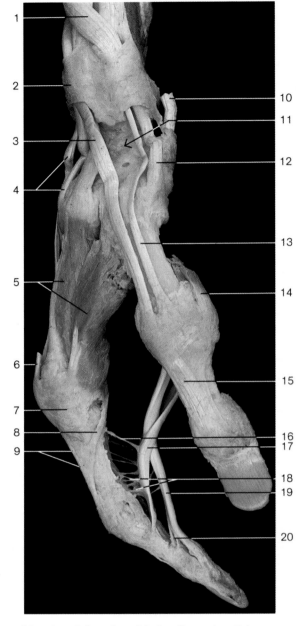

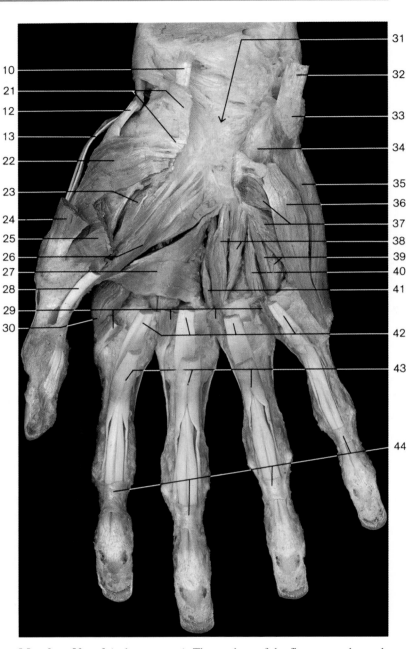

**Muscles of thumb and index finger** (medial aspect). The tendons of the extensor muscles of the thumb and the insertion of the flexor tendons of the index finger are displayed.

**Muscles of hand** (palmar aspect). The tendons of the flexor muscles and parts of the thumb muscles have been removed. The carpal tunnel has been opened.

1  Tendons of extensor pollicis brevis and abductor pollicis longus muscle
2  Extensor retinaculum
3  Tendon of extensor pollicis longus muscle
4  Tendons of extensor carpi radialis longus and brevis muscles
5  First dorsal interosseous muscle
6  Tendon of extensor digitorum muscle for index finger
7  Location of metacarpophalangeal joint
8  Tendon of lumbrical muscle
9  Extensor expansion of index finger
10  Tendon of flexor carpi radialis muscle (cut)
11  Anatomical snuffbox
12  Tendon of abductor pollicis longus muscle
13  Tendon of extensor pollicis brevis muscle
14  Tendon of abductor pollicis brevis muscle

15  Extensor expansion of extensor of thumb
16  Vinculum longum
17  Tendons of flexor digitorum superficialis muscle dividing to allow passage of deep tendons
18  Vincula of flexor tendons
19  Tendon of flexor digitorum profundus muscle
20  Vinculum breve
21  Radial carpal eminence (cut edge of flexor retinaculum)
22  Opponens pollicis muscle
23  Deep head of flexor pollicis brevis muscle
24  Abductor pollicis brevis muscle (cut)
25  Superficial head of flexor pollicis brevis muscle (cut)
26  Oblique head of adductor pollicis muscle
27  Transverse head of adductor pollicis muscle
28  Tendon of flexor pollicis longus muscle (cut)

29  Lumbrical muscles (cut)
30  First dorsal interosseous muscle
31  Position of carpal tunnel
32  Tendon of flexor carpi ulnaris muscle
33  Location of pisiform bone
34  Hook of hamate bone
35  Abductor digiti minimi muscle
36  Flexor digiti minimi brevis muscle
37  Opponens digiti minimi muscle
38  Second palmar interosseous muscle
39  Third palmar interosseous muscle
40  Fourth dorsal interosseous muscle
41  Third dorsal interosseous muscle
42  Tendon of flexor digitorum profundus muscle (cut)
43  Tendons of flexor digitorum superficialis muscle (cut)
44  Fibrous flexor sheaths

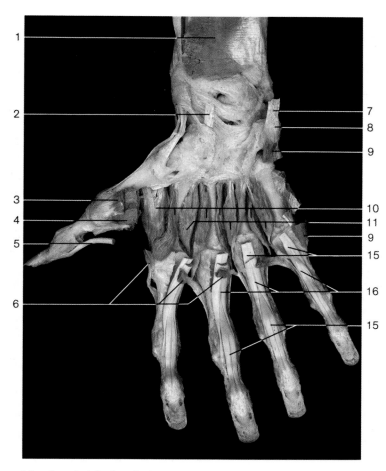

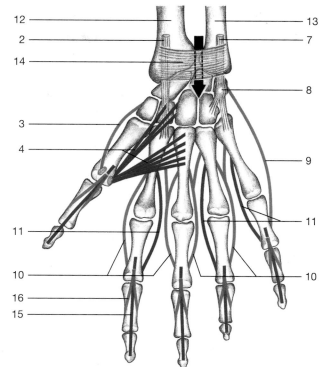

**Muscles of right hand,** deep layer (palmar aspect). The thenar and hypothenar muscles have been removed to display the interosseous muscles.

**Actions of interosseous muscles** in abduction and adduction of fingers (palmar aspect).
(Schematic drawing.) Arrow: carpal tunnel.
Red = abduction
(dorsal interosseous, abductor digiti minimi, and abductor pollicis brevis muscles).
Blue = adduction
(palmar interosseous muscles, adductor pollicis muscle).

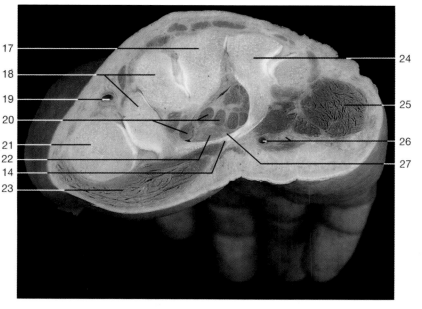

**Transverse section through the right hand,** showing the carpal tunnel (canalis carpi).

1   Pronator quadratus muscle
2   Tendon of flexor carpi radialis muscle
3   Abductor pollicis brevis muscle (divided)
4   Adductor pollicis muscle (divided)
5   Tendon of flexor pollicis longus muscle
6   Lumbrical muscles (cut)
7   Tendon of flexor carpi ulnaris muscle
8   Pisiform bone
9   Abductor digiti minimi muscle (divided)
10  Dorsal interosseous muscles
11  Palmar interosseous muscles
12  Radius
13  Ulna
14  Flexor retinaculum
15  Tendons of flexor digitorum
    profundus muscle
16  Tendons of flexor digitorum
    superficialis muscle
17  Capitate bone
18  Trapezium bone and trapezoid bone
19  Radial artery
20  Tendon of flexor muscles
21  First metacarpal bone
22  Median nerve
23  Thenar muscles
24  Hamate bone
25  Hypothenar muscles
26  Ulnar artery and nerve
27  Carpal tunnel (canalis carpi)

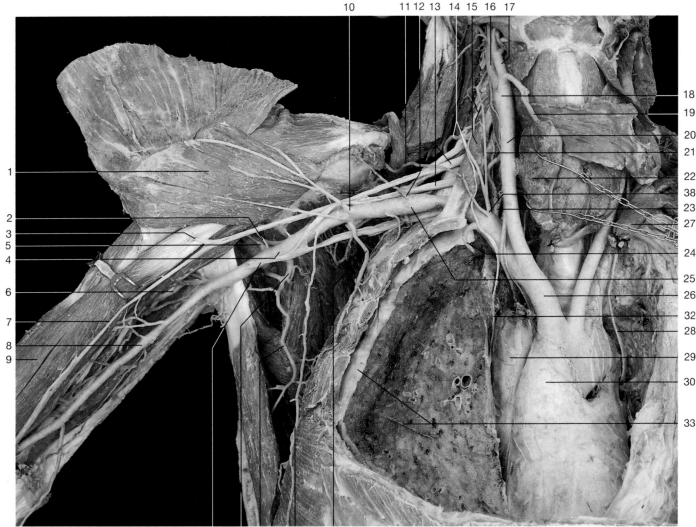

**Main branches of right subclavian and axillary arteries** (anterior aspect). Pectoralis muscles have been reflected, clavicle and anterior wall of thorax removed, and right lung divided. Left lung with pleura and thyroid gland have been reflected laterally to display aortic arch and common carotid artery with their branches.

| | | |
|---|---|---|
| 1 Pectoralis minor muscle (reflected) | 22 Thyroid gland | 43 Radial collateral artery |
| 2 Anterior circumflex humeral artery | 23 Inferior thyroid artery | 44 Radial recurrent artery |
| 3 Musculocutaneous nerve (divided) | 24 Internal thoracic artery | 45 Radial artery |
| 4 Axillary artery | 25 Right subclavian artery | 46 Anterior and posterior interosseous |
| 5 Posterior circumflex humeral artery | 26 Brachiocephalic trunk | arteries |
| 6 Profunda brachii artery | 27 Left brachiocephalic vein (divided) | 47 Princeps pollicis artery |
| 7 Median nerve (var.) | 28 Left vagus nerve | 48 Deep palmar arch |
| 8 Brachial artery | 29 Superior vena cava (divided) | 49 Common palmar digital arteries |
| 9 Biceps brachii muscle | 30 Ascending aorta | 50 Ulnar recurrent artery |
| 10 Thoraco-acromial artery | 31 Median nerve (divided) | 51 Recurrent interosseous artery |
| 11 Suprascapular artery | 32 Phrenic nerve | 52 Common interosseous artery |
| 12 Descending scapular artery | 33 Right lung (divided) and pulmonary pleura | 53 Ulnar artery |
| 13 Brachial plexus (middle trunk) | 34 Thoracodorsal artery | 54 Superficial palmar arch |
| 14 Transverse cervical artery | 35 Subscapular artery | 55 Median nerve and brachial artery |
| 15 Scalenus anterior muscle and phrenic nerve | 36 Lateral mammary branches (variant) | 56 Biceps brachii muscle |
| 16 Right internal carotid artery | 37 Lateral thoracic artery | 57 Ulnar nerve |
| 17 Right external carotid artery | 38 Thyrocervical trunk | 58 Flexor pollicis longus muscle |
| 18 Carotid sinus | 39 Superior thoracic artery | 59 Palmar digital arteries |
| 19 Superior thyroid artery | 40 Superior ulnar collateral artery | 60 Anterior interosseous artery |
| 20 Right common carotid artery | 41 Inferior ulnar collateral artery | 61 Flexor carpi ulnaris muscle |
| 21 Ascending cervical artery | 42 Middle collateral artery | 62 Superficial palmar branch of radial artery |

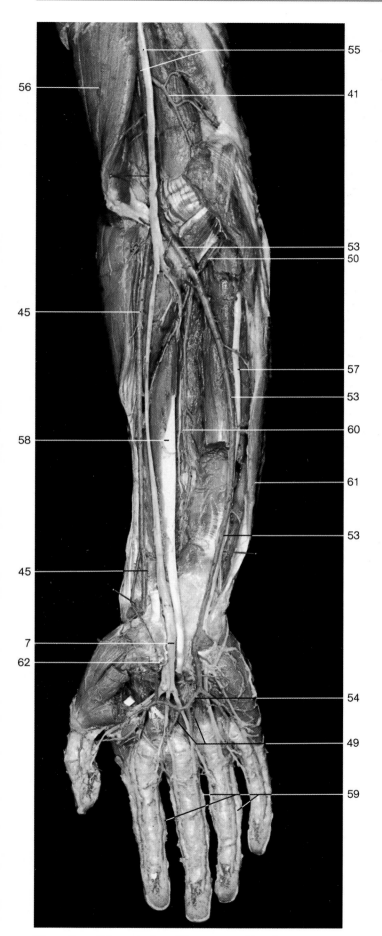

55
41
56
53
50
45
57
53
60
58
61
53
45
7
62
54
49
59

**Dissection of the arteries of forearm and hand.**
The superficial flexor muscles have been removed,
the carpal tunnel opened, and the flexor retinaculum cut.
The arteries have been filled with colored resin.

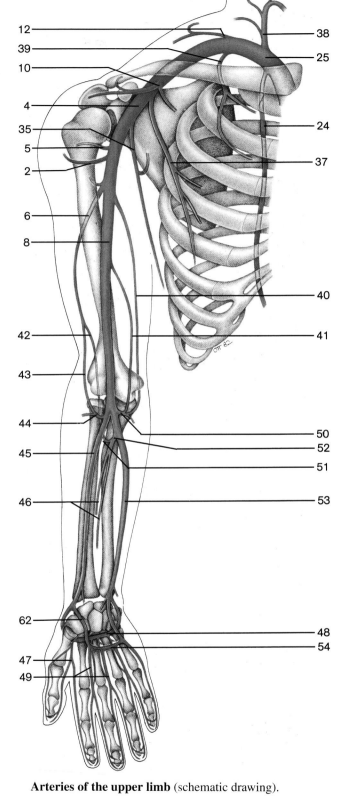

12
39
10
4
35
5
2
6
8
42
43
44
45
46
62
47
49

38
25
24
37
40
41
50
52
51
53
48
54

**Arteries of the upper limb** (schematic drawing).

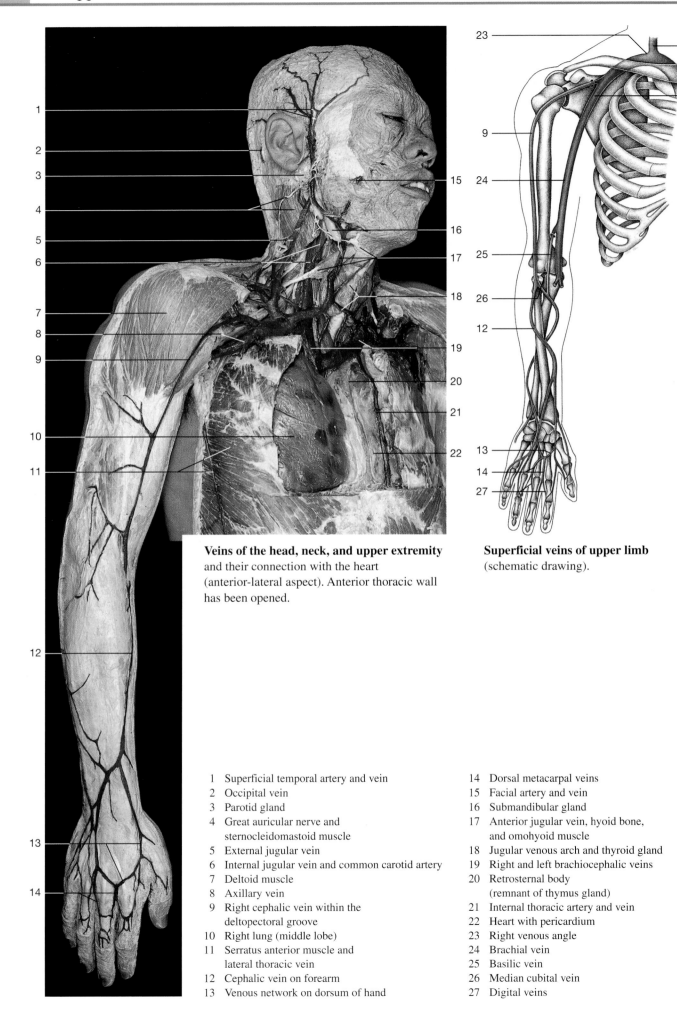

**Veins of the head, neck, and upper extremity** and their connection with the heart (anterior-lateral aspect). Anterior thoracic wall has been opened.

**Superficial veins of upper limb** (schematic drawing).

1  Superficial temporal artery and vein
2  Occipital vein
3  Parotid gland
4  Great auricular nerve and sternocleidomastoid muscle
5  External jugular vein
6  Internal jugular vein and common carotid artery
7  Deltoid muscle
8  Axillary vein
9  Right cephalic vein within the deltopectoral groove
10  Right lung (middle lobe)
11  Serratus anterior muscle and lateral thoracic vein
12  Cephalic vein on forearm
13  Venous network on dorsum of hand

14  Dorsal metacarpal veins
15  Facial artery and vein
16  Submandibular gland
17  Anterior jugular vein, hyoid bone, and omohyoid muscle
18  Jugular venous arch and thyroid gland
19  Right and left brachiocephalic veins
20  Retrosternal body (remnant of thymus gland)
21  Internal thoracic artery and vein
22  Heart with pericardium
23  Right venous angle
24  Brachial vein
25  Basilic vein
26  Median cubital vein
27  Digital veins

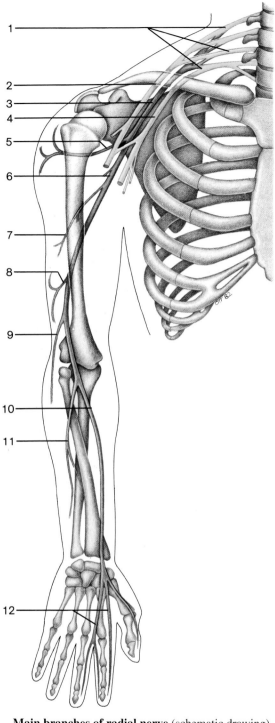

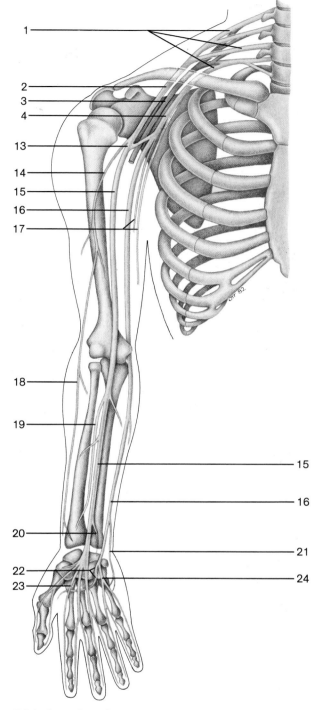

**Main branches of radial nerve** (schematic drawing).
Posterior divisions of trunks and posterior cord and
its branches are indicated in green.

**Main branches of musculocutaneous, median, and
ulnar nerves** (schematic drawing).
Anterior divisions of the trunks and all the components
arising from them are indicated in yellow.

| | |
|---|---|
| 1 Brachial plexus | 13 Roots of median nerve |
| 2 Lateral cord of brachial plexus | 14 Musculocutaneous nerve |
| 3 Posterior cord of brachial plexus | 15 Median nerve |
| 4 Medial cord of brachial plexus | 16 Ulnar nerve |
| 5 Axillary nerve | 17 Medial cutaneous nerves of arm and forearm |
| 6 Radial nerve | 18 Lateral cutaneous nerve of forearm |
| 7 Posterior cutaneous nerve of arm | 19 Anterior interosseous nerve |
| 8 Lower lateral cutaneous nerve of arm | 20 Palmar branch of median nerve |
| 9 Posterior cutaneous nerve of forearm | 21 Dorsal branch of ulnar nerve |
| 10 Superficial branch of radial nerve | 22 Deep branch of ulnar nerve |
| 11 Deep branch of radial nerve | 23 Common palmar digital nerves of median nerve |
| 12 Dorsal digital nerves | 24 Superficial branch of ulnar nerve |

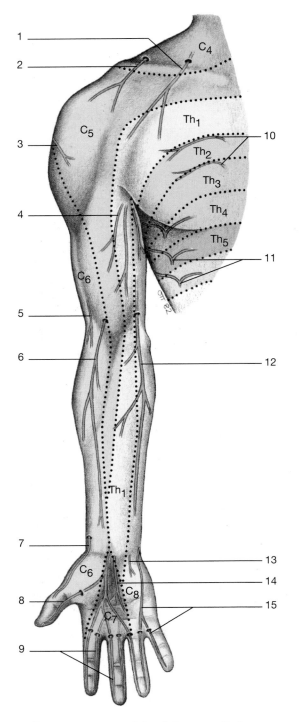

**Cutaneous nerves of the right upper limb**
(ventral aspect). (Semischematic drawing.)

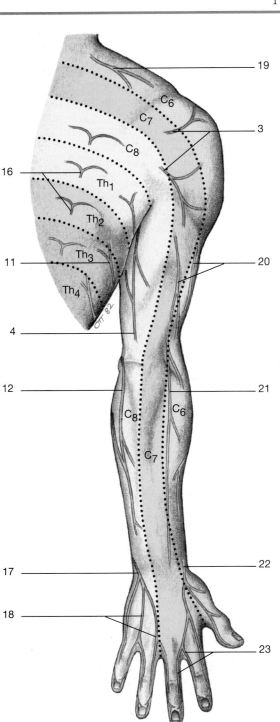

**Cutaneous nerves of the right upper limb**
(dorsal aspect). (Semischematic drawing.)

| | | | |
|---|---|---|---|
| 1 | Medial supraclavicular nerve | 13 | Palmar cutaneous branch of ulnar nerve |
| 2 | Intermediate supraclavicular nerve | 14 | Palmar branch of median nerve |
| 3 | Upper lateral cutaneous nerve of arm | 15 | Palmar digital branches of ulnar nerve |
| 4 | Terminal branches of intercostobrachial nerves | 16 | Cutaneous branches of dorsal rami of spinal nerves |
| 5 | Lower lateral cutaneous nerve of arm | 17 | Dorsal branch of ulnar nerve |
| 6 | Lateral cutaneous nerve of forearm | 18 | Dorsal digital nerves |
| 7 | Terminal branch of superficial branch of radial nerve | 19 | Posterior supraclavicular nerve |
| 8 | Palmar digital nerve of thumb (branch of median nerve) | 20 | Posterior cutaneous nerve of arm |
| 9 | Palmar digital branches of median nerve | 21 | Posterior cutaneous nerve of forearm |
| 10 | Anterior cutaneous branches of intercostal nerves | 22 | Superficial branch |
| 11 | Lateral cutaneous branches of intercostal nerves | 23 | Dorsal digital branches |
| 12 | Medial cutaneous nerve of forearm | | |

20–23 from radial nerve

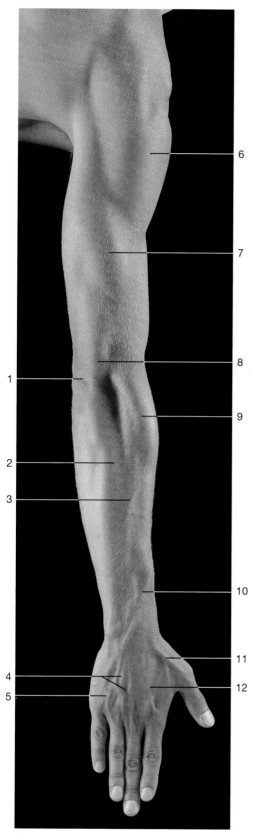

**Surface anatomy of the right arm, fore-arm, and hand** (dorsal aspect).

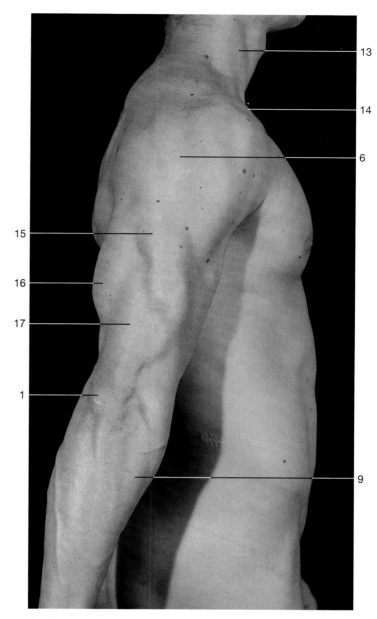

**Surface anatomy of the right arm** (lateral aspect).
Triceps brachii muscle is strongly contracted.

| | | | |
|---|---|---|---|
| 1 | Olecranon | 11 | Tendon of abductor pollicis longus muscle |
| 2 | Extensor muscles of forearm | | |
| 3 | Accessory cephalic vein | 12 | Tendon of extensor indicis muscle |
| 4 | Tendons of extensor digitorum muscle | 13 | Sternocleidomastoid muscle |
| 5 | Dorsal venous network of hand | 14 | Clavicle |
| | | 15 | Lateral head of triceps brachii muscle |
| 6 | Deltoid muscle | | |
| 7 | Triceps brachii muscle | 16 | Medial head of triceps brachii muscle |
| 8 | Lateral epicondyle of humerus | | |
| 9 | Brachioradialis muscle | 17 | Tendon of triceps brachii muscle |
| 10 | Cephalic vein | | |

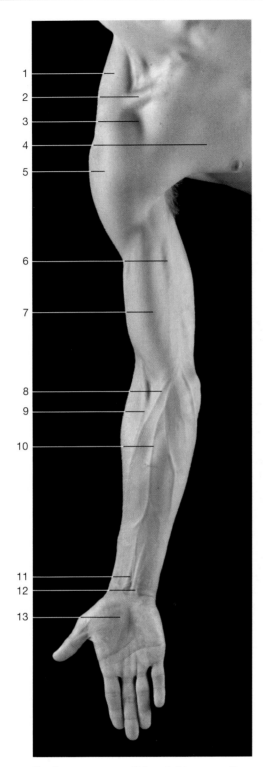

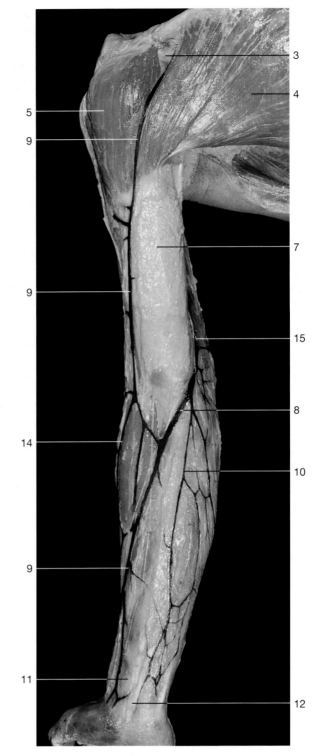

**Surface anatomy of the right arm and hand** (anterior aspect).

**Superficial veins of the right arm,** injected with blue gelatine (anterior aspect).

| | | | |
|---|---|---|---|
| 1 | Trapezius muscle | 8 | Median cubital vein |
| 2 | Clavicle | 9 | Cephalic vein |
| 3 | Deltopectoral triangle | 10 | Median vein of forearm |
| 4 | Pectoralis major muscle | 11 | Tendon of flexor carpi radialis |
| 5 | Deltoid muscle | 12 | Tendon of palmaris longus muscle |
| 6 | Brachial vein | 13 | Location of adductor pollicis muscle |
| 7 | Biceps brachii muscle | 14 | Accessory cephalic vein |
| | | 15 | Basilic vein |

crop1 crop2 crop3

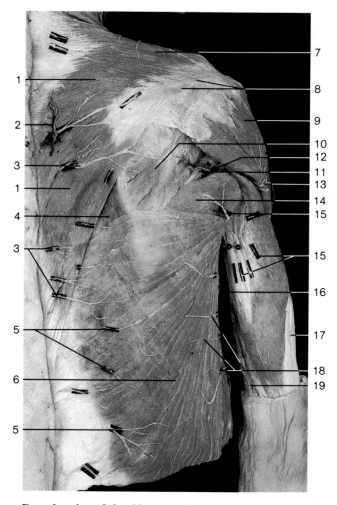

**Dorsal region of shoulder,** superficial layer. Note the segmental arrangement of the cutaneous nerves of the back.

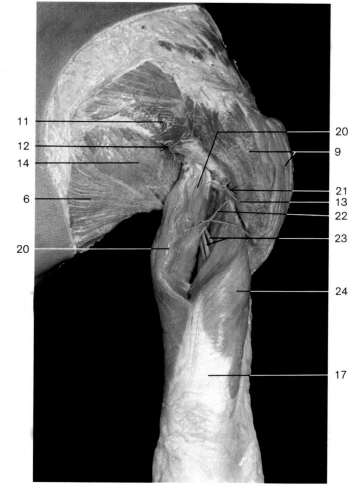

**Shoulder and arm** (dorsal aspect). Dissection of the quadrangular and triangular spaces of the axillary region.

1 Trapezius muscle
2 Dorsal branches of posterior intercostal artery and vein (medial cutaneous branches)
3 Medial branches of dorsal rami of spinal nerves
4 Rhomboid major muscle
5 Lateral branches of dorsal rami of spinal nerves
6 Latissimus dorsi muscle
7 Posterior supraclavicular nerves
8 Spine of scapula
9 Deltoid muscle
10 Infraspinatus muscle
11 Teres minor muscle
12 Triangular space with circumflex scapular artery and vein
13 Upper lateral cutaneous nerve of arm with artery
14 Teres major muscle
15 Terminal branches of intercostobrachial nerve
16 Medial cutaneous nerve of arm
17 Tendon of triceps brachii muscle
18 Lateral cutaneous branches of intercostal nerves
19 Medial cutaneous nerve of forearm
20 Long head of triceps brachii muscle
21 Quadrangular space with axillary nerve and posterior humeral circumflex artery
22 Anastomosis between profunda brachii artery and posterior humeral circumflex artery
23 Course of radial nerve and profunda brachii artery
24 Lateral head of triceps brachii muscle
25 Course of descending scapular artery and dorsal scapular nerve
26 Course of suprascapular nerve, artery, and vein

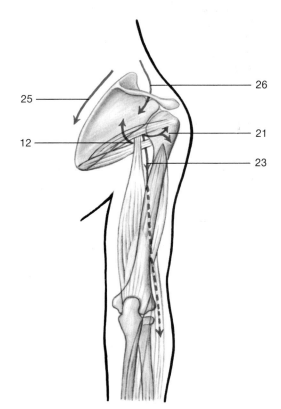

**Course of vessels and nerves to shoulder and upper limb** (schematic drawing).

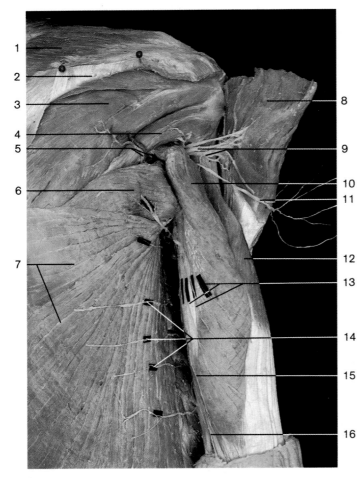

**Scapular region, arm and shoulder,** deep layer (dorsal aspect). Part of deltoid muscle has been cut and reflected to display the quadrangular and triangular spaces of the axillary region.

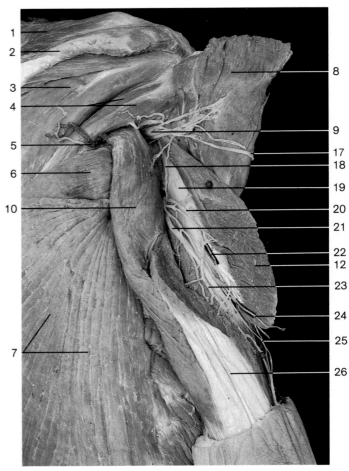

**Scapular region and posterior brachial region, arm and shoulder,** deep layer (dorsal aspect). The lateral head of the triceps brachii muscle has been cut to display the radial nerve and accompanying vessels.

1   Trapezius muscle
2   Spine of scapula
3   Infraspinatus muscle
4   Teres minor muscle
5   Triangular space containing circumflex scapular artery and vein
6   Teres major muscle
7   Latissimus dorsi muscle
8   Deltoid muscle (cut and reflected)
9   Quadrangular space containing axillary nerve and posterior circumflex humeral artery and vein
10  Long head of triceps brachii muscle
11  Cutaneous branch of axillary nerve
12  Lateral head of triceps brachii muscle
13  Terminal branches of intercostobrachial nerve

14  Lateral cutaneous branches of intercostal nerves
15  Medial cutaneous nerve of arm
16  Medial cutaneous nerve of forearm
17  Upper lateral cutaneous nerve of arm
18  Anastomosis between profunda brachii artery and posterior humeral circumflex artery
19  Humerus
20  Profunda brachii artery
21  Radial nerve
22  Radial collateral artery
23  Middle collateral artery
24  Lower lateral cutaneous nerve of arm
25  Posterior cutaneous nerve of forearm
26  Tendon of triceps brachii muscle

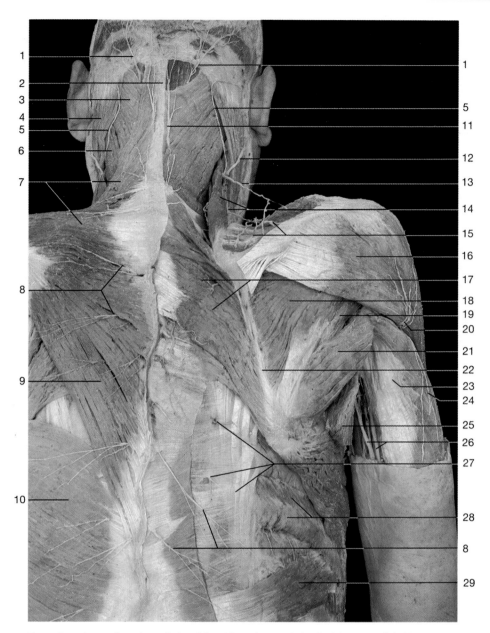

**Dorsal regions of neck and shoulder** (dorsal aspect). Left side: superficial layer. Right side: trapezius and latissimus dorsi muscles have been removed. Dissection of dorsal branches of spinal nerves.

1   Greater occipital nerve
2   Ligamentum nuchae
3   Splenius capitis muscle
4   Sternocleidomastoid muscle
5   Lesser occipital nerve
6   Splenius cervicis muscle
7   Descending and transverse fibers of trapezius muscle
8   Medial cutaneous branches of dorsal rami of spinal nerves
9   Ascending fibers of trapezius muscle
10  Latissimus dorsi muscle
11  Cutaneous branch of third occipital nerve
12  Great auricular nerve
13  Accessory nerve (n. XI)
14  Posterior supraclavicular nerve and levator scapulae muscle
15  Branches of suprascapular artery

16  Deltoid muscle
17  Rhomboid major muscle
18  Infraspinatus muscle
19  Teres minor muscle
20  Upper lateral cutaneous nerve of arm (branch of axillary nerve)
21  Teres major muscle
22  Medial margin of scapula
23  Long head of triceps muscle
24  Posterior cutaneous nerve of arm (branch of radial nerve)
25  Latissimus dorsi muscle (divided)
26  Ulnar nerve and brachial artery
27  Lateral cutaneous branches of dorsal rami of spinal nerves and iliocostalis thoracis muscle
28  External intercostal muscle and seventh rib
29  Serratus posterior inferior muscle

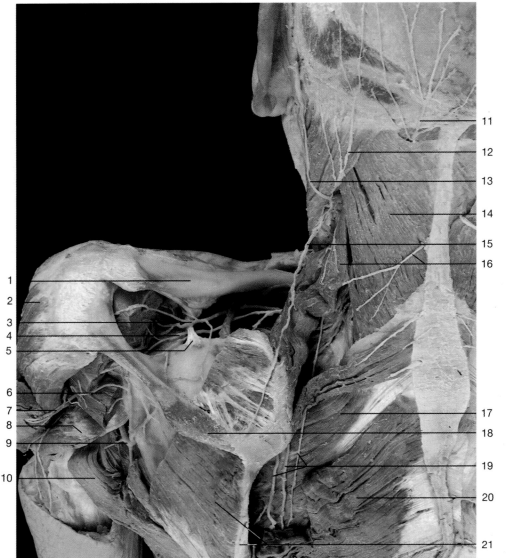

1   Clavicle
2   Deltoid muscle
3   Suprascapular artery
4   Suprascapular nerve
5   Superior transverse scapular
    ligament
6   Teres minor muscle
7   Axillary nerve and posterior
    circumflex humeral artery
8   Long head of triceps muscle
9   Circumflex scapular artery
10  Teres major muscle
11  Greater occipital nerve
12  Lesser occipital nerve
13  Great auricular nerve
14  Splenius capitis muscle
15  Accessory nerve (n. XI)
16  Third occipital nerve and
    levator scapulae muscle
17  Serratus posterior superior
    muscle
18  Spine of scapula
19  Descending scapular artery
    and dorsal scapular nerve
20  Rhomboid major muscle
21  Infraspinatus muscle and
    medial margin of scapula
22  Radial nerve and profunda
    brachii artery
23  Thoracodorsal artery
24  Thyrocervical trunk
25  Roots of brachial plexus

**Dorsal region of shoulder,** deepest layer. Rhomboid and scapular muscles fenestrated; posterior part of deltoid muscle reflected.

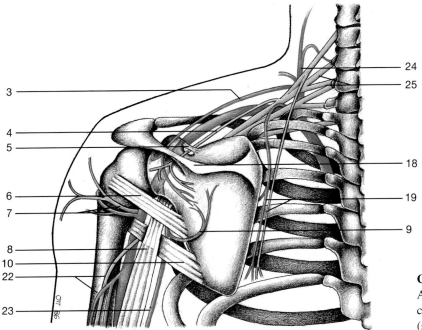

**Collateral circulation of shoulder.**
Anastomosis of suprascapular and circumflex scapular arteries (semischematic drawing).

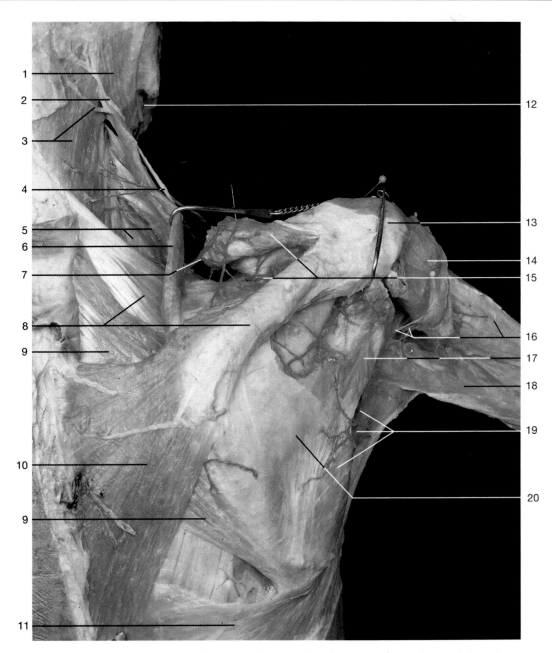

**Scapular region, arm, and shoulder** (dorsal aspect). Arteries of scapular region are injected. Trapezius, deltoid, and infraspinatus muscles are partially removed or reflected.

1  Sternocleidomastoid muscle
2  Lesser occipital nerve
3  Splenius capitis muscle and third occipital nerve
4  Accessory nerve (n. XI)
5  Splenius cervicis muscle and transverse cervical artery (deep branch)
6  Levator of scapula muscle
7  Transverse cervical artery (superficial branch)
8  Spine of scapula and serratus posterior superior muscle
9  Rhomboid major muscle

10  Trapezius muscle
11  Latissimus dorsi muscle
12  Facial artery
13  Acromion
14  Deltoid muscle
15  Suprascapular artery and supraspinatus muscle (reflected)
16  Axillary nerve, posterior circumflex humeral artery, and lateral head of triceps brachii muscle
17  Teres minor muscle
18  Long head of triceps brachii muscle
19  Circumflex scapular artery and teres major
20  Infraspinatus muscle

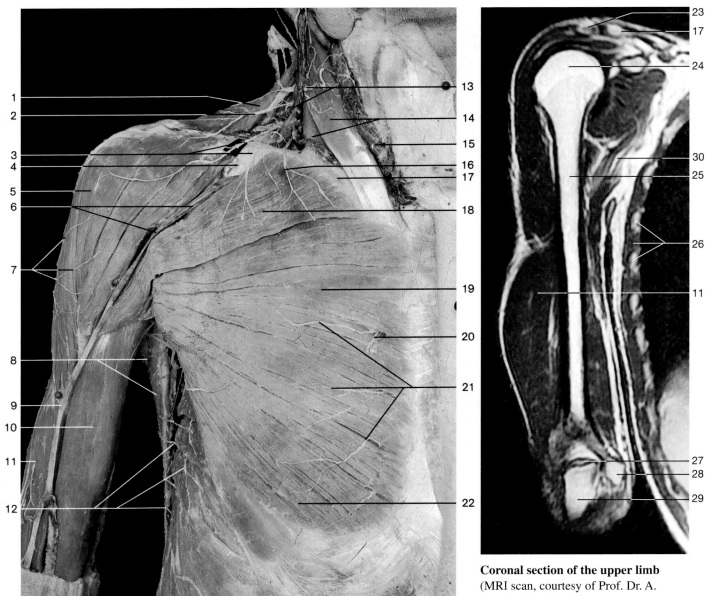

**Coronal section of the upper limb** (MRI scan, courtesy of Prof. Dr. A. Heuck, Munich).

**Right shoulder and thoracic wall,** superficial layer (anterior aspect). Dissection of the cutaneous nerves and veins.

1  Trapezius muscle
2  Posterior supraclavicular nerve
3  Middle supraclavicular nerve
4  Deltopectoral triangle
5  Deltoid muscle
6  Cephalic vein within the deltopectoral groove
7  Upper lateral cutaneous nerve of arm
   (branch of axillary nerve)
8  Latissimus dorsi muscle
9  Cephalic vein
10  Biceps brachii muscle
11  Triceps brachii muscle
12  Lateral cutaneous branches of intercostal nerves
13  Transverse cervical nerve and external jugular vein
14  Sternocleidomastoid muscle
15  Anterior jugular vein

16  Anterior supraclavicular nerve
17  Clavicle
18  Clavicular part of pectoralis major muscle
19  Sternocostal part of pectoralis major muscle
20  Perforating branch of internal thoracic artery
21  Anterior cutaneous branches of intercostal nerves
22  Abdominal part of pectoralis major muscle
23  Acromion
24  Head of humerus
25  Humerus
26  Ribs and intercostal muscles
27  Humero-ulnar joint
28  Head of radius
29  Ulna
30  Brachial artery

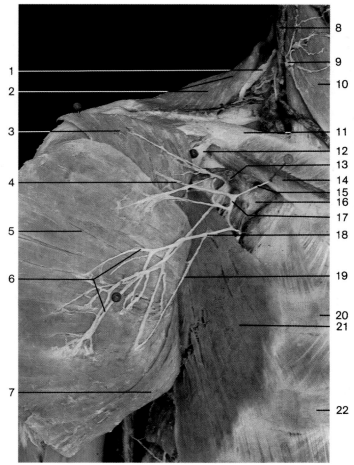

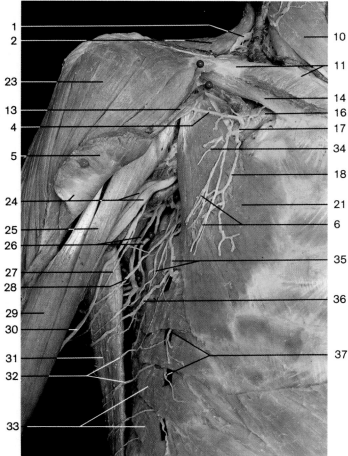

**Right deltopectoral triangle, infraclavicular region**
(anterior aspect). The pectoralis major muscle has been cut
and reflected.

**Thoracic wall and shoulder,** deep layer. **Right axillary
region** (anterior aspect). The pectoralis major muscle has
been cut and partly removed.

1   Accessory nerve
2   Trapezius muscle
3   Pectoralis major muscle (clavicular part)
4   Acromial branch of thoraco-acromial artery
5   Pectoralis major muscle
6   Lateral pectoral nerves
7   Abdominal part of pectoralis major muscle
8   External jugular vein
9   Cutaneous branches of cervical plexus
10  Sternocleidomastoid muscle
11  Clavicle
12  Clavipectoral fascia
13  Cephalic vein
14  Subclavius muscle
15  Clavicular branch of thoraco-acromial artery
16  Subclavian vein
17  Thoraco-acromial artery
18  Pectoral branch of thoraco-acromial artery
19  Medial pectoral nerve
20  Second rib

21  Pectoralis minor muscle
22  Third rib
23  Deltoid muscle
24  Pectoralis major muscle (reflected), brachial artery, and
    median nerve
25  Short head of biceps brachii muscle
26  Thoracodorsal artery and nerve
27  Medial cutaneous nerve of arm
28  Intercostobrachial nerve ($T_2$)
29  Long head of biceps brachii muscle
30  Medial cutaneous nerve of forearm
31  Latissimus dorsi muscle
32  Lateral cutaneous branches of intercostal nerves
    (posterior branches)
33  Serratus anterior muscle
34  Medial pectoral nerve
35  Long thoracic nerve and lateral thoracic artery
36  Intercostobrachial nerve ($T_3$)
37  Lateral cutaneous branches of intercostal nerves
    (anterior branches)

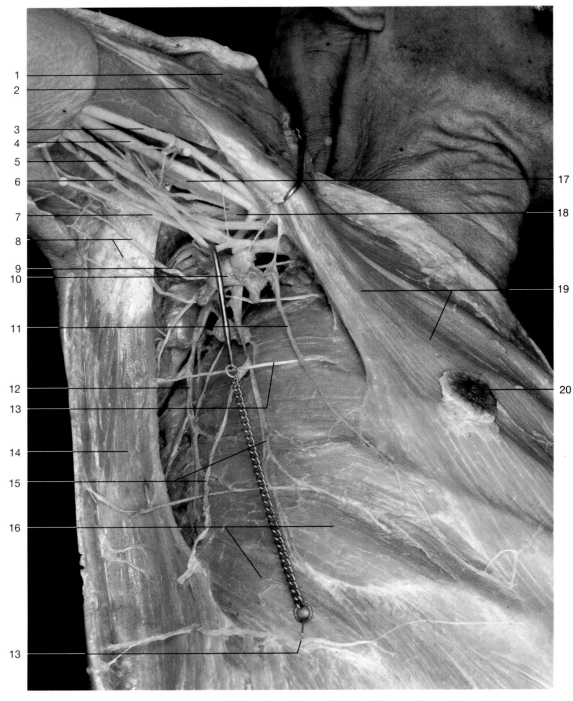

**Right axillary region** (inferior aspect). **Dissection of superficial axillary nodes and lymphatic vessels.** The pectoralis major muscle has been slightly elevated.

| | | | |
|---|---|---|---|
| 1 | Deltoid muscle | 12 | Thoracodorsal artery |
| 2 | Cephalic vein | 13 | Lateral cutaneous branch of intercostal nerve |
| 3 | Median nerve | 14 | Latissimus dorsi muscle |
| 4 | Brachial artery | 15 | Thoraco-epigastric vein |
| 5 | Medial cutaneous nerves of arm and forearm | 16 | Serratus anterior muscle |
| 6 | Ulnar nerve | 17 | Musculocutaneous nerve |
| 7 | Basilic vein | 18 | Radial nerve |
| 8 | Intercostobrachial nerves | 19 | Pectoralis major muscle |
| 9 | Circumflex scapular artery | 20 | Nipple |
| 10 | Superficial axillary nodes | | |
| 11 | Lateral thoracic artery | | |

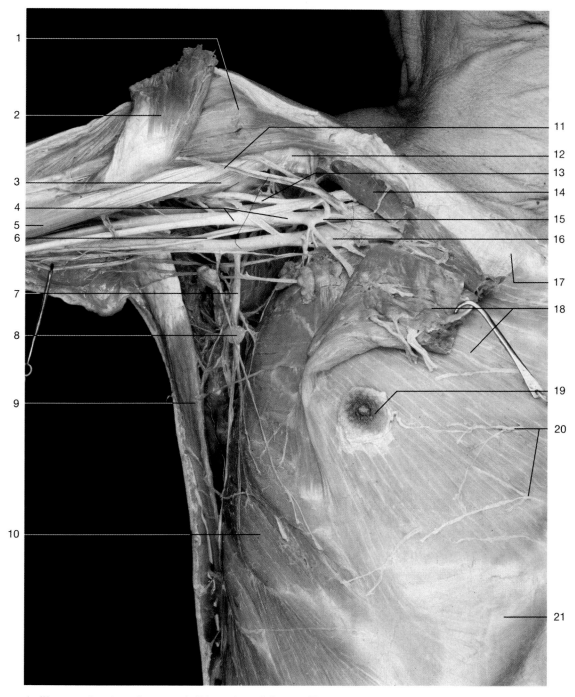

**Axillary region** (anterior aspect). **Dissection of deep axillary nodes.** Pectoralis major and minor muscles divided and reflected. Shoulder girdle and arm elevated and reflected.

1  Deltoid muscle
2  Insertion of pectoralis major muscle
3  Coracobrachialis muscle
4  Roots of median nerve, axillary artery
5  Short head of biceps brachii muscle
6  Ulnar nerve and medial cutaneous nerve
    of forearm
7  Thoraco-epigastric vein
8  Deep axillary node
9  Latissimus dorsi muscle
10  Serratus anterior muscle

11  Cephalic vein
12  Insertion of pectoralis minor muscle (coracoid process)
13  Musculocutaneous nerve
14  Subclavius muscle
15  Thoraco-acromial artery
16  Axillary vein
17  Clavicle
18  Pectoralis major and minor muscles (reflected)
19  Nipple
20  Anterior cutaneous branches of intercostal nerves
21  Anterior layer of rectus sheath

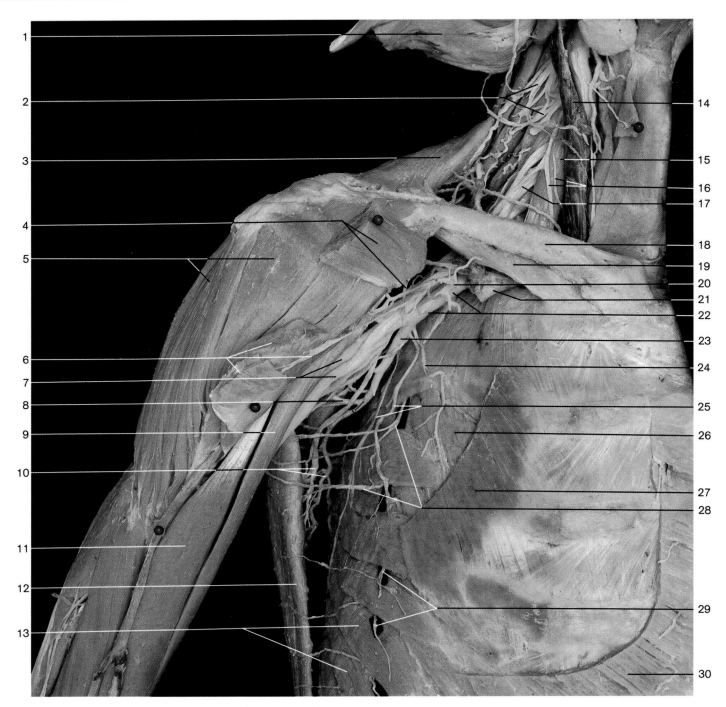

**Right axillary region** (anterior aspect). The pectoralis major and minor muscles have been cut and reflected to display the vessels and nerves of the axilla.

1  Sternocleidomastoid muscle (cut and reflected)
2  Cervical plexus
3  Trapezius muscle
4  Pectoralis minor muscle and medial pectoral nerve
5  Deltoid muscle
6  Pectoralis major muscle and lateral pectoral nerve
7  Median nerve and brachial artery
8  Circumflex scapular artery
9  Short head of biceps brachii muscle
10  Thoracodorsal artery and nerve
11  Long head of biceps brachii muscle
12  Latissimus dorsi muscle
13  Serratus anterior muscle
14  Internal jugular vein
15  Scalenus anterior muscle

16  Phrenic nerve and ascending cervical artery
17  Brachial plexus (at the levels of the trunks)
18  Clavicle
19  Subclavius muscle
20  Thoraco-acromial artery
21  Subclavian vein (cut)
22  Axillary artery
23  Subscapular artery
24  Superior thoracic artery
25  Lateral thoracic artery and long thoracic nerve
26  External intercostal muscle
27  Insertion of pectoralis minor muscle
28  Intercostobrachial nerves
29  Lateral cutaneous branches of intercostal nerves
30  Insertion of pectoralis major muscle

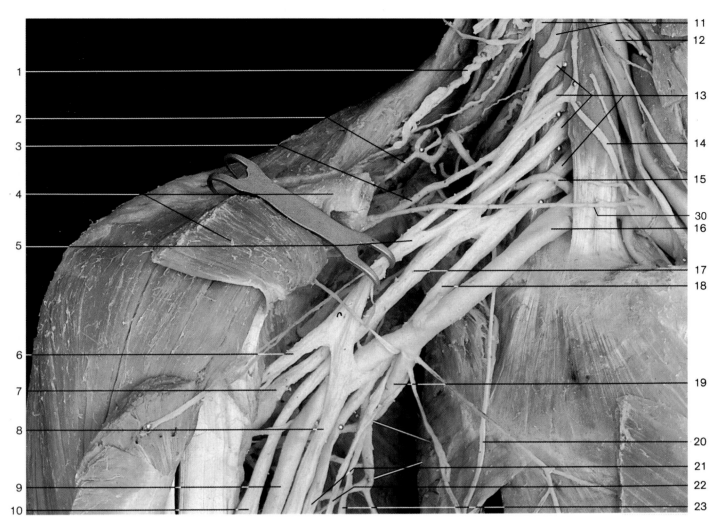

**Brachial plexus** (anterior aspect). Clavicle and the two pectoralis muscles have been partly removed.

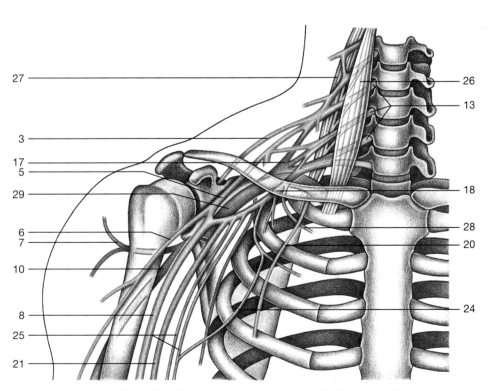

**Main branches of brachial plexus.** Posterior cord in purple, lateral cord in orange, and medial cord in green (schematic drawing).

1  Accessory nerve
2  Dorsal scapular artery
3  Suprascapular nerve
4  Clavicle and pectoralis minor muscle
5  Lateral cord of brachial plexus
6  Musculocutaneous nerve
7  Axillary nerve
8  Median nerve
9  Brachial artery
10  Radial nerve
11  Cervical plexus
12  Common carotid artery
13  Roots of brachial plexus ($C_5$–$T_1$)
14  Phrenic nerve
15  Transverse cervical artery
16  Subclavian artery
17  Posterior cord of brachial plexus
18  Medial cord of brachial plexus
19  Subscapular artery
20  Long thoracic nerve
21  Ulnar nerve
22  Medial cutaneous nerve of forearm
23  Thoracodorsal nerve
24  Intercostobrachial nerve
25  Medial cutaneous nerves of arm and forearm
26  Scalenus anterior muscle
27  Scalenus medius muscle
28  Intercostal nerve ($T_1$)
29  Axillary artery
30  Suprascapular artery

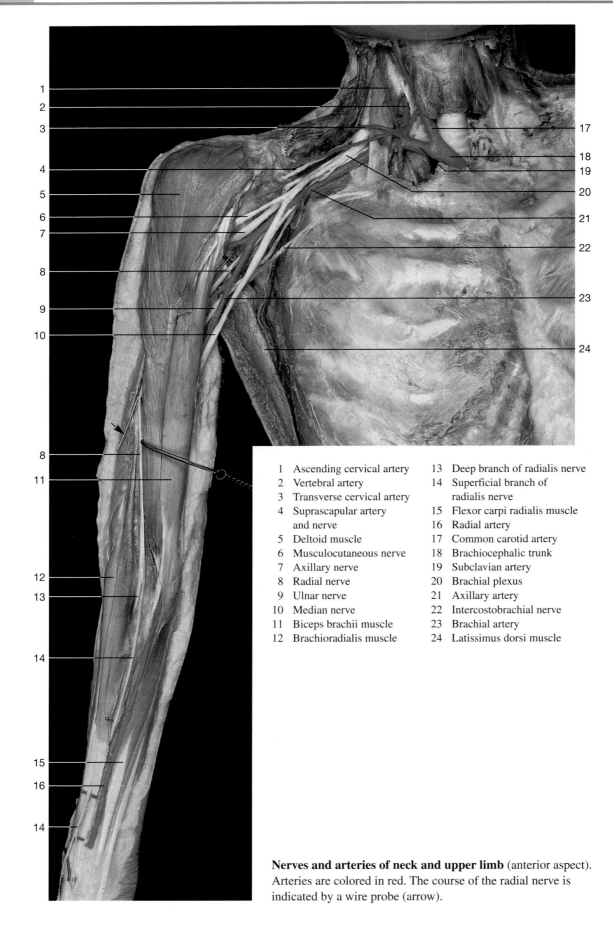

| | | | |
|---|---|---|---|
| 1 | Ascending cervical artery | 13 | Deep branch of radialis nerve |
| 2 | Vertebral artery | 14 | Superficial branch of |
| 3 | Transverse cervical artery | | radialis nerve |
| 4 | Suprascapular artery | 15 | Flexor carpi radialis muscle |
| | and nerve | 16 | Radial artery |
| 5 | Deltoid muscle | 17 | Common carotid artery |
| 6 | Musculocutaneous nerve | 18 | Brachiocephalic trunk |
| 7 | Axillary nerve | 19 | Subclavian artery |
| 8 | Radial nerve | 20 | Brachial plexus |
| 9 | Ulnar nerve | 21 | Axillary artery |
| 10 | Median nerve | 22 | Intercostobrachial nerve |
| 11 | Biceps brachii muscle | 23 | Brachial artery |
| 12 | Brachioradialis muscle | 24 | Latissimus dorsi muscle |

**Nerves and arteries of neck and upper limb** (anterior aspect).
Arteries are colored in red. The course of the radial nerve is
indicated by a wire probe (arrow).

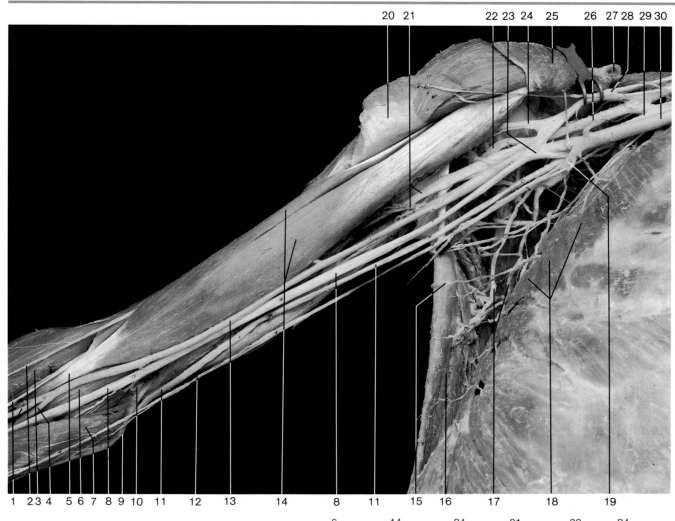

20 21    22 23 24   25    26 27 28 29 30

1  2 3 4   5 6 7  8 9 10  11    12    13    14    8    11    15  16    17    18    19

**Right arm. Dissection of vessels and nerves** (medial aspect). Shoulder girdle has been reflected slightly.

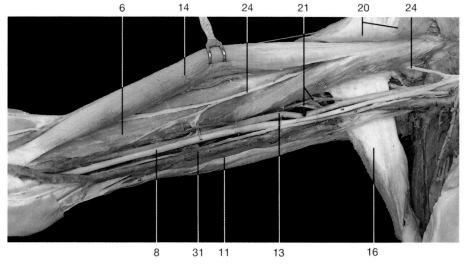

6    14    24    21    20    24

8    31   11    13    16

**Right arm. Dissection of vessels and nerves,** deeper layer. Biceps muscle has been reflected.

| | | | |
|---|---|---|---|
| 1 | Radial artery and superficial branch of radial nerve | 8 | Median nerve |
| 2 | Lateral cutaneous nerve of forearm | 9 | Medial epicondyle of humerus |
| 3 | Brachioradialis muscle | 10 | Inferior ulnar collateral artery |
| 4 | Ulnar artery | 11 | Ulnar nerve |
| 5 | Tendon of biceps brachii muscle | 12 | Medial cutaneous nerve of forearm |
| 6 | Brachialis muscle | 13 | Brachial artery |
| 7 | Pronator teres muscle | 14 | Biceps brachii muscle |
| | | 15 | Intercostobrachial nerve (T₃) |
| | | 16 | Latissimus dorsi muscle |

17  Thoracodorsal nerve and artery
18  Serratus anterior muscle
19  Subscapular artery
20  Pectoralis major muscle (reflected) and lateral pectoral nerve
21  Radial nerve and profunda brachii artery
22  Axillary nerve
23  Roots of the median nerve with axillary artery

24  Musculocutaneous nerve
25  Pectoralis minor muscle (reflected) and medial pectoral nerve
26  Posterior cord of brachial plexus
27  Clavicle (cut)
28  Lateral cord of brachial plexus
29  Medial cord of brachial plexus
30  Subclavian artery
31  Brachial vein

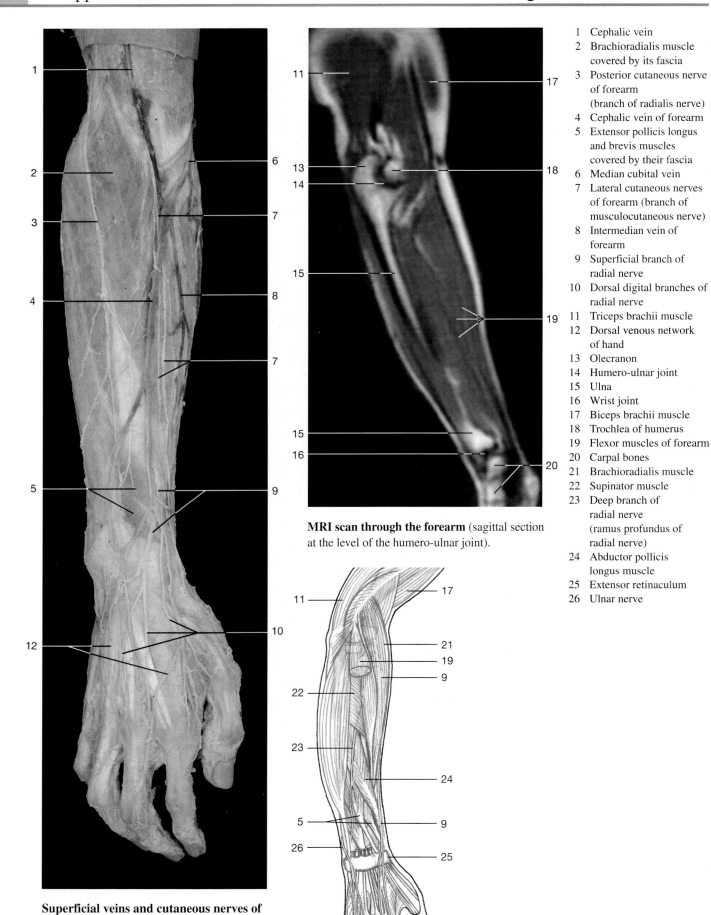

1   Cephalic vein
2   Brachioradialis muscle
    covered by its fascia
3   Posterior cutaneous nerve
    of forearm
    (branch of radialis nerve)
4   Cephalic vein of forearm
5   Extensor pollicis longus
    and brevis muscles
    covered by their fascia
6   Median cubital vein
7   Lateral cutaneous nerves
    of forearm (branch of
    musculocutaneous nerve)
8   Intermedian vein of
    forearm
9   Superficial branch of
    radial nerve
10  Dorsal digital branches of
    radial nerve
11  Triceps brachii muscle
12  Dorsal venous network
    of hand
13  Olecranon
14  Humero-ulnar joint
15  Ulna
16  Wrist joint
17  Biceps brachii muscle
18  Trochlea of humerus
19  Flexor muscles of forearm
20  Carpal bones
21  Brachioradialis muscle
22  Supinator muscle
23  Deep branch of
    radial nerve
    (ramus profundus of
    radial nerve)
24  Abductor pollicis
    longus muscle
25  Extensor retinaculum
26  Ulnar nerve

**MRI scan through the forearm** (sagittal section
at the level of the humero-ulnar joint).

**Superficial veins and cutaneous nerves of
forearm and hand** (anteromedial aspect).

**Course of the nerves to forearm and hand**
(dorsal aspect).

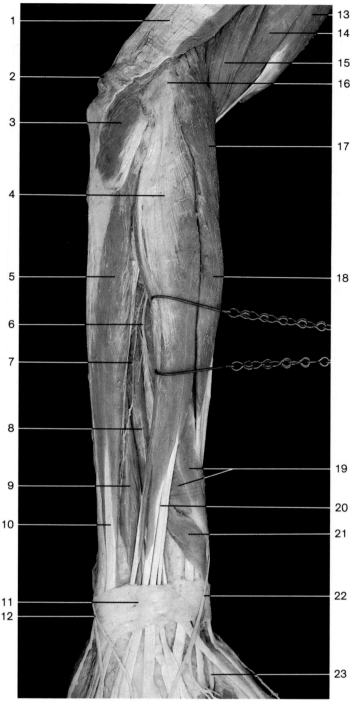

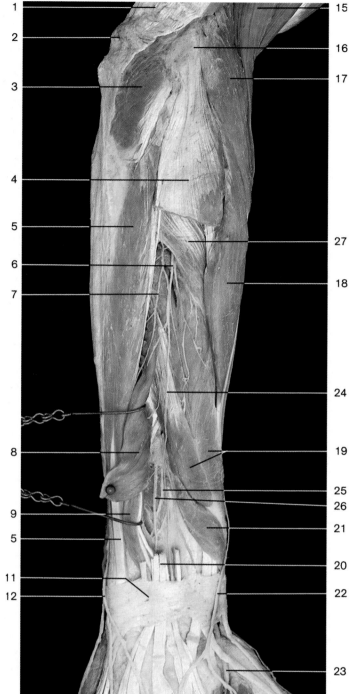

**Vessels and nerves of right forearm,** superficial layer
(dorsal aspect).

**Vessels and nerves of right forearm,** deep layer
(dorsal aspect).

1  Tendon of triceps brachii muscle
2  Olecranon
3  Anconeus muscle
4  Extensor digitorum muscle
5  Extensor carpi ulnaris muscle
6  Deep branch of radial nerve
7  Posterior interosseous artery
8  Extensor pollicis longus muscle
9  Extensor indicis muscle
10  Tendon of extensor carpi ulnaris muscle

11  Extensor retinaculum
12  Dorsal branch of ulnar nerve
13  Biceps brachii muscle
14  Brachialis muscle
15  Brachioradialis muscle
16  Lateral epicondyle of humerus
17  Extensor carpi radialis longus muscle
18  Extensor carpi radialis brevis muscle
19  Abductor pollicis longus muscle
20  Tendons of extensor digitorum muscle

21  Extensor pollicis brevis muscle
22  Superficial branch of radial nerve
23  Radial artery
24  Posterior interosseous nerve
25  Posterior interosseous branch of
    radial nerve
26  Posterior branch of anterior
    interosseous artery
27  Supinator muscle

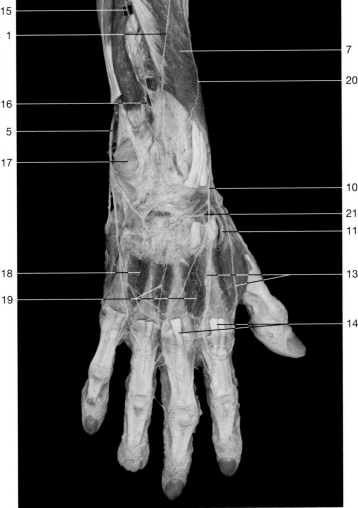

**Cutaneous nerves and veins of forearm and hand** (superficial layer, dorsal aspect).

**Dorsal region of forearm and hand** (deeper layer). Extensor digitorum muscle has been partly removed.

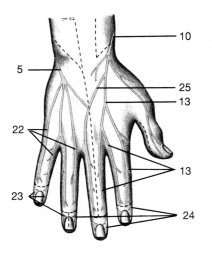

**Innervation pattern of dorsal surfaces of hand**

2½ digits by radial nerve, 2½ digits by ulnar nerve. Note that the terminal branches to the dorsal surfaces of the distal phalanges are derived from the palmar digital nerves. The cutaneous distribution varies; often 3½ digits are innervated by the radial and 1½ digits by the ulnar nerve.

1   Posterior cutaneous nerve of forearm (branch of radial nerve)
2   Extensor digitorum muscle
3   Tendon of extensor carpi ulnaris muscle
4   Extensor retinaculum
5   Ulnar nerve
6   Dorsal venous network of hand
7   Abductor pollicis longus muscle
8   Cephalic vein
9   Extensor pollicis brevis muscle
10   Radial nerve, superficial branch
11   Radial artery
12   Tendon of extensor pollicis longus muscle
13   Dorsal digital branches of radial nerve
14   Tendons of extensor digitorum muscle with intertendinous connections
15   Posterior interosseus nerve (branch of the deep radial nerve)
16   Posterior interosseous artery
17   Styloid process of ulna
18   Dorsal interosseus muscle IV
19   Dorsal carpal branch of radial artery
20   Lateral cutaneous nerve of forearm (branch of musculocutaneous nerve)
21   Dorsal metacarpal artery
22   Proper dorsal digital branches of ulnar nerve
23   Regions supplied by palmar digital nerves (ulnar nerve)
24   Regions supplied by palmar digital nerves (median nerve)
25   Communicating branch with ulnar nerve

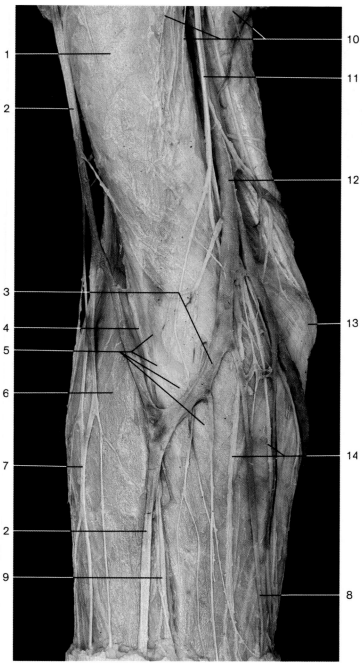

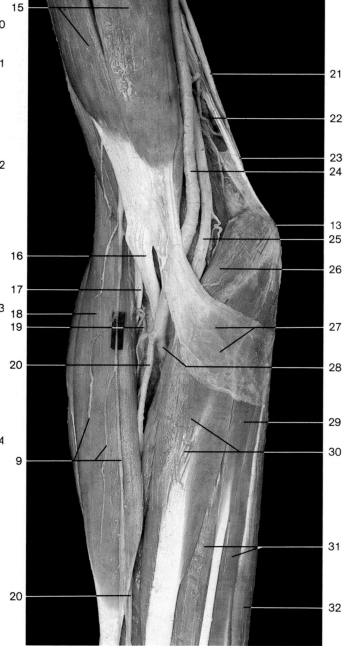

**Cubital region** (anterior aspect), dissection of cutaneous nerves and veins.

**Cubital region,** superficial layer (anterior aspect).
The fasciae of the muscles have been removed.

1   Biceps brachii muscle with fascia
2   Cephalic vein
3   Median cubital vein
4   Lateral cutaneous nerve of forearm
5   Tendon and aponeurosis of biceps brachii muscle
    (covered by the antebrachial fascia)
6   Brachioradialis muscle with fascia
7   Accessory cephalic vein
8   Median vein of forearm
9   Branches of lateral cutaneous nerve of forearm
10  Terminal branches of medial cutaneous nerve of arm
11  Medial cutaneous nerve of forearm
12  Basilic vein
13  Medial epicondyle of humerus
14  Terminal branches of medial cutaneous nerve
    of forearm
15  Biceps brachii muscle

16  Tendon of biceps brachii muscle
17  Radial nerve
18  Brachioradialis muscle
19  Radial recurrent artery
20  Radial artery
21  Ulnar nerve
22  Superior ulnar collateral artery
23  Medial intermuscular septum
24  Brachial artery
25  Median nerve
26  Pronator teres muscle
27  Bicipital aponeurosis
28  Ulnar artery
29  Palmaris longus muscle
30  Flexor carpi radialis muscle
31  Flexor digitorum superficialis muscle
32  Flexor carpi ulnaris muscle

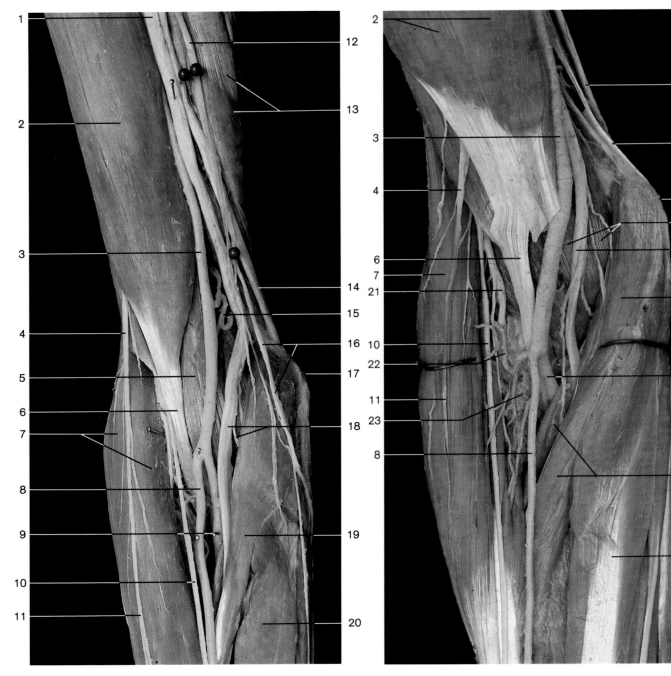

**Cubital region,** middle layer (anterior aspect).
The bicipital aponeurosis has been removed.

**Cubital region,** middle layer (anterior aspect).
The pronator teres and brachioradialis muscles
have been slightly reflected.

| | |
|---|---|
| 1  Median nerve | 13  Triceps brachii muscle |
| 2  Biceps brachii muscle | 14  Ulnar nerve |
| 3  Brachial artery | 15  Inferior ulnar collateral artery |
| 4  Lateral cutaneous nerve of forearm | 16  Anterior branch of medial cutaneous nerve of forearm |
|    (terminal branch of musculocutaneous nerve) | 17  Medial epicondyle of humerus |
| 5  Brachialis muscle | 18  Median nerve with branches to pronator teres muscle |
| 6  Tendon of biceps brachii muscle | 19  Pronator teres muscle |
| 7  Brachioradialis muscle | 20  Flexor carpi radialis muscle |
| 8  Radial artery | 21  Deep branch of radial nerve |
| 9  Ulnar artery | 22  Radial recurrent artery |
| 10  Superficial branch of radial nerve | 23  Supinator muscle |
| 11  Lateral cutaneous nerve of forearm | 24  Medial intermuscular septum of arm |
| 12  Medial cutaneous nerve of forearm | |

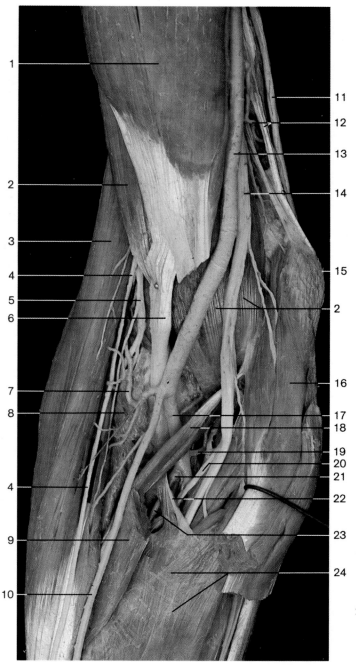

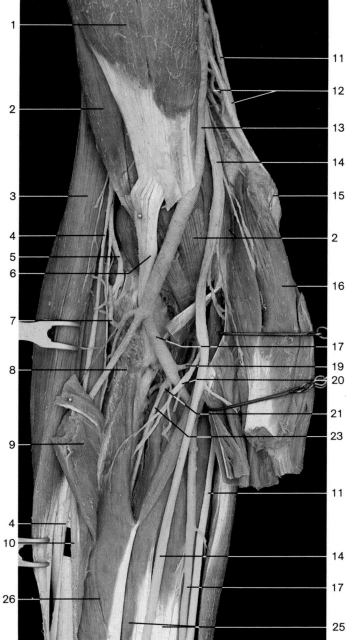

**Cubital region,** deep layer (anterior aspect). The pronator teres and flexor carpi ulnaris muscles have been cut and reflected.

**Cubital region,** deepest layer (anterior aspect). The flexor digitorum superficialis and the ulnar head of the pronator teres have been cut and reflected.

| | |
|---|---|
| 1   Biceps brachii muscle | 14   Median nerve |
| 2   Brachialis muscle | 15   Medial epicondyle of humerus |
| 3   Brachioradialis muscle | 16   Humeral head of pronator teres muscle |
| 4   Superficial branch of radial nerve | 17   Ulnar artery |
| 5   Deep branch of radial nerve | 18   Ulnar head of pronator teres muscle |
| 6   Tendon of biceps brachii muscle | 19   Ulnar recurrent artery |
| 7   Radial recurrent artery | 20   Anterior interosseous nerve |
| 8   Supinator muscle | 21   Common interosseous artery |
| 9   Insertion of pronator teres muscle | 22   Tendinous arch of flexor digitorum superficialis muscle |
| 10   Radial artery | 23   Anterior interosseous artery |
| 11   Ulnar nerve | 24   Flexor digitorum superficialis muscle |
| 12   Medial intermuscular septum of arm and | 25   Flexor digitorum profundus muscle |
|         superior ulnar collateral artery | 26   Flexor pollicis longus muscle |
| 13   Brachial artery | |

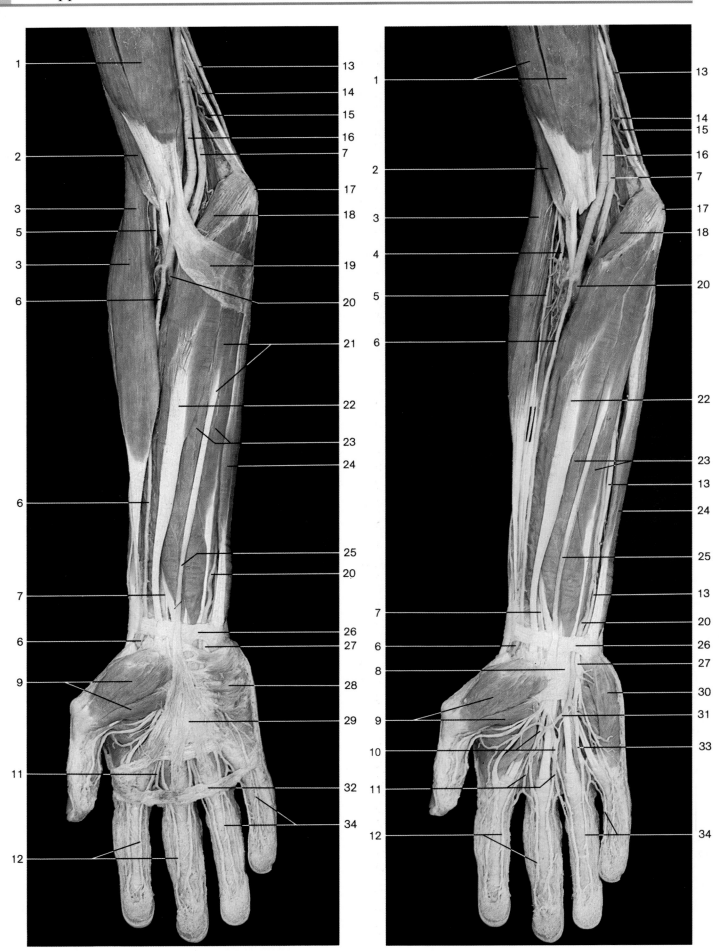

**Vessels and nerves of right forearm and hand,** superficial layer (palmar aspect).

**Vessels and nerves of right forearm and hand,** superficial layer (palmar aspect). The palmar aponeurosis of the hand and the bicipital aponeurosis have been removed.

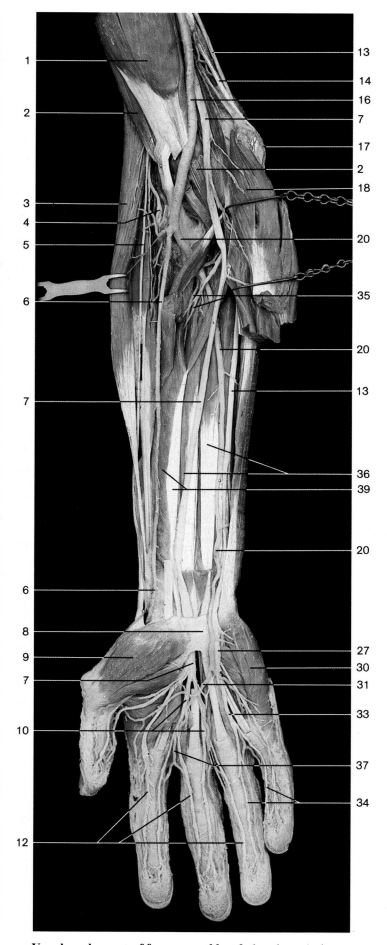

1  Biceps brachii muscle
2  Brachialis muscle
3  Brachioradialis muscle
4  Deep branch of radial nerve
5  Superficial branch of radial nerve
6  Radial artery
7  Median nerve
8  Flexor retinaculum
9  Thenar muscles
10  Common palmar digital branches of median nerve
11  Common palmar digital arteries
12  Proper palmar digital nerves (median nerve)
13  Ulnar nerve
14  Medial intermuscular septum of arm
15  Superior ulnar collateral artery
16  Brachial artery
17  Medial epicondyle of humerus
18  Pronator teres muscle
19  Bicipital aponeurosis
20  Ulnar artery
21  Palmaris longus muscle
22  Flexor carpi radialis muscle
23  Flexor digitorum superficialis muscle
24  Flexor carpi ulnaris muscle
25  Tendon of palmaris longus muscle
26  Remnant of antebrachial fascia
27  Superficial branch of ulnar nerve
28  Palmaris brevis muscle
29  Palmar aponeurosis
30  Hypothenar muscles
31  Superficial palmar arch
32  Superficial transverse metacarpal ligament
33  Common palmar digital branch of ulnar nerve
34  Proper palmar digital branches of ulnar nerve
35  Anterior interosseous artery and nerve
36  Flexor digitorum profundus muscle
37  Common palmar digital arteries
38  Palmar branch of median nerve
39  Flexor pollicis longus muscle
40  Palmar branch of ulnar nerve

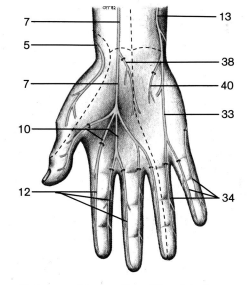

**Cutaneous innervation of hand** (palmar aspect).
(Schematic drawing.)
Cutaneous innervation of palmar surface:
3½ digits by median nerve,
1½ digits by ulnar nerve.

**Vessels and nerves of forearm and hand,** deep layer (palmar aspect). The superficial layer of the flexor muscles has been removed.

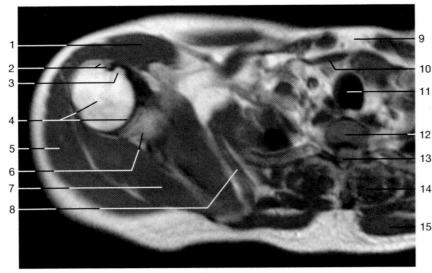

**Horizontal section through the right shoulder joint** (section 1; MRI scan; inferior aspect).

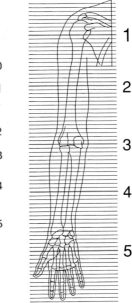

**Upper extremity, location of sections 1–5** (MRI scans, courtesy of Prof. Dr. A. Heuck, Munich, Germany).

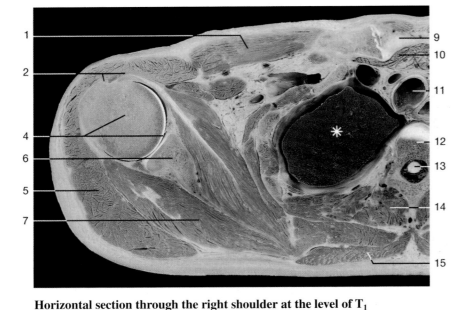

**Horizontal section through the right shoulder at the level of $T_1$** (section 1; inferior aspect). * = Upper lobe of lung.

1   Pectoralis major muscle
2   Greater tubercle and tendon of biceps muscle
3   Lesser tubercle
4   Head of humerus and articular cavity of shoulder joint
5   Deltoid muscle
6   Scapula
7   Infraspinatus muscle
8   Serratus anterior muscle
9   Sternum
10  Infrahyoid muscles
11  Trachea
12  Body of thoracic vertebra
13  Vertebral canal and spinal cord
14  Deep muscles of the back
15  Trapezius muscle
16  Brachialis muscle
17  Radial nerve and profunda brachii vessels

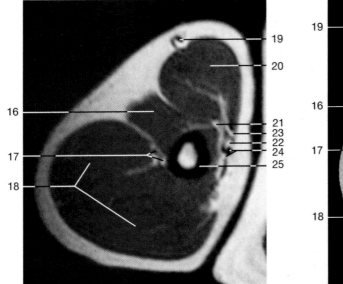

**Axial section through the middle of the right arm** (section 2; MRI scan; inferior aspect).

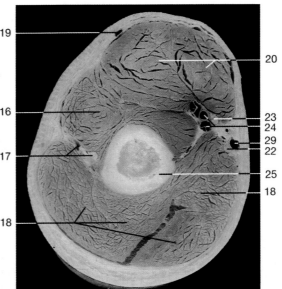

**Axial section through the middle of the right arm** (section 2; inferior aspect).

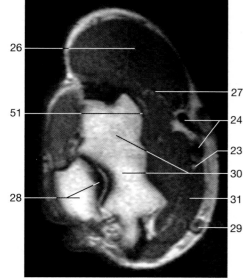

18  Triceps brachii muscle
19  Cephalic vein
20  Biceps brachii muscle
21  Musculocutaneous nerve
22  Ulnar nerve
23  Medianus nerve
24  Brachial artery and vein
25  Shaft of humerus
26  Brachioradialis muscle
27  Radial nerve
28  Olecranon and articular cavity
    of elbow joint
29  Basilic vein
30  Humerus
31  Pronator teres muscle
32  Extensor muscles of forearm
33  Ramus profundus of
    radialis nerve
34  Anterior interosseus
    vessels and nerve
35  Interosseous membrane
36  Ulna
37  Radius
38  Radial artery and superficial
    branch of radial nerve
39  Flexor pollicis longus muscle
40  Flexor digitorum
    superficialis and profundus
    muscles
41  Ulnar nerve, ulnar artery, and
    vein
42  Flexor carpi ulnaris muscle
43  Radial artery
44  Metacarpal bones III and IV
45  Carpal canal with tendons of
    flexor digitorum muscles
46  Hypothenar muscle
47  Median nerve
48  Interosseous muscles
49  First metacarpal bone
50  Thenar muscles
51  Articular cavity of
    humeroradial joint

**Axial section through the right elbow joint** (section 3; MRI scan; courtesy of Prof. W. Bautz and R. Janka, M. D., University of Erlangen, Germany.).

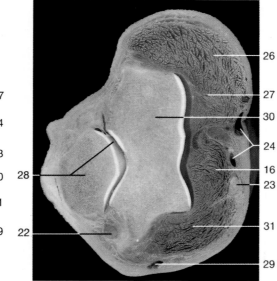

**Axial section through the right elbow joint** (section 3; inferior aspect).

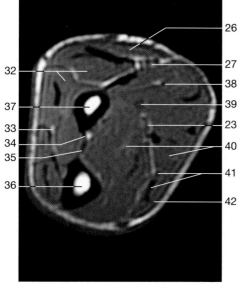

**Axial section through the middle of the right forearm** (section 4; MRI scan; courtesy of Prof. W. Bautz and R. Janka, M. D., University of Erlangen, Germany.).

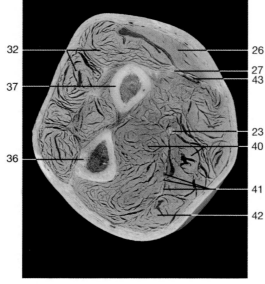

**Axial section through the middle of the right forearm** (section 4; inferior aspect).

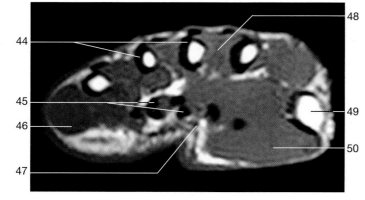

**Axial section through the right hand** (section 5; MRI scan; courtesy of Prof. W. Bautz and R. Janka, M. D., University of Erlangen, Germany.).

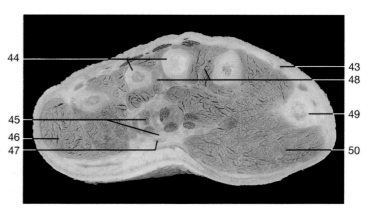

**Axial section through the right hand at the level of the metacarpus** (section 5; inferior aspect).

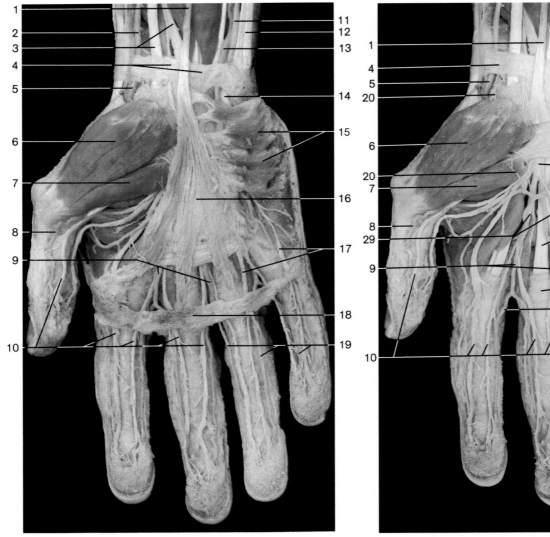

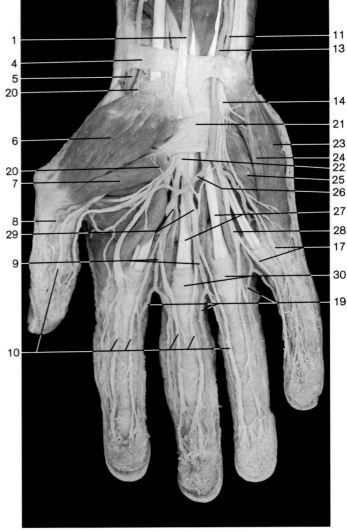

**Right hand,** superficial layer, dissection of vessels and nerves (palmar aspect).

**Right hand,** superficial layer, dissection of vessels and nerves (palmar aspect). The palmar aponeurosis has been removed to display the superficial palmar arch.

1   Tendon of palmaris longus muscle
2   Radial artery
3   Tendon of flexor carpi radialis muscle and median nerve
4   Distal part of antebrachial fascia
5   Radial artery passing into the anatomical snuffbox
6   Abductor pollicis brevis muscle
7   Superficial head of flexor pollicis brevis muscle
8   Palmar digital artery of thumb
9   Common palmar digital arteries
10  Proper palmar digital nerves (median nerve)
11  Ulnar nerve
12  Tendon of flexor carpi ulnaris muscle
13  Ulnar artery
14  Superficial branch of ulnar nerve
15  Palmaris brevis muscle
16  Palmar aponeurosis

17  Palmar digital nerves (ulnar nerve)
18  Superficial transverse metacarpal ligament
19  Proper palmar digital arteries
20  Superficial palmar branch of radial artery
    (contributing to the superficial palmar arch)
21  Flexor retinaculum
22  Median nerve
23  Abductor digiti minimi muscle
24  Flexor digiti minimi brevis muscle
25  Opponens digiti minimi muscle
26  Superficial palmar arch
27  Tendons of flexor digitorum superficialis muscle
28  Common palmar digital branch of ulnar nerve
29  Common palmar digital branch of median nerve
30  Fibrous sheath of flexor tendons

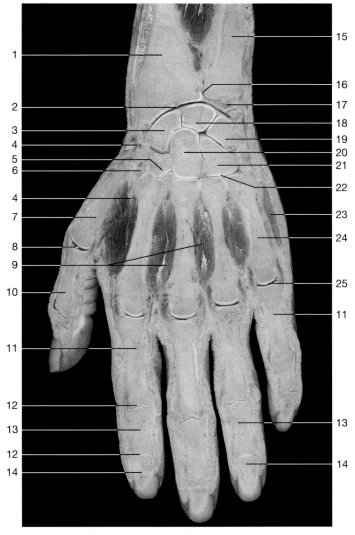

**Coronal section through the right hand** (palmar aspect).

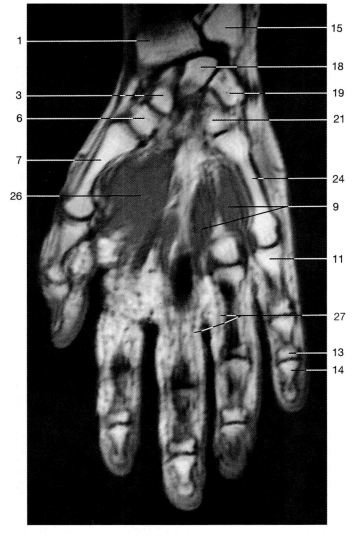

**Coronal section through the right hand** (palmar aspect)
(MRI scan, courtesy of Prof. Dr. A. Heuck, Munich).

| | |
|---|---|
| 1 Radius | 15 Ulna |
| 2 Wrist joint | 16 Distal radio-ulnar joint |
| 3 Scaphoid (navicular) bone | 17 Articular disc |
| 4 Radial artery | 18 Lunate bone |
| 5 Trapezoid bone | 19 Triangular bone |
| 6 Trapezium bone | 20 Capitate bone |
| 7 First metacarpal bone | 21 Hamate bone |
| 8 Metacarpophalangeal joint of thumb | 22 Carpometacarpal joints |
| 9 Interosseous muscles | 23 Abductor digiti minimi muscle |
| 10 Proximal phalanx of thumb | 24 Fifth metacarpal bone |
| 11 Proximal phalanx of fingers | 25 Metacarpophalangeal joint |
| 12 Interphalangeal joints | 26 Adductor pollicis muscle |
| 13 Middle phalanx | 27 Proper palmar digital arteries |
| 14 Distal phalanx | |

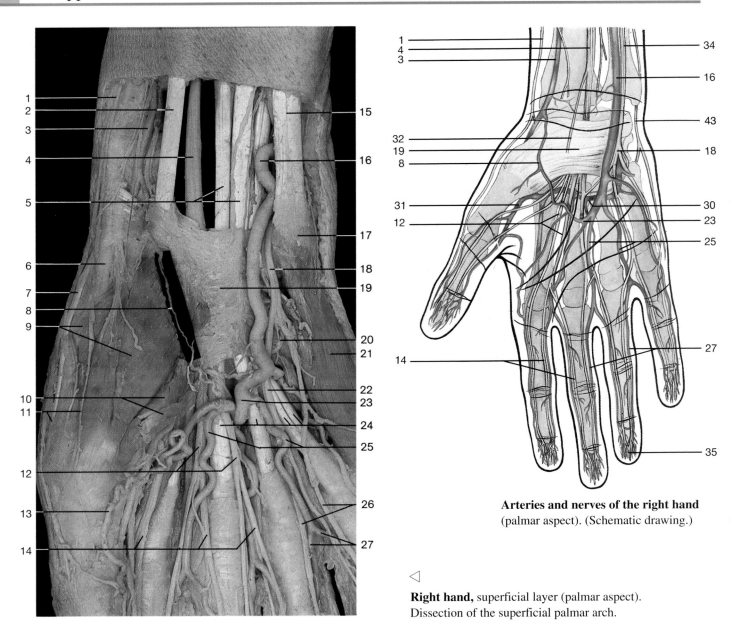

1
2
3
4
5
6
7
8
9
10
11
12
13
14

15
16
17
18
19
20
21
22
23
24
25
26
27

1
4
3

32
19
8

31
12

14

34
16
43
18
30
23
25
27
35

**Arteries and nerves of the right hand**
(palmar aspect). (Schematic drawing.)

◁

**Right hand,** superficial layer (palmar aspect).
Dissection of the superficial palmar arch.

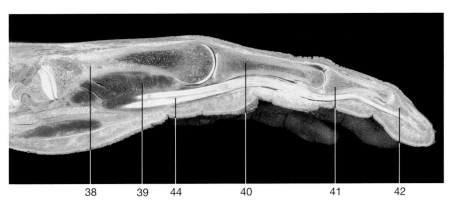

38    39    44    40    41    42

**Longitudinal section through the hand**
at the level of the third finger.

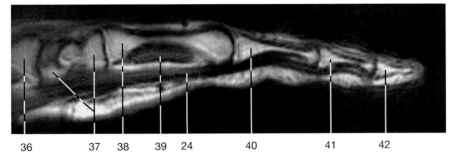

36    37    38    39    24    40    41    42

**Longitudinal section through the hand**
at the level of the third finger (MRI scan,
courtesy of Prof. Dr. A. Heuck, Munich).

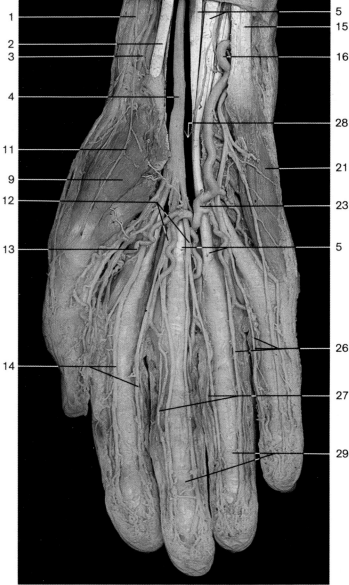

**Right hand,** middle layer (palmar aspect). The flexor retinaculum has been removed.

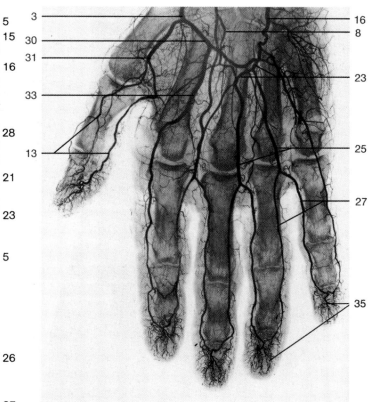

**Arteriogram of the right hand** (palmar aspect).

1   Superficial branch of radial nerve
2   Tendon of flexor carpi radialis muscle
3   Radial artery
4   Median nerve
5   Tendon of flexor digitorum superficialis muscle
6   Tendon of abductor pollicis longus muscle
7   Tendon of extensor pollicis brevis muscle
8   Superficial palmar branch of radial artery
9   Abductor pollicis brevis muscle
10  Superficial head of flexor pollicis brevis muscle
11  Terminal branches of superficial branch of radial nerve
12  Common palmar digital nerves (median nerve)
13  Proper palmar digital arteries of thumb
14  Proper palmar digital nerves (median nerve)
15  Tendon of flexor carpi ulnaris muscle
16  Ulnar artery
17  Position of pisiform bone
18  Superficial branch of ulnar nerve
19  Flexor retinaculum
20  Deep branch of ulnar nerve

21  Abductor digiti minimi muscle
22  Common palmar digital nerves (ulnar nerve)
23  Superficial palmar arch
24  Tendons of flexor digitorum muscles
25  Common palmar digital arteries
26  Palmar digital nerves (ulnar nerve)
27  Proper palmar digital arteries
28  Carpal tunnel
29  Fibrous sheaths for the tendons of flexor digitorum
    muscles
30  Deep palmar arch
31  Princeps pollicis artery
32  Palmar branch of median nerve
33  Common digital palmar artery
34  Ulnar nerve
35  Capillary network of finger
36  Radius
37  Carpal bones
38  Metacarpal bone
39  Interosseous muscles
40  Proximal phalanx
41  Middle phalanx
42  Distal phalanx
43  Dorsal branch of ulnar nerve
44  Tendons of flexor digitorum profundus (upper)
    and superficialis (lower) muscles

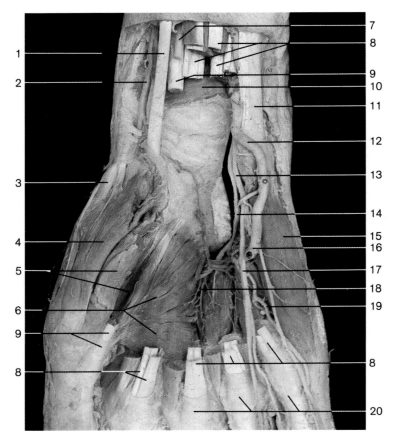

1  Tendon of flexor carpi radialis muscle
2  Radial artery
3  Tendon of abductor pollicis longus muscle
4  Abductor pollicis brevis muscle
5  Superficial and deep heads of flexor pollicis
   brevis muscle
6  Oblique and transverse heads of adductor
   pollicis muscle
7  Median nerve
8  Tendons of flexor digitorum superficialis and
   profundus muscles
9  Tendon of flexor pollicis longus muscle
10 Pronator quadratus muscle
11 Tendon of flexor carpi ulnaris muscle
12 Ulnar artery
13 Superficial branch of ulnar nerve
14 Deep branch of ulnar nerve
15 Abductor digiti minimi muscle
16 Superficial palmar arch (cut end)
17 Common palmar digital nerves (ulnar nerve)
18 Palmar metacarpal arteries of deep palmar arch
19 Palmar digital artery of the fifth finger
20 Fibrous sheaths of tendons of flexor muscles
21 Palmar interosseous muscles
22 Opponens pollicis muscle (cut)
23 Deep palmar arch
24 First dorsal interosseous muscle
25 First lumbrical muscle

**Right hand,** deep layer (palmar aspect). The carpal tunnel has
been opened, the tendons of the flexor muscles have been removed,
and the superficial palmar arch has been cut.

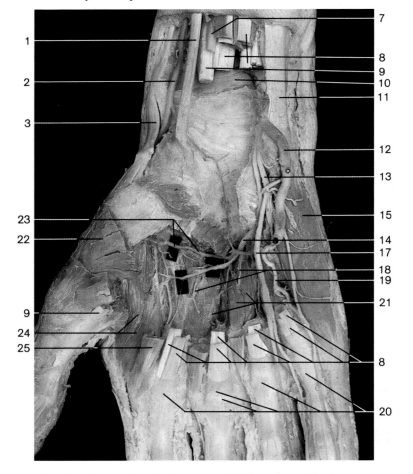

**Right hand,** deep layer (palmar aspect). Dissection of the deep
palmar arch.

# 8  Lower Limb

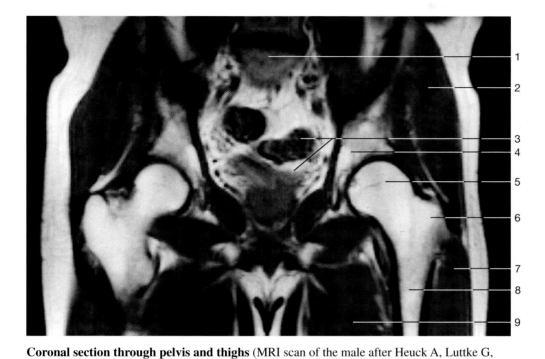

1   Sacral promontory
2   Gluteus medius muscle
3   Small intestine and urinary bladder
4   Acetabulum
5   Head of femur
6   Greater trochanter of femur
7   Vastus lateralis muscle
8   Femur
9   Adductor muscles
10  Knee joint with menisci
11  Tibia
12  Soleus muscle
13  Tibialis anterior muscle
14  Distal tibiofibular joint
15  Ankle joint
16  Fibula (lateral malleolus)

**Coronal section through pelvis and thighs** (MRI scan of the male after Heuck A, Luttke G, Rohen JW. MR-Atlas der Extremitäten. Stuttgart: Schattauer, 1994).

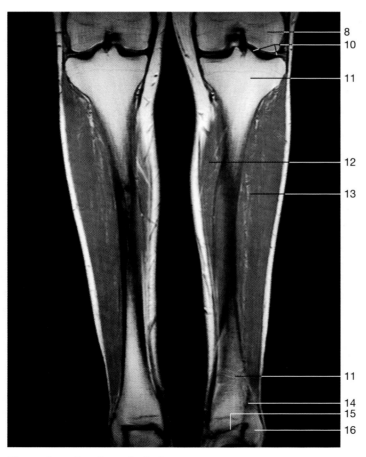

**Coronal section through the legs**
(MRI scan after Heuck A, Luttke G, Rohen JW, 1994).

The lower limb (extremity) is specialized for support of the upright posture, locomotion, and maintaining balance. In contrast to the upper limb, the lower limb is more restricted in its movements, and the joints are tighter and fixed by strong ligaments. The hip joint is a ball-and-socket type of synovial joint between the head of the femur and acetabulum. The knee joint is a hinge type of synovial joint that permits only limited rotation. The talocrural joint is a hinge joint between the talus, fibula, and tibia, only allowing movements of flexion and extension. The long axis of the foot is at a right angle to that of the leg, thus forming an effective arch for the upright stance of man.

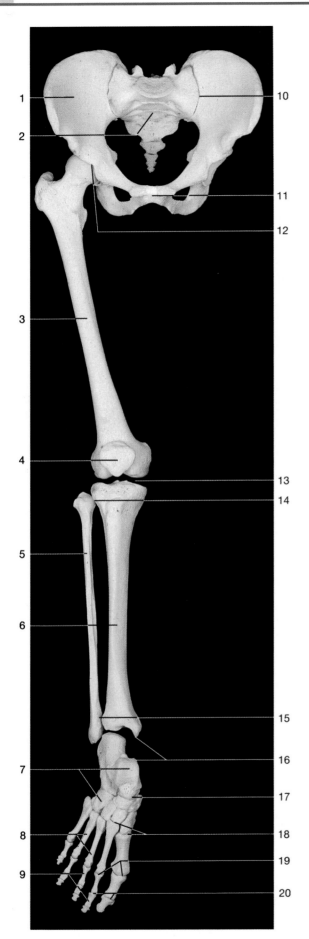

**Skeleton of pelvic girdle and lower limb**
(anterior aspect). The ankle joint has been dislocated.

| A | Pelvic girdle | 9 | Phalanges |
|---|---|---|---|
| B | Thigh | 10 | Sacro-iliac joint |
| C | Leg | 11 | Pubic symphysis |
| D | Foot | 12 | Hip joint |
| 1 | Right hip bone | 13 | Knee joint |
| 2 | Sacrum | 14 | Proximal tibiofibular joint |
| 3 | Femur | 15 | Distal tibiofibular joint |
| 4 | Patella | 16 | Ankle joint |
| 5 | Fibula | 17 | Talocalcaneonavicular joint |
| 6 | Tibia | 18 | Tarsometatarsal joints |
| 7 | Tarsal bones | 19 | Metatarsophalangeal joints |
| 8 | Metatarsal bones | 20 | Interphalangeal joints |

The pelvic girdle is firmly connected to the vertebral column at the sacro-iliac joint. Therefore, the body can be kept upright more easily even if only one limb is used for support (as in walking). The mobility of the lower limb is more limited than that of the upper limb.

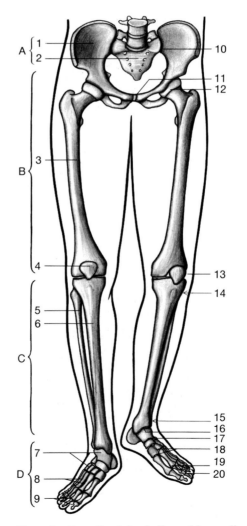

**Organization of pelvic girdle and lower limb.**

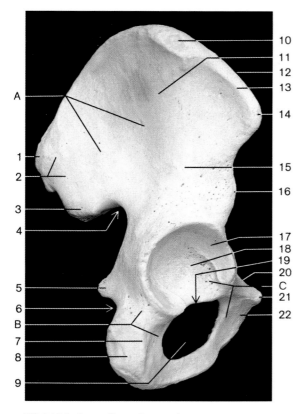

**Right hip bone** (lateral aspect).

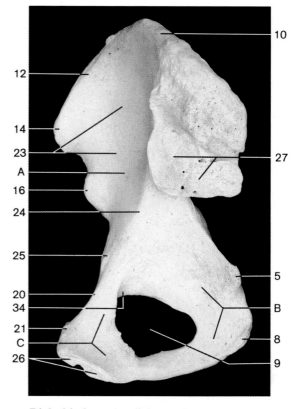

**Right hip bone** (medial aspect).

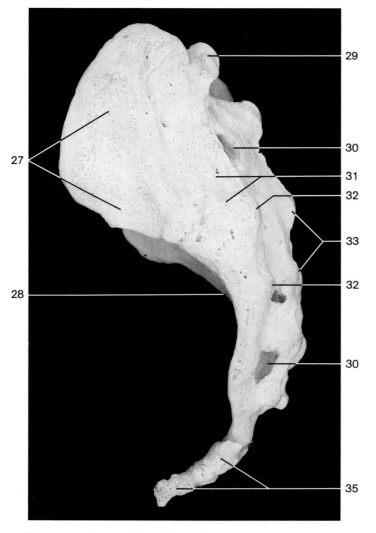

**Sacrum and coccyx** (lateral aspect).

A  Ilium
B  Ischium
C  Pubis

1  Posterior superior iliac spine
2  Posterior gluteal line
3  Posterior inferior iliac spine
4  Greater sciatic notch
5  Ischial spine
6  Lesser sciatic notch
7  Body of ischium
8  Ischial tuberosity
9  Obturator foramen
10  Iliac crest
11  Anterior gluteal line
12  Internal lip of iliac crest
13  External lip of iliac crest
14  Anterior superior iliac spine
15  Inferior gluteal line
16  Anterior inferior iliac spine
17  Lunate surface of acetabulum
18  Acetabular fossa
19  Acetabular notch
20  Pecten pubis
21  Pubic tubercle
22  Body of pubis
23  Iliac fossa
24  Arcuate line
25  Iliopubic eminence
26  Symphysial surface of pubis
27  Auricular surface
28  Pelvic surface of sacrum
29  Superior articular process of sacrum
30  Dorsal sacral foramina
31  Sacral tuberosity
32  Lateral sacral crest
33  Median sacral crest
34  Obturator groove
35  Coccyx

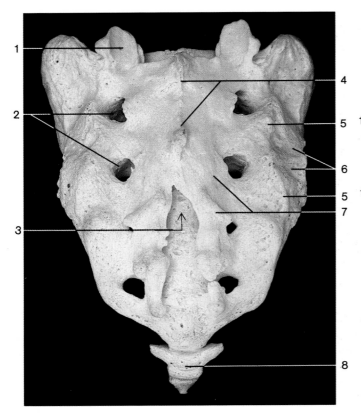

**Sacrum** (posterior aspect).

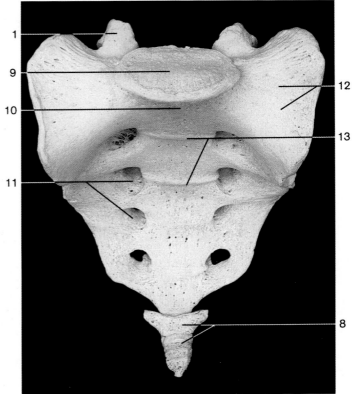

**Sacrum** (anterior aspect).

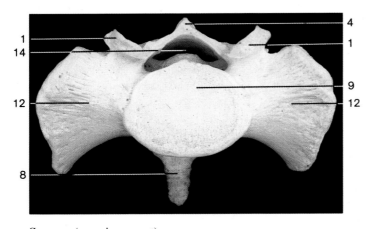

**Sacrum** (superior aspect).

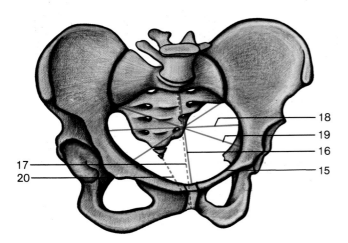

**Diameters of pelvis** (oblique superior aspect).
(Schematic drawing.)

1  Superior articular process of sacrum
2  Dorsal sacral foramina
3  Sacral hiatus
4  Median sacral crest
5  Lateral sacral crest
6  Sacral tuberosity
7  Intermediate sacral crest
8  Coccyx
9  Base of sacrum
10  Sacral promontory
11  Anterior sacral foramina
12  Lateral part of sacrum (ala)
13  Transverse line of sacrum
14  Sacral canal
15  Linea terminalis
16  True conjugate
17  Diagonal conjugate
18  Transverse diameter
19  Oblique diameter
20  Inferior pelvic aperture or outlet

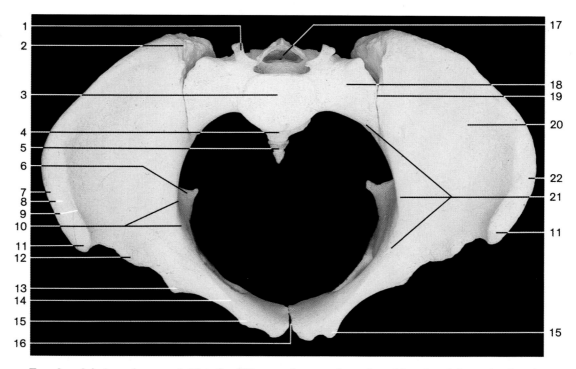

**Female pelvis** (superior aspect). Note the differences between the male and female pelvis, predominantly in the form and dimensions of the sacrum, the superior and inferior apertures, and the alae of the ilium.

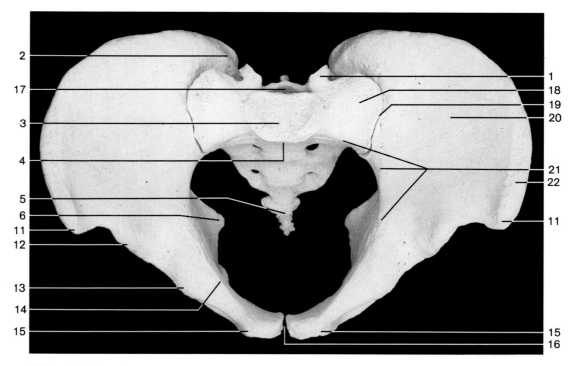

**Male pelvis** (superior aspect). Compare with the female pelvis (depicted above).

| | | | |
|---|---|---|---|
| 1 | Superior articular process of sacrum | 12 | Anterior inferior iliac spine |
| 2 | Posterior superior iliac spine | 13 | Iliopubic eminence |
| 3 | Base of sacrum | 14 | Pecten pubis |
| 4 | Sacral promontory | 15 | Pubic tubercle |
| 5 | Coccyx | 16 | Pubic symphysis |
| 6 | Ischial spine | 17 | Sacral canal |
| 7 | External lip | 18 | Ala of sacrum |
| 8 | Intermediate line    } of iliac crest | 19 | Position of sacro-iliac joint |
| 9 | Internal lip | 20 | Iliac fossa |
| 10 | Arcuate line | 21 | Linea terminalis |
| 11 | Anterior superior iliac spine | 22 | Iliac crest |

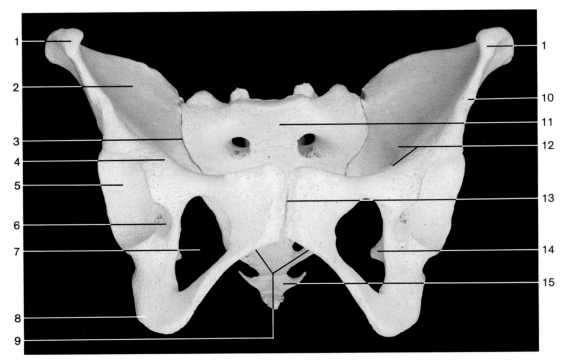

**Female pelvis** (anterior aspect). Note the differences between the form and dimensions of the male and female pelvis. The female pubic arch is wider than the male. The obturator foramen in the female pelvis is triangular, while that in the male pelvis is ovoid.

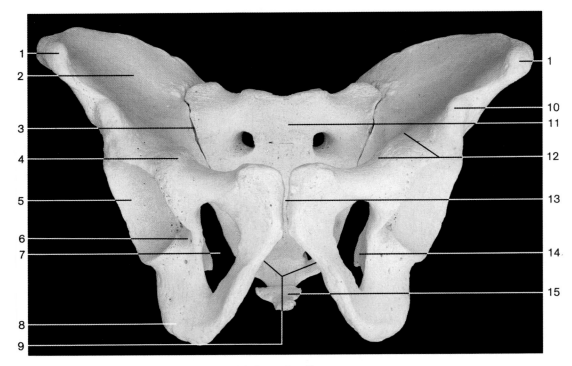

**Male pelvis** (anterior aspect). Compare with foregoing figure.

| | | | |
|---|---|---|---|
| 1 | Anterior superior iliac spine | 9 | Pubic arch |
| 2 | Iliac fossa | 10 | Anterior inferior iliac spine |
| 3 | Position of sacro-iliac joint | 11 | Sacrum |
| 4 | Iliopubic eminence | 12 | Linea terminalis (at margin of superior aperture) |
| 5 | Lunate surface of acetabulum | 13 | Pubic symphysis |
| 6 | Acetabular notch | 14 | Ischial spine |
| 7 | Obturator foramen | 15 | Coccyx |
| 8 | Ischial tuberosity | | |

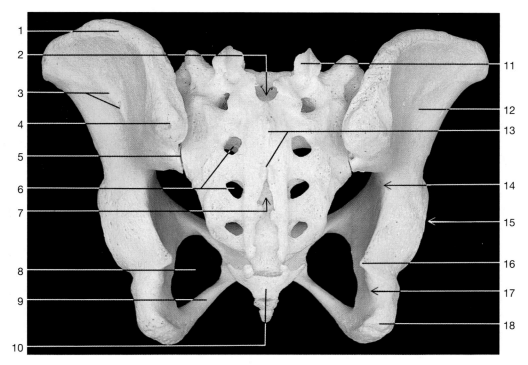

**Female pelvis** (posterior aspect). Note the differences between the female and male pelvis, especially with respect to the inferior aperture, the shape of the sacrum, the two sciatic notches, and the pubic arch.

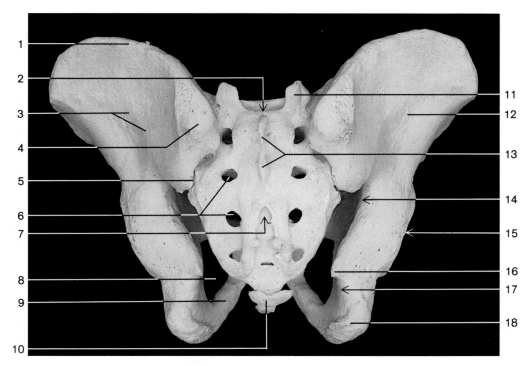

**Male pelvis** (posterior aspect). Compare with the female pelvis (depicted above).

| | |
|---|---|
| 1 Iliac crest | 10 Coccyx |
| 2 Sacral canal | 11 Superior articular process of sacrum |
| 3 Posterior gluteal line | 12 Gluteal surface of ilium |
| 4 Posterior superior iliac spine | 13 Median sacral crest |
| 5 Position of sacro-iliac joint | 14 Greater sciatic notch |
| 6 Dorsal sacral foramina | 15 Position of acetabulum |
| 7 Sacral hiatus | 16 Ischial spine |
| 8 Obturator foramen | 17 Lesser sciatic notch |
| 9 Ramus of ischium | 18 Ischial tuberosity |

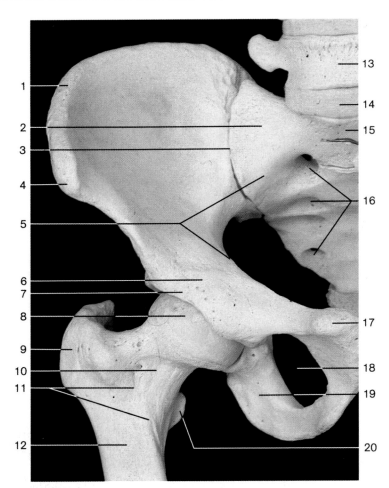

**Bones of right hip joint** (anterior aspect).

1   Iliac crest
2   Lateral part of sacrum (ala)
3   Position of sacro-iliac joint
4   Anterior superior iliac spine
5   Linea terminalis
6   Iliopubic eminence
7   Bony margin of acetabulum
8   Head of femur
9   Greater trochanter
10  Neck of femur
11  Intertrochanteric line
12  Shaft of femur
13  Fifth lumbar vertebra
14  Imitation intervertebral disc between fifth lumbar
    vertebra and sacrum
15  Sacral promontory
16  Anterior sacral foramina
17  Pubic tubercle
18  Obturator foramen
19  Ramus of ischium
20  Lesser trochanter
21  Dorsal sacral foramina
22  Greater sciatic notch
23  Ischial spine
24  Pubic symphysis
25  Pubis
26  Ischial tuberosity
27  Intertrochanteric crest
28  Symphysial surface

**Diameters of the pelvis**
A   True conjugate (11–11.5 cm) (Conjugata vera)
B   Diagonal conjugate (12.5–13 cm)
C   Largest diameter of pelvis
D   Inferior pelvic aperture
E   Pelvic inclination (60°)

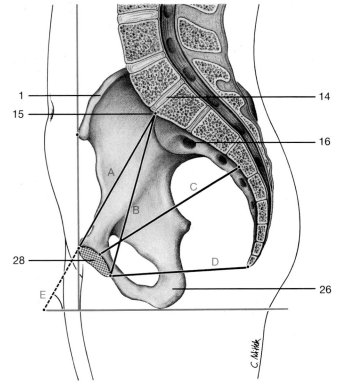

**Inclination and diameters of the female pelvis,**
right half (medial aspect).

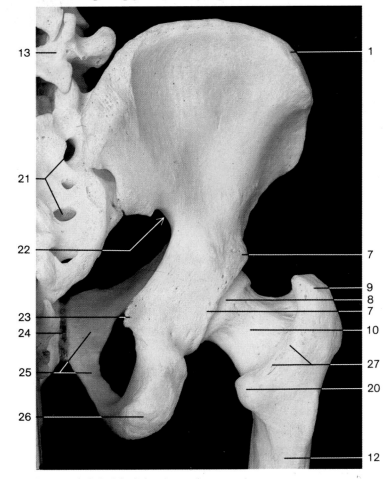

**Bones of right hip joint** (posterior aspect).

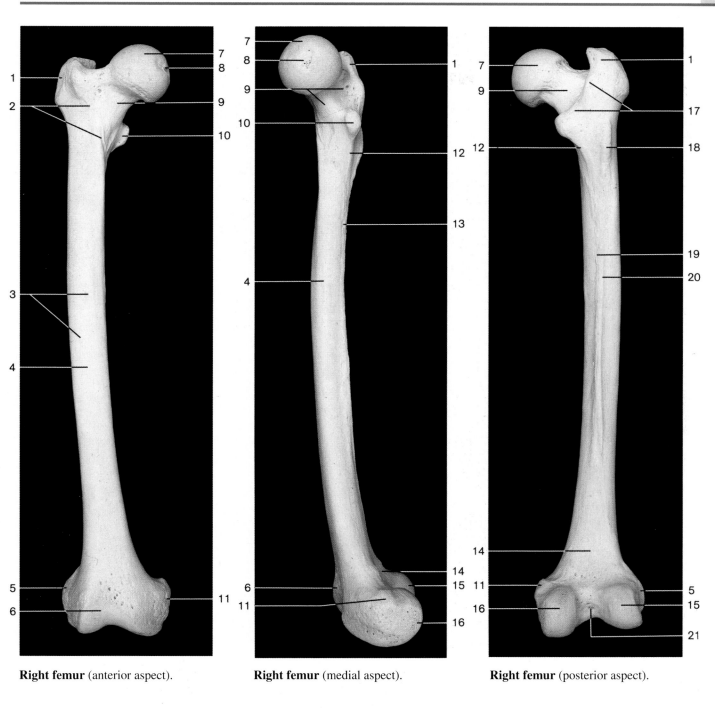

**Right femur** (anterior aspect).

**Right femur** (medial aspect).

**Right femur** (posterior aspect).

1  Greater trochanter
2  Intertrochanteric line
3  Nutrient foramina
4  Shaft of femur (diaphysis)
5  Lateral epicondyle
6  Patellar surface
7  Head

8  Fovea of head
9  Neck
10  Lesser trochanter
11  Medial epicondyle
12  Pectineal line
13  Linea aspera
14  Popliteal surface

15  Lateral condyle
16  Medial condyle
17  Intertrochanteric crest
18  Third trochanter
19  Medial lip of linea aspera
20  Lateral lip of linea aspera
21  Intercondylar fossa

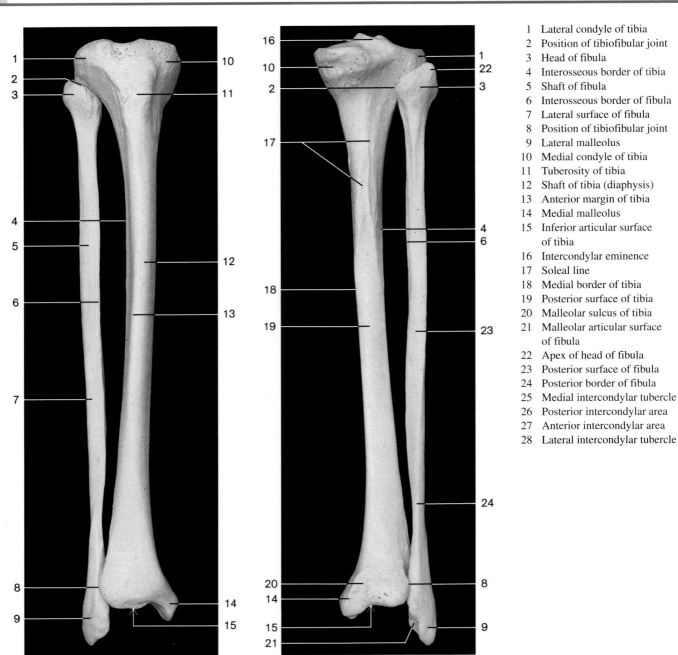

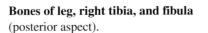

1  Lateral condyle of tibia
2  Position of tibiofibular joint
3  Head of fibula
4  Interosseous border of tibia
5  Shaft of fibula
6  Interosseous border of fibula
7  Lateral surface of fibula
8  Position of tibiofibular joint
9  Lateral malleolus
10 Medial condyle of tibia
11 Tuberosity of tibia
12 Shaft of tibia (diaphysis)
13 Anterior margin of tibia
14 Medial malleolus
15 Inferior articular surface
   of tibia
16 Intercondylar eminence
17 Soleal line
18 Medial border of tibia
19 Posterior surface of tibia
20 Malleolar sulcus of tibia
21 Malleolar articular surface
   of fibula
22 Apex of head of fibula
23 Posterior surface of fibula
24 Posterior border of fibula
25 Medial intercondylar tubercle
26 Posterior intercondylar area
27 Anterior intercondylar area
28 Lateral intercondylar tubercle

**Bones of leg, right tibia, and fibula**
(anterior aspect).

**Bones of leg, right tibia, and fibula**
(posterior aspect).

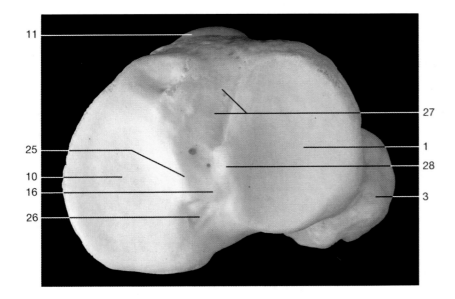

**Upper end of right tibia with fibula**
(from above), anterior margin of tibia above.
Superior articular surface of tibia.

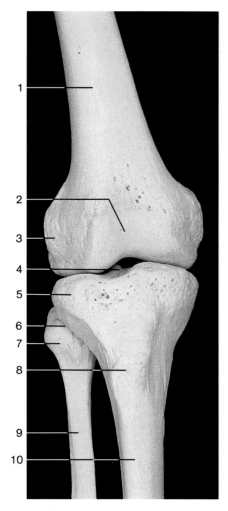

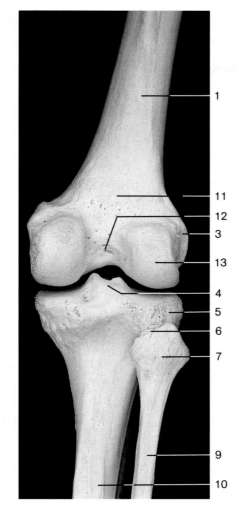

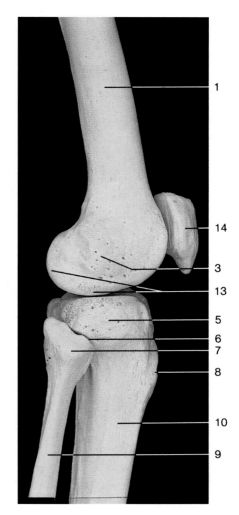

**Bones of right knee joint**
(anterior aspect).

**Bones of right knee joint**
(posterior aspect).

**Bones of right knee joint**
(lateral aspect).

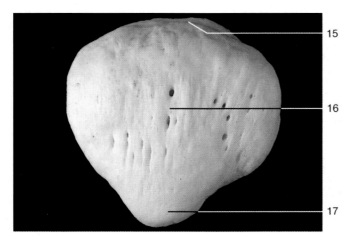

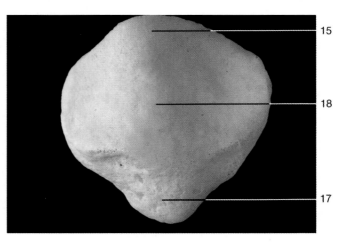

**Right patella** (anterior aspect).

**Right patella** (posterior aspect).

| | |
|---|---|
| 1 Femur | 10 Shaft of tibia |
| 2 Patellar surface of femur | 11 Popliteal surface of femur |
| 3 Lateral epicondyle of femur | 12 Intercondylar fossa of femur |
| 4 Intercondylar eminence of tibia | 13 Lateral condyle of femur |
| 5 Lateral condyle of tibia | 14 Patella |
| 6 Position of tibiofibular joint | 15 Base of patella |
| 7 Head of fibula | 16 Anterior surface of patella |
| 8 Tuberosity of tibia | 17 Apex of patella |
| 9 Fibula | 18 Articular surface of patella |

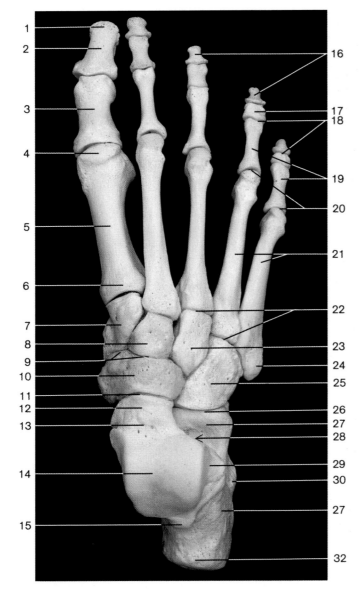

**Bones of right foot** (dorsal aspect).

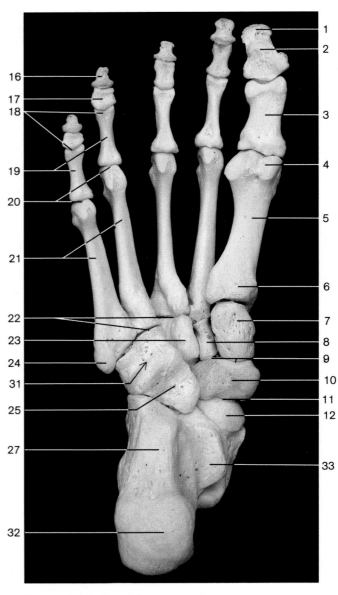

**Bones of right foot** (plantar aspect).

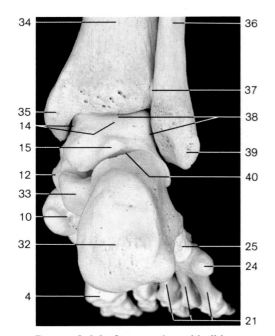

**Bones of right foot** together with tibia
and fibula (posterior aspect).

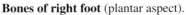

1   Tuberosity of distal phalanx of great toe
2   Distal phalanx of great toe
3   Proximal phalanx of great toe
4   Head of first metatarsal bone
5   First metatarsal bone
6   Base of first metatarsal bone
7   Medial cuneiform bone
8   Intermediate cuneiform bone
9   Position of cuneonavicular joint
10  Navicular bone

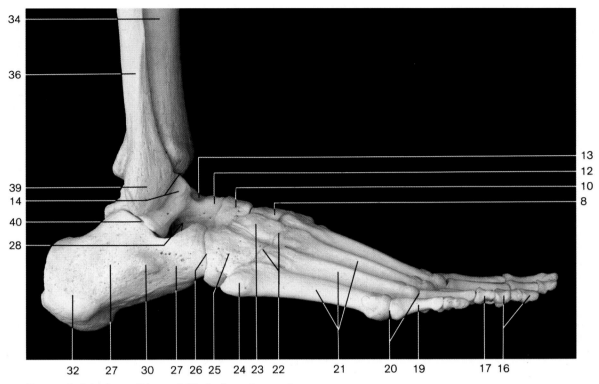

**Bones of right foot, tibia, and fibula** (lateral aspect).

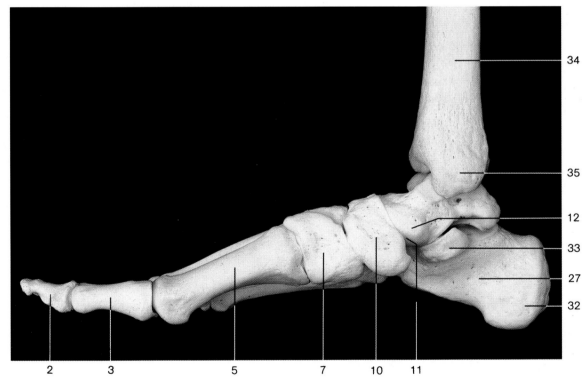

**Bones of right foot, tibia, and fibula** (medial aspect).

| | | | | |
|---|---|---|---|---|
| 11 | Position of talocalcaneonavicular joint | 21 | Metatarsal bones | 31 Groove for tendon of peroneus longus |
| 12 | Head of talus | 22 | Position of tarsometatarsal joints | 32 Calcaneal tuberosity |
| 13 | Neck of talus | 23 | Lateral cuneiform bone | 33 Sustentaculum tali |
| 14 | Trochlea of talus | 24 | Tuberosity of fifth metatarsal bone | 34 Tibia |
| 15 | Posterior talar process | 25 | Cuboid bone | 35 Medial malleolus |
| 16 | Distal phalanges | 26 | Position of calcaneocuboid joint | 36 Fibula |
| 17 | Middle phalanges | 27 | Calcaneus | 37 Position of tibiofibular syndesmosis |
| 18 | Position of interphalangeal joints | 28 | Tarsal sinus | 38 Position of ankle joint |
| 19 | Proximal phalanges | 29 | Lateral malleolar surface of talus | 39 Lateral malleolus |
| 20 | Position of metatarsophalangeal joints | 30 | Peroneal trochlea of calcaneus | 40 Position of subtalar joint |

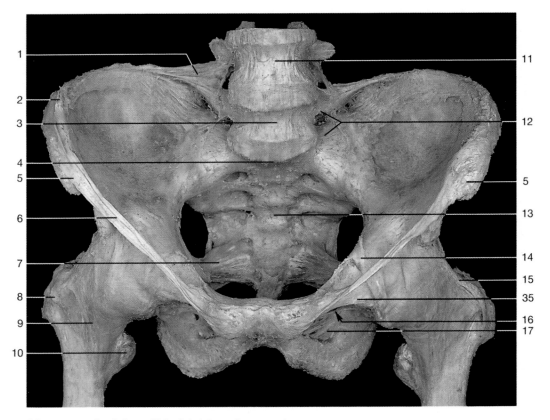

**Ligaments of pelvis and hip joint** (anterior aspect).

| | | |
|---|---|---|
| 1 Iliolumbar ligament | 13 Sacrum | 26 Articular capsule of hip joint |
| 2 Iliac crest | 14 Iliopectineal arch | 27 Dorsal sacro-iliac ligaments |
| 3 Fifth lumbar vertebra | 15 Iliofemoral ligament (horizontal band) | 28 Coccyx with superficial dorsal |
| 4 Sacral promontory | 16 Obturator canal | sacrococcygeal ligament |
| 5 Anterior superior iliac spine | 17 Obturator membrane | 29 Head of femur |
| 6 Inguinal ligament | 18 Greater sciatic foramen | 30 Articular cartilage of head of femur |
| 7 Sacrospinous ligament | 19 Sacrospinous ligament | 31 Articular cavity of hip joint |
| 8 Greater trochanter | 20 Sacrotuberous ligament | 32 Acetabular lip |
| 9 Iliofemoral ligament (vertical band) | 21 Lesser sciatic foramen | 33 Spongy bone |
| 10 Lesser trochanter | 22 Ischial tuberosity | 34 Ligament of head of femur |
| 11 Fourth lumbar vertebra | 23 Ischiofemoral ligament | 35 Pubofemoral ligament |
| 12 Iliolumbar and ventral sacro-iliac | 24 Intertrochanteric crest | 36 Zona orbicularis |
| ligaments | 25 Femur | |

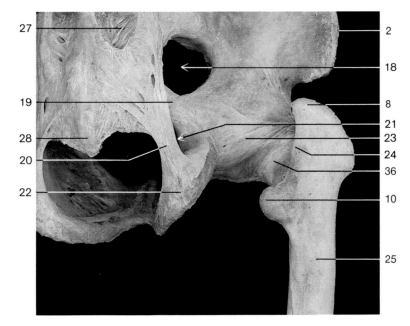

**Ligaments of pelvis and hip joint** (right posterior aspect).

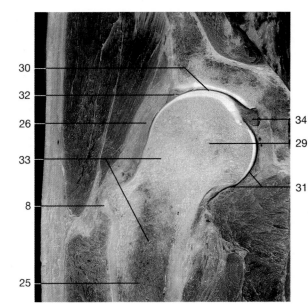

**Coronal section of right hip joint** (anterior view).

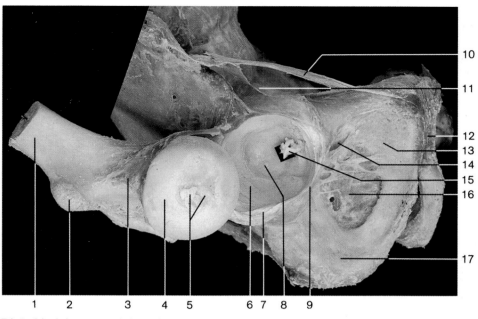

1  Femur
2  Lesser trochanter
3  Neck of femur
4  Head of femur
5  Fovea of head with cut edge of
   ligament of head
6  Lunate surface of acetabulum
7  Acetabular lip
8  Acetabular fossa
9  Transverse acetabular ligament
10 Inguinal ligament
11 Iliopectineal arch
12 Pubic symphysis
13 Pubic bone
14 Obturator canal
15 Ligament of head of femur
16 Obturator membrane
17 Ischium
18 Anterior longitudinal ligament
   (level of fifth lumbar vertebra)
19 Sacral promontory
20 Iliolumbar ligament
21 Iliac crest
22 Anterior superior iliac spine
23 Iliofemoral ligament (horizontal
   band)
24 Iliofemoral ligament (vertical
   band)
25 Greater trochanter
26 Pubofemoral ligament
27 Anterior inferior iliac spine
28 Ventral sacro-iliac ligaments
29 Sacrospinous ligament
30 Sacrotuberous ligament
31 Intertrochanteric line
32 Ischiofemoral ligament
33 Zona orbicularis

**Right hip joint,** opened (lateral anterior aspect). The ligament of the head of the femur has been divided, and the femur has been posteriorly reflected.

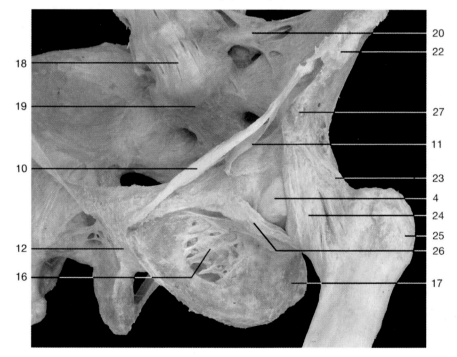

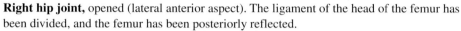

◁ **Ligaments of the pelvis and hip joint** (anterolateral aspect).

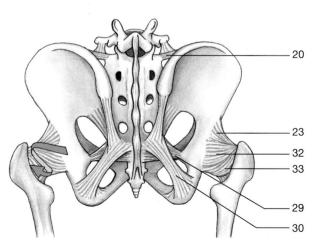

**Ligaments of hip joint** (anterior aspect). (Schematic drawing.)

**Ligaments of hip joint** (posterior aspect). (Schematic drawing.)

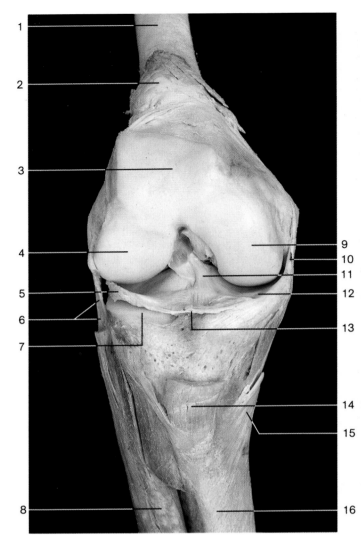

**Right knee joint** (opened) **with ligaments** (anterior aspect). The patella and articular capsule have been removed and the femur slightly flexed.

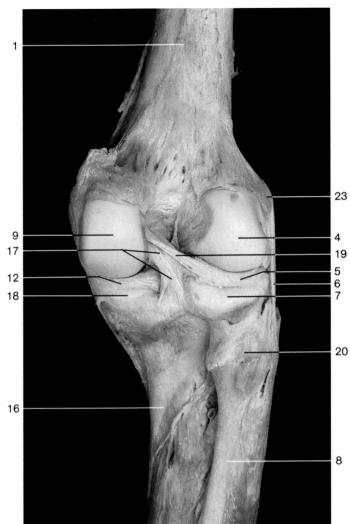

**Right knee joint with ligaments** (posterior aspect). The joint is extended and the articular capsule has been removed.

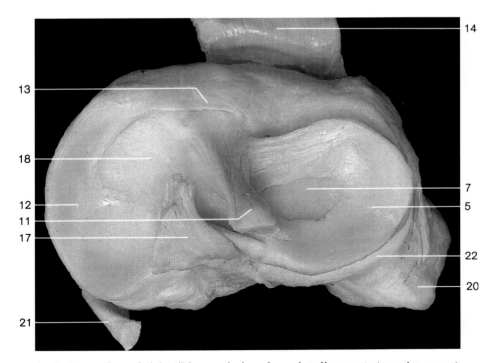

**Articular surface of right tibia, menisci, and cruciate ligaments** (superior aspect). Anterior margin of tibia above.

1   Femur
2   Articular capsule with suprapatellar bursa
3   Patellar surface
4   Lateral condyle of femur
5   Lateral meniscus of knee joint
6   Fibular collateral ligament
7   Lateral condyle of tibia (superior articular surface)
8   Fibula
9   Medial condyle of femur
10  Tibial collateral ligament
11  Anterior cruciate ligament
12  Medial meniscus of knee joint
13  Transverse ligament of knee
14  Patellar ligament
15  Common tendon of sartorius, semitendinosus, and gracilis muscles
16  Tibia
17  Posterior cruciate ligament
18  Medial condyle of tibia (superior articular surface)
19  Posterior meniscofemoral ligament
20  Head of fibula
21  Tendon of semimembranosus muscle
22  Posterior attachment of articular capsule of knee joint
23  Lateral epicondyle of femur

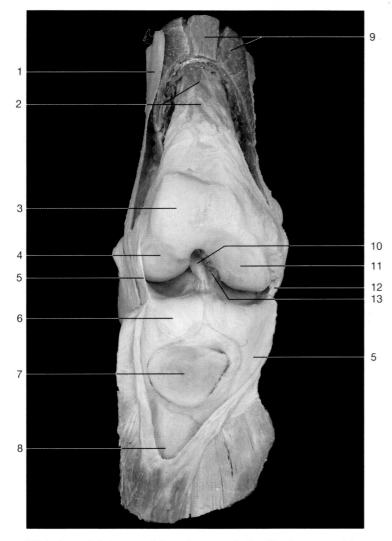

1    Iliotibial tract
2    Articular muscle of knee
3    Patellar surface
4    Lateral condyle of femur
5    Articular capsule
6    Infrapatellar fat pad
7    Patella (articular surface)
8    Suprapatellar bursa
9    Quadriceps muscle of thigh (divided)
10    Anterior cruciate ligament
11    Medial condyle of femur
12    Fibular collateral ligament
13    Posterior cruciate ligament
14    Medial epicondyle of femur
15    Intercondylar fossa of femur
16    Tibial collateral ligament
17    Medial meniscus of knee joint
18    Medial intercondylar tubercle
19    Femur
20    Lateral epicondyle of femur
21    Lateral meniscus of knee joint
22    Epiphysial line of tibia
23    Tibia

**Right knee joint,** opened (anterior aspect). Patellar ligament with patella reflected.

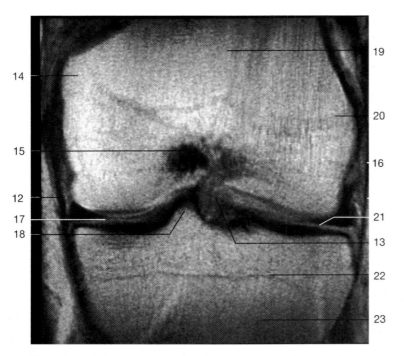

**Right knee joint.** Frontal section through the central part of the joint (posterior aspect, MRI scan). (See also p. 10.)

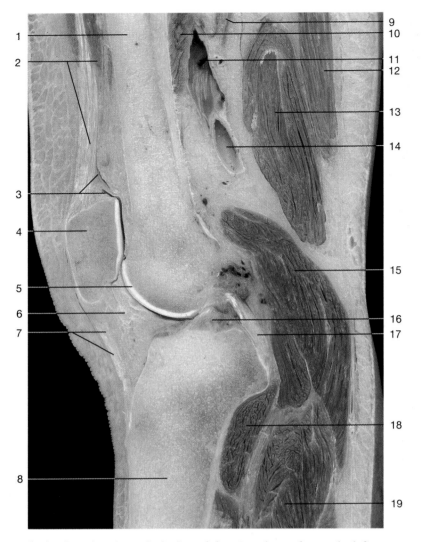

1   Femur
2   Quadriceps femoris muscle
3   Suprapatellar bursa and articular cavity
4   Patella
5   Patellar surface (articular cartilage)
6   Infrapatellar fat pad
7   Patellar ligament
8   Tibia
9   Tibial nerve
10  Adductor magnus muscle
11  Popliteal vein
12  Semitendinosus muscle
13  Semimembranosus muscle
14  Popliteal artery
15  Gastrocnemius muscle
16  Anterior cruciate ligament
17  Posterior cruciate ligament
18  Popliteus muscle
19  Soleus muscle
20  Deep flexor muscles of leg
21  Calcaneal tendon
22  Epiphysial line of tibia
23  Calcaneus
24  Ankle joint
25  Talus
26  Lateral meniscus
27  Epiphysial line of femur

**Sagittal section through the knee joint.** Anterior surface to the left.

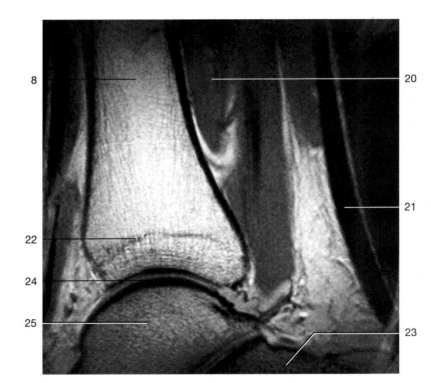

**Ankle joint.** Sagittal section; anterior part to the left. (MRI scan.)

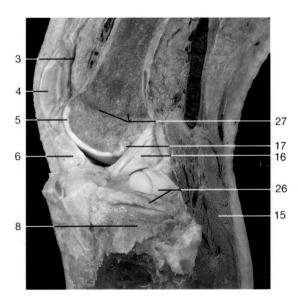

**Left knee joint.** Anterior cruciate ligament (lateral aspect).

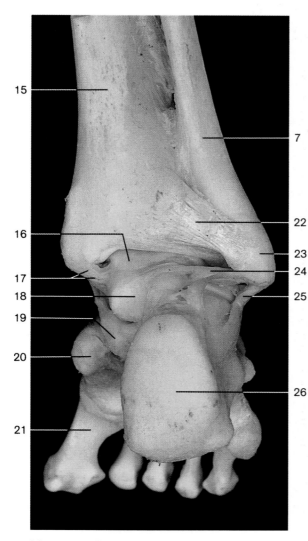

**Ligaments of ankle joint,** right leg (posterior aspect).

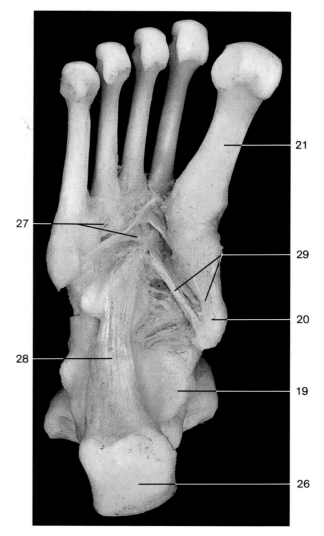

**Deep ligaments of the foot,** right foot (plantar aspect). The toes have been removed.

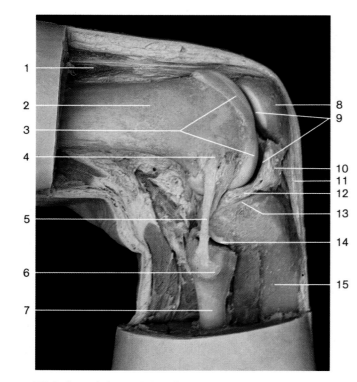

**Right knee joint and tibiofibular joint with ligaments.** Note the position of the lateral meniscus.

1   Quadriceps femoris muscle
2   Femur
3   Patellar surface
4   Lateral epicondyle of femur
5   Fibular collateral ligament
6   Head of fibula
7   Fibula
8   Patella
9   Articular cavity of knee joint
10  Infrapatellar fat pad
11  Patellar ligament
12  Lateral meniscus of knee joint
13  Lateral condyle of tibia (superior articular facet)
14  Tibiofibular joint
15  Tibia
16  Trochlea of talus (superior surface)
17  Deltoid ligament of ankle (posterior tibiotalar part)
18  Talus
19  Sustentaculum tali
20  Navicular bone
21  First metatarsal bone
22  Posterior tibiofibular ligament
23  Lateral malleolus
24  Posterior talofibular ligament
25  Calcaneofibular ligament
26  Calcaneal tuberosity
27  Plantar tarsometatarsal ligaments
28  Long plantar ligament
29  Plantar cuneonavicular ligaments

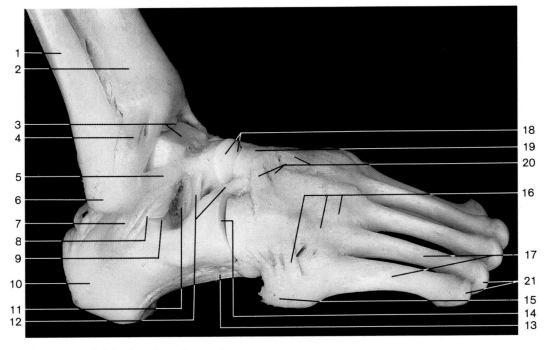

**Ligaments of right foot** (lateral aspect).

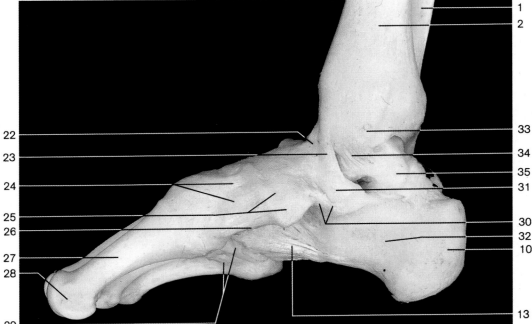

**Ligaments of right foot** (medial aspect).

 1  Fibula
 2  Tibia
 3  Trochlea of talus and ankle joint
 4  Anterior tibiofibular ligament
 5  Anterior talofibular ligament
 6  Lateral malleolus
 7  Calcaneofibular ligament
 8  Lateral talocalcaneal ligament
 9  Subtalar joint
10  Tuber calcanei
11  Interosseous talocalcaneal ligament
12  Bifurcate ligament
13  Long plantar ligament
14  Calcaneocuboid joint
15  Tuberosity of fifth metatarsal bone
16  Dorsal tarsometatarsal ligaments
17  Metatarsal bones

18  Head of talus and talocalcaneonavicular joint
19  Navicular bone
20  Dorsal cuneonavicular ligaments
21  Heads of metatarsal bones
22  Medial or deltoid ligament of ankle (tibionavicular part)
23  Medial or deltoid ligament of ankle (tibiocalcaneal part)
24  Dorsal cuneonavicular ligaments
25  Navicular bone
26  Plantar cuneonavicular ligament
27  First metatarsal bone
28  Head of first metatarsal bone
29  Plantar tarsometatarsal ligaments
30  Plantar calcaneonavicular ligament
31  Sustentaculum tali
32  Calcaneus
33  Medial malleolus
34  Medial or deltoid ligament of ankle (posterior part)
35  Talus

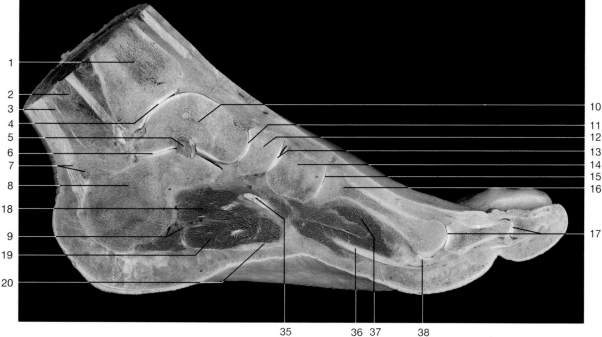

**Longitudinal section through the foot at the level of first phalanx.**

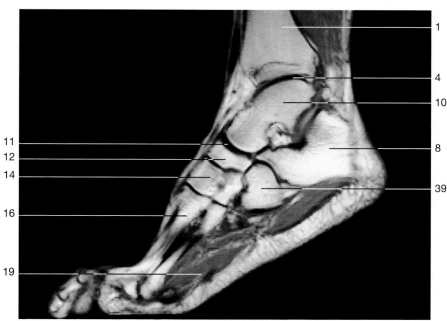

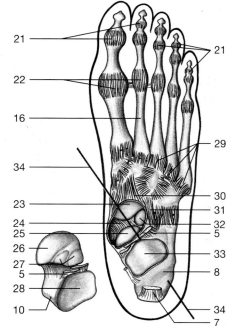

**Sagittal section through the foot** (MRI scan after Heuck A, Luttke G, Rohen JW; 1994).

**Talocalcaneonavicular joint.** The talus has been rotated to show the articular surfaces of the joint.

| | | | |
|---|---|---|---|
| 1 | Tibia | 17 | Metatarsophalangeal and interphalangeal joints |
| 2 | Deep flexor muscles | 18 | Quadratus plantae muscle with flexor tendons |
| 3 | Superficial flexor muscles | | |
| 4 | Ankle joint | 19 | Flexor digitorum brevis muscle |
| 5 | Interosseous talocalcaneal ligament | 20 | Plantar aponeurosis |
| 6 | Subtalar joint | 21 | Articular capsules of interphalangeal joints |
| 7 | Calcaneal or Achilles tendon and bursa | | |
| 8 | Calcaneus | 22 | Articular capsules of metatarsophalangeal joints |
| 9 | Vessels and nerves of foot | | |
| 10 | Talus | 23 | Articular surface of navicular bone |
| 11 | Talocalcaneonavicular joint | 24 | Plantar calcaneonavicular ligament |
| 12 | Navicular bone | 25 | Middle talar articular surface of calcaneus |
| 13 | Cuneonavicular joint | 26 | Navicular articular surface of talus |
| 14 | Intermediate cuneiform bone | 27 | Anterior and middle calcaneal surfaces of talus |
| 15 | Tarsometatarsal joints | | |
| 16 | Metatarsal bones | | |

| | |
|---|---|
| 28 | Posterior calcaneal surface of talus |
| 29 | Dorsal tarsometatarsal ligaments |
| 30 | Talonavicular ligament |
| 31 | Bifurcate ligament |
| 32 | Anterior talar articular surface of calcaneus |
| 33 | Posterior talar articular surface of calcaneus |
| 34 | Axis for inversion and eversion |
| 35 | Tendon of tibialis posterior muscle |
| 36 | Tendon of flexor hallucis longus muscle |
| 37 | Flexor hallucis brevis muscle |
| 38 | Sesamoid bone |
| 39 | Cuboid bone |

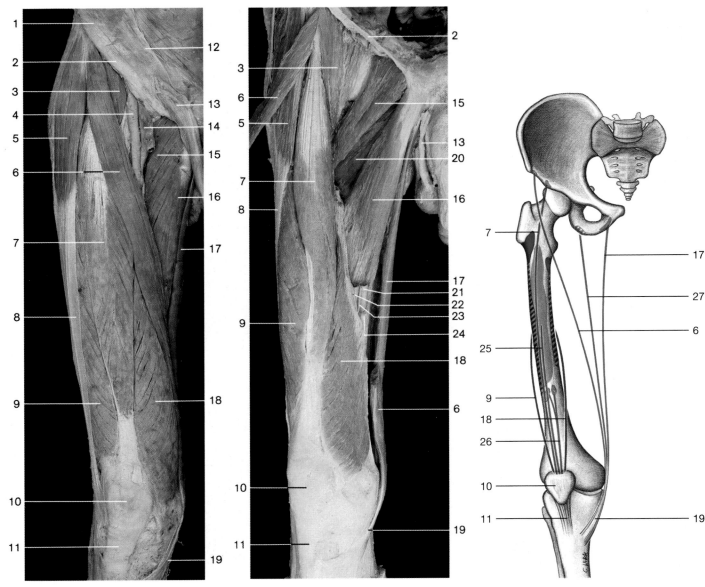

**Extensor and adductor muscles of thigh,** right thigh (anterior aspect).

**Quadriceps muscle and superficial layer of adductor muscles,** right thigh (anterior aspect). The sartorius muscle has been divided.

**Course of extensor muscles of thigh** and muscles inserting with common tendon on tibia.

1   Anterior superior iliac spine
2   Inguinal ligament
3   Iliopsoas muscle
4   Femoral artery
5   Tensor fasciae latae muscle
6   Sartorius muscle
7   Rectus femoris muscle
8   Iliotibial tract
9   Vastus lateralis muscle
10  Patella
11  Patellar ligament
12  Aponeurosis of external abdominal oblique muscle
13  Spermatic cord
14  Femoral vein

15  Pectineus muscle
16  Adductor longus muscle
17  Gracilis muscle
18  Vastus medialis muscle
19  Common tendon of sartorius, gracilis, and semitendinosus muscles (pes anserinus)
20  Adductor brevis muscle
21  Femoral artery      ⎫
22  Femoral vein        ⎬  entering the adductor canal
23  Saphenous nerve     ⎭
24  Fascia of adductor canal
25  Vastus intermedius muscle
26  Articularis genus muscle
27  Semitendinosus muscle

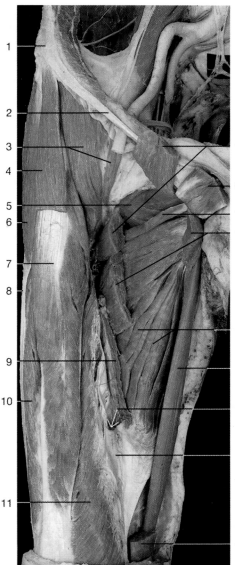

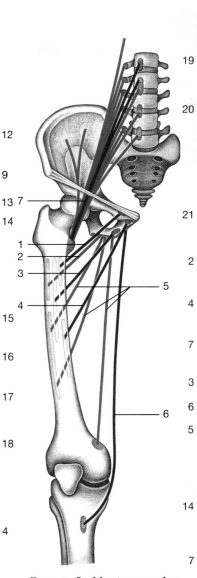

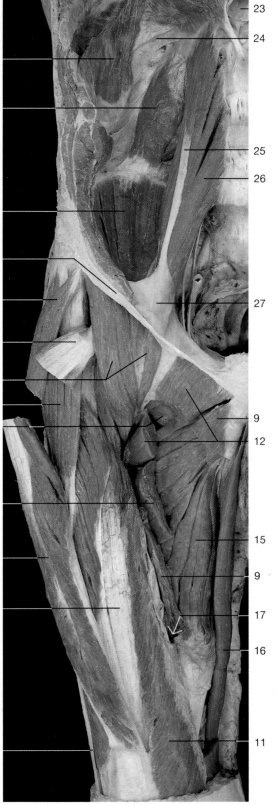

**Deep layer of adductor muscles.**
**Adductor magnus muscle** (anterior aspect). Pectineus, adductor longus, and brevis muscles have been divided.

**Course of adductor muscles**
(schematic drawing).

1 Pectineus muscle (blue)
2 Adductor minimus muscle (red)
3 Adductor brevis muscle (blue)
4 Adductor longus muscle (blue)
5 Adductor magnus muscle (red)
6 Gracilis muscle (blue)
7 Iliopsoas muscle (red/blue)

**Iliopsoas and adductor muscles,** deepest layer (anterior aspect). Pectineus, adductor longus and brevis, and rectus femoris muscles have been divided.

| | |
|---|---|
| 1 Anterior superior iliac spine | 15 Adductor magnus muscle |
| 2 Inguinal ligament | 16 Gracilis muscle |
| 3 Iliopsoas muscle | 17 Adductor hiatus |
| 4 Sartorius muscle | 18 Vasto-adductor membrane |
| 5 Obturator externus muscle | 19 Diaphragm |
| 6 Tensor fasciae latae muscle | 20 Quadratus lumborum |
| 7 Rectus femoris muscle | muscle |
| 8 Iliotibial tract | 21 Iliacus muscle |
| 9 Adductor longus muscle (divided) | 22 Vastus intermedius muscle |
| 10 Vastus lateralis muscle | 23 Aorta in aortic hiatus |
| 11 Vastus medialis muscle | 24 Twelfth rib |
| 12 Pectineus muscle (divided) | 25 Psoas minor muscle |
| 13 Adductor minimus muscle | 26 Psoas major muscle |
| 14 Adductor brevis muscle (cut) | 27 Iliopectineal arch |

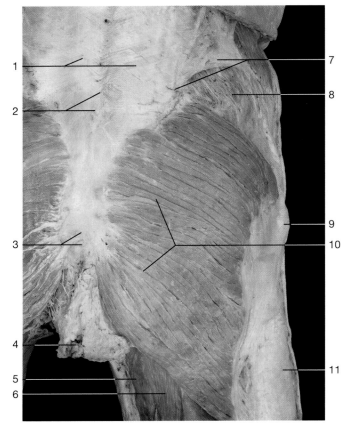

1
2

3

4
5
6

7
8

9
10

11

**Gluteal muscles, superficial layer** (posterior aspect).

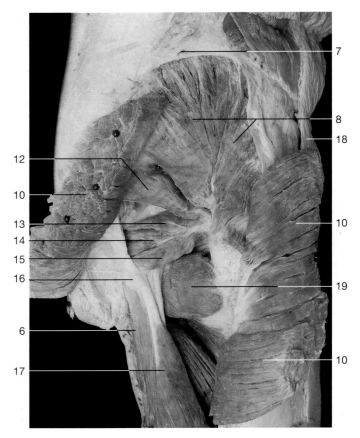

12
10
13
14
15
16

6
17

7

8
18

10

19

10

**Gluteal muscles, deeper layer** (posterior aspect).

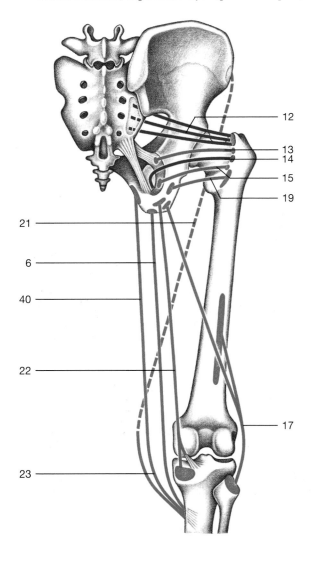

12

13
14

15
19

21

6

40

22

23

17

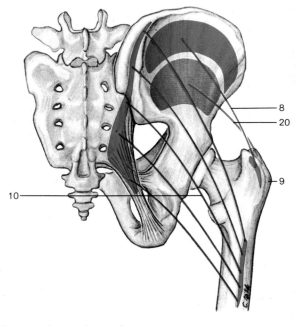

8
20

9

10

**Course of gluteal muscles**
(posterior aspect; schematic drawing).

◁

**Course of gluteal muscles** (deeper layer) **and of
ischiocrural muscles** (posterior aspect).
Sartorius muscle is indicated by dotted line (schematic
drawing).

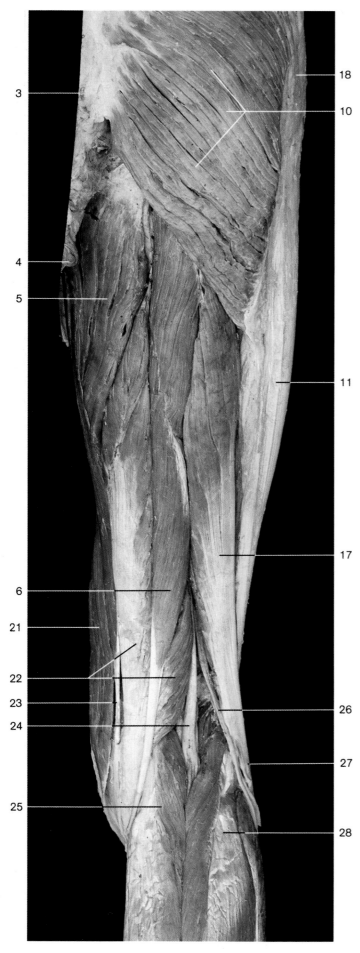

1  Thoracolumbar fascia
2  Spinous processes of lumbar vertebrae
3  Coccyx
4  Anus
5  Adductor magnus muscle
6  Semitendinosus muscle
7  Iliac crest
8  Gluteus medius muscle
9  Greater trochanter
10  Gluteus maximus muscle
11  Iliotibial tract
12  Piriformis muscle
13  Superior gemellus muscle
14  Obturator internus muscle
15  Inferior gemellus muscle
16  Ischial tuberosity
17  Biceps femoris muscle
18  Tensor fasciae latae muscle
19  Quadratus femoris muscle
20  Gluteus minimus muscle
21  Sartorius muscle
22  Semimembranosus muscle
23  Tendon of gracilis muscle
24  Tibial nerve
25  Medial head of gastrocnemius muscle
26  Common peroneal nerve
27  Tendon of biceps femoris muscle
28  Lateral head of gastrocnemius muscle
29  Rectus femoris muscle
30  Vastus medialis muscle
31  Vastus intermedius muscle
32  Vastus lateralis muscle
33  Sciatic nerve
34  Gluteus maximus muscle (insertion)
35  Great saphenous vein
36  Femoral artery
37  Femoral vein
38  Adductor longus muscle
39  Femur
40  Gracilis muscle
41  Septum between semitendinosus
    and semimembranosus muscles

**Flexors of the right thigh, superficial layer** (dorsal aspect).

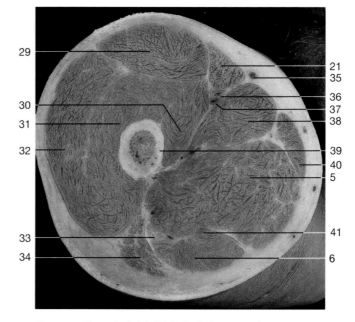

**Cross section of right thigh** (inferior aspect).
Anterior side on top.

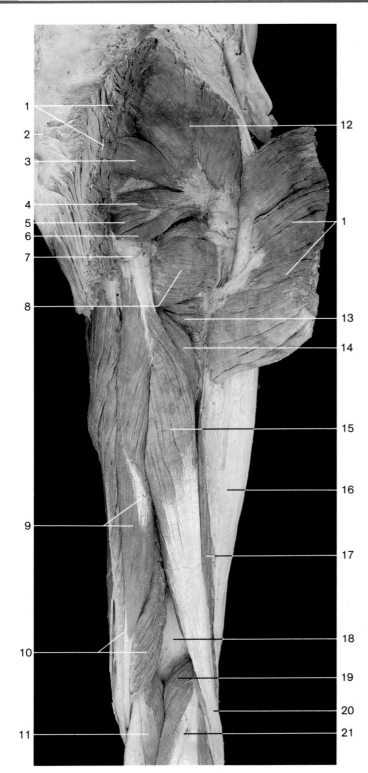

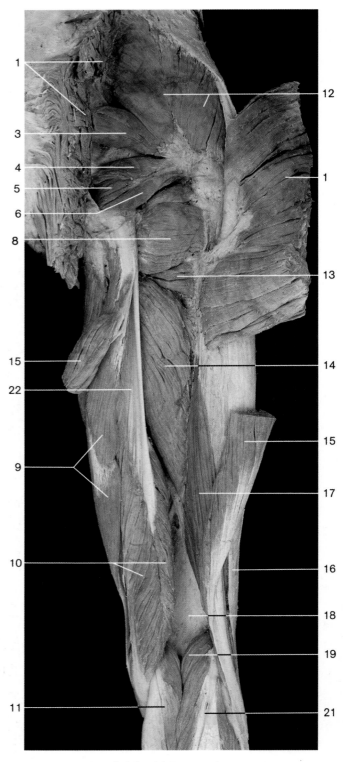

**Dorsal muscles of right thigh** (posterior aspect).
The gluteus maximus muscle has been cut and reflected.

**Dorsal muscles of right thigh** (posterior aspect).
The gluteus maximus muscle and the long head of biceps femoris muscle have been divided and displaced.

| | | | | |
|---|---|---|---|---|
| 1 | Gluteus maximus muscle (divided) | 9 | Semitendinosus muscle with intermediate tendon | 17 Short head of biceps femoris muscle |
| 2 | Position of coccyx | 10 | Semimembranosus muscle | 18 Popliteal surface of femur |
| 3 | Piriformis muscle | 11 | Medial head of gastrocnemius muscle | 19 Plantaris muscle |
| 4 | Superior gemellus muscle | 12 | Gluteus medius muscle | 20 Tendon of biceps femoris muscle |
| 5 | Obturator internus muscle | 13 | Adductor minimus muscle | 21 Lateral head of gastrocnemius muscle |
| 6 | Inferior gemellus muscle | 14 | Adductor magnus muscle | 22 Membranous part of |
| 7 | Ischial tuberosity | 15 | Long head of biceps femoris muscle |    semimembranosus muscle |
| 8 | Quadratus femoris muscle | 16 | Iliotibial tract | |

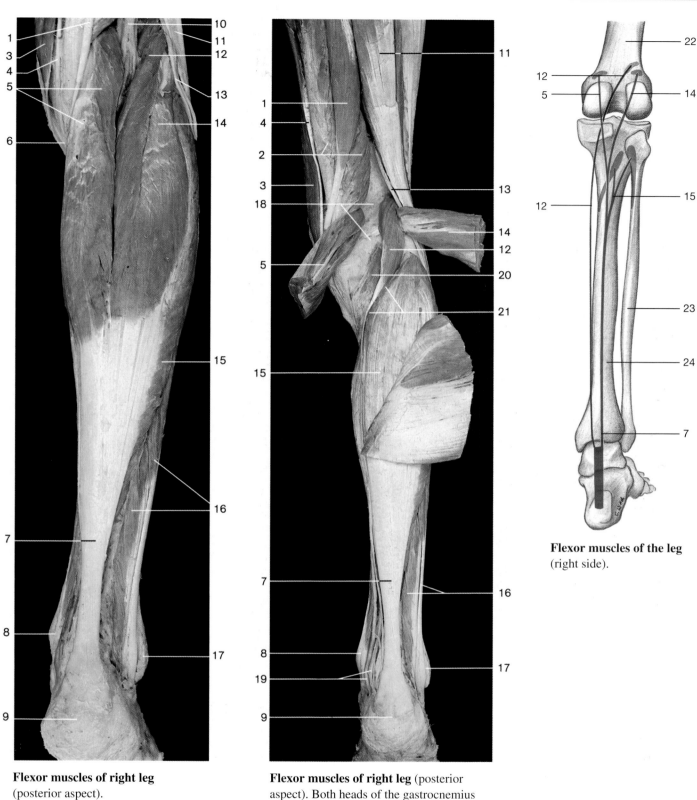

**Flexor muscles of right leg**
(posterior aspect).

**Flexor muscles of right leg** (posterior
aspect). Both heads of the gastrocnemius
muscle have been cut and reflected.

**Flexor muscles of the leg**
(right side).

| | | |
|---|---|---|
| 1   Semitendinosus muscle | 9   Calcaneal tuberosity | 18   Popliteal fossa |
| 2   Semimembranosus muscle | 10   Tibial nerve | 19   Tibial nerve and posterior tibial |
| 3   Sartorius muscle | 11   Biceps femoris muscle | artery |
| 4   Tendon of gracilis muscle | 12   Plantaris muscle | 20   Popliteus muscle |
| 5   Medial head of gastrocnemius muscle | 13   Common peroneal nerve | 21   Tendinous arch of soleus muscle |
| 6   Common tendon of gracilis, | 14   Lateral head of gastrocnemius muscle | 22   Femur |
| sartorius, and semitendinosus muscles | 15   Soleus muscle | 23   Fibula |
| 7   Calcaneal or Achilles tendon | 16   Peroneus longus and brevis muscles | 24   Tibia |
| 8   Medial malleolus | 17   Lateral malleolus | |

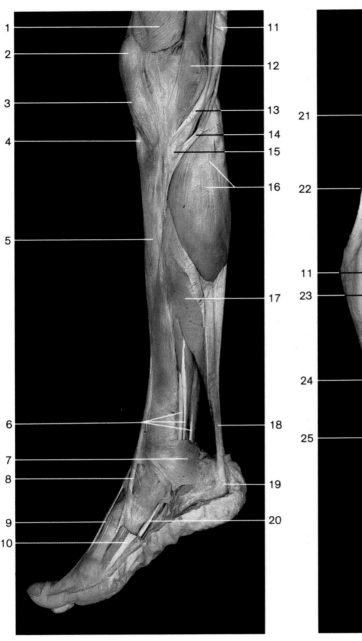

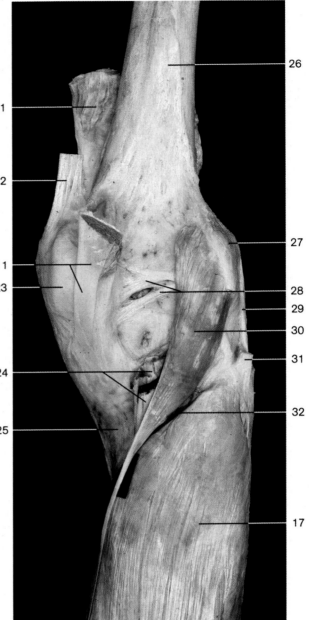

**Muscles of right leg and foot** (medial aspect).

**Popliteal region with plantaris and soleus,** right side (dorsal aspect). Notice the insertion of the tendon of semimembranosus.

1  Vastus medialis muscle
2  Patella
3  Patellar ligament
4  Tibial tuberosity
5  Tibia
6  Tendons of deep flexor muscles (from anterior to posterior: 1. tibialis posterior; 2. flexor digitorum longus; 3. flexor hallucis longus muscles)
7  Flexor retinaculum
8  Tendon of tibialis anterior muscle
9  Tendon of extensor hallucis longus muscle
10  Abductor hallucis muscle
11  Semimembranosus muscle
12  Sartorius muscle
13  Tendon of gracilis muscle
14  Tendon of semitendinosus muscle
15  Common tendon of gracilis, semitendinosus, and sartorius muscles

16  Medial head of gastrocnemius muscle
17  Soleus muscle
18  Calcaneal or Achilles tendon
19  Calcaneus muscle
20  Tendon of flexor hallucis longus muscle
21  Quadriceps femoris muscle (divided)
22  Tendon of adductor magnus muscle (divided)
23  Medial condyle of femur
24  Popliteal artery and vein, tibial nerve
25  Tibia
26  Femur
27  Lateral epicondyle of femur
28  Oblique popliteal ligament
29  Lateral (fibular) collateral ligament
30  Plantaris muscle
31  Tendon of biceps femoris muscle (divided)
32  Tendinous arch of soleus muscle

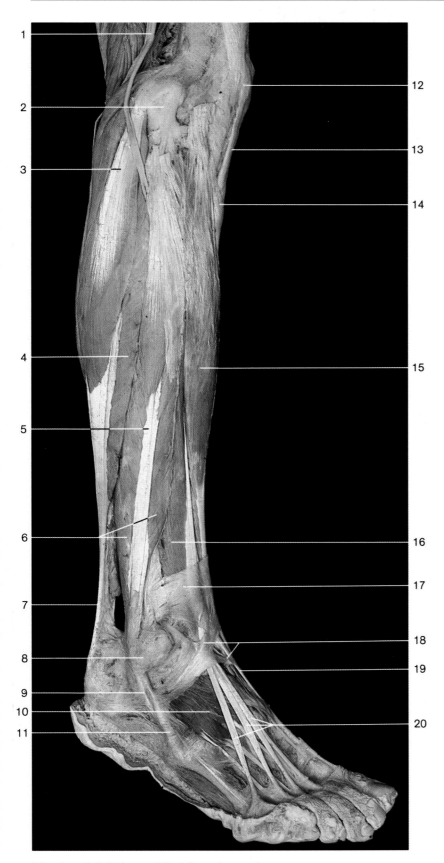

**Muscles of right leg and foot** (lateral aspect).

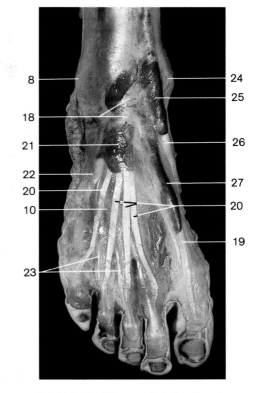

**Right foot with synovial sheaths of extensor muscles** (dorsal aspect). The synovial sheaths have been injected with blue solution.

1   Common peroneal nerve
2   Head of fibula
3   Lateral head of gastrocnemius muscle
4   Soleus muscle
5   Peroneus longus muscle
6   Peroneus brevis muscle
7   Calcaneal or Achilles tendon
8   Lateral malleolus muscle
9   Tendon of peroneus longus muscle
10  Extensor digitorum brevis muscle
11  Tendon of peroneus brevis muscle
12  Patella
13  Patellar ligament
14  Tuberosity of tibia
15  Tibialis anterior muscle
16  Extensor digitorum longus muscle
17  Superior extensor retinaculum
18  Inferior extensor retinaculum
19  Tendon of extensor hallucis longus muscle
20  Tendons of extensor digitorum longus muscle
21  Common synovial sheath of extensor digitorum longus muscle
22  Tendon of peroneus tertius muscle to the lateral margin of foot
23  Tendons of extensor digitorum brevis muscle
24  Medial malleolus
25  Synovial sheath of tendon of tibialis anterior muscle
26  Tendon of tibialis anterior muscle
27  Synovial sheath of tendon of extensor hallucis longus muscle

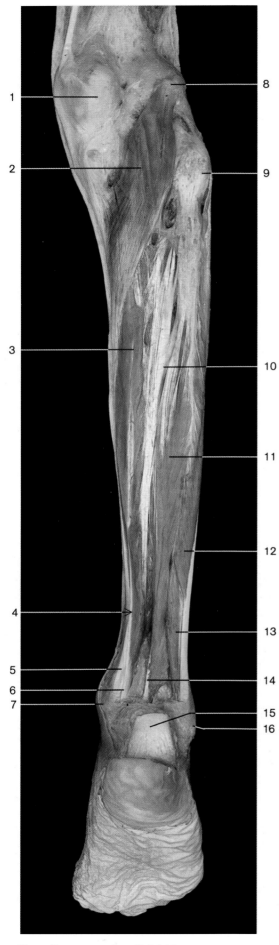

1   Medial condyle of femur
2   Popliteus muscle
3   Flexor digitorum longus muscle
4   Crossing of tendons in leg
5   Tendon of tibialis posterior muscle
6   Tendon of flexor digitorum longus muscle
7   Medial malleolus
8   Lateral condyle of femur
9   Head of fibula
10  Tibialis posterior muscle
11  Flexor hallucis longus muscle
12  Peroneus longus muscle
13  Peroneus brevis muscle
14  Tendon of flexor hallucis longus muscle
15  Calcaneal tendon (divided)
16  Lateral malleolus

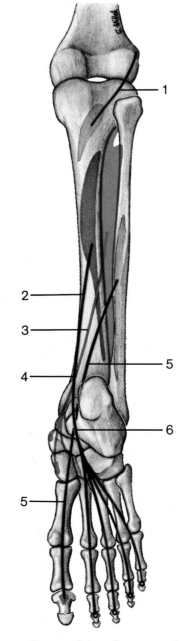

1   Popliteus muscle (blue)
2   Flexor digitorum longus muscle (blue)
3   Tibialis posterior muscle (red)
4   Crossing of tendons in leg
5   Flexor hallucis longus muscle (blue)
6   Crossing of tendons in sole

**Deep flexor muscles of right leg**
(posterior aspect).

**Course of deep flexor muscles of leg** (schematic drawing).

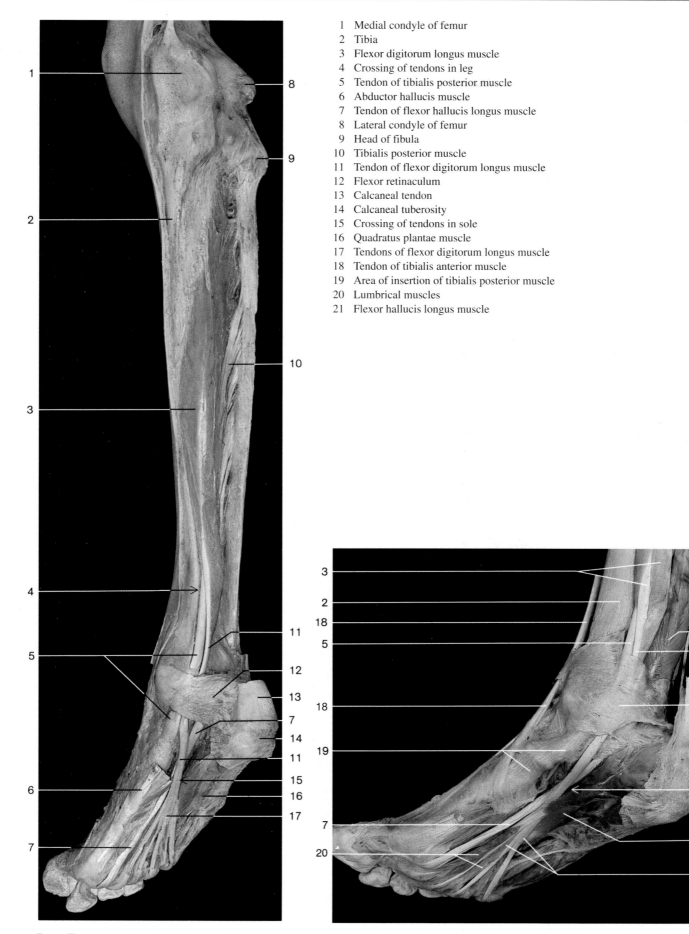

1  Medial condyle of femur
2  Tibia
3  Flexor digitorum longus muscle
4  Crossing of tendons in leg
5  Tendon of tibialis posterior muscle
6  Abductor hallucis muscle
7  Tendon of flexor hallucis longus muscle
8  Lateral condyle of femur
9  Head of fibula
10  Tibialis posterior muscle
11  Tendon of flexor digitorum longus muscle
12  Flexor retinaculum
13  Calcaneal tendon
14  Calcaneal tuberosity
15  Crossing of tendons in sole
16  Quadratus plantae muscle
17  Tendons of flexor digitorum longus muscle
18  Tendon of tibialis anterior muscle
19  Area of insertion of tibialis posterior muscle
20  Lumbrical muscles
21  Flexor hallucis longus muscle

**Deep flexor muscles of right leg and foot**
(posterior oblique medial aspect). Flexor
digitorum brevis and flexor hallucis longus
muscles have been removed.

**Sole of foot; tendons of long flexor muscles** (oblique medial and inferior
aspect).

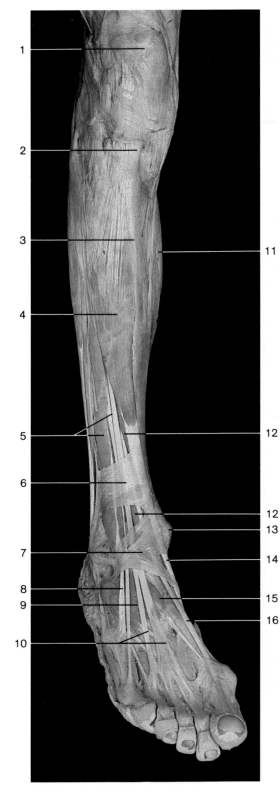

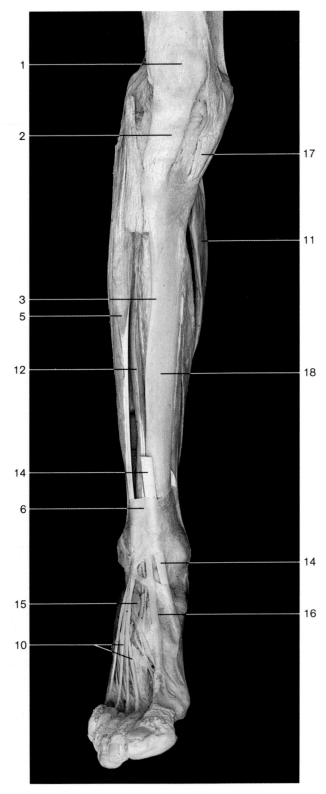

**Extensor muscles of right leg and foot**
(oblique anterolateral aspect).

**Extensors of the right leg and foot** (anterior aspect).
Part of the tibialis anterior muscle has been removed.

| | | | |
|---|---|---|---|
| 1 | Patella | 8 | Tendon of peroneus tertius muscle |
| 2 | Patellar ligament | 9 | Extensor digitorum brevis muscle |
| 3 | Anterior margin of tibia | 10 | Tendons of extensor digitorum |
| 4 | Tibialis anterior muscle | | longus muscle |
| 5 | Extensor digitorum longus muscle | 11 | Gastrocnemius muscle |
| 6 | Superior extensor retinaculum | 12 | Extensor hallucis longus muscle |
| 7 | Inferior extensor retinaculum | 13 | Medial malleolus |

| | |
|---|---|
| 14 | Tendon of tibialis anterior muscle |
| 15 | Extensor hallucis brevis muscle |
| 16 | Tendon of extensor hallucis |
| | longus muscle |
| 17 | Common tendon of gracilis, |
| | semitendinosus, and sartorius muscles |
| 18 | Tibia |

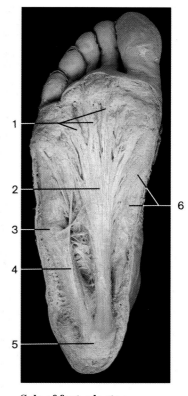

Sole of foot, plantar
aponeurosis (from below).

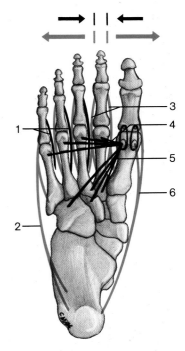

Course of abductor and adductor
muscles of foot (schematic drawing).
Red arrows = abduction.
Black arrows = adduction.

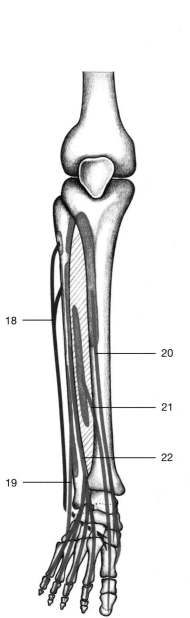

Extensor muscles of the
leg (right side).

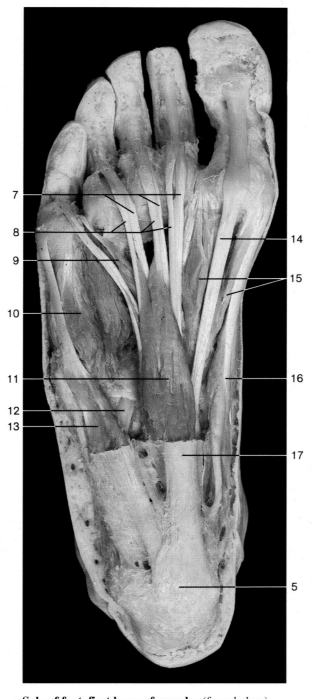

Sole of foot, first layer of muscles (from below).
The plantar aponeurosis and the fasciae of the
superficial muscles have been removed.

| | | | |
|---|---|---|---|
| 1 | Longitudinal bands of plantar aponeurosis | 12 | Tendon of peroneus longus muscle |
| 2 | Plantar aponeurosis | 13 | Abductor digiti minimi muscle |
| 3 | Position of tuberosity of fifth metatarsal bone | 14 | Tendon of flexor hallucis longus muscle |
| 4 | Muscles of fifth toe with fascia | 15 | Flexor hallucis brevis muscle |
| 5 | Calcaneal tuberosity | 16 | Abductor hallucis muscle |
| 6 | Muscles of great toe with fascia | 17 | Plantar aponeurosis (cut) |
| 7 | Tendons of flexor digitorum longus muscle | 18 | Peroneus longus muscle |
| 8 | Tendons of flexor digitorum brevis muscle | 19 | Peroneus brevis muscle |
| 9 | Lumbrical muscle | 20 | Tibialis anterior muscle |
| 10 | Flexor digiti minimi brevis muscle | 21 | Extensor hallucis longus muscle |
| 11 | Flexor digitorum brevis muscle | 22 | Extensor digitorum longus muscle |

1 Plantar interossei muscles (black)
2 Abductor digiti minimi muscle (red)
3 Dorsal interosseous muscles (red)
4 Transverse head of adductor
  muscle (black)
5 Oblique head of adductor
  muscle (black)
6 Abductor hallucis muscle (red)

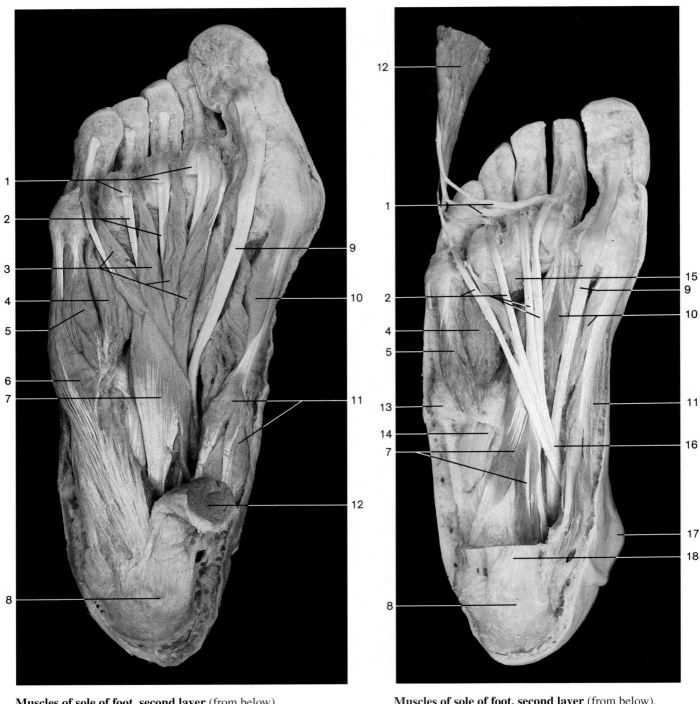

**Muscles of sole of foot, second layer** (from below).
The flexor digitorum brevis muscle has been divided.

**Muscles of sole of foot, second layer** (from below).
The tendons of the flexor muscles and the crossing of
tendons are displayed. The flexor digitorum brevis
muscle has been divided and reflected.

| | | |
|---|---|---|
| 1 | Tendons of flexor digitorum brevis muscle | |
| 2 | Tendons of flexor digitorum longus muscle | |
| 3 | Lumbrical muscles | |
| 4 | Interossei muscles | |
| 5 | Flexor digiti minimi brevis muscle | |

6　Abductor digiti minimi muscle
7　Quadratus plantae muscle
8　Calcaneal tuberosity
9　Tendon of flexor hallucis longus muscle
10　Flexor hallucis brevis muscle
11　Abductor hallucis muscle
12　Flexor digitorum brevis muscle (divided)

13　Tuberosity of fifth metatarsal bone
14　Tendon of peroneus longus muscle
15　Transverse head of adductor hallucis muscle
16　Crossing of tendons in sole of foot
17　Medial malleolus
18　Plantar aponeurosis (divided)

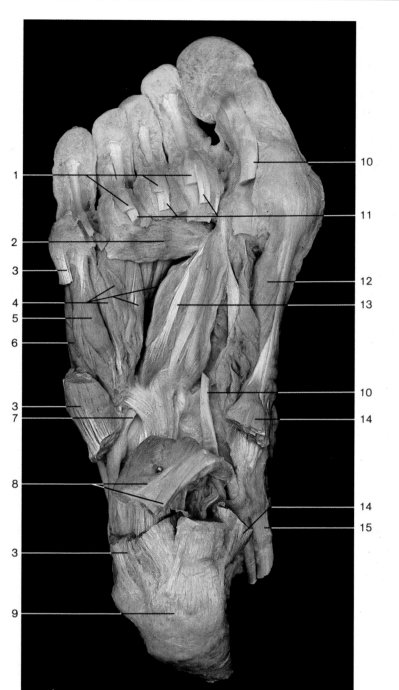

**Muscles of sole of foot, third layer** (from below). The flexor digitorum brevis muscle has been removed, and the quadratus plantae, abductor hallucis, and digiti minimi muscles have been divided.

**Muscles of sole of foot, fourth layer** (from below). The interosseous muscles and the canal for the tendon of peroneus longus muscle are shown.

1 Tendons of flexor digitorum brevis muscle
2 Transverse head of adductor hallucis muscle
3 Abductor digiti minimi muscle
4 Interossei muscles
5 Flexor digiti minimi brevis muscle
6 Opponens digiti minimi muscle
7 Tendon of peroneus longus muscle

8 Quadratus plantae muscle with tendon of flexor digitorum longus muscle
9 Calcaneal tuberosity
10 Tendons of flexor hallucis longus muscle (divided)
11 Tendon of flexor digitorum longus muscle
12 Flexor hallucis brevis muscle
13 Oblique head of adductor hallucis muscle
14 Abductor hallucis muscle (cut)

15 Tendon of tibialis posterior muscle
16 Dorsal interossei muscles
17 Plantar interossei muscles
18 Tuberosity of fifth metatarsal bone
19 Tendon of flexor digitorum longus muscle (crossing of plantar tendons)
20 Long plantar ligament

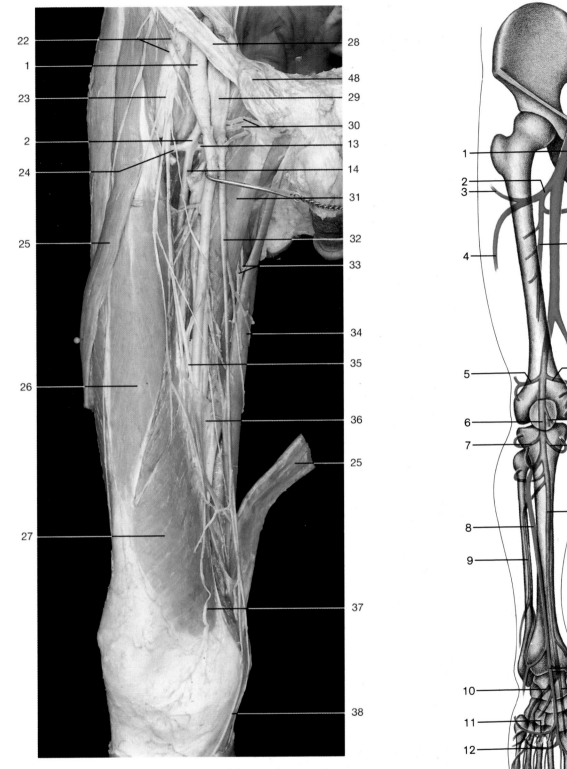

**Main arteries and nerves of right thigh** (anterior aspect).
Sartorius muscle has been divided and reflected. The femoral
vein has been partly removed to show the deep femoral
artery. Notice: the vessels enter the adductor canal to reach
the popliteal fossa.

**Main arteries of lower extremity,** right side (ventral aspect).
(Schematic drawing.)

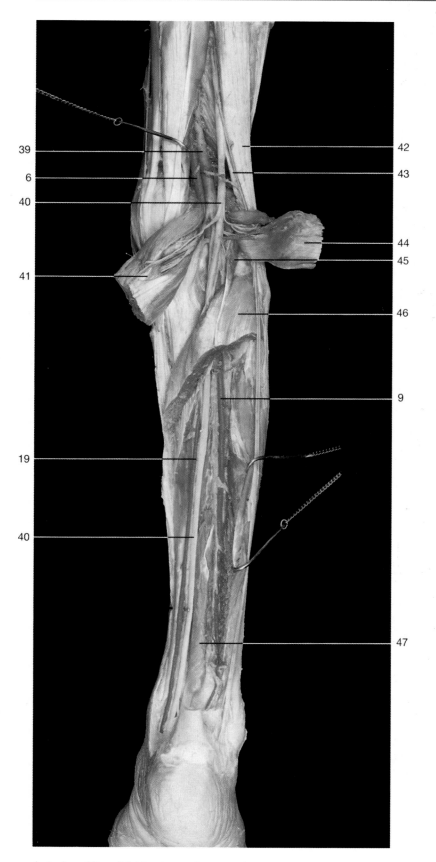

**Arteries of the right leg** (posterior aspect).

1 Femoral artery
2 Profunda femoris artery
3 Ascending branch of lateral circumflex femoral artery
4 Descending branch of lateral circumflex femoral artery
5 Lateral superior genicular artery
6 Popliteal artery
7 Lateral inferior genicular artery
8 Anterior tibial artery
9 Peroneal artery
10 Lateral plantar artery
11 Arcuate artery with dorsal metatarsal arteries
12 Plantar arch with plantar metatarsal arteries
13 Medial circumflex femoral artery
14 Profunda femoris artery with perforating arteries
15 Descending genicular artery
16 Medial superior genicular artery
17 Middle genicular artery
18 Medial inferior genicular artery
19 Posterior tibial artery
20 Dorsalis pedis artery
21 Medial plantar artery
22 Superficial and deep circumflex iliac arteries
23 Femoral nerve
24 Lateral circumflex femoral artery
25 Sartorius muscle (cut and reflected)
26 Rectus femoris muscle
27 Vastus medialis muscle
28 Inguinal ligament
29 Femoral vein (cut)
30 External pudendal artery and vein
31 Adductor longus muscle
32 Great saphenous vein
33 Obturator artery and nerve
34 Gracilis muscle
35 Saphenous nerve
36 Tendinous wall of adductor canal
37 Anterior cutaneous branch of femoral nerve
38 Infrapatellar branch of saphenous nerve
39 Popliteal vein
40 Tibial nerve
41 Medial head of gastrocnemius muscle
42 Biceps femoris muscle
43 Common peroneal nerve
44 Lateral head of gastrocnemius muscle
45 Plantaris muscle
46 Soleus muscle
47 Flexor hallucis longus muscle
48 Spermatic cord

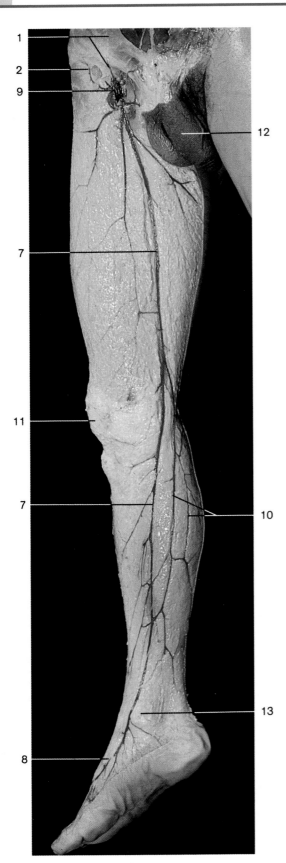

**Superficial veins of lower limb,** right side (medial anterior aspect). The veins have been injected with red solution.

**Medial malleolar region.** Dissection of ▷ tibial nerve, posterior tibial vessels, and great saphenous vein (veins injected with blue resin).

**Main veins of lower limb,** right side (anterior aspect). (Schematic drawing.)

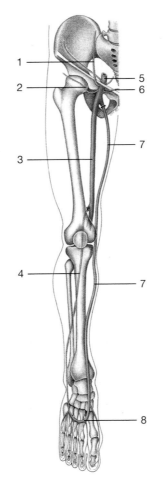

1   Superficial epigastric vein
2   Superficial circumflex iliac vein
3   Femoral vein
4   Small saphenous vein
5   External iliac vein
6   External pudendal vein
7   Great saphenous vein
8   Dorsal venous arch
9   Saphenous opening with femoral vein
10  Venous anastomoses of small saphenous vein with great saphenous vein
11  Patella
12  Penis
13  Medial malleolus
14  Popliteal fossa
15  Perforating veins
16  Lateral malleolus
17  Dorsal digital veins of foot
18  Dorsal venous arch of foot
19  Dorsal metatarsal veins of foot
20  Anterior tibial artery and veins
21  Tibia
22  Posterior tibial artery and veins
23  Fibula
24  Peroneal artery and vein
25  Deep layer of crural fascia
26  Superficial layer of crural fascia
27  Perforating veins I–III (of Cockett)
28  Tibial nerve
29  Arcuate vein
30  Saphenous nerve
31  Medial dorsal cutaneous nerve (branch of superficial peroneal nerve)
32  Posterior tibial vein

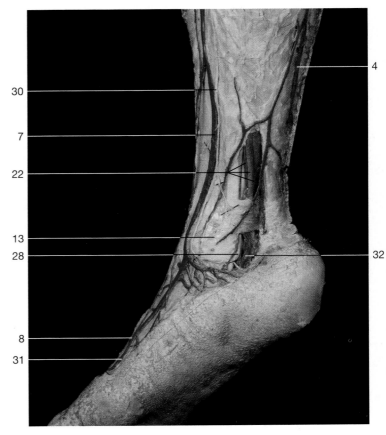

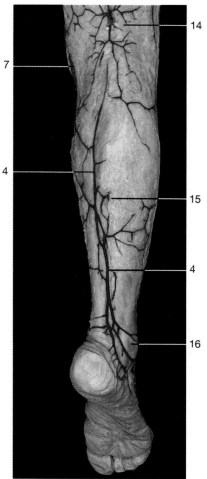

**Superficial veins of leg** (posterior aspect; injected with blue resin).

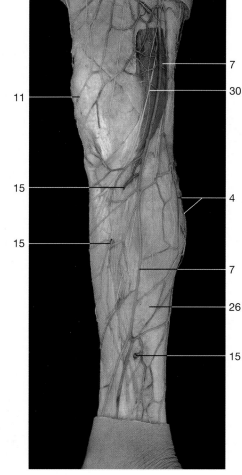

**Superficial veins of leg.** The perforating veins of Cockett have been dissected (left side, medial aspect).

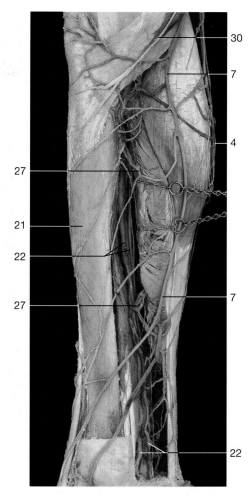

**Veins of leg.** The anastomoses between superficial and deeper veins are dissected (left side, medial aspect).

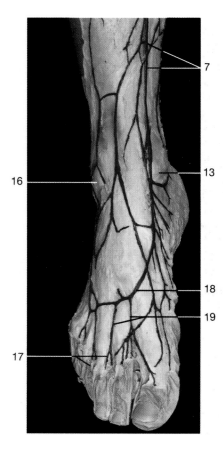

**Superficial veins on dorsum of foot** (injected with blue resin).

**Anastomoses between superficial and deep veins of the leg** (after Aigner). (Schematic drawing.) Arrows: directions of blood flow.

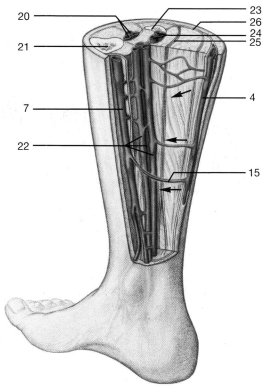

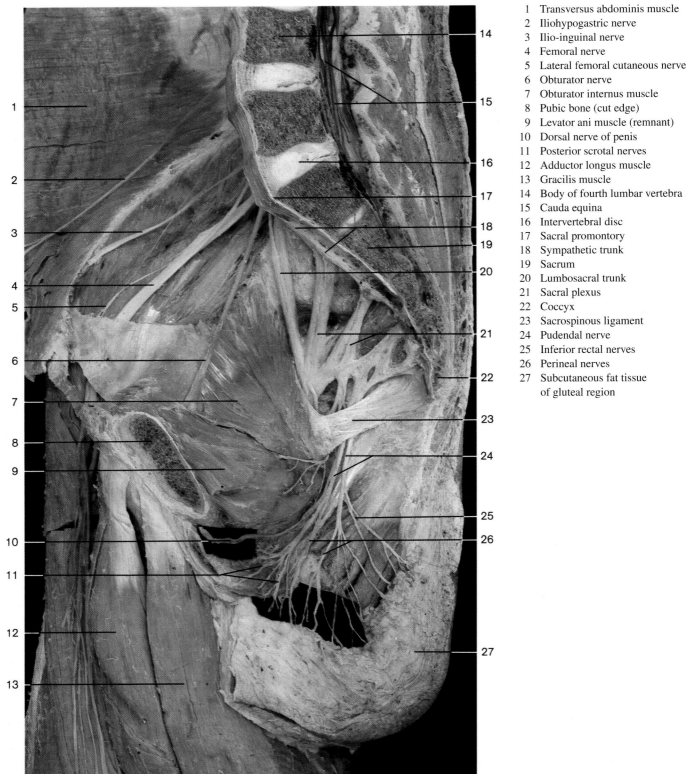

1   Transversus abdominis muscle
2   Iliohypogastric nerve
3   Ilio-inguinal nerve
4   Femoral nerve
5   Lateral femoral cutaneous nerve
6   Obturator nerve
7   Obturator internus muscle
8   Pubic bone (cut edge)
9   Levator ani muscle (remnant)
10  Dorsal nerve of penis
11  Posterior scrotal nerves
12  Adductor longus muscle
13  Gracilis muscle
14  Body of fourth lumbar vertebra
15  Cauda equina
16  Intervertebral disc
17  Sacral promontory
18  Sympathetic trunk
19  Sacrum
20  Lumbosacral trunk
21  Sacral plexus
22  Coccyx
23  Sacrospinous ligament
24  Pudendal nerve
25  Inferior rectal nerves
26  Perineal nerves
27  Subcutaneous fat tissue
    of gluteal region

**Lumbosacral plexus in situ,** right side (medial aspect).
Pelvic organs with peritoneum and part of the levator ani muscle have been removed.

1 Subcostal nerve
2 Iliohypogastric nerve
3 Ilio-inguinal nerve
4 Lateral femoral cutaneous nerve
5 Genitofemoral nerve
6 Pudendal nerve
7 Femoral nerve
8 Obturator nerve
9 Sciatic nerve
10 Lumbar plexus (L$_1$–L$_4$) ⎤
11 Sacral plexus (L$_4$–S$_4$) ⎬ lumbosacral plexus
12 "Pudendal" plexus (S$_2$–S$_4$) ⎦
13 Inferior cluneal nerves
14 Posterior femoral cutaneous nerve
15 Common peroneal nerve
16 Tibial nerve
17 Lateral sural cutaneous nerve
18 Medial and lateral plantar nerves
19 Saphenous nerve
20 Infrapatellar branch of saphenous nerve
21 Deep peroneal nerve
22 Superficial peroneal nerve
23 Anterior cutaneous branch of iliohypogastric nerve
24 Lateral cutaneous branch of iliohypogastric nerve
25 Femoral branch of genitofemoral nerve
26 Lateral cutaneous branches of intercostal nerve
27 Anterior cutaneous branches of intercostal nerve
28 Genital branch of genitofemoral nerve
29 Anterior scrotal nerve

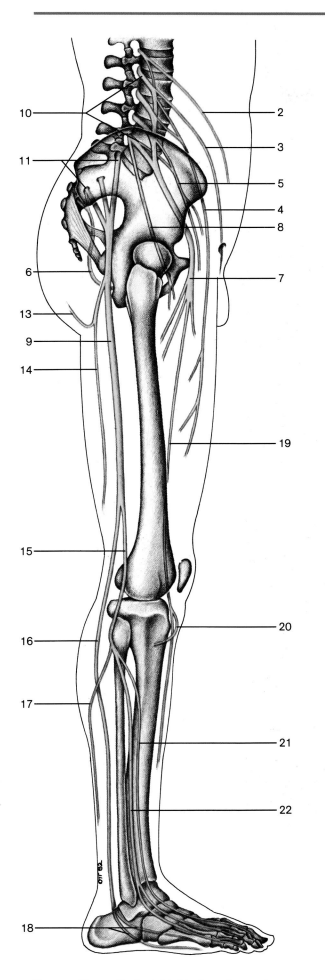

**Nerves of lower limb,** right side (lateral aspect).
(Schematic drawing.)

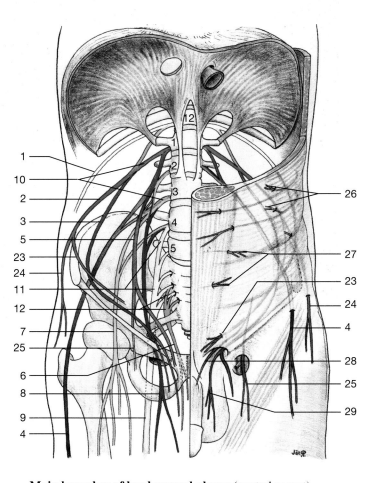

**Main branches of lumbosacral plexus** (ventral aspect).
(Schematic drawing.)

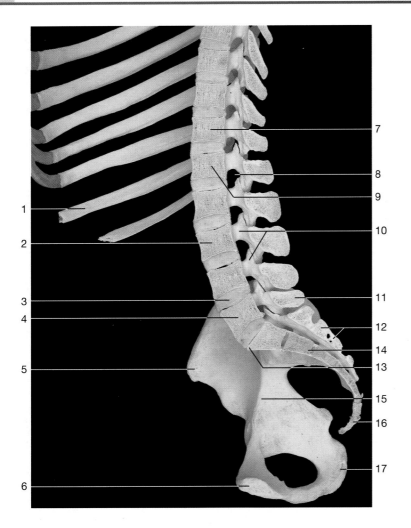

**Lumbar part of vertebral column with pelvis**
(sagittal section, medial aspect).

1  Eleventh rib
2  Body of third lumbar vertebra
3  Intervertebral disc
4  Body of fifth lumbar vertebra
5  Anterior superior iliac spine
6  Symphysial surface
7  Body of twelfth thoracic vertebra
8  Intervertebral foramen
9  Body of first lumbar vertebra
10  Vertebral canal
11  Spinous process of fifth lumbar vertebra
12  Sacrum (median sacral crest)
13  Promontory (promontorium)
14  Sacrum
15  Arcuate line
16  Coccyx
17  Ischial tuberosity
18  Sympathetic trunk with ganglia
19  Ureter
20  Iliohypogastric nerve (Th$_{12}$, L$_1$)
21  Ilio-inguinal nerve (L$_1$)
22  Femoral nerve (L$_2$–L$_4$)
23  Genitofemoral nerve (L$_1$, L$_2$)
24  Inferior hypogastric plexus
25  Ductus deferens
26  Urinary bladder
27  Medullary cone of spinal cord
28  Root filaments of spinal nerves
29  Subarachnoidal cavity
       (filled with cerebrospinal fluid) (blue)
30  Terminal filament of spinal cord
31  Sacral plexus
32  Pelvic splanchnic nerves (nervi erigentes)
33  Rectum

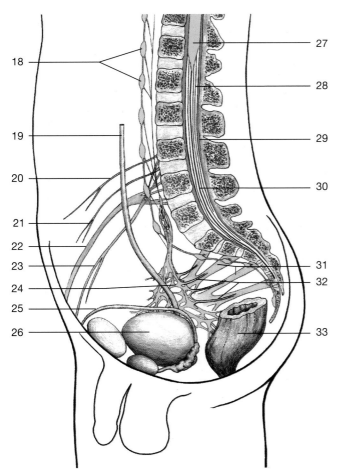

**Vertebral canal with spinal cord and root filaments.**
Note the high location of the medullary cone. Sacral plexus and inferior hypogastric plexus are schematically shown.

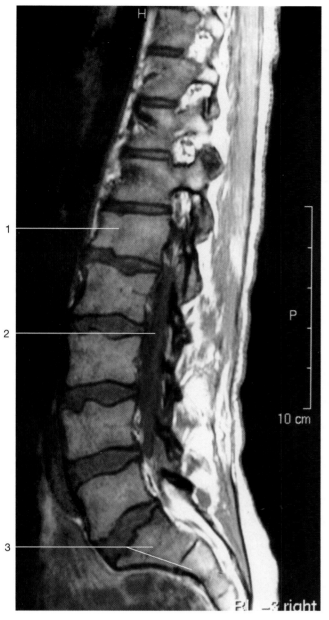

**MRI scan of lumbar part of vertebral canal** (paramedian section).

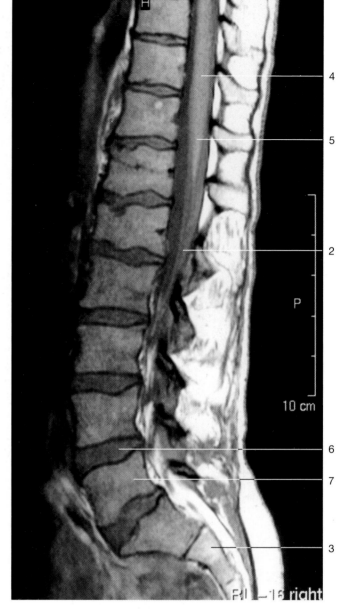

**MRI scan of lumbar part of vertebral canal at the level of the medullary cone** (median section).

1   First lumbar vertebra
2   Root filaments of spinal nerves
3   Sacrum
4   Spinal cord
5   Medullary cone of spinal cord
6   Intervertebral disc between fourth and fifth lumbar vertebra
7   Fifth lumbar vertebra

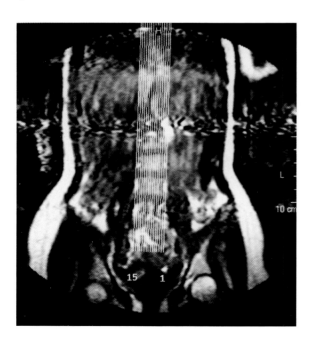

**Location of the sagittal sections through the vertebral canal.** (Sections 7 and 11 are depicted above; courtesy of Prof. W. Bautz, Erlangen, Germany).

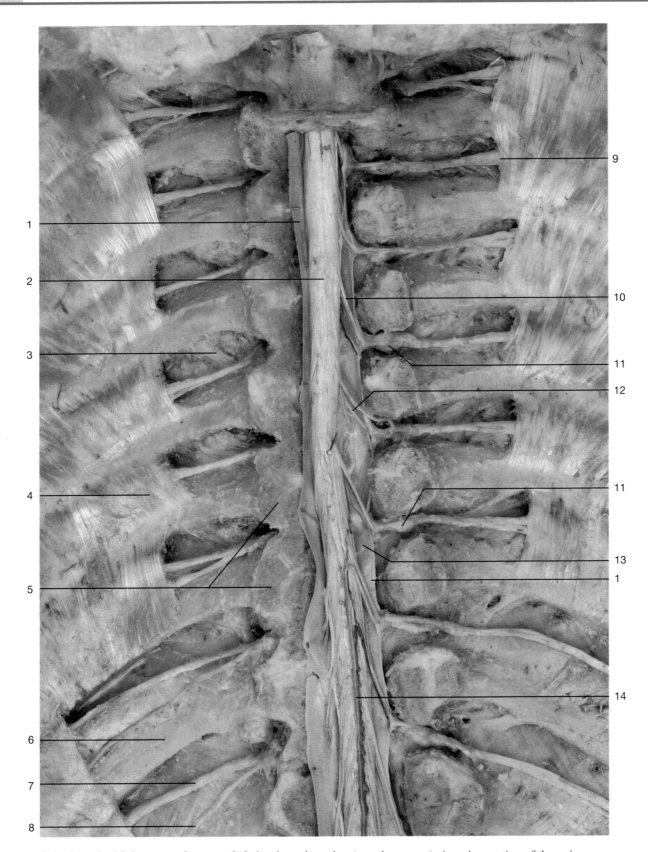

**Spinal cord with intercostal nerves.** Inferior thoracic region (anterior aspect). Anterior portion of thoracic vertebrae removed, dural sheath opened, and spinal cord slightly reflected to the right to display the dorsal and ventral roots.

| | | |
|---|---|---|
| 1   Dura mater | 6   Eleventh rib | 10   Anterior root filaments |
| 2   Spinal cord | 7   Intercostal nerve | 11   Spinal (dorsal root) ganglion |
| 3   Costotransverse ligament | 8   Collateral branch of intercostal nerve | 12   Posterior root filaments |
| 4   Innermost intercostal muscle | 9   Intercostal nerve (entering the | 13   Arachnoid mater and denticulate ligament |
| 5   Vertebral arches (cut surfaces) | intermuscular interval) | 14   Anterior spinal artery |

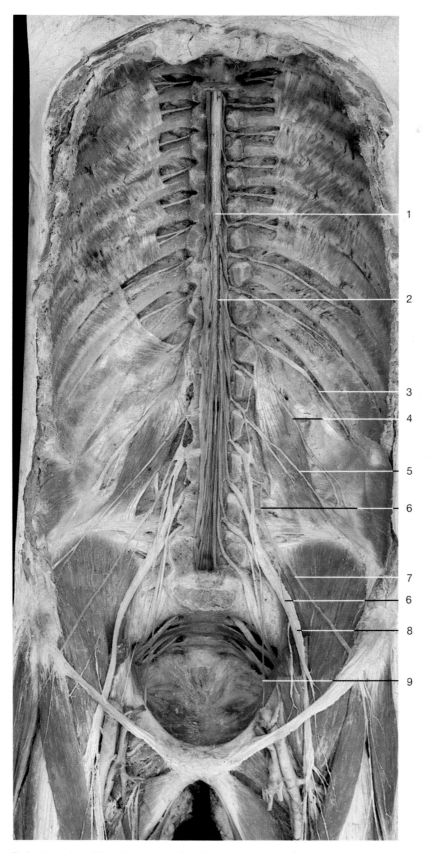

**Spinal cord and lumbar plexus in situ** (anterior aspect).

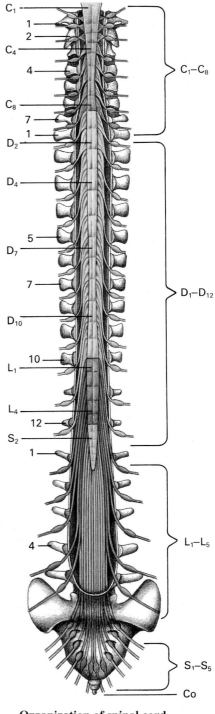

**Organization of spinal cord segments** in relation to the vertebral column (anterior aspect). C = cervical; D = thoracic; L = lumbar; S = sacral segments; Co = coccygeal bone. Numbers indicate the related vertebrae.

| | | | |
|---|---|---|---|
| 1 | Conus medullaris | 6 | Genitofemoral nerve |
| 2 | Filum terminale | 7 | Lateral femoral cutaneous nerve |
| 3 | Subcostal nerve | 8 | Femoral nerve |
| 4 | Iliohypogastric nerve | 9 | Obturator nerve |
| 5 | Ilio-inguinal nerve | | |

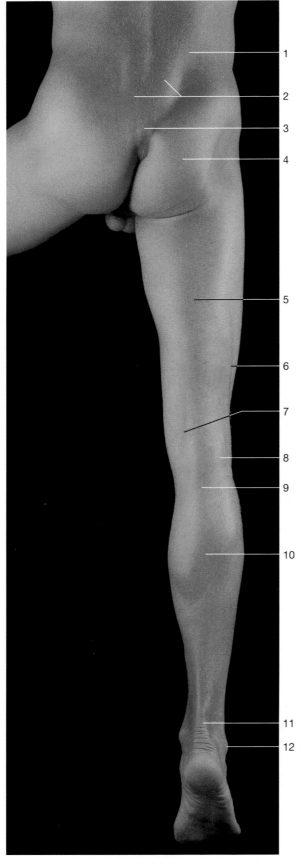

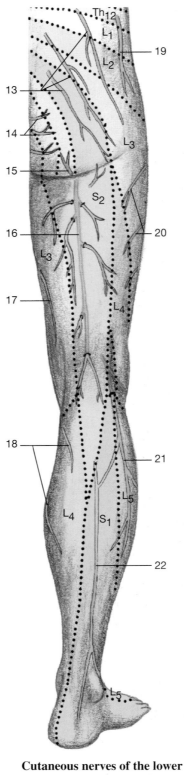

1  Iliac crest
2  Sacrum
3  Coccyx
4  Gluteus maximus muscle
5  Dorsal muscles of the leg
6  Iliotibial tract
7  Tendon of semimembranosus
   muscle
8  Tendon of biceps femoris
   muscle
9  Popliteal fossa
10 Triceps surae muscle
11 Calcaneal or Achilles
   tendon
12 Lateral malleolus
13 Superior cluneal nerves
14 Middle cluneal nerves
15 Inferior cluneal nerves
16 Posterior femoral cutaneous
   nerve
17 Obturator nerve
18 Saphenous nerve
19 Iliohypogastric nerve
20 Branch of lateral femoral
   cutaneous nerves
21 Common peroneal nerve
22 Sural nerve

**Cutaneous nerves of the lower limb** (dorsal aspect).
Dotted lines = border of segments.

**Surface anatomy of the right leg** (dorsal aspect).
Gluteal muscles contracted.

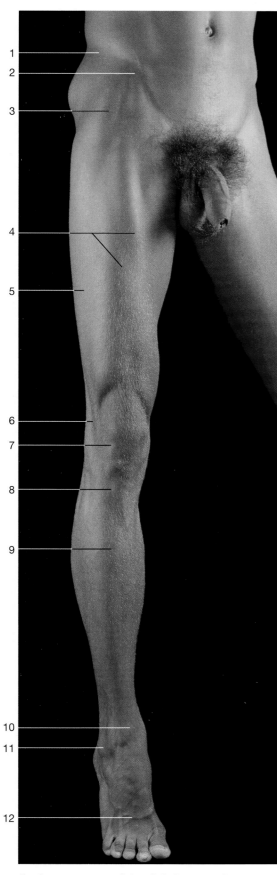

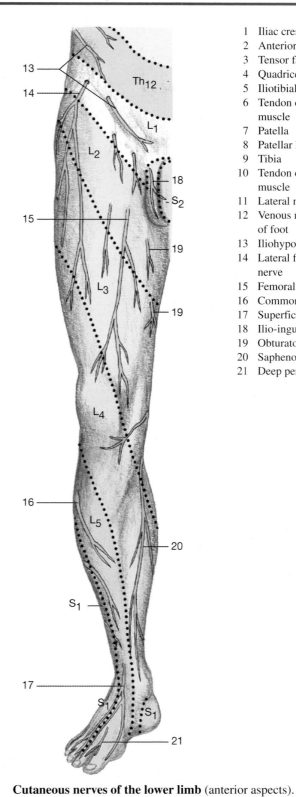

1   Iliac crest
2   Anterior superior iliac spine
3   Tensor fasciae latae muscle
4   Quadriceps femoris muscle
5   Iliotibial tract
6   Tendon of biceps femoris
    muscle
7   Patella
8   Patellar ligament
9   Tibia
10  Tendon of tibialis anterior
    muscle
11  Lateral malleolus
12  Venous network of dorsum
    of foot
13  Iliohypogastric nerve
14  Lateral femoral cutaneous
    nerve
15  Femoral nerve
16  Common peroneal nerve
17  Superficial peroneal nerve
18  Ilio-inguinal nerve
19  Obturator nerve
20  Saphenous nerve
21  Deep peroneal nerve

**Cutaneous nerves of the lower limb** (anterior aspects).
Dotted lines = border of segments.

**Surface anatomy of the right leg** (anterior aspect).

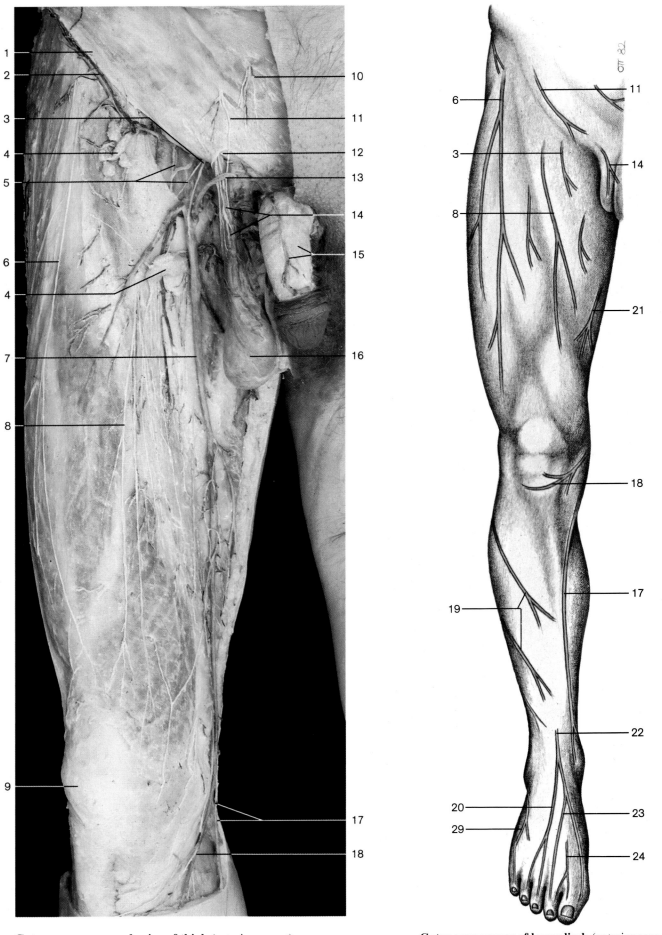

**Cutaneous nerves and veins of thigh** (anterior aspect).

**Cutaneous nerves of lower limb** (anterior aspect).
(Schematic drawing.)

1   Inguinal ligament
2   Superficial circumflex iliac vein
3   Femoral branch of genitofemoral nerve
4   Superficial inguinal lymph nodes
5   Saphenous opening with femoral artery and vein
6   Lateral femoral cutaneous nerve
7   Great saphenous vein
8   Anterior cutaneous branches of femoral nerve
9   Patella
10  Terminal branches of subcostal nerve
11  Terminal branches of iliohypogastric nerve
12  Superficial inguinal ring
13  External pudendal vein
14  Spermatic cord with genital branch of genitofemoral
    nerve
15  Penis with superficial dorsal vein of penis
16  Testis and its coverings
17  Saphenous nerve
18  Infrapatellar branch of saphenous nerve
19  Lateral sural cutaneous nerves
20  Intermediate dorsal cutaneous branch of superficial
    peroneal nerve
21  Cutaneous branch of obturator nerve
22  Superficial peroneal nerve
23  Medial dorsal cutaneous branch of superficial
    peroneal nerve
24  Deep peroneal nerve
25  Femoral nerve
26  Femoral artery
27  Superficial epigastric vein
28  Femoral vein
29  Lateral dorsal cutaneous branch of sural nerve
30  Inguinal nodes (enlarged)
31  Lympathic vessels
32  Sartorius muscle

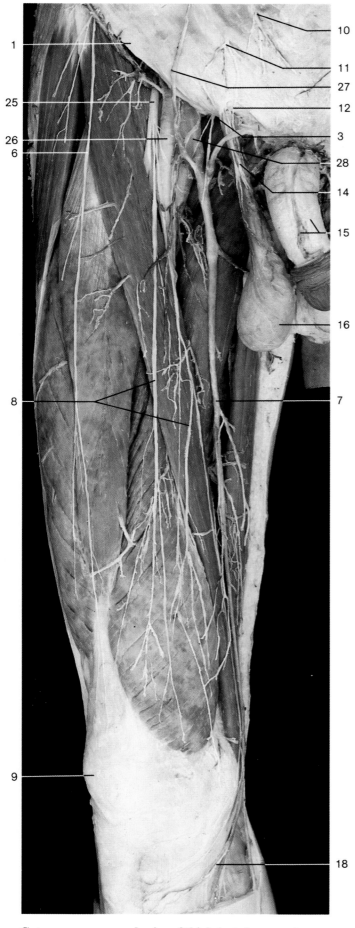

**Cutaneous nerves and veins of thigh** (anterior aspect).
The fascia lata and fasciae of the thigh muscles have been
removed.

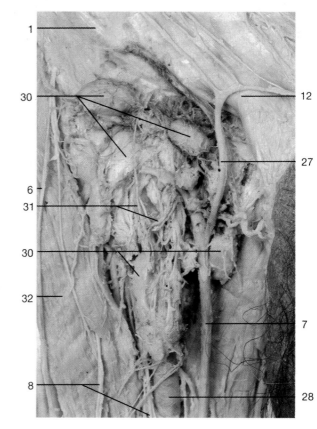

**Inguinal nodes with lymphatic vessels**
(anterior aspect).

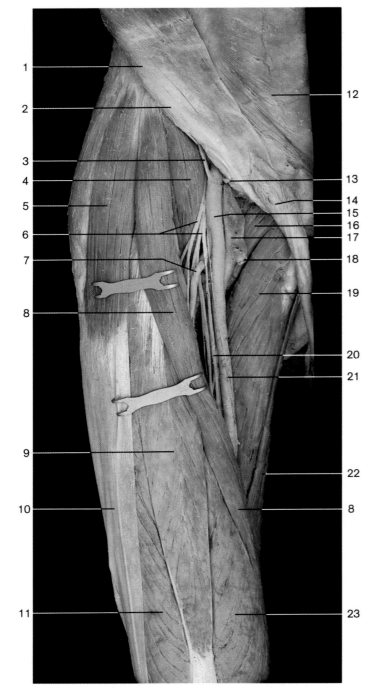

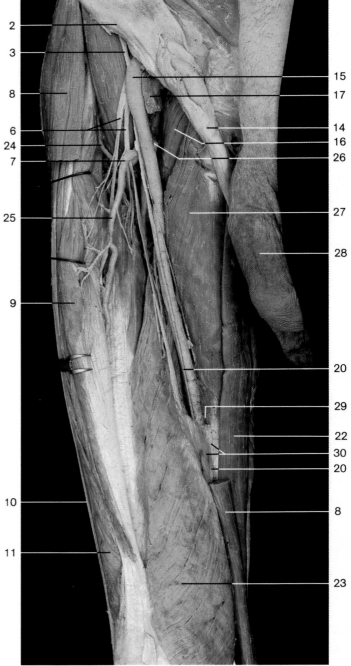

**Anterior region of right thigh** (anterior aspect).
The fascia lata has been removed, and the sartorius muscle has been slightly reflected.

**Anterior region of right thigh** (anterior aspect).
The fascia lata has been removed, and the sartorius muscle has been divided.

| | |
|---|---|
| 1   Anterior superior iliac spine | 16   Pectineus muscle |
| 2   Inguinal ligament | 17   Femoral vein |
| 3   Deep circumflex iliac artery | 18   Great saphenous vein (divided) |
| 4   Iliopsoas muscle | 19   Adductor longus muscle |
| 5   Tensor fasciae latae muscle | 20   Saphenous nerve |
| 6   Femoral nerve | 21   Muscular branch of femoral nerve |
| 7   Lateral circumflex femoral artery | 22   Gracilis muscle |
| 8   Sartorius muscle | 23   Vastus medialis muscle |
| 9   Rectus femoris muscle | 24   Ascending branch of lateral circumflex femoral artery |
| 10   Iliotibial tract | 25   Descending branch of lateral circumflex femoral artery |
| 11   Vastus lateralis muscle | 26   Medial circumflex femoral artery |
| 12   Anterior sheath of rectus abdominis muscle | 27   Adductor longus muscle |
| 13   Inferior epigastric artery | 28   Penis |
| 14   Spermatic cord | 29   Entrance to adductor canal |
| 15   Femoral artery | 30   Vasto-adductor membrane of fascia beneath sartorius muscle |

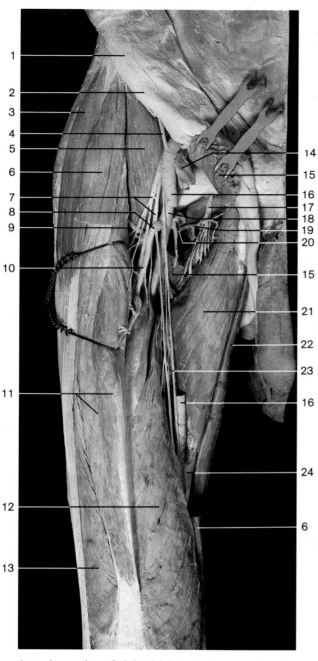

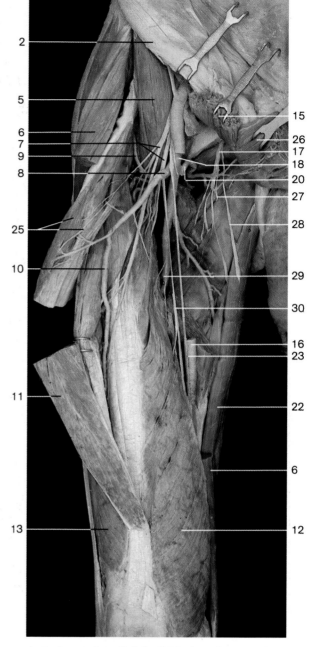

**Anterior region of right thigh** (anterior aspect).
The fascia lata has been removed. Sartorius muscle, pectineus muscle, and femoral artery have been cut to display the deep femoral artery with its branches. The rectus femoris muscle has been slightly reflected.

1  Anterior superior iliac spine
2  Inguinal ligament
3  Tensor fasciae latae muscle
4  Deep circumflex iliac artery
5  Iliopsoas muscle
6  Sartorius muscle (cut)
7  Femoral nerve
8  Lateral circumflex femoral artery
9  Ascending branch of lateral circumflex femoral artery
10  Descending branch of lateral circumflex femoral artery
11  Rectus femoris muscle
12  Vastus medialis muscle
13  Vastus lateralis muscle
14  Femoral vein
15  Pectineus muscle (cut)
16  Femoral artery (cut)

**Anterior region of right thigh** (anterior aspect).
The sartorius, pectineus, adductor longus, and rectus femoris muscles have been divided and reflected. The greater part of the femoral artery has been removed.

17  Obturator nerve
18  Profunda femoris artery
19  Ascending branch of medial circumflex femoral artery
20  Medial circumflex femoral artery
21  Adductor longus muscle
22  Gracilis muscle
23  Saphenous nerve
24  Distal part of vasto-adductor membrane
25  Rectus femoris muscle with muscular branch of femoral nerve
26  Adductor longus muscle (divided)
27  Posterior branch of obturator nerve
28  Anterior branch of obturator nerve
29  Point at which perforating artery branches off from profunda femoris artery
30  Muscular branch of femoral nerve to vastus medialis muscle

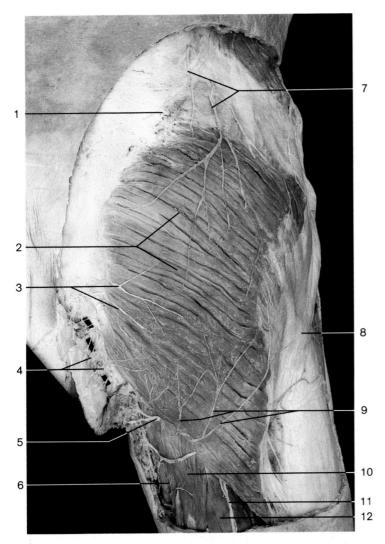

**Gluteal region,** right side (posterior aspect).

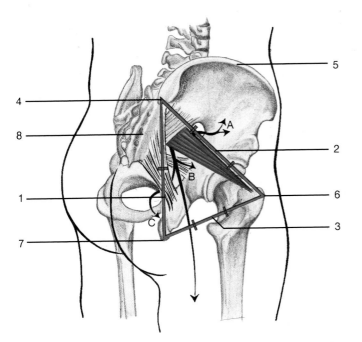

**Gluteal region,** right side (posterolateral aspect). Location of sciatic foramina in relation to the bones (schematic drawing).

1  Iliac crest
2  Gluteus maximus muscle
3  Middle cluneal nerves
4  Anococcygeal nerves
5  Perineal branch of posterior femoral cutaneous nerve
6  Adductor magnus muscle
7  Superior cluneal nerves
8  Position of greater trochanter
9  Inferior cluneal nerves
10  Semitendinosus muscle
11  Posterior femoral cutaneous nerve
12  Long head of biceps femoris muscle

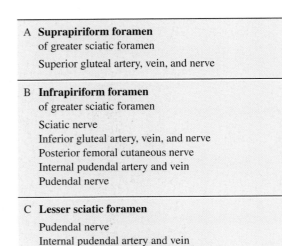

A  **Suprapiriform foramen**
   of greater sciatic foramen

   Superior gluteal artery, vein, and nerve

B  **Infrapiriform foramen**
   of greater sciatic foramen

   Sciatic nerve
   Inferior gluteal artery, vein, and nerve
   Posterior femoral cutaneous nerve
   Internal pudendal artery and vein
   Pudendal nerve

C  **Lesser sciatic foramen**

   Pudendal nerve
   Internal pudendal artery and vein

**Red lines**

1  Spine-tuber line:
   the infrapiriform foramen is situated in the middle of this line
2  Spine-trochanter line:
   the suprapiriform foramen is located in the upper third
3  Tuber-trochanter line:
   the ischiadic nerve can be found between the middle and posterior third

**Other structures**

4  Posterior superior iliac spine
5  Iliac crest
6  Greater trochanter
7  Ischial tuberosity
8  Sacrum

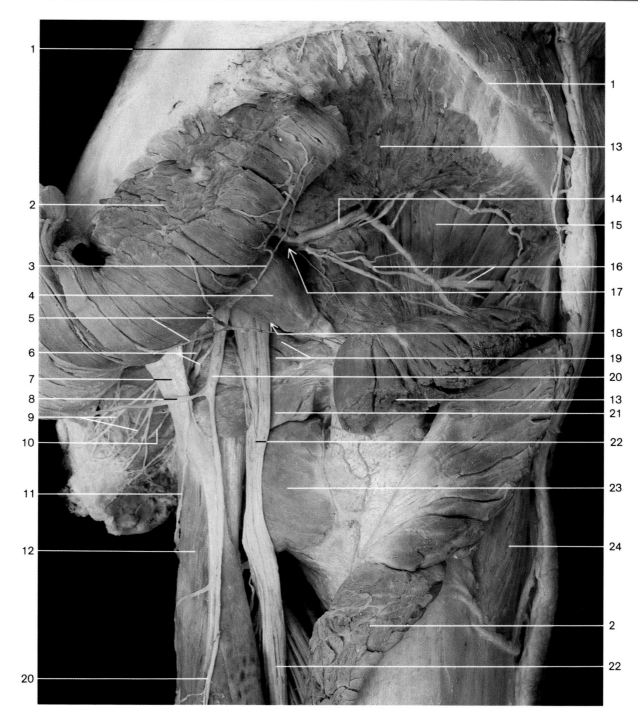

**Gluteal region,** right side (dorsal aspect). The gluteus maximus and gluteus medius muscles have been divided and reflected. Notice the position of the foramina above and below the piriformis muscle and the lesser sciatic foramen.

1  Iliac crest
2  Gluteus maximus muscle (cut)
3  Inferior gluteal nerve
4  Piriformis muscle
5  Muscular branches of inferior gluteal artery
6  Pudendal nerve and internal pudendal artery within the lesser sciatic foramen (entrance to the pudendal canal)
7  Sacrotuberous ligament
8  Inferior cluneal nerve
9  Inferior rectal nerves
10  Inferior rectal arteries
11  Perforating cutaneous nerve
12  Long head of biceps femoris muscle

13  Gluteus medius muscle (cut)
14  Deep branch of superior gluteal artery
15  Gluteus minimus muscle
16  Superior gluteal nerve
17  Suprapiriform foramen  } greater sciatic foramen
18  Infrapiriform foramen
19  Tendon of obturator internus and superior gemellus muscles
20  Posterior femoral cutaneous nerve
21  Inferior gemellus muscle
22  Sciatic nerve
23  Quadratus femoris muscle
24  Tensor fasciae latae muscle

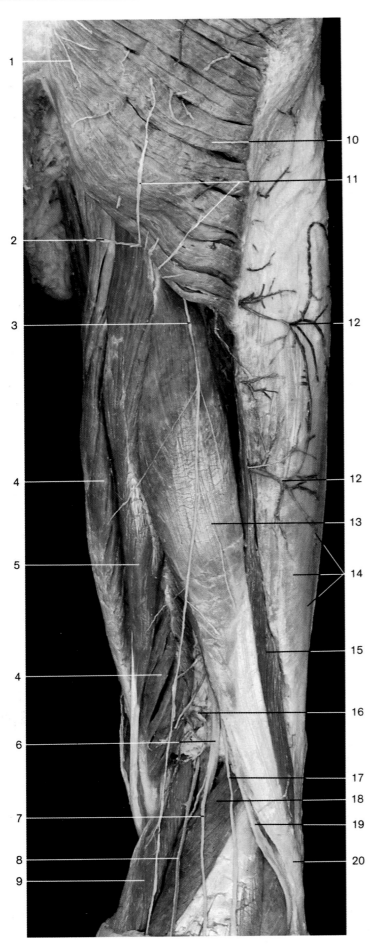

1  Middle cluneal nerves
2  Perineal branch of posterior femoral cutaneous nerve
3  Posterior femoral cutaneous nerve
4  Semimembranosus muscle
5  Semitendinosus muscle
6  Tibial nerve
7  Medial sural cutaneous nerve
8  Small saphenous vein
9  Medial head of gastrocnemius muscle
10  Gluteus maximus muscle
11  Inferior cluneal nerves
12  Cutaneous veins
13  Long head of biceps femoris muscle
14  Iliotibial tract
15  Short head of biceps femoris muscle
16  Popliteal fossa
17  Lateral sural cutaneous nerve
18  Lateral head of gastrocnemius muscle
19  Common peroneal nerve
20  Tendon of biceps femoris muscle
21  Inferior gluteal nerve
22  Sacrotuberous ligament
23  Inferior rectal branches of pudendal nerve
24  Anus
25  Gluteus medius muscle
26  Piriformis muscle
27  Sciatic nerve
28  Inferior gluteal artery
29  Gluteus maximus muscle (cut)
30  Quadratus femoris muscle
31  Sciatic nerve dividing into its two branches: the common peroneal nerve and the tibial nerve
32  Muscular branches of sciatic nerve to hamstring muscles
33  Popliteal artery
34  Popliteal vein
35  Small saphenous vein (cut)
36  Long head of biceps femoris muscle (cut)
37  Superficial peroneal nerve

**Cutaneous nerves of thigh** (posterior aspect).
The fascia lata and the fasciae of muscles have been removed.

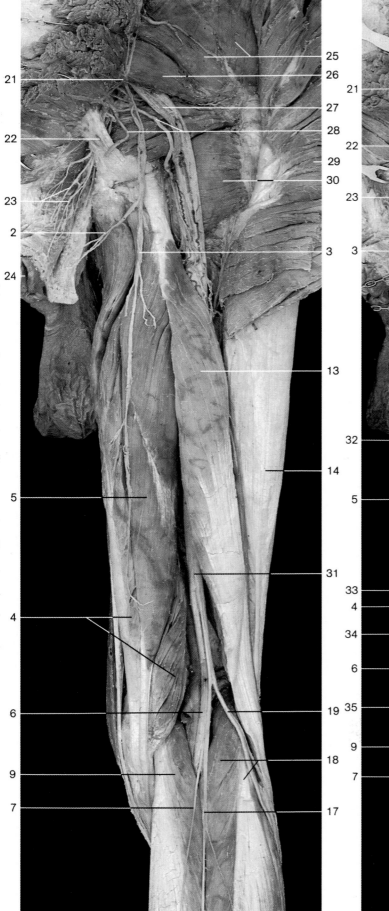

**Posterior femoral region and gluteal region,** right side (posterior aspect). The gluteus maximus muscle has been divided and reflected.

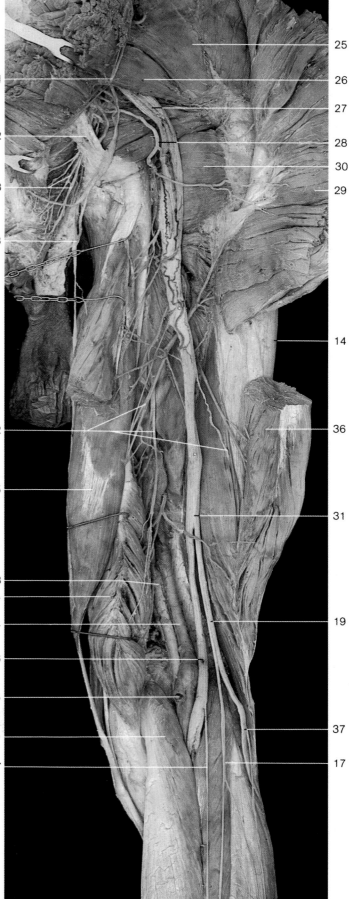

**Posterior femoral region and gluteal region,** right side (posterior aspect). The gluteus maximus muscle and the long head of the biceps femoris muscle have been divided and reflected.

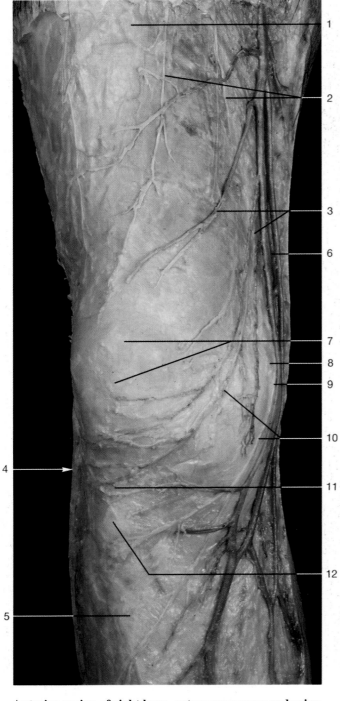

**Anterior region of right knee, cutaneous nerves and veins** (anterior aspect).

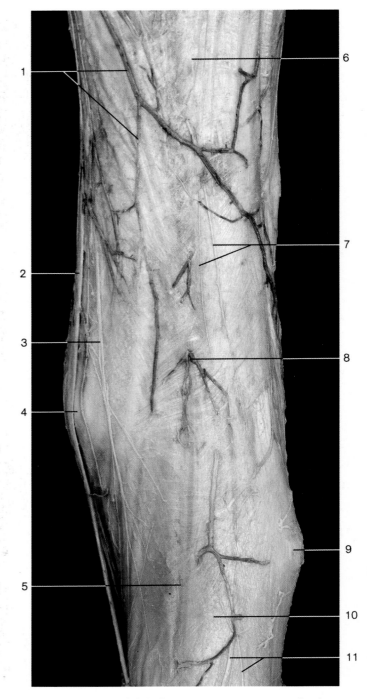

**Posterior region of right knee, cutaneous nerves and veins** (posterior aspect).

1    Fascia lata
2    Terminal branches of anterior cutaneous branches
     of femoral nerve
3    Venous network around knee
4    Position of head of fibula
5    Superficial crural fascia
6    Great saphenous vein
7    Patella
8    Position of medial epicondyle of femur
9    Saphenous nerve
10   Infrapatellar branches of saphenous nerve
11   Patellar ligament
12   Position of tuberosity of tibia

1    Cutaneous veins (tributaries of great saphenous vein)
2    Great saphenous vein
3    Cutaneous branch of femoral nerve
4    Position of medial epicondyle of femur
5    Position of small saphenous vein
6    Fascia lata
7    Terminal branches of posterior femoral cutaneous nerve
8    Cutaneous veins of popliteal fossa
9    Position of head of fibula
10   Superficial layer of fascia cruris
11   Lateral sural cutaneous nerve

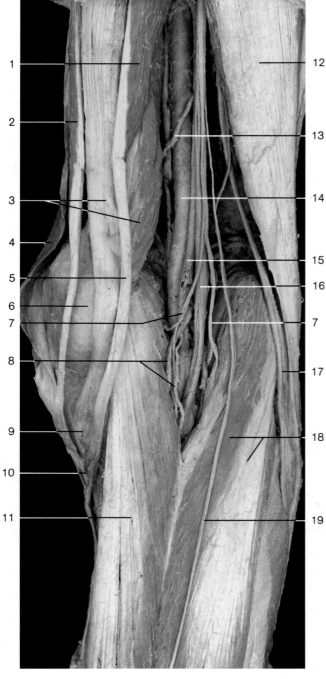

**Right leg, posterior crural region** (posterior aspect).
The gastrocnemius muscle has been divided and reflected.

**Right leg, posterior crural region,** deep layer (posterior aspect).
The gastrocnemius and the soleus muscles have been divided and reflected.

1  Semitendinosus muscle
2  Gracilis muscle
3  Semimembranosus muscle
4  Sartorius muscle
5  Tendon of semitendinosus muscle
6  Position of medial condyle of femur
7  Muscular branches of tibial nerve
8  Sural arteries and veins
9  Tendon of semimembranosus muscle
10  Common tendon of gracilis, semitendinosus, and sartorius
    muscles
11  Medial head of gastrocnemius muscle
12  Biceps femoris muscle
13  Muscular branch of popliteal artery

14  Popliteal artery
15  Popliteal vein
16  Tibial nerve
17  Common peroneal nerve
18  Lateral head of gastrocnemius muscle
19  Medial sural cutaneous nerve
20  Medial superior genicular artery
21  Medial head of gastrocnemius muscle (cut and reflected)
22  Medial inferior genicular artery
23  Soleus muscle
24  Tendon of plantaris muscle
25  Lateral superior genicular artery
26  Lateral inferior genicular artery
27  Plantaris muscle

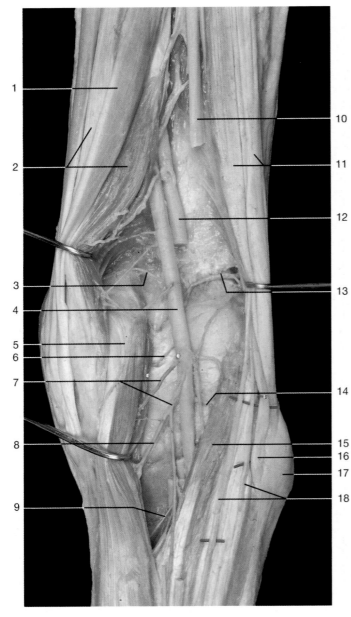

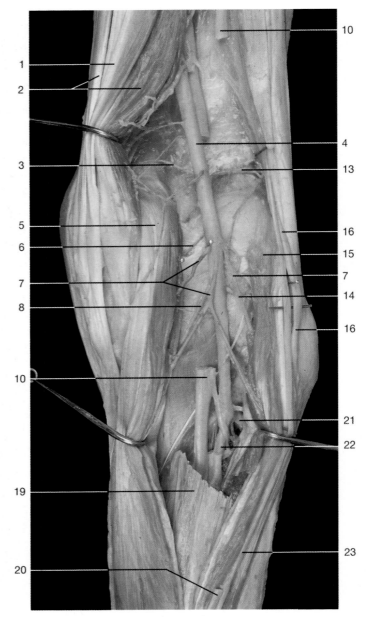

**Right leg, popliteal fossa,** deep layer (posterior aspect).
The muscles have been reflected to display the genicular
arteries.

**Right leg, popliteal fossa,** deepest layer (posterior aspect).
Tibial nerve and popliteal vein have been partly removed
and a portion of the soleus muscle was cut away to display
the anterior tibial artery.

| | |
|---|---|
| 1   Semitendinosus muscle | 12   Popliteal vein (cut) |
| 2   Semimembranosus muscle | 13   Lateral superior genicular artery |
| 3   Medial superior genicular artery | 14   Lateral inferior genicular artery |
| 4   Popliteal artery | 15   Lateral head of gastrocnemius muscle |
| 5   Medial head of gastrocnemius muscle | 16   Common peroneal nerve |
| 6   Middle genicular artery | 17   Head of fibula |
| 7   Muscular branches | 18   Lateral sural cutaneous nerves |
| 8   Medial inferior genicular artery | 19   Soleus muscle |
| 9   Tendon of plantaris muscle | 20   Medial sural cutaneous nerve |
| 10   Tibial nerve (cut) | 21   Anterior tibial artery |
| 11   Biceps femoris muscle | 22   Posterior tibial artery |
| | 23   Lateral sural cutaneous nerve |

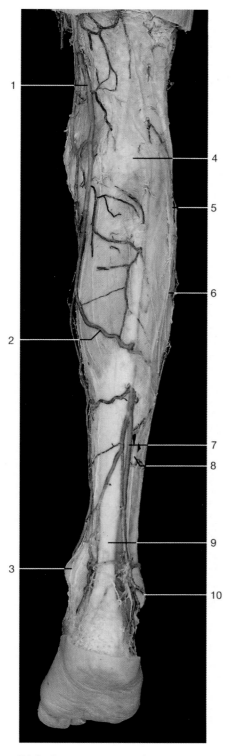

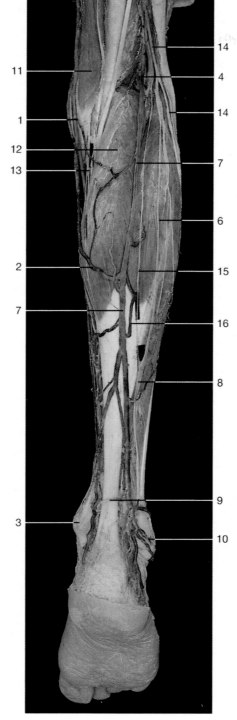

**Right leg, cutaneous veins and nerves** (posterior aspect).

**Right leg, cutaneous nerves and veins** (posterior aspect). The superficial layer of the crural fascia has been removed.

**Right leg, cutaneous veins and nerves** (anterior-medial aspect; veins are colored).

1   Great saphenous vein
2   Venous anastomosis between small and great saphenous veins
3   Medial malleolus
4   Popliteal fossa
5   Position of head of fibula
6   Lateral sural cutaneous nerve
7   Small saphenous vein

8   Sural nerve
9   Calcaneal tendon
10  Lateral malleolus
11  Semitendinosus muscle
12  Medial head of gastrocnemius muscle
13  Saphenous nerve
14  Common peroneal nerve
15  Medial sural cutaneous nerve

16  Perforating veins
17  Superficial peroneal nerve
18  Dorsal venous arch
19  Intermediate dorsal cutaneous nerve
20  Infrapatellar branches of saphenous nerve
21  Terminal branches of saphenous nerve
22  Medial dorsal cutaneous nerve

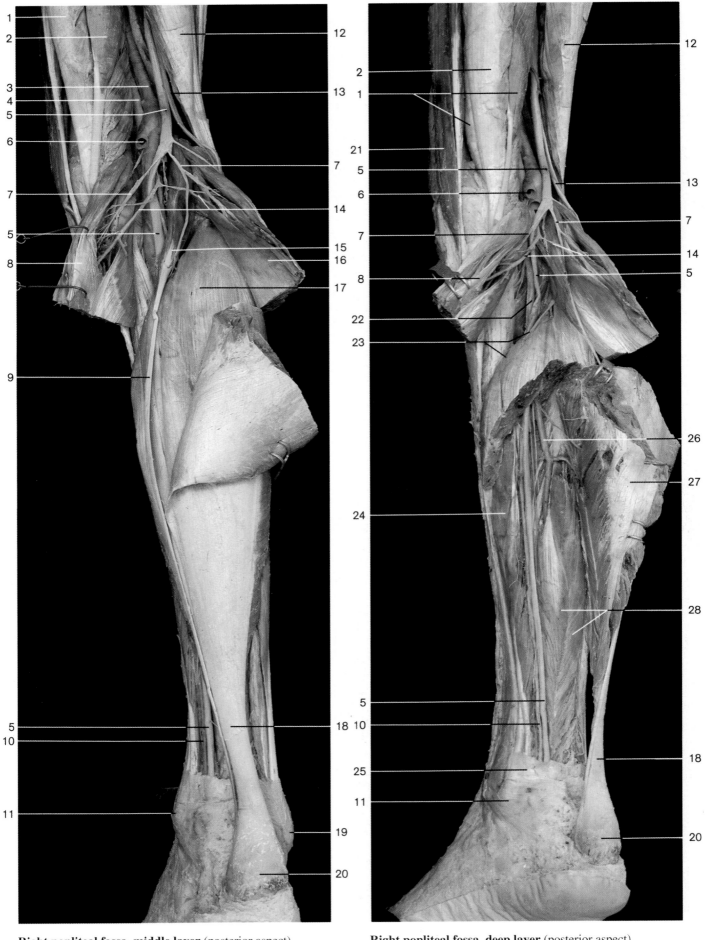

**Right popliteal fossa, middle layer** (posterior aspect).
The cutaneous veins and nerves have been removed.

**Right popliteal fossa, deep layer** (posterior aspect).
The medial head of gastrocnemius muscle has been divided
and reflected.

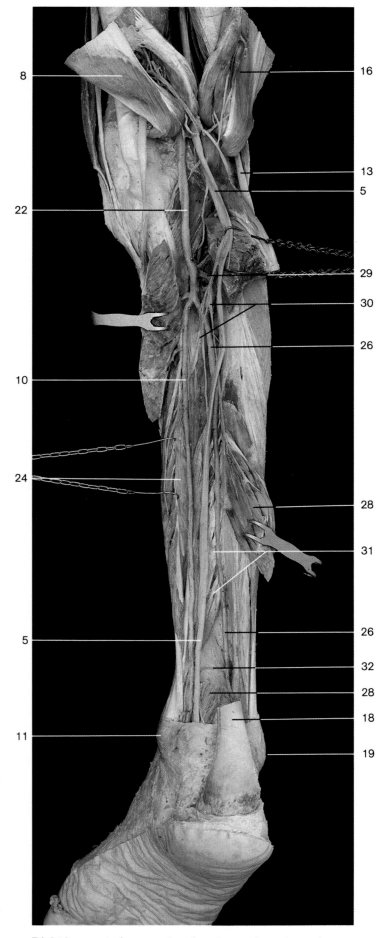

1 Semimembranosus muscle
2 Semitendinosus muscle
3 Popliteal vein
4 Popliteal artery
5 Tibial nerve
6 Small saphenous vein (cut)
7 Muscular branch of tibial nerve
8 Medial head of gastrocnemius muscle
9 Tendon of plantaris muscle
10 Posterior tibial artery
11 Medial malleolus
12 Biceps femoris muscle
13 Common peroneal nerve
14 Sural arteries
15 Plantaris muscle
16 Lateral head of gastrocnemius muscle
17 Soleus muscle
18 Calcaneal tendon
19 Lateral malleolus
20 Calcaneal tuberosity
21 Sartorius muscle
22 Popliteal artery
23 Tendinous arch of soleus muscle
24 Flexor digitorum longus muscle
25 Flexor retinaculum
26 Peroneal artery
27 Soleus muscle
28 Flexor hallucis longus muscle
29 Anterior tibial artery
30 Muscular branches of tibial nerve
31 Tibialis posterior muscle
32 Communicating branch of peroneal artery
33 Tendon of tibialis anterior muscle
34 Tibia
35 Tendon of extensor hallucis longus muscle
36 Tendons of extensor digitorum longus muscle
37 Anterior tibialis artery
38 Fibula
39 Tendons of peroneus longus and brevis muscles

**Right leg, posterior crural region,** deepest layer (posterior aspect). Triceps surae (gastrocnemius and soleus) and flexor hallucis longus muscles have been cut and reflected.

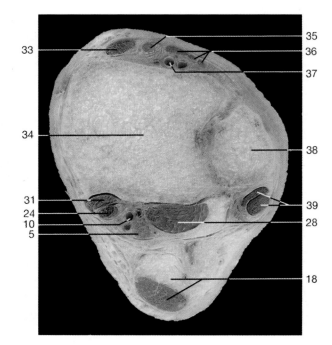

**Cross section of the leg, superior to the malleoli** (from below).

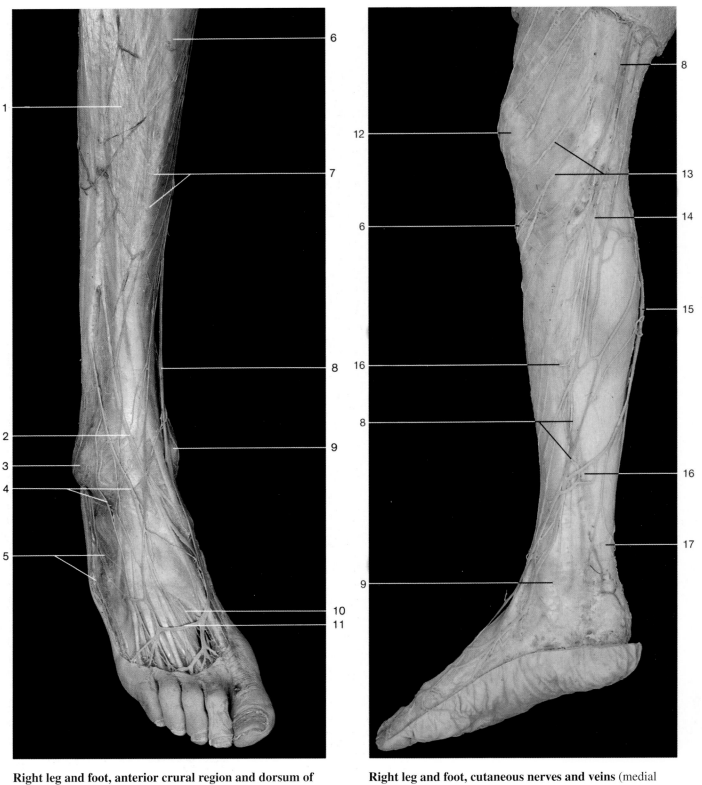

**Right leg and foot, anterior crural region and dorsum of foot, cutaneous nerves and veins** (anterior aspect).

**Right leg and foot, cutaneous nerves and veins** (medial aspect).

1   Superficial crural fascia
2   Medial cutaneous branch of superficial peroneal nerve
3   Lateral malleolus
4   Lateral cutaneous branch of superficial peroneal nerve
5   Cutaneous branch of sural nerve
6   Position of tuberosity of tibia
7   Anterior margin of tibia
8   Great saphenous vein
9   Medial malleolus

10   Deep peroneal nerve
11   Venous arch of dorsum of foot
12   Position of patella
13   Infrapatellar branches of saphenous nerve
14   Saphenous nerve
15   Small saphenous vein
16   Perforating vein
17   Calcaneal tendon

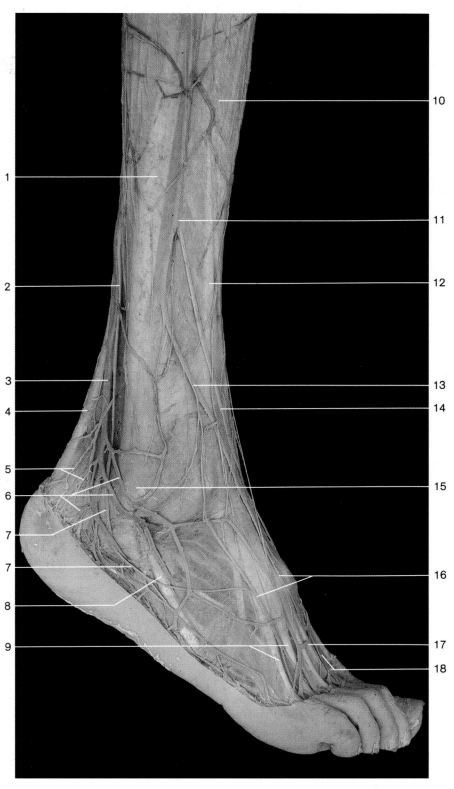

**Right leg and dorsum of foot, cutaneous nerves and veins** (lateral aspect).

1  Position of fibula
2  Sural nerve
3  Small saphenous vein
4  Calcaneal tendon
5  Lateral calcaneal branches of
   sural nerve
6  Venous network at lateral malleolus
7  Cutaneous branch of sural nerve
8  Tendon of peroneus brevis muscle
9  Tendons of extensor digitorum
   longus muscle

10  Fascia cruris
11  Superficial peroneal nerve
12  Position of tibia
13  Lateral cutaneous branch ⎤ of superficial
14  Medial cutaneous branch ⎦ peroneal nerve
15  Lateral malleolus
16  Dorsal digital nerves
17  Dorsal venous arch
18  Deep peroneal nerve

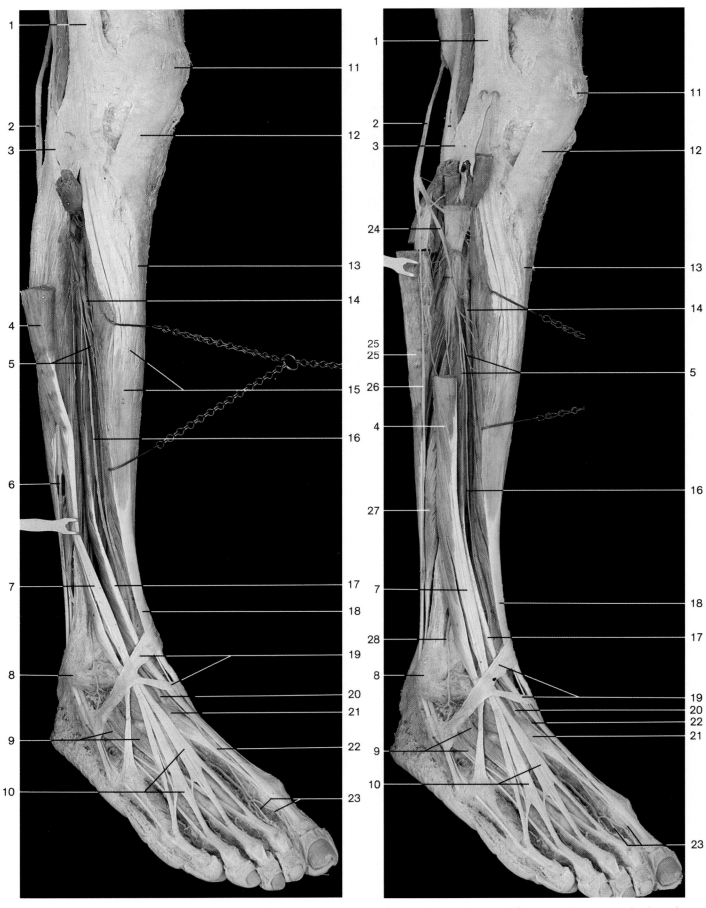

**Right leg and dorsum of foot, middle layer** (anterior lateral aspect). The extensor digitorum longus muscle has been divided and reflected laterally.

**Right leg and dorsum of foot, deep layer** (anterior lateral aspect). The extensor digitorum longus and peroneus longus muscles have been divided or removed. The common peroneal nerve has been elevated to show its course around the head of fibula.

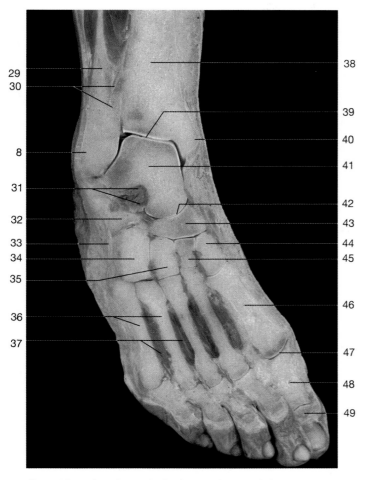

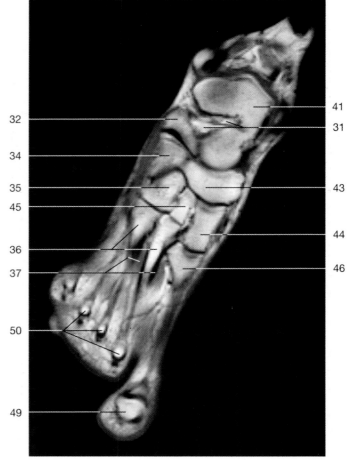

**Coronal section through the foot and ankle joint**
(anterior aspect).

**Coronal section through the foot**
(MRI scan after Heuck A, Luttke G, Rohen JW; 1994).

| | |
|---|---|
| 1 Iliotibial tract | 26 Superficial peroneal nerve (with peroneal muscles laterally reflected) |
| 2 Common peroneal nerve | 27 Peroneus brevis muscle |
| 3 Position of head of fibula | 28 Lateral anterior malleolar artery |
| 4 Extensor digitorum longus muscle | 29 Fibula |
| 5 Muscular branches of deep peroneal nerve | 30 Distal tibiofibular joint (syndesmosis) |
| 6 Superficial peroneal nerve | 31 Talocalcaneal interosseous ligament |
| 7 Tendon of extensor digitorum longus muscle | 32 Calcaneus |
| 8 Lateral malleolus | 33 Tendon of peroneus brevis muscle |
| 9 Extensor digitorum brevis muscle | 34 Cuboid bone |
| 10 Tendons of extensor digitorum longus muscle | 35 Lateral cuneiform bone |
| 11 Patella | 36 Metatarsal bones |
| 12 Patellar ligament | 37 Dorsal interosseous muscles |
| 13 Anterior margin of tibia | 38 Tibia |
| 14 Anterior tibial artery | 39 Ankle joint |
| 15 Tibialis anterior muscle | 40 Medial malleolus |
| 16 Deep peroneal nerve | 41 Talus |
| 17 Extensor hallucis longus muscle | 42 Talocalcaneonavicular joint |
| 18 Tendon of tibialis anterior muscle | 43 Navicular bone |
| 19 Extensor retinaculum | 44 Medial cuneiform bone |
| 20 Dorsalis pedis artery | 45 Intermediate cuneiform bone |
| 21 Extensor hallucis brevis muscle | 46 First metatarsal bone |
| 22 Deep peroneal nerve (on dorsum of foot) | 47 Metatarsophalangeal joint of great toe |
| 23 Dorsal digital nerves (terminal branches of deep peroneal nerve) | 48 Proximal phalanx of great toe |
| 24 Deep peroneal nerve | 49 Distal phalanx of great toe |
| 25 Peroneus longus muscle (cut) | 50 Heads of metatarsal bones II–IV |

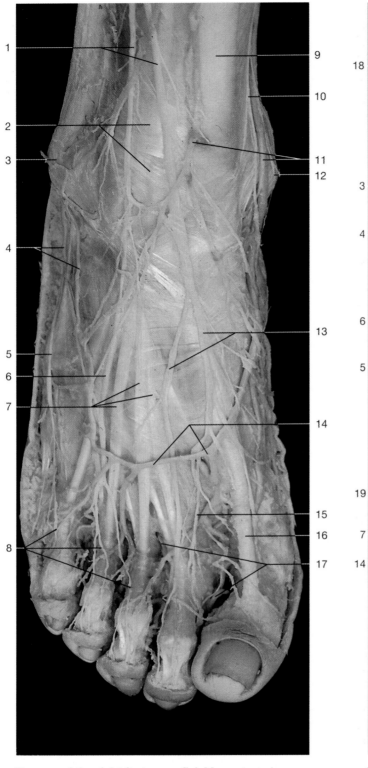

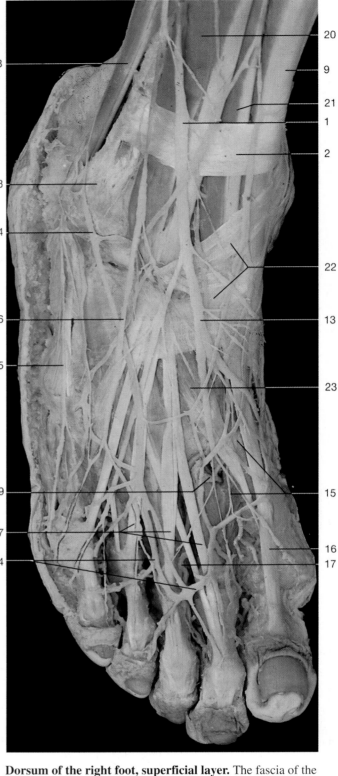

**Dorsum of the right foot, superficial layer** (anterior aspect).

**Dorsum of the right foot, superficial layer.** The fascia of the dorsum has been removed.

1 Superficial peroneal nerve
2 Superior extensor retinaculum
3 Lateral malleolus
4 Venous network of lateral malleolus and tributaries of small saphenous vein
5 Lateral dorsal cutaneous nerve (branch of sural nerve)
6 Intermediate dorsal cutaneous nerve
7 Tendons of extensor digitorum longus muscle
8 Dorsal digital nerves

9 Tendon of tibialis anterior muscle
10 Saphenous nerve
11 Venous network of medial malleolus and tributaries of great saphenous vein
12 Medial malleolus
13 Medial dorsal cutaneous nerves
14 Dorsal venous arch
15 Dorsal digital nerve (of deep peroneal nerve)
16 Tendon of extensor hallucis longus muscle

17 Dorsal digital arteries
18 Peroneal muscles
19 Deep plantar branch of dorsalis pedis artery anastomosing with plantar arch
20 Extensor digitorum longus muscle
21 Extensor hallucis longus muscle
22 Inferior extensor retinaculum
23 Extensor hallucis brevis muscle

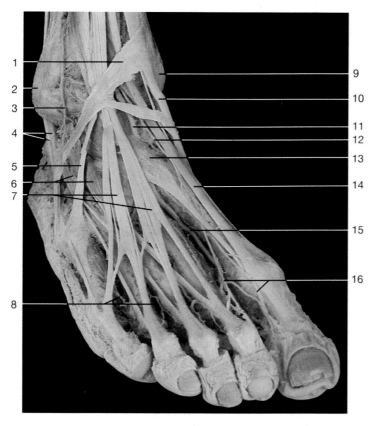

1  Extensor retinaculum
2  Lateral malleolus
3  Lateral anterior malleolar artery
4  Tendons of peroneal muscles
5  Tendon of peroneus tertius muscle
6  Extensor digitorum brevis muscle
7  Tendons of extensor digitorum longus muscle
8  Dorsal metatarsal arteries
9  Medial malleolus
10 Tendon of tibialis anterior muscle
11 Dorsalis pedis artery
12 Deep peroneal nerve (on dorsum of foot)
13 Extensor hallucis brevis muscle
14 Tendon of extensor hallucis longus muscle
15 Dorsalis pedis artery with deep plantar branch to
   the plantar arch
16 Dorsal digital nerves (terminal branches of deep
   peroneal nerve)
17 Lateral tarsal artery
18 Extensor digitorum brevis muscle (divided)
19 Arcuate artery
20 Dorsal interosseous muscles
21 Deep peroneal nerve
22 Medial cuneiform and first metatarsal bone
23 Tendon of peroneus longus muscle
24 Abductor hallucis and flexor hallucis brevis muscles
25 Medial plantar artery, vein, and nerve
26 Fourth and fifth metatarsal bone
27 Adductor hallucis muscle (oblique head)
28 Tendons of flexor digitorum longus muscle
29 Lateral plantar artery, vein, and nerve
30 Flexor digitorum brevis muscle
31 Plantar aponeurosis

**Dorsum of right foot, middle layer** (anterior lateral aspect).
The cutaneous nerves have been removed.

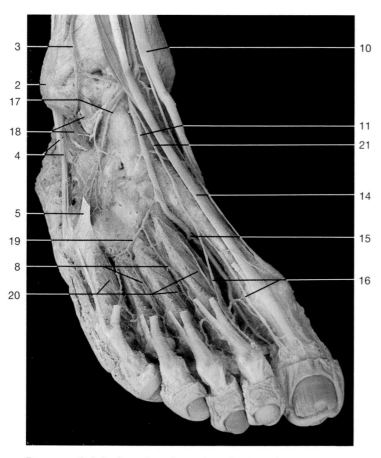

**Dorsum of right foot, deep layer** (anterior lateral aspect).
The extensor digitorum and hallucis breves muscles have
been removed.

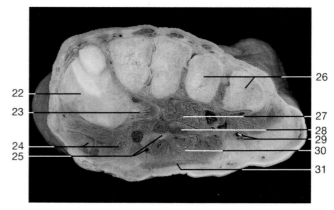

**Cross section of the right foot** at the level of the
metatarsal bones (posterior aspect).

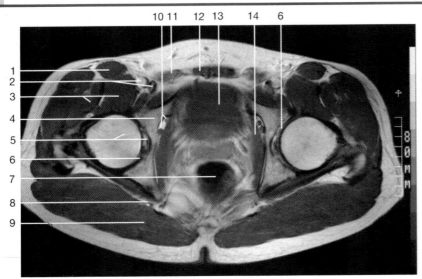

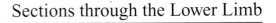

**Axial section through the pelvis and the hip joints** (section 1; MRI scan; inferior aspect).

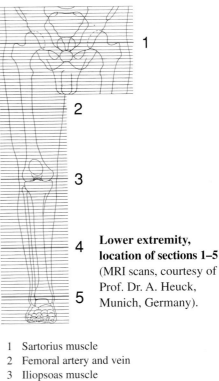

**Lower extremity, location of sections 1–5** (MRI scans, courtesy of Prof. Dr. A. Heuck, Munich, Germany).

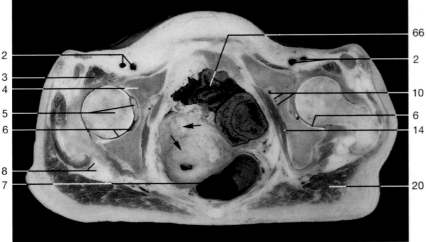

**Axial section through the pelvis and the hip joints in the female** (section 1; inferior aspect). (Arrows: uterus, myometrium with myoma.)

1   Sartorius muscle
2   Femoral artery and vein
3   Iliopsoas muscle
4   Pubis (os pubis)
5   Femoral head with ligament of femoral head
6   Articular cavity
7   Rectum
8   Sciatic nerve and accompanying artery
9   Gluteus maximus muscle
10  Obturator vessels and obturator nerve
11  Rectus abdominis muscle
12  Pyramidalis muscle
13  Urinary bladder
14  Obturator internus muscle
15  Rectus femoris muscle
16  Vastus intermedius and vastus lateralis of quadriceps femoris muscle

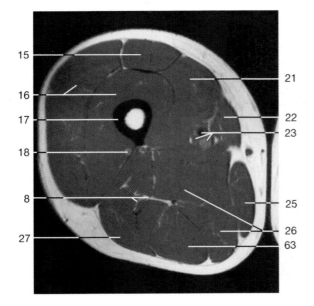

**Axial section through the middle of the right thigh** (section 2; MRI scan; inferior aspect).

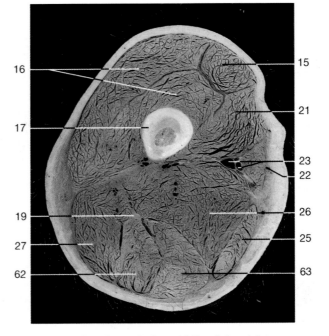

**Axial section through the middle of the right thigh** (section 2; inferior aspect).

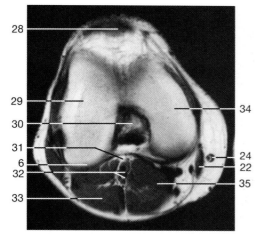

**Axial section through the right knee joint** (section 3; MRI scan; inferior aspect).

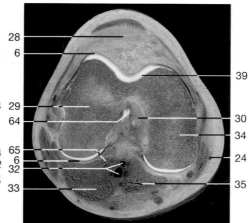

**Axial section through the right knee joint** (section 3; inferior aspect).

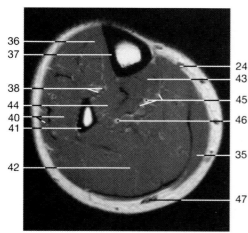

**Axial section through the middle of the right leg** (section 4; MRI scan; inferior aspect).

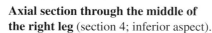

**Axial section through the middle of the right leg** (section 4; inferior aspect).

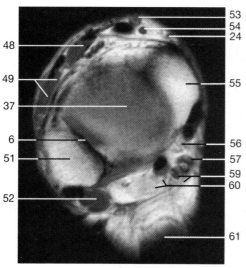

**Axial section through the end of the right leg** (section 5; MRI scan; inferior aspect).

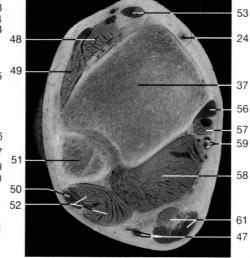

**Axial section through the end of the right leg** (section 5; inferior aspect).

17  Femur
18  Perforating artery
19  Sciatic nerve
20  Gluteus maximus muscle (insertion)
21  Vastus medialis muscle
22  Sartorius muscle
23  Femoral artery and vein
24  Great saphenous vein
25  Gracilis muscle
26  Adductor muscles
27  Biceps femoris muscle
28  Patellar ligament
29  Lateral condyle of femur
30  Posterior cruciate ligament
31  Tibial nerve
32  Popliteal artery and vein
33  Lateral head of gastrocnemius muscle
34  Medial condyle of femur
35  Medial head of gastrocnemius muscle
36  Tibialis anterior muscle
37  Tibia
38  Deep peroneal nerve, anterior tibial artery, and vein
39  Patellar surface
40  Peroneus longus and brevis muscles
41  Fibula
42  Soleus muscle
43  Flexor digitorum longus muscle
44  Tibialis posterior muscle
45  Posterior tibial artery and vein and tibial nerve
46  Peroneal artery
47  Small saphenous vein and sural nerve
48  Extensor hallucis longus muscle
49  Extensor digitorum longus muscle
50  Tendon of peroneus longus muscle
51  Lateral malleolus (fibula)
52  Peroneus brevis muscle
53  Tibialis anterior muscle (tendon)
54  Dorsalis pedis artery
55  Medial malleolus (tibia)
56  Tibialis posterior muscle (tendon)
57  Flexor digitorum longus muscle (tendon with synovial sheath)
58  Flexor hallucis longus muscle
59  Posterior tibial artery and vein
60  Lateral and medial plantar nerves
61  Calcaneal tendon
62  Semitendinosus muscle
63  Semimembranosus muscle
64  Anterior cruciate ligament
65  Plantaris muscle
66  Small intestine

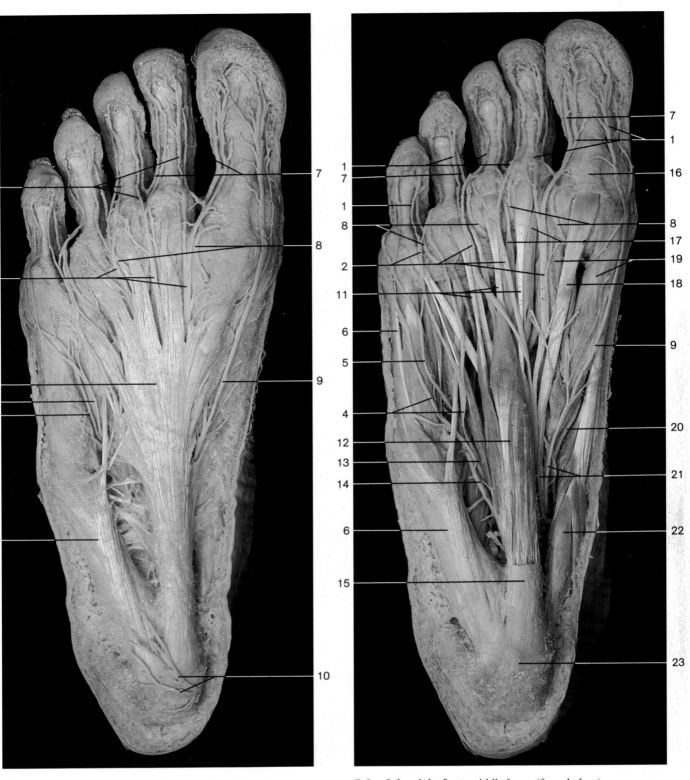

1
7
1

2

3
4
5

6

7

8

9

10

1
7
1
8
2
11
6
5
4
12
13
14
6
15

7
1
16
8
17
19
18
9

20
21
22

23

**Sole of the right foot,** superficial layer (from below).
Dissection of cutaneous nerves and vessels.

**Sole of the right foot,** middle layer (from below).
The plantar aponeurosis has been removed.

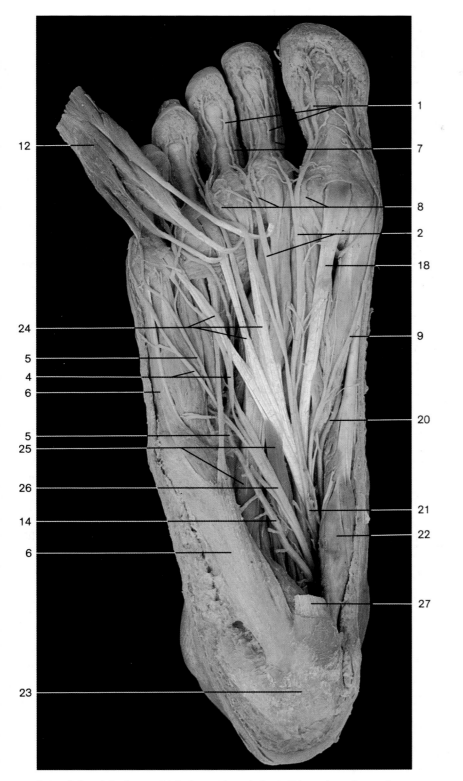

1 Proper plantar digital nerves
2 Common plantar digital nerves
3 Plantar aponeurosis
4 Superficial branch of lateral plantar nerve
5 Superficial branch of lateral plantar artery
6 Abductor digiti minimi
7 Proper plantar digital arteries
8 Common plantar digital arteries
9 Digital branch of medial plantar nerve to great toe
10 Medial calcaneal branches
11 Tendons of flexor digitorum brevis muscle
12 Flexor digitorum brevis muscle
13 Superficial branch of lateral plantar nerve
14 Lateral plantar artery
15 Plantar aponeurosis (remnant)
16 Digital synovial sheath
17 Lumbrical muscles
18 Tendon of flexor hallucis longus muscle
19 Flexor hallucis brevis muscle
20 Medial plantar artery
21 Medial plantar nerve
22 Abductor hallucis muscle
23 Calcaneal tuberosity
24 Tendons of flexor digitorum longus muscle
25 Quadratus plantae muscle
26 Lateral plantar nerve
27 Flexor digitorum brevis muscle (cut)
28 Synovial sheaths
29 Plantar arch

**Sole of the right foot,** middle layer (from below). Dissection of vessels and nerves. The flexor digitorum brevis muscle has been divided and anteriorly reflected.

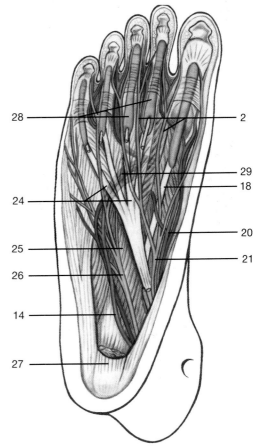

**Sole of the right foot.** Synovial sheaths of flexor tendons indicated in light blue (schematic drawing).

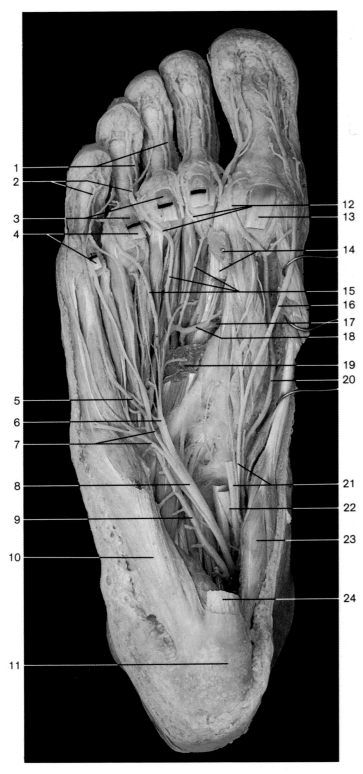

1   Proper plantar digital arteries
2   Proper plantar digital nerves
3   Tendons of flexor digitorum brevis muscle
4   Tendons of flexor digitorum longus muscle
5   Superficial branch of lateral plantar artery
6   Deep branch of lateral plantar nerve
7   Superficial branch of lateral plantar nerve
8   Lateral plantar nerve
9   Lateral plantar artery
10   Abductor digiti minimi muscle
11   Calcaneal tuberosity
12   Common plantar digital arteries
13   Tendon of flexor hallucis longus muscle
14   Insertion of both heads of adductor hallucis muscle
15   Plantar metatarsal arteries
16   Medial plantar nerve of great toe
17   Deep plantar branch of dorsalis pedis artery
      (perforating branch)
18   Plantar arch
19   Oblique head of adductor hallucis muscle (cut)
20   Medial plantar artery
21   Medial plantar nerve
22   Crossing of tendons in sole of foot (flexor hallucis
      longus and flexor digitorum longus muscles)
23   Abductor hallucis muscle
24   Origin of flexor digitorum brevis muscle

**Sole of the right foot,** deep layer (from below). Dissection of vessels and nerves. The flexor digitorum brevis muscle, the quadratus plantae muscle with the tendons of the flexor digitorum longus muscle, and some branches of the medial plantar nerve have been removed. The flexor hallucis brevis and adductor hallucis muscles have been cut and portions removed to show the somewhat atypical course of the medial plantar artery and deep muscles of the foot.

# Index

Page numbers in **bold** indicate main discussions.

Page numbers in **bold** indicate main discussions.

Page numbers in **bold** indicate main discussions.

Page numbers in **bold** indicate main discussions.

Page numbers in **bold** indicate main discussions.

Page numbers in **bold** indicate main discussions.

Page numbers in **bold** indicate main discussions.

Page numbers in **bold** indicate main discussions.

Page numbers in **bold** indicate main discussions.

Page numbers in **bold** indicate main discussions.

Page numbers in **bold** indicate main discussions.

Page numbers in **bold** indicate main discussions.

Page numbers in **bold** indicate main discussions.

Page numbers in **bold** indicate main discussions.

Page numbers in **bold** indicate main discussions.

Page numbers in **bold** indicate main discussions.

Page numbers in **bold** indicate main discussions.

Page numbers in **bold** indicate main discussions.

Page numbers in **bold** indicate main discussions.

Page numbers in **bold** indicate main discussions.

Page numbers in **bold** indicate main discussions.

Page numbers in **bold** indicate main discussions.

Page numbers in **bold** indicate main discussions.

Page numbers in **bold** indicate main discussions.

Page numbers in **bold** indicate main discussions.

Page numbers in **bold** indicate main discussions.

Page numbers in **bold** indicate main discussions.

Page numbers in **bold** indicate main discussions.

Page numbers in **bold** indicate main discussions.

Page numbers in **bold** indicate main discussions.